W9-DAJ-585

Introduction to
Communicative Disorders

Introduction to Communicative Disorders

THIRD EDITION

M. N. Hegde

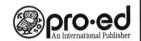
pro·ed
An International Publisher

8700 Shoal Creek Boulevard
Austin, Texas 78757-6897
800/897-3202   Fax 800/397-7633
www.proedinc.com

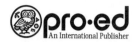

© 2001, 1995 by PRO-ED, Inc.
8700 Shoal Creek Boulevard
Austin, Texas 78757-6897
800/897-3202   Fax 800/397-7633
www.proedinc.com

Library of Congress Cataloging-in-Publication Data

Hegde, M. N. (Mahabalagiri N.), 1941–
    Introduction to communicative disorders / M. N. Hegde.—3rd ed.
        p.   cm.
    Includes bibliographical references and index.
    ISBN 0-89079-863-X—ISBN 0-89079-864-8 (Inst man)—ISBN 0-89079-865-6 (stud csbk)
    1. Communicative disorders   I. Title.
RC423 .H3828 2001
616.8'55—dc21

                                                                00-045872
                                                                CIP

This book is designed in Sabon and Futura.

Printed in the United States of America

    3   4   5   6   7   8   9   10   05   04

Contents

CHAPTER 9
Neurologically Based Communicative Disorders   *319*

CHAPTER 10
Hearing and Its Disorders   *373*

Preface

Our social behavior is essentially communicative behavior. To communicate is to care, share, and connect with each other. Human life is as rich and varied as it is because of our ability to communicate with our fellow human beings. An individual whose communicative ability is hampered is socially and emotionally isolated. Communicative handicaps in modern societies create serious personal, social, educational, and occupational difficulties for an individual. Therefore, human communication and its disorders is an important discipline that touches all of us.

This book is an introduction to both the science of communication and the profession of communicative disorders. It is written for the student who wishes to find out if the science and disorders of communication is his or her field as well as for the student who has decided that it is. The profession of communicative disorders is based on the science of hearing, speech, language, and other forms of communication. It tries to show how the field has evolved into a major scientific discipline and a health care profession.

Communicative disorders is a rapidly growing science and profession. Being interdisciplinary, it draws from such diverse fields as physics, biology, psychology, linguistics, medicine, sociology, and philosophy. This is part of the reason why it is an exciting field.

The field is exciting also because the speech–language pathologist or the audiologist helps restore a vital link of existence that may be broken in some individuals: the ability to communicate. It is a profession that is simultaneously challenging and immensely rewarding. If this book is able to give the beginning student a flavor for this engrossing science and helping profession, it will have served its purpose. I will be especially pleased if the book also prompts the student to seriously consider majoring in communicative disorders.

Since the first edition of this book was published in 1991 and the second edition in 1995, many instructors have offered extensive comments about its coverage and writing style. The feedback has been overwhelmingly positive and has come from numerous instructors across the country. Instructors have repeatedly stated that the book reflects the current knowledge and that its coverage is both extensive and uniform across issues and topics. They have found the book an effective teaching tool because of its organization and simple writing style that avoids jargon. The feedback suggests that these characteristics have prompted the instructors to use the book as the primary text in their courses. This third edition retains and enhances these characteristics.

This text has two companion volumes to enhance teaching and learning. The first is the *Instructor's Coursebook* and the second is the *Student's Coursebook*. Both contain essentially the same information: an outline of the textbook chapters, definition of basic terms, summaries of important information, clinical procedures, and so forth. The *Instructor's Coursebook* contains complete examinations and answer keys, while the *Student's Coursebook* contains only typical questions and their answers. Both coursebooks leave the right half of each page blank. On this blank space, instructors can make their own notes and students can take class notes. This makes it possible for students to integrate information from the text, instructor's lectures, and outside reading materials into a single, coherent source. Students have found the coursebooks especially helpful.

I have revised all chapters for this edition to improve or refine the coverage and update information as needed. Chapter 9 has been expanded to include information on dementia, right hemisphere syndrome, traumatic brain injury, and dysphagia. Chapter 11 on culture, communication, diversity, and disorders has been completely rewritten to include an overview of primary dialects of English as spoken around the world and a section on Native American languages.

My thanks are due to Dr. Stephen McFarlane, professor of speech–language pathology and associate dean of the Medical School, University of Nevada, Reno. He has graciously provided several pictures that are used in Chapter 7. I also thank Shriram Ramamurthy who has helped me in preparing many figures for this edition. As always, I am thankful to my wife Prema's continued support and encouragement for my commitment to scientific and professional writing.

Communication and Its Disorders

Communication is vital to both biological and social existence. **Communication** is exchange of information. Information may be exchanged between cells, body parts, individuals, and groups of persons. Nerve impulses travel across cell bodies. As body parts, the eye and the ear inform the brain about the environmental events that stimulate them. The brain in turn communicates with the peripheral organs of the body by issuing commands to move and act in various ways. Communication at these biological levels is mostly an electro-chemical event. It is the communication between individuals and groups that is of special interest to us.

Human and Animal Communication

Human communication is social interaction among people. In this sense, communication is a social event; it is action that often affects other people. Communication that has no effect on other people is no communication at all. Typically, communication has an effect only in a social context. Therefore, **communication** may be simply defined as a form of social behavior.

Most if not all organisms have some form of social communication. Animals at all levels communicate with each other. However, the animal communication is primarily instinctive because it serves the need for survival. The bees, with their different patterns of movement, communicate to their fellow bees the distance, direction, amount, and quality of pollen they have found. Wild animals sense and communicate an imminent danger to the other members of the herd by movement, vocalization, and gesture. Lower organisms communicate information regarding the location of food, as ants do. Cats and dogs tell us that they are hungry or thirsty.

Although natural animal communication is instinctive, researchers have shown that it is possible to teach limited social communication to some animals. For example, chimpanzees have been taught words expressed in the form of manual signs (as in the American Sign Language). Chimpanzees also have learned to use plastic tokens that stand for words. There is even limited evidence that chimpanzees can combine symbols (such as plastic tokens) to form simple sentence-like expressions. Nonetheless, the research so far falls short of showing that animals can learn to recombine what they have learned to form an infinite variety of messages as humans do when they communicate. Besides, nonhuman organisms are obviously not capable of spoken language. Their laryngeal and speech production mechanism has not evolved to an advanced and flexible stage where learning a form of oral language is possible. The neural (brain) structure that controls this mechanism in animals also falls short of the complex capabilities of the human brain.

Human beings have the most elaborate, sophisticated, versatile, and creative means of communication. The more complex neurophysiological mechanism present in humans makes this unprecedented level and type of communication possible. This highly flexible mechanism, which includes the breathing and the voicing structures, the brain, and the peripheral nerves, has made the emergence of language possible. This mechanism is sensitive to environmental influences that help shape a language or other forms of complex communication (e.g., varied sign languages).

Language and Communication

It is _language_ that makes people so much more efficient at communication. A language may be defined either linguistically or behaviorally. A common _linguistic_ definition of **language** is that it is a system of symbols and codes used in communication. A _behavioral_ definition is that **language** is a form of social behavior, shaped and maintained by a verbal community. In later sections, we will try to understand these definitions fully; for the present, we may think of language as a means of communication and as a form of social behavior.

People generally think of language as a form of spoken or written communication. A spoken language also is called an ʾoral language. But note that as defined earlier, language need not be spoken or oral, in which case it is non-oral. Oral language is spoken with words, whereas ʾnon-oral language is expressed through gestures, symbols, or both. Whereas any spoken language is an example of an oral language, American Sign Language is an example of a non-oral language. There are other forms of non-oral language, which may include gestural and symbolic communication. The complexity and diversity of human languages are responsible for much of the human social interaction, culture, arts, and sciences that are typically equated with unique human accomplishments.

Anatomical structures and how they help produce speech are described in **Chapter 3.**

Unlike the animal modes of communication, human languages also are remarkably free from the needs of survival. That an opera singer sings to survive is only a metaphoric expression. People need not sing or even talk to survive biologically. However, the sophisticated neurophysiological mechanisms that are used in oral language are linked to biological survival. For example, although an air supply from the lungs is essential for oral communication, the primary functions of the lungs are biological. Similarly, although vocal fold vibrations are essential for normal oral language, those folds have evolved to serve biological functions (e.g., protecting the airway passage to the lungs). Talking is most efficient only when the biological functions are satisfied or not severely interrupted. When breathing is interrupted, one does not think of speech.

Once freed from the restraints of biological survival, communication through language became a powerful tool for social, cultural, artistic, and scientific accomplishments. Language is creative mostly because it is not exclusively tied to instinctual and biological needs. Humans have created special forms of culture by unique use of language as in poetry, play, and other forms of literature. Because most of what is considered uniquely human is in some way related to language, language and communication are considered the essence of human existence.

Communication and Social Survival

Language and communication have assumed such great importance in modern societies that in an ironic fashion, communication is essential for **social survival.** Without communication or language, a human may survive as an organism but will have difficulty thriving as a social person. Such a person may be deprived of success and satisfaction that come from many forms of human accomplishments that are rooted in language and communication. Lack of communication in one form or the other may lead to social isolation.

As societies have become more complex, organized, and interrelated both within and among themselves, effective communication has gained increasingly greater importance. Language and communication are now crucial for even mundane occupational success or survival as vocations have become more sophisticated, complex, and interrelated.

The advanced technology of modern societies has given a new meaning to communication. Constant and rapid exchange of information has become a new cornerstone of modern societies. Through the Internet, people in far corners of the world can achieve instant communication and exchange of information. Mechanical means of information storage, retrieval, and transfer with the help of computers have created a new age of communication. This new age is making even greater demands upon individuals to communicate more frequently, faster, and more efficiently. A by-product of this technology is a new kind of help that is now available for persons with communicative disorders. Computerized means of communication can now help people who are severely physically handicapped communicate more efficiently and more fully than before.

The Study of Human Communication

The scientific study of human communication is somewhat recent. In fact, the interest in the disorders of communication has played a major role in promoting a more intensive study of communicative behaviors, systems, and processes.

Because of its complexity, scientists have analyzed communication by breaking it into different aspects or components. Unfortunately, the same complexity also has led to theoretical differences. Scientists have not always agreed on how to analyze language and what components to emphasize. Another reason for theoretical differences is that many disciplines target language or communication for their study. For example, philosophers, linguists, psychologists, biologists, neurologists, engineers, sociologists, anthropologists, literary people, speech–language pathologists, and various other professionals are interested in the study of communication. Inevitably, their diverse training and outlook have produced contrasting viewpoints.

To facilitate our later understanding of the disorders of communication, I shall describe five basic aspects or components of communication. These five aspects have their corresponding disorders of communication: voice, articulation, language, fluency, and hearing. Figure 1.1 shows these components of human communication.

Voice

Voice is an essential element of *oral* communication. Without voice, there is no vocal communication except for whispered speech, which does not require voice. Although many species of animals can make vocal sounds (sounds of voice), only humans are capable of making a wide range of vocal sounds that are used in oral communication. Humans have achieved this because of their dynamic vocal mechanism. Without voice, communication is *nonvocal* and takes the form of signs and symbols.

The most important structure that lays the foundation for oral communication is the **larynx,** a structure in the neck. The larynx contains **vocal folds,** which are a pair of thin muscles and associated tissue that vibrate when air from the lungs passes over them.

The vibrations of the vocal folds are the source of human voice. The lungs supply the necessary power to set the folds into vibration. The vibrating vocal

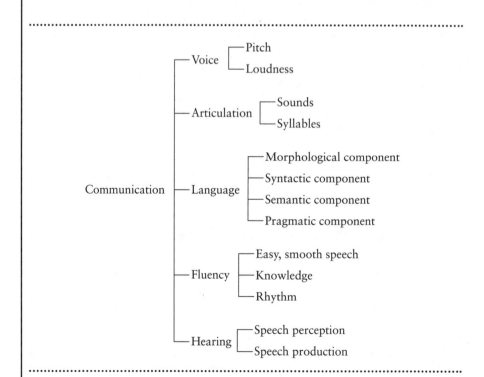

Figure 1.1. Components of human communication.

folds also open and close. When the folds open and close regularly, they produce pleasant and normal voice. Irregular openings and closings cause unpleasant and disordered voice.

The human voice is capable of variations that create diversity in communication as well as many aesthetic effects. The pitch and loudness of voice vary across individuals and speaking situations within the same individual. The human voice can give information over and beyond the words spoken. The voice itself carries some message value. The *tone* with which someone says something is often as important, if not more important, than what is said. The voice can express anger, resentment, disappointment, joy, enthusiasm, or love without using words that express such emotions.

The structures of the throat, the mouth, and the nose modify the sound the larynx produces. This modification is known as **resonance**. Various structures, including the tongue and the lips, **articulate** the modified laryngeal sound into speech sounds. Without articulation, we do not have speech; we have only the undifferentiated sound of the vibrating vocal folds.

Articulation

Articulation means movement. In the context of speech, articulation is the movement of the speech mechanism to produce the sounds of speech. The various structures of the speech mechanism, including the soft palate, the tongue, and the lips, come together, move apart, and change their shapes to create the sounds of speech.

The study of speech sounds and sound patterns used to create words is called **phonology**. Phonology is the domain of both linguists and speech–language pathologists. Phonology is a relatively new term. In the past, much of the information about speech sounds, their classification, production, and perception was included under **phonetics** and **articulation**. Currently, phonetics and phonology are closely related. Generally speaking, **phonetics** describes the production, perception, and classification of speech sounds. *Phonology* is primarily concerned with the broader rules and processes that govern the patterns of sound, their acquisition, use, and the knowledge that underlies the use of sound systems. Because of its broader concern with how sounds are organized into patterns that underlie language, phonology is a part of the study of language. The earlier study of articulation of individual speech sounds did not bear such a direct relation to the study of language.

Specialists prefer to use the terms *phone* and *phoneme* to describe various sounds of speech. A **phone** is a single speech sound. For instance, a speaker's single production of /k/ is described as a phone. However, when the same speaker produces the same sound several times in a row, each production will differ somewhat from each other, though they all are perceived as /k/. Such multiple productions of a single phone is called a phoneme. Therefore, a **phoneme** is defined as a *group* of speech sounds. Phonemes are important for meaning; when you change a phoneme in a word, often the meaning changes. For example, the two words, *kit* and *bit* mean different things, precisely because of the different initial phonemes the letters *k* and *b* represent; the other phonemes of the two words are the same.

The phonemes are combined to form syllables and words. **Syllables** are either vowels or vowels combined with consonants. When a syllable consists of an initial and a final consonant, as in the word *Tom,* the middle vowel is its nucleus. The initial consonant helps *release* the syllable and the final consonant *arrests* it. Each language has certain permissible combinations of phonemes that form words. Other combinations may be uncommon or nonexistent. By observing the ways in which phonemes are normally combined in a language, phonologists derive rules of phoneme combinations.

Because phonemes help form syllables and words, they are the building blocks of speech. In a narrower sense, **speech** is the production of phonemes; articulated sounds and syllables constitute speech.

Language

Earlier, language was defined as either a system of codes and symbols or as a form of social behavior. Such a definition applies equally well to oral and non-oral means of communication. When the production of speech sounds is organized into a higher level of words and sentences that generates meaning, we call it **oral language.** In a well-known form of non-oral language, American Sign Language, manual signs are organized into a higher system of communication, just as the oral language is organized. In either case, language is a larger, more abstract system than speech. One can articulate speech sounds without producing oral language, but one cannot produce oral language without articulating speech sounds. Therefore, speech is the essential component of oral language.

Language also may be expressive or receptive. **Expressive** language is language *produced;* speaking is expressive. **Receptive** language is language *understood;* listening is receptive. In essence, expressive language involves production skills and receptive language involves listening and understanding skills.

Unless otherwise specified, in this and most other sections, our main emphasis will be on oral language. As noted before, specialists in many disciplines have studied oral language. Speech–language pathologists have joined the team in recent years. There are many approaches to the study of language, but my description will be limited to the linguistic and the behavioral approaches because of their direct influence on speech–language pathology. The main elements of these two approaches are illustrated in Figure 1.2.

The Linguistic Study of Language

Linguistics is the study of language, its structure, and the rules that govern that structure. **Linguists** are specialists in linguistics.

There is no universally accepted linguistic definition of language. A definition offered earlier, that language is a code or a system used to communicate, is a linguistic definition. According to linguists, the system of codes or symbols helps represent objects, events, and relationships. A verbal community arbitrarily selects the codes or symbols. Words of each language and the signs or gestures of a manual system of communication mean something specific only because the verbal community has agreed upon them. For example, there is no inherent reason why the word *apple* should stand for what it does in the English language. Linguists also tend to describe language as a mental or cognitive system of rules. It is generally believed that the rules help formulate acceptable sentences of language and their social use.

Linguists have described several components of language. Apart from the phonological component, they have described morphologic, syntactic, and semantic components. In recent years, a pragmatic component has been added

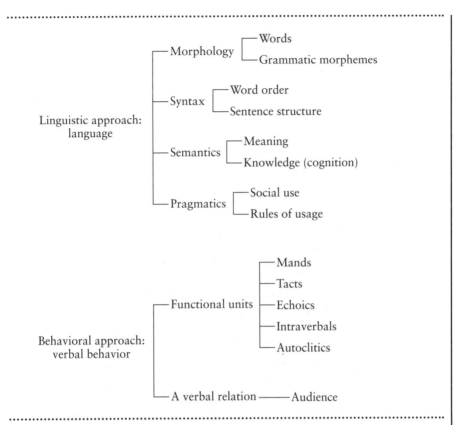

Figure 1.2. Approaches to the study of language.

to this list. We shall take a brief look at each of these components. Most of these components are associated with a specialized study. For example, *morphology* studies the morphologic component. We shall start with this study.

Morphology of Language. **Morphology** means the study of *structures*. Biologists and anatomists use the term in describing how the body parts and organs are formed. In linguistics, morphology means the study of word structures. Morphology describes how words are formed out of more basic elements of language, called morphemes. The morphologic component is a part of grammar.

A **morpheme** is the smallest meaningful unit of a language. Each morpheme is different from the other because each signals a distinct meaning. Morphemes are used to form words. Morphemes take different forms. A whole word consists of at least one morpheme; it may consist of two or more morphemes. A word like *book* is counted as a single morpheme; you cannot break it into smaller parts and still signal some meaning. But the word *books* has two morphemes: *book* and the plural inflection *s*. Although the *s* is described as a phoneme (a sound of speech) in the context of phonology, it is a morpheme in this context because it can be added or deleted from words and thus change the meaning. The plural inflection *s* means *more than one*; therefore, it is a morpheme. Similarly, while *go* is a single morpheme, *going* has two morphemes. The present progressive *ing*, when added to *go* changes the meaning of that word.

In each language, longer words, more complex words, and words that mean different things are created by combining different morphemes. These combinations are not random; there are patterns. Words that cannot be broken down into smaller units (and still retain meaning) but to which other morphemes can be added are called the **base** or **root morphemes.** Other morphemes can be added to these base morphemes. However, base morphemes can take other morphemes at their beginning or their end. This creates two additional classes of morphemes.

A morpheme added at the beginning of a base morpheme is called a **prefix.** Prefixes increase the number of morphemes of a base morpheme (word). For instance, the morpheme *pre* is a frequently used prefix in English. The word *prearranged* has three morphemes: *pre, arrange,* and the past inflection *ed.* Another frequently used prefix is *un* (*understate*, two morphemes; *understated,* three morphemes). Many prefixes can be combined with several base morphemes. Table 1.1 shows a few additional examples of base morphemes, prefixes, and their combined forms.

A morpheme added at the end of a base morpheme (word) is called a **suffix.** Suffixes, too, increase the number of morphemes in a word. For example, the present progressive *ing* is a common English suffix. It is typically added to such verbs as *do* (do*ing*) and *walk* (walk*ing*), creating longer words with altered meanings. Table 1.2 shows a few additional examples of base morphemes, suffixes, and their combined forms.

A morpheme may be *free* or *bound*. A **free** morpheme can stand alone and mean something. All base or root words are free morphemes. Words such as *cat, man, child, go, bad, good,* and *host* are free morphemes. They cannot be reduced to smaller units without destroying their meaning. Produce only a part of these words and you will know why they cannot be broken down without destroying their meaning.

A **bound** morpheme cannot convey meaning by itself; it must be joined with a free morpheme to do so. For instance, the past tense inflection *ed* means something only when added to a free morpheme (such as *bake*). If you produced only *ed,* it does not have the same meaning as it does when it is joined to a free morpheme. Most bound morphemes are the small elements of grammar. Therefore, they are also called **grammatic morphemes.** Among many others, the following bound morphemes also are examples of grammatic morphemes:

ing	The present progressive (*coming, going*)
s	The regular plural morpheme (*books, cats*)
's	The possessive inflection (*man's, lady's*)
s	The third-person singular verb (*smiles, begs*)
ed	The regular past tense (*walked, combed*)

Table 1.1

Examples of English Prefixes

Prefix	Base Morpheme	Combined Form
Anti	establishment	*Anti*establishment
	social	*Anti*social
Re	view	*Re*view
	form	*Re*form
Un	equal	*Un*equal
	employment	*Un*employment

Table 1.2

Examples of English Suffixes

Suffix	Base Morpheme	Combined
ize	Memory	Memor*ize*
	Modern	Modern*ize*
ly	Slow	Slow*ly*
	Wise	Wise*ly*
ism	Native	Nativ*ism*
	Social	Social*ism*

As you can see from the examples, morphemes are means of modifying word structures to change meaning. The morphology of a given language describes the rules of such modifications. It describes what kinds of morphemic combinations are permissible in a given language. Because sounds (phonemes) and syllables are the building blocks of morphemes, morphology is closely related to phonology. Also, morphology is related to the study of meaning (semantics) because morphemic changes alter meanings of words. Therefore, it is good to remember at all times that different components of language are closely interrelated. They are separated only to simplify the analysis of language.

The Syntax of Language. The basic meaning of the word *syntax* is to join, to put together. In language, syntax is one of the two parts of grammar; the other part, as noted before, is the morphologic aspect of language. In the study of language, **syntax** is the arrangement of words to form meaningful sentences. The word order and the overall structure of a sentence are its syntax.

Syntax also is a collection of rules. These rules specify the ways and order in which words may be combined to form sentences in a particular language. The syntactic rules of one language may not completely apply to another language, although some rules may be applicable to many if not all of the languages. At the least, all languages have their own acceptable word order.

Language is creative mostly because its elements (the words) can be arranged and rearranged in many different ways. The syntax of a language rules out random and meaningless word order. For example, the following group of words means nothing, though the individual words themselves are perfectly meaningful: "didn't was going he he to said come but." Rearranged, this meaningless jumble of words makes perfect sense: "He said he was going to come, but didn't."

Linguists do not make the rules of syntax, they only derive the rules from the way people arrange words to form meaningful sentences. Acceptable word orders within a language may be arbitrary to begin with. Soon such orders become a matter of social convention that the individual speakers of the language learn. Radical deviations from the long-established conventional word order confuse people. Therefore, a habitual order also becomes a syntactic rule of the language.

CHOMSKY'S THEORY OF SYNTAX. An influential theory of syntax proposed by Noam Chomsky in the 1950s introduced some new concepts into the study of languages. His theory also revived some very old concepts. The theory has had a significant effect on linguistics and speech–language pathology as well.

Chomsky's theory is variously known as the **transformational generative theory** and the **government and binding theory.**

Criticizing the traditional linguistic approach of merely describing language as being limited, Chomsky proposed a new theory of language (1957, 1965). He stated that syntactic structures are the essence of language. He believed that language is a product of the unique human mind. Chomsky suggested that there are universal rules of grammar that apply to all languages.

Chomsky made a distinction between language competence and language performance. He described **language competence** as the innate and perfect knowledge of the rules of the universal grammar, which apply to all languages. Such a knowledge is already available at the time of birth. He believed that unless the child is born with a knowledge of the rules of grammar, a young child of limited mental capacity would not acquire language, which is a highly complex system of codes and rules.

Language performance is the actual production of language. Though the speakers of a language have a perfect knowledge of the rules of grammar, the production itself may be imperfect because of such factors as fatigue and distraction. Chomsky was not very interested in language production. His theory concentrated heavily on the linguistic competence, because Chomsky considered the knowledge of grammar central to an understanding of language.

A few other concepts Chomsky introduced include the surface and deep structure of language. The **surface structure** (or the **S-Structure**) is the actual arrangement of words in a syntactic order. It is the phrase or the sentence you can see or hear. Underlying this surface structure is the abstract **deep structure** (or the **D-Structure**), which primarily holds the rules of sentence formation.

If the language has two structures, how are they related? Chomsky's answer was the concept of grammatic transformations. A **transformation** is an operation that relates the deep and the surface structures and yields different forms of sentences. It is a process by which you arrange and rearrange words to change sentences. Grammatic transformations involve deleting, substituting, adding, and rearranging words to change meaning. Consider the following examples:

The boy kicked the ball.
Who kicked the ball? (a question-transformation)
Did the boy kick the ball? (another question-transformation)
The ball was not kicked by the boy. (the negative-transformation)
The ball was kicked by the boy. (the passive-transformation)

Each of the examples involves a *transformation* of either adding, deleting, substituting, or rearranging words to form different kinds of sentences. These transformations account for the creative nature of language. Chomsky believed that such creative transformation of sentence forms is the essence of language. Therefore, his theory is often called the transformational generative theory of grammar. He stated that with the help of the knowledge of the rules of grammar and transformations, speakers can *generate* an endless variety of sentences.

Although revised periodically, Chomsky's theory (1957, 1965, 1981) has retained its basic assumption that language is due to a special linguistic ability and that grammar is the essence of language. Chomsky further believed that language development is not due to learning. Because the essence of language—the knowledge of the rules of universal grammar—is innate, language development is due largely to innate mechanisms.

Semantics. The study of meaning in language is called **semantics.** The **semantic component** refers to meaning that words, phrases, and sentences convey. **Semanticists,** the specialists who study meaning, believe that meaning is the essence of language and communication. Anything said may be meaningful, but if listeners do not find it, the communication is likely to stop abruptly.

The two most difficult and interrelated questions in semantics are What is meaning? and Where do you find it? Is meaning the content of language, the referents of language, a concept, a cognitive process, an indescribable mental event, or an appropriate response of a listener?

A theory that is currently popular in speech–language pathology is that the structure or form of language has a content, which is its meaning. For instance, a word which has a structure holds meaning within it. Similarly, such other structures as phrases and sentences hold their meanings. A problem with this theory is that if a structure of language, say a word, contained its own meaning, then we should have no difficulty understanding meaning of utterances in all conditions, as long as we knew the meaning of the individual words used. But sometimes, in spite of knowing what the words mean, a listener may not understand the meaning of utterances. A friend approaches you Monday morning on the campus and asks, "What happened last night?" and you are puzzled. You know the meaning of all of the words, but you still do not understand the meaning of the question.

Some theorists have proposed that the meaning of a word is the object, person, or event it refers to. According to this theory, the meaning of the word *chair* is the object chair. This is the **referent theory of meaning.** Critics of this theory point out that there are many words for which there is no clear reference (*sure, perhaps, but,* just to name a few). The theory works fine for some concrete words, but the meanings of abstract words remain elusive in this theory.

Another theory states that meaning is in the concepts we have about what we talk about. According to this theory, the meaning of the word *chair* is not the object chair, but the concept a person has gained about chairs. There are many variations of this basic position. One variation states that meaning is a **cognitive process.** Accordingly, meaning is the sum total of mental images, ideas, and thoughts that language evokes in listeners or readers. The main problem with these theories is that it is hard to study meaning objectively when it is described as a private mental event.

Some psychologists have proposed that meaning is the appropriate response of listeners. If you asked for "cookie" and you received a piece of candy, or much worse, the listener did not understand you at all, then no meaning was conveyed. We know that the meaning of an utterance was grasped only when the listener responds in some way. However, the main problem with this theory is that one can understand the meaning of an utterance but not give an overt response. In such cases, we may conclude erroneously that no meaning was conveyed.

Researchers of child language acquisition have categorized meanings that children seem to acquire. These semantic categories or relations (Gleason, 2001; McLauglin, 1998; Owens, 1996) are contrasting units of meaning. The different units of meaning are expressed in different forms of words, phrases, and sentences. For example, a child who learns to say "my hat" is showing that he or she understands the semantic notion called *possession;* the child who simply names objects has acquired the semantic notion called *nomination;* the child who says "Daddy cut the grass" has acquired the notion of *agent* (person who did the cutting), and so on. Researchers on child language have studied the sequence in which children acquire many semantic notions.

Pragmatics. In the past, language was often analyzed with no regard to its social use. The grammar of a language can be described without paying much attention to how people talk in natural settings. The rules of grammar are fixed and formal; the rules can ignore who speaks what, why, and under what conditions. This approach has been criticized by those who think of language as a tool that people use in social interactions.

Pragmatics is the study of the rules that govern the use of language in social situations. Therefore, pragmatics places greater emphasis on **functions** or use of language than on its structure. What do people do with their language? How does social context affect what is said? How do children learn what to say and when to say it? What kinds of intentions do children have behind their utterances? How can we classify language utterances in terms of their intentions or effects on other people? How are the social skills of communication, including taking turns in conversation, maintaining a topic of discussion, and narrating a story, learned? These are the kinds of questions the experts in pragmatics try to answer.

There is no single theory of pragmatics of language. In an early pragmatic theory, every utterance is a **speech act,** which means that utterances influence listeners, and, therefore, saying also is doing (Austin, 1962; Searle, 1969). It was suggested that speech acts are the basic units of communication, not morphemes, words, or sentences.

Although pragmatists generally agree that language use or function is more important than its structure, they do not agree on the kinds or number of functions a language serves. According to one theory, language serves such functions as instrumental, regulatory, and interactional (Halliday, 1975). Through the **instrumental** function of language, we try to get what we want. Most of our verbal requests through which we get our needs satisfied are instrumental (e.g., "Could I have some water, please?"). Through the **regulatory** function, we try to get others to do what we want them to do; when we command something (e.g., "Do as I tell you"), we use the regulatory function of language. Through the **interactional** function, we engage others in social interaction (e.g., "Let us play tennis this afternoon").

Pragmatists have pointed out that children acquire language in specific social contexts. Even to understand the meaning of an utterance, we need to know its physical and social context. For example, a child pointing to the spilled milk and saying "milk" probably means something totally different from the same child saying "milk" while reaching for the milk bottle.

In recent years, researchers also have looked at the rules of conversation. It has been suggested that speakers somehow follow the rules of taking turns and not interrupting the speaker, maintaining eye contact, and maintaining topics of conversation. When these rules are violated, we have pragmatic language disorders.

The Behavioral Study of Language

Psychologists have offered theories of language that are different from those the linguists have offered. Just as there are many linguistic theories of language, there are many psychological theories as well. In this section, I shall describe only one of the theories to give you a sample of a nonlinguistic approach to the study of language.

The behavioral psychologist B. F. Skinner (1957) proposed a theory that is most nonlinguistic in its orientation. Skinner was not interested in language as a mental or cognitive system because he considered such a view would preclude an experimental study of the subject matter. Therefore, he reformulated language as verbal behavior so it could be studied with the techniques he considered most appropriate.

Skinner (1957) defined **verbal behavior** as a form of social behavior maintained by the actions of a verbal community. He did not analyze language in terms of such structural units as phonemes, morphemes, syllables, words, phrases, and sentences. Instead, he analyzed functional units of verbal behaviors. A **functional unit** is a class or a group of verbal responses all of which are produced under similar circumstances and receive similar consequences. A functional unit has similar causes and the responses within the unit tend to have similar effects on the listener.

In the case of verbal behavior, a **consequence** is what a listener or listeners say or do. One kind of consequence is called a reinforcer. A **reinforcer** is an event that follows a response and thereby makes that response more likely in the future. Another kind of consequence is called a punisher. A **punisher** is an event that follows a response and thereby makes that response less likely in the future. A functional unit (a class of verbal responses) may have one type of consequence. A different functional unit may have a different type of consequence. A teenager, for example, brags in the presence of some friends who have paid attention in the past (reinforcer). Thus, his or her bragging has received a reinforcing consequence from friends and, therefore, is more likely in their presence. However, the same teenager may not brag in the presence of his or her parents, who may have discouraged (punished) it. Thus, the teenager's bragging will have received a different consequence from parents and, therefore, is less likely in their presence.

Verbal behavior is characteristically produced under social stimulation. Obviously, and for the most part, overt speaking behavior requires the presence of other persons who serve as the audience. **Audience** in Skinner's analysis refers to a relation between the speaker and the listener. The audience sets the stage for speech. In some cases, a physiological need such as thirst or hunger stimulates speech (e.g., "Do you have something to eat?"). Needs of this sort cause various kinds of requests, commands, and demands. Skinner called them **mands,** which are reinforced by food and other biologically satisfying events and are caused by states of deprivation or motivation.

In many cases, physical objects and events stimulate speaking. Verbal responses of this kind are called tacts. A **tact** is a group of verbal responses that describe and comment on the things and events around us. Tacts are reinforced socially. A smile, a nod of approval, and similar statements by a listener may all reinforce a tact. For example, when you say "What a beautiful sunset!" someone may smile or say "It's gorgeous!"

Tacts and mands help clarify the statement made earlier that functional units with different causes and different consequences are the basic units in Skinner's analysis of verbal behavior. Mands are functional units in the sense that there are different kinds of mands, but all are made when something is needed and are reinforced similarly. For example, "May I have something to drink?" or "May I have something to eat?" are both mands and are reinforced similarly: both statements are reinforced with something to drink or eat. Similarly, "Here are two chairs" or "There goes a monkey" are both tacts caused by environmental objects or events and are reinforced by some kind of social response from one or more listeners. This also illustrates that each functional unit contains a variety of responses.

Other functional units Skinner described include echoics, intraverbals, and autoclitics. **Echoics** are imitative verbal responses whose stimuli are the speech

> By and large, Skinner's view of verbal behavior and the pragmatic view of language share common grounds.

of another person. Reinforcement for an echoic is based on a close resemblance between the stimulus and the response. Clinicians who teach language to children with language disorders typically model the target responses, which the children imitate. The clinician reinforces only when the child's imitations at least approximate the clinician's modeled response.

We all know that once we begin talking, we may just go on. What causes such continuous talking when we cannot point to some motivational and physical stimuli? The causes of such talking is talking itself. Prior verbal responses stimulate subsequent verbal responses. The fact that you said something, for whatever the reason, can make you say more. Verbal responses so caused are intraverbals. **Intraverbals** are a group of verbal responses that are stimulated by the speaker's own prior verbal responses. Much of our conversational speech is made up of tacts and intraverbals.

Skinner does not think that grammar is primary in verbal behavior in the sense that it comes first in verbal learning or that it is all-important. Children do not learn grammatic morphemes before they learn other aspects of verbal behavior. The question of syntax emerges only when the child has acquired certain words to be put in order. Therefore, grammar is secondary to such primary verbal responses as mands and tacts. Skinner's term for grammar and related responses is autoclitics. **Autoclitics** are secondary verbal responses which help point out the causes of primary verbal responses. In this sense, Skinner's interpretation of grammar is radically different from that of linguists.

To understand Skinner's definition of an autoclitic, we must ask, What do grammatical features do? Why do we use a grammatical feature, say a plural s or a possessive 's or an auxiliary is? Are they produced for the benefit of the speaker or the listener? In other words, who needs grammatical features? In the following utterances, what do the underlined features do?

I see two book*s* on the table.
Mommy's hat.

The underlined parts are traditionally described as grammatical morphemes and are described as autoclitics in the behavioral analysis: the plural and the possessive s inflection, the article *the,* and the preposition *on.* These autoclitics point to some aspects of the stimulus situation that caused the speaker to say what he or she said. By using the plural s in the first utterance, the speaker tells the listener that the cause of his or her statement is more than one book; by using the preposition *on,* the speaker is pointing to the relation between the book and the table, also a part of the causative stimuli; and by using the article *the,* the speaker is specifying which of the several tables is part of the stimuli that prompted the response. In the second utterance, the child is specifying the relationship between the mother and a hat. The possessive 's tells the listener that the stimuli for the verbal response include the mother and her hat.

The examples make it clear that autoclitics are a way of clarifying for the listener some aspects of the stimuli that prompted the verbal response. Grammar is for the benefit of the listener, not the speaker. This may be the reason why speakers with language disorders are often surprised when people do not fully understand them because of the missing grammatical features. Those speakers know what they are talking about. But what causes them to say what they say (or aspects of stimuli that prompted a response) is not clear to the listeners.

> # A Comparative Summary of the Approaches to the Study of Language
>
> ## Linguistic Approaches
>
> - Linguists are concerned mainly with the structure of language.
>
> - Language is defined as a mental system of codes, symbols, and rules that are used in communication.
>
> - The approach identifies phonological, morphological, syntactic, semantic, and pragmatic components.
>
> - The phonological component refers to the speech sounds and their patterns.
>
> - The morphological component consists of word structures and grammatic morphemes.
>
> - The syntactic component consists of word order and sentence structure. The semantic component is the meaning in language.
>
> - The pragmatic aspect is the use of language in social contexts.
>
> ## Behavioral Approach
>
> - The behavioral scientists are concerned mainly with the cause–effect (functional) units, not structures of language. They prefer to describe language as verbal behavior.
>
> - Verbal behavior is defined as a form of social behavior shaped and maintained by the members of a verbal community.
>
> - Verbal behavior is broken down into such functional units as mands and tacts that are caused by a different set of factors. Responses belonging to a functional unit are reinforced by similar consequences that follow them.
>
> - Functional units are learned under specific conditions of internal (motivational) or external stimulation and specific consequences that follow them.
>
> - Grammar is not primary; it is secondary to primary functional units and helps point out the reasons or causes of those primary responses.

Fluency

Normal voice and the acquisition of speech and language are not sufficient to communicate effectively. Effective communication requires fluency. Fluency is a characteristic of both speech and language. One can say a word fluently or struggle while saying it, giving an impression of lack of fluency. Most often, however, fluency is best judged when the speaker talks continuously. In this sense, language production is a better indicator of fluency than isolated speech production.

Fluency is easy, smooth, flowing, and effortless speech. To the listener, fluent speech gives an impression of a rhythmic flow. To the speaker, fluent speech feels easy to produce and requires less effort, struggle, and muscular tension. Fluency facilitates communication. While nonfluent speech does not necessarily suggest a lack of language competence, fluent speech, especially when it makes sense, almost always suggests a high level of competence.

Nonfluent speech is not a necessary indication of lack of knowledge. People who have disorders of fluency, such as stuttering, or those who speak a foreign language with difficulty, may be knowledgeable but may not be fluent. However, fluent speech on a topic may be an indication of a high degree of knowledge. Compared to a person who knows little about a topic, a person who knows more about the topic can speak with greater fluency. While knowledge can lead to fluent speech, knowledge is not necessary to be fluent, at least for short durations. To listeners' dismay, some people are fluent without much knowledge. However, extended, sensible, and fluent speech on a topic almost always requires good knowledge of whatever is talked about.

Fluent speech flows perhaps because speech also can stimulate more speech. In the flowing, fluent speech, one word leads to another, one sentence prompts another, and one thought stimulates another thought. Prior speech of the speaker evokes subsequent speech in a chainlike fashion. In a well-formed sentence, every word and sentence may be a stimulus for the next word and sentence. When this happens, the speech or the speaker seems to move smoothly from one segment of speech to the next.

The chainlike characteristic of fluent speech may be due to the intraverbal nature of talking. Intraverbals, as you recall from the behavioral analysis of language, are verbal behaviors whose causes are the speaker's own prior verbal behaviors. When we say one word leads to another, we suggest the intraverbal flow of speech. Therefore, it is possible that, among other factors, intraverbals make fluent speech possible.

Fluency also is closely related to another aspect of communication called prosody. **Prosody** refers to variations in rate, pitch, loudness, stress, intonation, and rhythm of continuous speech. Prosody is a quality of both voice and fluency. Speech that lacks variations in pitch and loudness is monotonous. Similarly, speech that is halting, dysfluent, and unusually slow or fast lacks the normal rhythm of fluency.

Hearing

Hearing is an important aspect of communication. Though not a component of speech or language, hearing is essential for normally acquired verbal communication. Therefore, hearing is closely related to speech and language.

Read more about the anatomy of the ear in **Chapter 3.**

The biological mechanism of human hearing includes the ear, the auditory nerve, and the brain. The ear is divided into three parts: the outer ear, the middle ear, and the inner ear. The outer ear includes the readily visible pinna (the structure that supports the frames of your eyeglasses) and the outer ear canal. The canal leads to the eardrum, which is the first structure of the middle ear. The sound waves travel through the canal and strike the eardrum, which vibrates and transmits sound to the three small bones in the middle ear. The inner ear is filled with fluids and an important structure called the cochlea. The vibrations of the middle ear bones cause movements in the fluids of the inner ear. These movements stimulate the structures within the cochlea. This stimulation is picked up by a nerve that specializes in carrying sound from the inner ear to the brain (the eighth cranial nerve). The brain interprets the meaning of the sound.

Normal hearing is essential for the typical acquisition of speech and language behaviors. Children acquire the language they hear. Normal hearing is essential for speech perception. If speech is not perceived by a young child, the acquisition of speech will be difficult. If speech is not perceived (or understood), communication is impaired at all age levels. Normal hearing also is essential for monitoring one's own speech production. We hear ourselves speak and make modifications in how we say what we say. In other words, the hearing mechanism gives us feedback on our speech performance. Based on this feedback we make modifications in our speech production.

Read more about audiology, the science of hearing, in **Chapter 10.**

Disorders of Communication

With an understanding of the basics of human communication and language, we are now ready to consider the disorders of communication. This discussion takes us into two professional realms: speech–language pathology and audiology. The profession of **speech–language pathology** is concerned with the study and understanding of human communication and its disorders, and assessment and treatment of those disorders. The twin profession of **audiology** is concerned with the study and understanding of normal and disordered hearing, and the rehabilitation of individuals with hearing impairments. The two professions are closely allied because of the interrelation between verbal communication and hearing.

Except for a few, very young children, persons who have disorders of communication know that they have a problem. Quite often, they can say what kind of a problem they have. Some individuals say they stutter, and others say they have a voice problem. Parents report that the child has a hearing problem, cannot say speech sounds correctly, or cannot talk in sentences.

There is no definition of disorders of communication that is satisfactory to all speech–language pathologists. For a long time, clinicians have used Van Riper's (1978) definition. Essentially, Van Riper said that **disordered speech** deviates from the speech of other persons, calls attention to itself, interferes with communication, and often causes distress in both the speaker and the listener.

Van Riper's definition of communication disorders emphasizes deviancy from the normal and the problem it creates for effective communication. The result is that not only the speaker is negatively affected, but also the listener. The definition, though widely used, is problematic because it is difficult to determine objectively how a speech disorder *interferes* with communication or how the speaker or the listener is *distressed*. It also is difficult to determine how and when speech calls attention to itself. In addition, it is hard to specify how often and to what extent speech should *call attention to itself* before it is diagnosed as defective. To complicate the matter further, exceptionally good speech may also call attention to itself.

Many clinicians prefer to describe disorders of communication in general terms and try to be as specific as possible in describing particular disorders. In general terms, people with disorders of communication may not be able to say what they wish to say; may not be able to say all they want to say; and may not be able to say what they wish as promptly or as smoothly as they want. Listeners may not understand some or most of what they say. The listeners may not know how to react to the speech that is defective and difficult to understand. Most listeners are embarrassed, whereas some listeners, some of the time, may express negative reactions. Some listeners tend to avoid people with communicative disorders. The speaker, because of all these reasons, may feel frustrated, embarrassed, and sometimes humiliated. The speaker may feel anxiety in speaking situations because of the past failures to communicate effectively, promptly, or fully. Some speakers with disordered speech may withdraw from speaking situations and interpersonal relationships.

In more specific terms, clinicians describe disorders of communication by pointing out a particular aspect of it that is problematic. For instance, a clinician might say that there is a voice problem or a fluency problem. Thus, a *classification* of disorders of communication directs our attention to specific disorders.

Classification of Communicative Disorders

Communicative disorders may be classified on the basis of either known or presumed causes, the age of onset, or different components of communication (voice, articulation, language, fluency, and hearing).

The classification based on known or presumed causes of disorders is **etiological. Etiology** means the study of causes of diseases and disorders. Physical diseases are often classified on the basis of their etiology. There are two broad etiological classifications of communicative disorders: the organic and the functional.

Organic disorders of communication are thought to be caused by some defect in the neurophysiological mechanism of speech. For example, a person who suffers a stroke and sustains damage to the left side of the brain is likely to lose some or most of his or her speaking ability. Called aphasia, this disorder of communication is a direct result of the brain damage. Similarly, children who are born with deafness or clefts of the palates, or who experience brain injury early in life, are likely to exhibit disorders of communication. Because of their physical basis, such disorders of communication are classified as organic or neurogenic.

Functional disorders of communication are those that do not have a demonstrable organic or neurologic cause. These disorders may also be called **idiopathic,** which means they are of unknown origin. It is presumed that functional disorders have an origin in faulty learning, environment, habits, emotional problems, and other unknown causes. It is a classification based on negative evidence: if an organic cause is not found, the disorder is thought to be functional or idiopathic. In many cases, there may be no positive evidence of a particular nonorganic cause. People who exhibit functional disorders of communication are physically healthy, their nervous system is normal, and their speech mechanism is free from defects. Nonetheless, they have a communicative disorder. For example, most people who stutter do not show serious organic deviations. Similarly, many children who have difficulty in producing speech sounds or learning language show no organic problems that could explain such difficulty.

The organic-functional classification of communicative disorders is not entirely satisfactory. The classification is etiological, but for many disorders, especially for the functional disorders, it is not possible to determine the causes. In most cases, the clinician cannot specify the cause or causes of stuttering, articulation difficulties, or language problems. That an organic cause was not found does not suggest that it does not exist. Our methods of detecting organic causes may be deficient. But more important, saying that something is not the cause of a disorder is not the same as pointing out its cause. After having diagnosed a functional disorder of communication, the clinician still does not know what caused it. The idea that functional disorders are habits or that they are due to emotional disorders is too vague to be useful.

Although specific causes of disorders are not always found, speech–language pathologists believe that all disorders of communication have causes. In recent years, research has suggested many potential causes. Currently, our knowledge about the causes of disorders applies mostly to groups of persons; it is difficult to say what caused a given disorder in a given individual.

The classification based on the age of onset yields two categories: congenital and acquired. **Congenital disorders** are noticed at the time of birth or soon thereafter. It is true that many speech–language disorders are not noticed at the time of or soon after birth because the newborn does not say much! However, many conditions that either cause or are associated with communicative disorders later may be noticed soon after birth or in very early infancy. These conditions include genetic syndromes that cause birth defects, physical deformities, brain damage, and mental retardation. Cleft palate is another congenital condition that may lead to speech and language problems. Similarly, deafness may be congenital; signs of deafness may be detected early in infancy.

A communicative disorder is **acquired** when there has been a period of normal communication. Some children and adults will have developed normal communicative behaviors before they become impaired for some reason. As noted before, a normally speaking adult may suffer a stroke and lose much of his or her ability to communicate. A child who was speaking normally may develop stuttering at age 5 or 7. An older person may lose much of his or her hearing, which may create difficulties in communication. In each of these and many similar cases of acquired communicative disorder, the individual will have had normal communicative behaviors prior to the onset.

The classification of congenital and acquired disorders, too, are not specific enough to be useful in planning treatment. The clinician needs to know what kind of disorder (acquired or congenital) a person has. An acquired or congenital problem of communication may affect speech, language, or both, as well as voice and fluency. If possible, the clinician would like to know what caused the disorder.

The classification based on the components of communication described earlier is illustrated in Figure 1.3. Any or all of the five components of communication—voice, articulation, language, fluency, and hearing—may be disordered. Thus we have disorders of voice, articulation, language, fluency, and hearing. This classification is **descriptive** (not etiological). In using this classification, the clinician looks at the particular aspect of communication that is disordered and describes the kinds of difficulties the person experiences.

While using a descriptive classification of disorders, the clinician still can make statements about the potential or actual causes when they are known. When the evidence justifies it, the clinician can make statements about the possible causes in given cases. Because this type of classification is most widely used in speech–language pathology, we shall use it in this book.

In the subsequent chapters of the book, you will read in detail about the various disorders of voice, articulation, language, fluency, and hearing. Therefore, our overview of the disorders will be brief and selective to illustrate their varied nature.

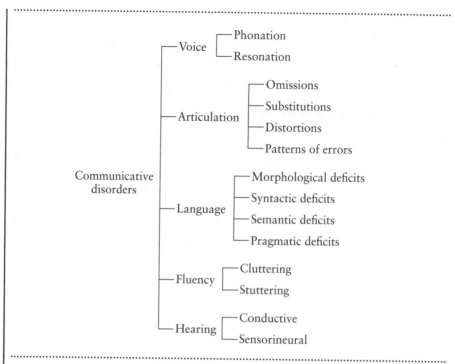

Figure 1.3. Major categories of communicative disorders.

Disorders of Voice

Disorders of voice
and their treatment
are described in
Chapter 7.

As a fundamental aspect of communication, normal and healthy voice is essential for socially acceptable oral communication. When the vocal mechanism does not work normally or the individual does not use that mechanism properly, we have disorders of voice. An extreme example of voice disorder is called **aphonia,** or total loss of voice. An aphonic person whispers to communicate. In some cases, aphonia is functional in the sense that there is no structural defect associated with the larynx. This kind of aphonia has a sudden onset possibly due to emotional trauma. In other cases, paralysis of the vocal folds can cause aphonia. This type of aphonia is organic.

Several voice disorders are due to vocally abusive behaviors of speakers. Excessive talking, shouting, cheering, and screaming are the primary abusive vocal behaviors that can cause vocal nodules and associated voice problems. **Vocal nodules,** more commonly seen in children, are small nodes that develop on the vocal folds and cause breathy and hoarse (rough) voice.

Disorders of Articulation (Phonological Disorders)

Most children learn the speech sounds of their language with ease and no special instruction. However, some children find this task extremely difficult and frustrating. In fact, problems of articulation in school-age children are among the most frequently treated disorders of communication.

Articulation is disordered when a person cannot correctly produce one or more of the phonemes of his or her language. Errors of many phonemes that form patterns or clusters are often described as **phonological disorders** (Peña-Brooks & Hegde, 2000).

Articulation disorders can pose a serious problem for the listeners. The speech of children who misarticulate multiple phonemes may be unintelligible to listeners. A few such children, especially when very young, talk freely with their multiple misarticulations. In such cases, the listeners have to constantly guess what the child says. A child, for example, may say, "Tum ba" for "Come back," or "Gi me um dum" for "Give me some gum." Not surprisingly, listeners find such a child difficult to understand.

Whereas most children's speech or articulation disorders are functional, speech disorders in adults, especially in those who have had normal speech, are usually due to some neurological problem. Such disorders are called **motor speech disorders.** The term *motor* suggests that it is the movement of the speech mechanism that is impaired due to nerve damage. The lips, tongue, jaw, and soft palate are not able to move swiftly and accurately to produce speech. People who have motor speech disorders may not show significant problems in language; that is, they can formulate grammatically correct sentences. However, they just cannot accurately produce what they can formulate because they have difficulty moving the speech structures as they wish.

Disorders of articulation and their treatment are described in **Chapter 4.**

Adult speech disorders of neurologic origin are described in **Chapter 9.**

Disorders of Language

A failure to acquire language in childhood or a loss of language in adulthood affects all aspects of life. In many respects, the language disorders found in children are different from those found in adults who have had normal communicative behaviors.

Language Disorders in Children

In children, difficulties in the acquisition of language are called **language disorders.** In the most extreme case, the child simply fails to acquire any oral language; the child does not speak at all. Such total lack of language acquisition is rare, however. Most children who experience difficulties in acquiring language do acquire some language. But these children do not acquire language at the same rate as others of their age. Some of them stop making much progress when other children of their age are still learning more complex aspects of language.

Language problems of the young child may be apparent at an early age. The child may be delayed in babbling, saying the first words, combining words into phrases, and producing grammatically correct sentences. Soon, the problems of the child with a language disorder become apparent in the morphologic, syntactic, semantic, and pragmatic aspects of language. The child may have a simple vocabulary consisting of basic and concrete words. The child may learn only one or two meanings of words that have many different meanings. For example, *food* may mean only dinner, and *cat* may mean only the family cat (Hegde, 1995).

Once some forms of sentences are learned, the child may fail to use various grammatic morphemes. The child's sentences may be simple or telegraphic in nature. Such grammatical elements as the articles, prepositions (e.g., *in, on*), and conjunctions (e.g., *and, but*) are typically missing in **telegraphic speech.** It tends to contain the most crucial words—nouns and verbs—while omitting less important, nonetheless required, features of language. Expressions like

Language acquisition and disorders are described in **Chapter 5.**

"Mommy come" for "Mommy *is* com*ing*" and "Me sick" for "*I am* sick" are commonly heard in the speech of children with language disorders.

The child with a language disorder tends to shy away from social situations. The child is less likely to use whatever language he or she has mastered. While talking, the child may fail to use the available language properly. The child may not know when to say what and to whom. In other words, the child will not have learned the social use of language. The child may not maintain eye contact during conversation. The child may change the topic of conversation abruptly and interrupt the speaker all the time.

Many children with language disorders are otherwise healthy and normal. However, in some cases, language disorders may be associated with mental retardation, hearing impairment, brain damage, or behavioral disorders including childhood schizophrenia and autism.

Many children who have language problems early in life can be expected to have academic difficulties when they enter grade school. Because most academic skills are language based, children with language disorders experience reading and writing problems. Those children may have difficulty in mastering abstract mathematical and scientific concepts. In school, children with language disorders may find themselves socially isolated as well.

Language Disorders in Adults

In some cases, the language disorders of childhood may persist into adulthood. Many people with mental retardation and congenitally deaf people continue to have oral language problems throughout their life span. However, for several reasons, many people experience language disorders for the first time as adults. Such individuals will have acquired language as usual and will have communicated normally for most of their lives. Then, in some cases, suddenly, and rather dramatically, adults may lose their language skills. In other cases, the language skills may deteriorate slowly over a period of time.

The sudden appearance of a language problem in adults has several causes. Most of these causes damage the brain, especially the left hemisphere of the brain, which is most responsible for language functions in a majority of people. As noted before, a frequent cause of adult language disorders is a **stroke,** which interrupts the flow of blood to various parts of the brain. When a group of brain cells do not receive blood, they may die from lack of oxygen. Other causes of adult language disorders include brain tumor and head injury. When the left hemisphere is damaged, most adults suffer a language disorder known as **aphasia,** which is a loss of language. Most people with aphasia, however, do not lose all of their speech; the degree of loss varies among individuals. Some individuals with aphasia are able to talk fluently, but their speech does not make sense. Most people with aphasia tend to have difficulties in speaking, understanding spoken language, and writing.

Adult language disorders of neurological origin are described in **Chapter 9.**

Adult loss of language also may be due to many neurologic diseases typically found in older people. A general term used to describe some of the progressive diseases of the nervous system in the aged is **dementia,** which is sometimes described as **senile dementia.** Alzheimer's disease, for example, is a form of dementia. The onset and development of this neurologic disease is a slow process. Eventually, patients are totally confused and they lose much of their memory of recent events. The patient is usually disoriented to time, place, and people. Speech and language functions deteriorate rapidly until the patient is unable to communicate altogether.

Disorders of Fluency

A person may have acquired the normal use of voice, articulation, and language but still may be vulnerable to problems of communication known as fluency disorders. The person who has a fluency disorder knows exactly what to say but cannot say it fluently.

There are at least two varieties of fluency disorders: cluttering and stuttering. **Cluttering** involves impaired fluency and rapid but disordered articulation, possibly combined with disorganized thought. Obviously, people differ in the rate at which they talk. Some talk slower than others and some talk at an unusually fast rate. Many speakers can talk relatively rapidly and yet be intelligible. However, when the rate is abnormally fast, the precision with which the sounds are articulated is lost. The speech then becomes unclear. This is cluttering.

Stuttering is the better known and the most researched of the fluency disorders. **Stuttering** is a disorder of fluency with excessive amounts or excessively long durations of dysfluency, which often are combined with tension, struggle, and related behaviors. People who stutter may repeat parts of words ("t-t-t-t-time") or whole words ("How, how, how are you today?"). They may prolong a sound ("sssssSaturday"). They may use excessive amounts of interjections such as *uh* and *um*. People who stutter may have long silent intervals in the middle of utterances. They often struggle to say the words, experience excessive muscle tension and hand and feet movements, and exhibit facial grimaces including knitting of the eyebrows, rapid eye blinks, and puckering of the lips, all associated with stuttering.

Stuttering typically starts in early childhood. It tends to run in families. Males are more frequently affected than females. If untreated, stuttering, in many cases, tends to persist into adult life. Some overcome stuttering without professional help. Severe forms of stuttering are emotionally debilitating to the individual. People who stutter tend to withdraw from social situations, avoid certain words that typically give them trouble, select occupations that do not require much talking, and are unhappy about all of these actions.

Disorders of fluency and their treatment are described in **Chapter 6.**

Hearing Impairment

We noted earlier that normal hearing is essential for the acquisition of oral speech and language behaviors. Therefore, impaired hearing is a frequent cause of a variety of communicative disorders.

The two major types of hearing impairment are conductive and sensorineural. In **conductive** hearing loss, the sound transmission from the outer or the middle ear to the inner ear is impaired. A frequent cause of conductive hearing loss in children is **otitis media,** or middle ear infection, due to cold, allergy, and other reasons. Due to such diseases of the middle ear, the sound is not efficiently transmitted to the inner ear. Conductive hearing loss also may be due to **otosclerosis,** in which the tiny bones of the middle ear do not vibrate normally because of soft, spongy growth on them. Once again, the sound is not efficiently transmitted to the inner ear. Less frequently, conductive hearing loss may be due to congenital malformations of the outer ear or the ear canal leading to the eardrum. The ear canal may be completely closed or the opening may be too small, thus blocking or greatly reducing the amount of sound that strikes the eardrum.

In **sensorineural** hearing loss, either the inner ear, or the auditory nerve that transmits sound to the brain, or both, may be impaired. The sensorineural hearing loss is in most cases congenital (present at birth) and in other cases hereditary. The cause may be prenatal, in that an infectious disease suffered by the pregnant mother may have damaged the fetal hearing mechanism. Maternal rubella (German measles) and mumps, among other diseases, are known to cause hearing loss in children. If the delivery of a baby is prolonged and distressed, the baby may suffer from **anoxia** (lack of oxygen), which can damage the hearing mechanism and cause sensorineural hearing loss.

Children who have normal hearing and communication may acquire sensorineural hearing loss. Such viral diseases as mumps, measles, or chicken pox in children may cause sensorineural hearing impairment.

The reduced hearing sensitivity of the older person also is sensorineural. This type of hearing loss is known as **presbycusis** and tends to be greater for higher frequency sounds than for lower frequency sounds.

Chapter 10 describes how audiologists measure hearing loss.

Regardless of the type of loss, the magnitude of its effect on communication depends on the degree of loss. Hearing loss varies from mild to profound. Even a mild conductive loss in early childhood can retard the process of speech and language acquisition. Significant delay in speech and language acquisition has been linked to chronic conductive hearing loss. Fortunately, surgical treatment of otitis media and otosclerosis is successful. Early treatment can prevent lasting effects of the conductive hearing loss on the acquisition of speech and language behaviors.

Hearing and its disorders are described in **Chapter 10**.

Sensorineural hearing loss tends to be much more severe than conductive hearing loss. Therefore, compared with conductive loss, sensorineural loss causes more serious problems of communication. Congenital sensorineural loss usually has marked effects on the acquisition of speech and language behaviors. A child with such a loss has difficulty learning the speech sounds. Numerous errors of articulation begin to appear. The child tends to distort, substitute, and omit many speech sounds. The child's voice will lack normal intonation and rhythm; the voice may also be of higher pitch. The acquisition of language is delayed in most cases. Children with moderate to profound loss may more readily learn manual signs and gestures than oral language skills. They tend to have limited vocabulary and have the greatest amount of difficulty with sentence structure and grammar of language.

Significant hearing loss affects both the production and the perception (understanding what others say) of speech. A person with a hearing impairment has difficulty monitoring his or her own speech, language, and voice. Limited communicative behaviors may lead to social isolation.

Prevalence of Communicative Disorders

It is often difficult to imagine the magnitude of a problem until we come across some statistics. How many people in the country are communicatively impaired? There is no conclusive answer to this question because no single research has focused on all kinds of communicative disorders in the entire population. Therefore, statements regarding the prevalence of communicative disorders are tentative. Most experts believe, however, that disorders of communication are more prevalent than most people think.

It is estimated that at least 17% of the U.S. population has a disorder of communication (Castrogiovanni, 1999b). This may even be a conservative estimate. The second highest of the handicapping conditions of school-age children are disorders of communication. Of all the school-age children receiving special educational services, in excess of 42% are classified as learning disabled and in excess of 25% are classified as speech or language impaired (Casby, 1989). It also is known that because of differing criteria for service delivery, many children who have less serious forms of communicative disorders may not be receiving services. Therefore, the prevalence data based on the number of children receiving services may not be accurate.

Communicative disorders are prevalent to a much higher degree in children who are otherwise disabled. In excess of 26% of all children with disabilities may have a disorder of communication (American Speech-Language-Hearing Association, 1984). About 2% of children with disabilities are hearing impaired. A majority of more than 6 million or so individuals with mental retardation in the country have speech and language problems.

Estimates of prevalence of specific disorders of communication are not entirely reliable, and the figures for all disorders may not add up to the total estimates. Roughly 3% of school-age children have articulation disorders and 4% of them stutter. The prevalence of stuttering in the general population is about 1%. The prevalence of voice disorders in the general population is estimated at 3% to 10%; it may be higher in school-age children and in older individuals (Castrogiovanni, 1999b). Language disorders are found in 8% to 12% of preschoolers. As children grow older, the prevalence of language disorders decreases. Largely due to neurological problems (e.g., strokes and dementia), 5% to 10% of the older population may experience language disorders (Bello, 1994; Castrogiovanni, 1999b). Consistent with increases in the number of older Americans, the prevalence of communicative disorders associated with aging also will reach higher levels. It is estimated that by the year 2040, there will be 65 million older Americans. Therefore, such problems as hearing loss and communicative disorders due to strokes and degenerative diseases of the brain (e.g., Alzheimer's disease) are expected to increase significantly in the coming decades.

In the general population, about 11% may have a hearing loss. Many of these people may also have a speech, voice, or language problem. As expected, the prevalence of hearing loss increases with age and is highest in the older populations. While only 1% to 2% of persons under 18 may have a hearing loss, nearly 32% of those 75 and older may have a hearing loss (Castrogiovanni, 1999a).

Prevalence refers to the number of individuals (or a percentage of the population) that currently have a particular disorder. Often, the prevalence of a disorder is based on the number of people who receive services in clinical and educational facilities. Unfortunately, many groups do not receive adequate services from speech–language pathologists and audiologists. Therefore, the prevalence of communicative disorders in such groups may be grossly underestimated. Communicative disorders of the mentally ill and those of the prison populations are probably in this category. Another major group that does not receive adequate services is the elderly in nursing homes and extended care facilities. A survey has shown that 60% of the elderly living in nursing homes may be communicatively impaired (Mueller & Peters, 1981). The same survey showed that 21% had voice disorders, 19% had articulation disorders (including

The term **incidence,** contrasted with prevalence, means the number of *new* cases that are likely to emerge in a population within a specified time period. Those who already have a disorder are excluded from this calculation.

dysarthria), 11% had aphasia, and 9% had hearing loss. Other surveys have shown that the prevalence of hearing loss in the age group of 70 to 79 years is about 70% (Ventry & Weinstein, 1983).

Effects of Communicative Disorders

Because communication is the essence of social existence, a serious disorder of communication has profound effects on the individual. The effects on social, emotional, and educational aspects of the child are considerable. Like communication, the disorder of communication also is an interactional process. Both the speaker with an impairment and his or her nonimpaired listeners are affected by the disorder.

Children with Communicative Disorders

A very young child who just began to stutter or misarticulate speech sounds may not be aware of his or her speech problem. But this lack of awareness does not last too long. Soon adults and children begin to react to the child's impaired communication. The child then begins to realize that there is something wrong with his or her way of talking.

That realization also is the beginning of much frustration, humiliation, embarrassment, social withdrawal, self-doubt, avoidance behaviors, feelings of shame, and many other emotional reactions. Children who have speech disorders can be an easy target for teasing by other children. Even when there is no explicit teasing, many children and even some adults cannot hide their negative reactions. People with communicative disorders may be deprived of opportunities to speak because of the belief that "they can't talk right." That they cannot talk right often translates into "they can't talk at all."

Many people believe that a child with a communicative disorder is less capable than children who speak normally. The child may sense this implicit or explicit assumption in strangers, neighbors, teachers, and others. Teachers may expect less from children with communicative disorders. Eventually, parents may also think that their child with a speech or language disorder cannot accomplish as much as other children. Finally, the child may come to believe that he or she is not, after all, as capable as other children with normal communicative skills.

Sometimes other people's good intentions do not work to the child's advantage. For example, a teacher who never calls on a child who stutters to answer questions or make oral presentations may be doing so to spare embarrassment for the child. But the child may feel completely left out and become increasingly more fearful of such assignments. More emotional damage may be caused by a teacher who abruptly terminates a child's oral presentation because the child who stutters is having a difficult time.

A child who is not able to articulate speech sounds or does not have adequate language skills may be frustrated in getting simple needs fulfilled. Parents also may be frustrated because they do not understand what their children with language disorders want. Some young children with language disorders cry and fuss all the time. They try to point to things, gesture, and lead the parents by hand to things they need. But when these strategies do not work—many times they do not—they have no other recourse. Some mothers of children with language disorders report that on occasion they spend so much time trying to figure out what their children want that both they and their children are frustrated and exhausted in the process. There are times when their attempts are totally futile.

As the child grows older, the untreated or unsuccessfully treated disorder of communication begins to take a greater toll on the life of the child. Schooling may be delayed because of a speech problem. In some cases, such a delay may not be justified. While a significant language disorder may justify delayed schooling, many instances of articulation and stuttering problems do not justify such a delay. Many children with these disorders have normal or superior intellectual abilities. Nonetheless, a misarticulating or stuttering child may be held back from the first or one of the subsequent grades. The negative feedback the child receives from such an action compounds the child's emotional responses and instills the belief that he or she is less capable than others simply because of the communication problem.

Adults with Communicative Disorders

The social problems the child with a communicative disability experiences may continue into the adolescent and adult years. However, the young adult with communicative disabilities faces additional problems, most of which center around social, educational, and occupational issues. The relationship with the opposite sex may pose special problems for the young adult. A young man whose voice is high pitched may sound immature and personally and socially unacceptable to females. The young man who lisps may find himself in a similar situation. A stutterer, because of past failures at communication, may cease all efforts at social interaction.

Young adults with a communication problem face dilemmas regarding educational and occupational choices. Because the occupational choices dictate the selection of educational programs, the two problems are closely related. People with communication problems think that they cannot enter certain occupations though they very much wish to. A college junior who stuttered told me that he really wanted to be a radio announcer but was terrified of taking courses in broadcasting and mass communication. He had decided to major in philosophy instead. He thought that philosophers are quiet thinkers, so philosophy would be kind to his disability. Another young woman who stuttered wanted to be a teacher but could not think of herself in front of the class talking to the kids. A high school senior who had a mild articulation problem wanted to be a physician but was not sure he would be accepted into medical school until his speech problem cleared. A woman who had an ambition of becoming a singer had second thoughts about it because of her frequent episodes of hoarse voice.

Many adults with communicative disorders eventually gain admission to various educational programs. Some are successfully treated by this time, others have improved to varying degrees, and some may still have the same problem. A few of the untreated go ahead with their first choices and still succeed against all odds. Others manage to complete their college education, first choice or not.

Many people, although disabled, find jobs in which they continue to have problems. I once treated a 28-year-old woman who stuttered and worked at the national head office of an insurance company. The main responsibility of her section in the office was to answer telephone inquiries from customers who had problems with their insurance. The young woman, whose stuttering was quite severe, had to take 100 or more phone calls a day from irate customers from all over the country. This is what she told me about her assignment:

> The night before I go on the toll-free phone line, I do not sleep well. The morning when I drive to work, I am sick in my stomach. If I stutter on the first phone call, I know I am going to stutter all day. These people are already irritated about some aspect of our service, and my stuttering does not help. I can't find another job until I get my high school diploma.

Adults who have had normal communicative skills but suddenly lose them experience some of the most disturbing effects of such loss. Stroke patients, for example, fall into this category. Most stroke patients will have planned on being productive for many more years. A severe stroke can change this expectation overnight. After the initial shock, the stroke patients realize that more than their dreams have been wiped out. They find out, much to their distress, that they cannot talk at all. Or, if they are able to say something, people just do not seem to understand them. The degree of frustration and sadness experienced by a stroke patient can be enormous, as indicated by the story of a physician who had communicative problems due to stroke but eventually recovered:

> There I was, lying in a hospital bed thinking what became of me. When my grandchildren came to see me, I just could not remember their names. One evening, I tried to tell my crying wife that I will be OK. No matter how hard I tried to say, 'Honey, I will come through this,' I just could not get the right words. My wife told me later that I kept fumbling and that I spoke only in jargon. Each of my attempts to say something was worse than my previous attempts. I did not know I was actually distressing my wife by confused mumbles. I didn't know that I didn't make any sense.

People whose larynx is surgically removed because of cancer lose their voice instantly. These individuals also suffer a great deal of emotional trauma the instant they find out that they are about to lose their natural voice forever. As we will find out in Chapter 7 of this book, they can learn alternative modes of communication. Nonetheless, the initial and unbearable thought is the prospect of a silent life in their later years.

Whether in children or adults, disorders of communication produce profound effects mainly because they drastically reduce the humans' ability to reach others through communication. Like touch and sight, communication, including hearing, is contact. Communication is more powerful than many other modes of contact because it can reach farther. This may be the reason why a disorder of communication affects people so deeply.

Summary

- Communication is a form of social behavior; it involves interaction among people.
- Language is defined either as a system of symbols and codes used in communication or as a form of social behavior shaped and maintained by a verbal community.

(continues)

- Communication is essential for social survival in modern societies.

- Communication is studied by examining its components, which include voice, articulation, language, fluency, and hearing.

- The various disorders of communication are studied by speech–language pathology and audiology.

- Communicative disorders often are classified into disorders of voice, disorders of articulation (phonological disorders), disorders of language, disorders of fluency, and disorders of hearing (hearing impairment).

- More than 17% of the U.S. population may have disorders of communication.

- Communicative disorders in children and adults affect all aspects of life.

Dialogue

Ms. Noledge-Hungry is an undergraduate student who is taking the introductory course in communicative disorders. Like many of her classmates, she is seriously considering the option of becoming a speech–language pathologist. Her instructor, Dr. Speech-Wisely has encouraged his students to visit him in his office and get issues and questions clarified. Therefore, Ms. Noledge-Hungry decided to see the professor and talk about human communication and its disorders.

For the student who reads this text, the dialogue at the end of each chapter serves three major purposes. First, the dialogue is a summary of the chapter written in the form of a conversation between the student and her professor. The student also offers summaries of information learned on the topic. Second, the dialogue is a study guide. It suggests areas that must be read in greater detail. Third, the dialogue gives a glimpse of the educational and professional future of a student who selects speech–language pathology (communicative disorders) as his or her major. The professor points out the kinds of courses a major in communicative disorders will take, the types of clinical practice the student will do, the settings in which the professionals work, and so on. In essence, the dialogue highlights the chapter information and gives the student an outlook on the education and profession.

N-H: Dr. Speech-Wisely, I am thinking about majoring in communicative disorders, and I found your lecture on human communication and its disorders very interesting.

S-W: I hope you are still interested after having suffered my lecture!

N-H: Oh yes, very much! In fact I am more interested now than before. But I do have a lot of questions. And I have only begun to find out what this field is all about.

S-W: Of course. But you will find answers as you move along.

N-H: I hope so! I guess the first task in summarizing what we have learned so far is to define communication and distinguish it from language. You defined communication in different ways. You said **communication** is exchange of information between two or more people.

S-W: Yes. I also defined **communication** as a form of social behavior. In these two senses, animals communicate with each other. Their communication is limited, instinctive, and related mostly to the needs of survival.

N-H: It is language that makes human communication different from animal communication. **Language** is more complex, versatile, and creative; it has been made possible by the evolution of a sophisticated neuromuscular mechanism found only in human beings.

S-W: That is correct. Because animals communicate without language and humans communicate with or without language, language and communication are closely related, but still different. **Language** is a means of communication; it can be oral or spoken, signed or manual, and it can be symbolic.

N-H: It was interesting to learn that neurophysiological mechanism—I have to work on this long expression—used in language evolved for biological reasons, not for language. All the same, it makes language possible at the human level.

S-W: Yes. Though language is not necessary for biological survival, it is for social survival. Effective communication with spoken and written language has become a crucial factor in modern societies. Now tell me, what are the five components of human communication?

N-H: Let me see. The five components are the **voice, articulation, language, fluency,** and **hearing.**

S-W: Very good! **Voice** is the production of sound by the vibrating vocal folds and modified by structures above the folds. Voice is basic to oral language.

N-H: The next component is **articulation** which is the movement of the speech mechanism in the production of speech sounds. The study of speech sounds is called **phonology.** A speech sound is technically described as a **phoneme,** which is a group of sounds. I am not so sure of the classification of speech sounds.

S-W: Well, there are many ways of classifying them. A basic distinction is made between vowels and consonants. Other classifications are based on whether the sound is voiced or not and on the place and manner of articulation.

N-H: The next component, **language,** is described as a mental system of codes and rules used in oral communication. There are two major approaches to the study of language: the **linguistic** and the **behavioral.** In the linguistic analysis, the morphologic, syntactic, semantic, and pragmatic components are identified.

S-W: That is right. You should be able to define each of them and identify the field of study associated with each except syntax. For example, the study of the morphologic component is morphology.

N-H: I know. The study of meaning or the semantic component is **semantics.** And the study of the use of language or the pragmatic component is **pragmatics.**

S-W: The **syntactic** component refers to sentence structure and word order. You should also know what a morpheme is and how they are classified.

N-H: OK, I will remember to study that more carefully. You also described the theory of Chomsky.

S-W: Yes. Chomsky made a distinction between **surface structure,** which is the arrangement of words into sentences that you can see or hear, and the **deep structure,** which is abstract and holds meaning. Can you define grammatic transformations?

N-H: That is a tough one. I think **grammatic transformations** are operations of relating the deep structure with the surface structure and creating different forms of sentences.

S-W: That is right. Chomsky also made a distinction between competence and performance. He defined **competence** as the knowledge of the rules of universal grammar and **performance** as the actual production of language. His theory had a great impact on the study of language within the linguistic approach. Now, tell me about the behavioral approach. Let me remind you, though, that you should be able to give brief descriptions of semantics and pragmatics.

N-H: OK. The behavioral approach of Skinner describes functional units of verbal behaviors. **Verbal behavior** is defined as a form of social behavior. A **functional unit** is a group of responses that have the same or similar causes and receive similar consequences. They are likely to have similar effects on the listener. Skinner defined several functional units such as **mands** and **tacts.**

S-W: You should be able to define each of the functional units. You should also be able to compare and contrast the linguistic and the behavioral approaches to the study of language. Now, tell me about fluency.

N-H: **Fluency** is described as easy, smooth, flowing, and effortless speech. It is related to knowledge or the intraverbal control, which is . . . how did you put it?

S-W: **Intraverbal control** means that fluency is partly controlled by a speaker's own prior speech. When you start talking, for whatever the reason, you keep going because your own speech is stimulus for more speech. Now, tell me about hearing.

N-H: **Hearing** is closely related to speech and language behaviors. Normal hearing is necessary for learning speech and language; it also is necessary for perception and production of speech and language.

S-W: That is correct. How do you classify disorders of communication?

N-H: There are different classifications. One classification includes **disorders of voice, articulation, language, fluency,** and **hearing.** A **congenital** problem, something the child is born with, may contribute to a disorder, or a disorder may be **acquired** later in life. A disorder may be **functional,** meaning that there is no **organic** basis, or it may be organic, meaning that some neurophysiological problem underlies it.

S-W: Very good! You will study various disorders in greater detail, but at this point you have gained a general idea of communicative disorders. We talked about voice disorders of phonation and resonance, a few conditions such as polyps and nodules that cause some voice problems, and disorders of articulation in children, which include omissions, substitutions, and distortions of speech sounds. We also discussed motor speech disorders called dysarthria and apraxia in adults which are due to neurological involvement. Then we discussed language disorders in both children and adults. The final speech disorder is that of fluency, which includes stuttering and cluttering.

N-H: We also discussed two kinds of hearing impairment: **conductive** and **sensorineural.** Both affect communication adversely. I am amazed to learn that more than 22 million people in the U.S. may have one or more disorders of communication.

S-W: Yes. Communicative disorders have profound effects on the social, emotional, personal, educational, and occupational life of the individual.

N-H: I find the stories of people with communicative disabilities very touching. Being able to help some of them must be wonderful.

S-W: Certainly. That is what this profession is all about: helping people who suffer, often silently, in verbal communities that are based on an ability to communicate. Lack of communication robs the essence of social existence. If you, as a professional, can help them communicate, you will have restored their membership in the verbal community. They can now relate to others.

N-H: What are you going to talk about next?

S-W: Next we will take a brief look at the people who call themselves speech–language pathologists and audiologists and see how they try to help people with disorders of communication. It will be a study in profiles of professional individuals. At a later time, we will discuss how these specialists are trained, how they do research, and how they are organized as a profession.

N-H: Sounds very interesting. I want to know how the specialists help people. I will have many questions about majoring in communicative disorders once I know a bit more.

S-W: OK. Take care and hit the books!

Study Questions

After studying the chapter, answer the following questions. If you are not sure, reread the material. Check your answers with the text and make sure you use technical words in your answers.

1. What is communication? Can you find it in animals?

2. Distinguish between communication and language.

3. What are the different kinds or forms of language? Give a brief description of each.

4. Write a paragraph about communication and social survival.

5. What are the four major aspects of communication?

6. Describe larynx and vocal folds.

7. Define articulation and phonology.

8. What is a phoneme? Give examples of two phonemes.

9. What are the two major approaches to the study of language?

10. Define morphology and morphemes.

11. What are grammatic morphemes?

12. Define syntax.

13. Briefly describe Chomsky's theory of syntax. Clearly distinguish between competence and performance, surface and deep structures, and grammatic transformations.

14. Define semantics. Describe two viewpoints of meaning: what it is and where it lies.

15. What is pragmatics? What functions does language serve according to one theory described in the text?

16. What is verbal behavior and what are its functional units in the behavioral analysis of language?

17. What are reinforcers?

18. Contrast *mands* and *tacts*.

19. Compare and contrast the linguistic and the behavioral analysis of language.

20. Describe fluency. What are the two major kinds of fluency disorders?

21. What is the role of normal hearing in communication?

22. Describe communicative disorders.

23. What are some of the listener reactions to disordered speech?

24. How are communicative disorders classified? Define the categories you identify.

25. Describe breathy and hoarse voice.

26. How are the errors of speech sounds classified?

27. What are motor speech disorders?

28. Describe language disorders. What is telegraphic speech?

29. What is aphasia and what causes it?

30. Distinguish between stuttering and cluttering.

31. Distinguish between conductive and sensorineural hearing loss.

32. How many people in the United States have communicative disorders?

33. What percentage of children receiving special educational services have speech or language impairments?

34. Describe some of the effects of communicative disorders on children.

35. Describe the effects of an acquired communicative disorder in an adult.

References

American Speech-Language-Hearing Association. (1984). Committee on prevention of communicative disorders. *Asha, 26,* 35–38.

Austin, J. (1962). *How to do things with words.* Cambridge: Harvard University Press.

Bello, J. (1994). Prevalence of speech, voice, and language disorders in the United States. *Communication facts, 1994 ed.* Rockville, MD: American Speech-Language-Hearing Association.

Casby, M. W. (1989). National data concerning communication disorders and special education. *Language, Speech, & Hearing Services in Schools, 20,* 22–30.

Castrogiovanni, A. (1999a). Incidence and prevalence of hearing impairment in the United States. *Communication facts, 1999 ed.* Rockville, MD: American Speech-Language-Hearing Association.

Castrogiovanni, A. (1999b). Incidence and prevalence of speech, voice, and language disorders in the United States. *Communication facts, 1999 ed.* Rockville, MD: American Speech-Language-Hearing Association.

Chomsky, N. (1957). *Syntactic structures.* The Hague: Mouton.

Chomsky, N. (1965). *Aspects of a theory of syntax.* Cambridge: MIT Press.

Chomsky, N. (1981). *Lectures on government and binding.* Dordrecht, Holland: Doris.

Gleason, J. B. (2001). *The development of language* (5th ed.). New York: Macmillan.

Halliday, M. A. K. (1975). *Learning how to mean.* London: Edward Arnold.

Hegde, M. N. (1995). *A coursebook on language disorders in children.* San Diego: Singular.

McLauglin, S. (1998). *Introduction to language development.* San Diego: Singular.

Mueller, P. B., & Peters, B. M. (1981). Needs and services in geriatric speech–language pathology and audiology. *Asha, 23,* 627–632.

Owens, R. (1996). *Language development: An introduction* (4th ed.). New York: Macmillan.

Peña-Brooks, A., & Hegde, M. N. (2000). *Assessment and treatment of articulation and phonological disorders in children.* Austin, TX: PRO-ED.

Searle, J. (1969). *Speech acts: An essay in the philosophy of language.* Cambridge: Harvard University Press.

Skinner, B. F. (1957). *Verbal behavior.* New York: Appleton-Century-Crofts.

Van Riper, C. (1978). *Speech correction: Principles and methods* (6th ed.). Englewood Cliffs, NJ: Prentice Hall.

Ventry, I. M., & Weinstein, B. (1983). Identification of elderly people with hearing loss. *Asha, 25,* 37–42.

Specialists in Communication and Its Disorders

- Speech–Language Pathologists
- Audiologists
- References

This book is about the science of communication, the disorders of communication, and the professions that help people with communicative disorders. The science of communication includes the speech and language science and the hearing science. The **speech science** is a study of speech, its anatomical and physiological bases, the formation and production of speech sounds, and the perception and understanding of speech. The **language science** is the study of the larger, more abstract, and organized system of verbal or nonverbal means of communication. The **hearing science** is the study of hearing, its anatomy and physiology, its perception and understanding, and its relation to communication.

All professions should be built on a solid knowledge base. The speech, language, and hearing sciences provide the knowledge base for the professions of communicative disorders. The twin professions in **communicative disorders** include speech–language pathology and audiology. **Speech–language pathology** is the scientific profession concerned with the disorders of human verbal and nonverbal communication, their assessment, and treatment. As the term suggests, the **speech–language pathologist** is a specialist in the study of speech and language, disorders of speech and language, and the assessment and treatment of speech and language disorders. **Audiology** is the profession concerned with the disorders of hearing and the rehabilitation of individuals with hearing impairment. An **audiologist** is a specialist in the study of hearing and hearing disorders, the assessment of hearing loss, and the rehabilitation of people with hearing impairment. This book also is about speech–language pathologists and audiologists.

Before we begin our understanding of human communication and its disorders, we shall take a look at these scientists and professionals as people who generate knowledge and help children and adults who have disordered communication. We shall take a glimpse at the kinds of work they do in a variety of settings.

Speech–Language Pathologists

 Pamela Benson, MA, CCC-SLP

Speech–Language Pathologist, Hudson Unified School District

Pamela Benson has worked for about 3 years as a speech–language pathologist at the Washington Elementary School in the central California town of Hudson. At age 28, Pamela is a productive and creative public school clinician.

Pamela always wanted to be a helping professional. As a high school student, she visited the university campus on a career day and was shown the department of communicative disorders and the speech and hearing clinic. Later, she visited the speech and hearing clinic on her own, saw a few treatment sessions, and talked with professors in the department. Subsequently, she also observed the work of a speech–language pathologist in an elementary school in town. The work of speech–language pathologists fascinated her. She found speech–language pathology to be the kind of helping profession she wanted to specialize in.

After she received her bachelor's degree in communicative disorders, she went on to graduate school and received her master's degree in speech–language pathology. Eventually, she received the **Certificate of Clinical Competence in Speech–Language Pathology (CCC-SLP)** issued by the American Speech-Language-Hearing Association. As soon as she graduated from the university, she was offered a position in the Hudson school district as a speech–language pathologist. She accepted the position because she liked working with children in an educational setting. She was assigned to two elementary schools within the district. She roughly divided her time between the two schools.

Pamela said,

> I screen children in selected grades at the beginning of the school year to find out who needs my help. When my screening procedures show that a child has a disorder of communication, I usually schedule that child for treatment. Other children I treat are referred to me by parents, classroom teachers, and special education specialists.

When a request for her service is received, Pamela makes an assessment of the child's communicative behaviors and makes a judgment about the need for services. If she decides that the child needs treatment, she then develops a treatment program for that child.

For the most part, Pamela treats children in small groups. In forming treatment groups, she makes every attempt to select children who have the same type of communicative disorder. "I may have three children who all have the same four speech sounds in error. I may have another treatment group consisting of children who stutter," said Pamela. Some children may be seen just once a week and others may be seen two times.

Pamela said that most of the children she treats have disorders of language or articulation. This is typical of most public school clinicians' case loads. Children who stutter and those who have voice problems also are often scheduled for treatment.

Compared to other countries, speech–language pathology in the United States is the biggest partly because of the large number of speech–language pathologists working in American public schools.

Historically, public schools in the United States have been a major setting for clinical speech–language services. This trend continues. This is partly because of Public Law (P.L.) 94-142, the Education for All Handicapped Children Act, passed by the U.S. Congress and signed into law in 1975. The law was amended in 1986 (Education of the Handicapped Act Amendments of 1986; P.L. 99-457). In 1990, the 1975 law was reauthorized and renamed as the Individuals with Disabilities Education Act (IDEA; P.L. 101-476). These laws require that children with disabilities, including infants and toddlers, and their families receive appropriate special educational services. Such special education services include speech, language, and hearing services to children with communicative disorders. In 1990, the U.S. Congress also passed the Americans with Disabilities Act of 1990 (P.L. 101-336), mandating reasonable access to public buildings, rest rooms, and assistance to deaf people with interpreters and special telecommunication devices.

Pamela said,

> As the law requires, I develop an **Individualized Education Program (IEP)** for each child I work with. In that IEP, I specify the child's current communicative behaviors, the target behaviors to be established, the treatment procedures to be used, and the tentative duration in which this will be accomplished. I also specify how the effects of the treatment program will be evaluated. I make sure that my treatment goals and procedures as well as the evaluative methods are written in objective terms.

In the case of children who are 2 years of age or younger, clinicians develop an **Individualized Family Service Plan** (IFSP).

She further stated that "At the end of a treatment program, I just cannot write that the child's communicative behaviors have improved. I should have some evidence to back up my statements."

Pamela enjoys her work with children and their parents. At the end of each semester, she sends a progress report to the parents of children who have been treated. She holds conferences with parents whenever practical. Teachers often call upon her expertise to help them with children who have problems of communication. She works closely with the teachers of her clients. She consults with special education specialists who may have children with disorders of communication. She said,

> When I work with a boy who has limited language, and I expand his vocabulary and teach him grammatically correct sentences, everybody notices the big change. The child's performance in the classroom improves. The child's social life is dramatically altered for the better. Both the teachers and the family recognize this. It is a wonderful feeling!

 ## Marge Hickson, MA, CCC-SLP

Speech–Language Pathologist, Lavall Community Hospital, Speech and Hearing Department

At age 36, Marge Hickson is an experienced clinician working in a hospital setting. Marge had previously worked in a public school for 5 years. When a position of a speech–language pathologist opened in the community hospital in town, she decided it was time for a change in her professional life, so she sought and got the job.

Marge is one of six speech–language pathologists working full time in the speech and hearing department of the hospital. The department also employs two audiologists. Marge and her colleagues work mostly with adults who have various disorders of communication. The speech and hearing department is housed within the hospital's physical rehabilitation department. Marge said,

> The rehabilitation department sees many people with physical disabilities including patients who have sustained head injuries. They also work with people who have orthopedic disabilities, including children. Children who have had cerebral palsy also are treated there. I work closely with all those patients who pose a tremendous challenge for the speech–language pathologist.

Aphasia, which is a sudden loss of language due to recent brain damage, is an emotionally debilitating disorder of communication. Communicative disorders associated with brain injury are described in **Chapter 9.**

Patients who have sustained head injury due to automobile, industrial, and other kinds of accidents tend to have impaired communication. Rehabilitation of these patients can be a slow and difficult process. In addition to these patients, Marge also works with patients who have had strokes and now have aphasia. Marge usually begins her work with these patients as soon as they are physically ready for treatment sessions. "My work with patients with aphasia is probably the most challenging aspect of my job, but it is also the most stimulating and rewarding," she said.

Even before the patients are ready for language treatment, Marge counsels the family members about the patient's communication problems and the prospects for improvement under treatment. Marge said,

> The family members of a stroke patient are often more saddened and confused than the patient. They are confused about the complicating physical problems and the language problem. The paralysis and the sudden loss of language are often the most visible and hence the most distressing problems they see. Counseling them about the relation between the stroke, the brain damage, and communication improves their understanding of the patient's problem. When I tell them that language treatment is available and can be very helpful, they are better able to cope with the situation.

In the initial stages of treatment, Marge treats most of her patients with aphasia in individual sessions, as shown in Figure 2.1. In subsequent sessions, she holds group treatment sessions to promote better social communication.

Chapter 9 describes electronic and other devices that help people with severe disabilities communicate.

Some individuals with severe physical disabilities cannot move their speech muscles to speak but can formulate sentences. In working with such individuals, Marge uses several means of nonverbal communication. One of them is an electronic communication board on which the patient arranges words to form sentences and thus communicates with others. A board also may contain symbols that stand for words and concepts. The patient then points to symbols in sequence to form "sentences." Marge stated,

> Though the treatment process is slow, the ability to form just a few sentences gives the patient hope. I am now using a computer that has a program that helps people with disabilities communicate. Patients learn to hit the right keys to call up stored words and phrases on the screen. This is an exciting area of work where we expect rapid technological advances.

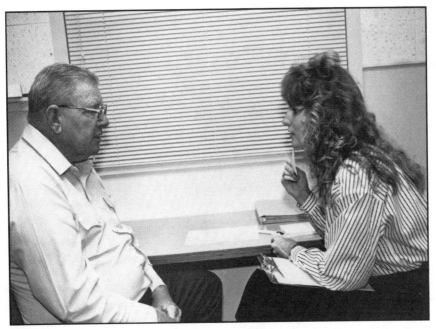

Figure 2.1. A patient with aphasia receives language treatment.

 Jean Tyson, MA, CCC-SLP

Speech–Language Pathologist, Tyson Speech and Language Clinic

At age 32, Jean Tyson owns her own speech and language clinic in a medium size Midwestern city. Before she opened her clinic, she had worked for 5 years as a speech–language pathologist in a state hospital speech and hearing department.

Most state hospitals for patients with mental illness and mental retardation have speech and hearing departments. Some of these departments serve the inpatients of the hospitals as well as people from the surrounding community on an outpatient basis. As a state hospital clinician, Jean treated people with a variety of mental or behavioral problems as well as many children and adults from the community who did not have any problem other than their disorder of communication.

People with mental illness and mental retardation exhibit a variety of speech and language problems. The speech–language pathologist who works in a state hospital develops speech and language treatment programs for people with mental illness or mental retardation. The clinician is usually a member of the interdisciplinary treatment team, which consists of a psychiatrist, a psychologist, a psychiatric nurse, a social worker, and other specialists. Together, the team makes an assessment of each client's problems and develops treatment programs. Each specialist then implements his or her treatment program.

After having worked for 5 years with a special and very challenging population seen in a mental hospital, Jean decided she needed a change. The town had no private speech and hearing clinic. She knew that private practice in speech and hearing is one of the fastest growing segments of the profession. In many medium to large cities across the country, enterprising speech–language pathologists have been opening private speech and language clinics. She also knew that many people, especially adults with communicative disorders, had no services available in her town. Therefore, she decided to open the town's first private speech and language clinic.

She opened her small clinic in a professional building, renting two rooms and hiring a receptionist/secretary. She said that,

> I knew very little about the business aspects of my profession. But when you start your own clinic, you learn fast. For about 2 years, I was the only clinician. But as my case load increased, I hired another speech–language pathologist to work in my clinic. As my practice grew, I added more professional staff. Right now I have six full-time and several part-time speech–language pathologists working in my clinic.

Jean and her clinicians treat both children and adults with communicative problems. Figure 2.2 shows typical treatment sessions involving a child and an adult.

Jean is the director of the clinic. In addition to the receptionist, Jean also has an office manager. The receptionist and the office manager work in the front office. Jean supervises the work of these two individuals. She also oversees the work of her professional staff.

Jean has the primary responsibility of marketing her clinic's services. By letters and telephone conversations, she keeps in touch with the area physicians who refer clients to the clinic. She said,

> An important part of my job is to secure contracts to provide professional speech and language services to area hospitals, nursing homes, and other agencies. The major hospital in town, a few nursing homes, the home health agency, and several extended care facilities do not have speech–language pathologists on their payroll. It is more practical for them to have an outside clinic contracted to provide services to their patients. I have such contracts with several agencies in this area.

Jean also contracts with many insurance companies including health maintenance organizations (HMOs) that offer health insurance for people. Many health insurance companies and HMOs now cover speech, language, and hearing services. Jean secures legal contracts from those companies and organizations to provide speech and language services to people insured by them.

Jean is a busy professional. She said,

> My goal is to offer the best quality service to our clients, manage my business prudently, and provide an exciting and stimulating professional environment for the speech–language pathologists who work for me. My clinic provides service to hundreds of adults and children who seek help for their communicative disorders. I think we are providing a valuable service to our community. I find my job both challenging and rewarding. As a private clinician, I set my own working hours and professional goals. I pick my own challenges. Owning a private clinic is not easy; you are always concerned about the client flow, the cash flow, and the expenses that are considerable. More important than anything is the concern you have about the people who work for you and the quality of service they offer their clients. Managing the personnel is one of the most difficult aspects of owning a business or professional practice. But I find all this very exciting.

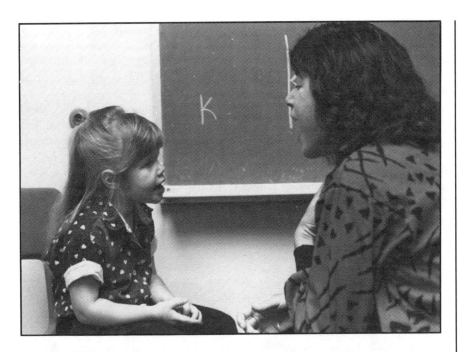

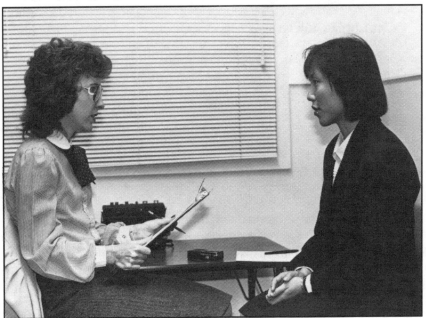

Figure 2.2. A child and an adult receive treatment for speech disorders.

 Lena Fisk, MA, CCC-SLP

Clinical Supervisor, Northern State University

Compared to a school speech–language pathologist or a private practitioner, Lena Fisk has a different kind of job. She is a clinical supervisor at a university

Chapter 12 describes the licenses, certificates, and other credentials required to work as a speech–language pathologist and audiologist.

speech and hearing clinic. Before she accepted this position, she worked as a speech–language pathologist in a community hospital speech and hearing clinic. But she liked the university atmosphere better, so when a clinical supervisor's position became available at the university speech and hearing clinic, she applied and got it.

Undergraduate or graduate students in speech–language pathology should work with people who have various disorders of communication under the supervision of a licensed and certified speech–language pathologist. Students should gain sufficient supervised clinical experience before they qualify for such credentials. Therefore, university speech and hearing clinics need professionally qualified speech–language pathologists who supervise student clinicians in the clinic to make sure that the students learn the various clinical procedures including assessment and treatment techniques.

Lena said,

> My job is very demanding because I have to take a graduate or an undergraduate student in the department who has no experience in working with people who have communicative disorders and help them become professional, competent clinicians. First-semester student clinicians will have met the academic requirement to enroll in clinical practicum. Through their academic courses, the clinicians will have acquired the basic information about assessment and treatment of communicative disorders, but the students are still totally inexperienced. Many students are naturally concerned about how they will do in the clinic. With guidance and supervision, most do fine, but they do not know that at the beginning. They are naturally concerned about this experience. I spend a lot of time talking with the students, going over the information about the clients they have been assigned to work with, and developing treatment plans for those clients.

Lena is in the speech and hearing clinic when her students are working with the clients. The treatment rooms at the university speech and hearing clinics are equipped with one-way mirrors. From inside the treatment room, the client and the student clinician see only a mirror on the wall. But from the other side of the wall, the supervisor can see through the mirror to observe what is going on inside the treatment room. The supervisor also can hear the conversation between the client and the student clinician through an audio system with a microphone placed inside the treatment room. As shown in Figure 2.3, the supervisor watches at least a portion of each session the student clinician holds with every client. Lena stated,

> I have to make judgments all the time about what I see through the mirror and what I hear through the headphones. I must make sure that the student is following an approved treatment plan for the client. I carefully listen to what the clinician says to the client. I watch closely how the clinician interacts with the client. Is the clinician behaving professionally? Is she effective? I also watch how the client is behaving. Is he or she feeling constantly uneasy, unsure? Are the client's communicative behaviors changing? Is the clinician documenting those changes by recording the client responses? These are some of the things I think about when I am watching a student clinician working with a client.

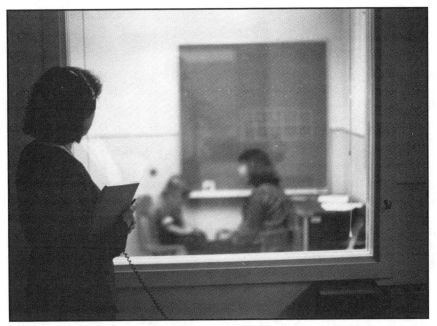

Figure 2.3. A clinical supervisor observes a student clinician in action.

The student clinician meets with Lena as often as necessary to discuss the client progress, treatment procedures, any changes that may have to be made, and the progress reports that must be written. During clinical practicum, the student clinician learns to write assessment reports, treatment plans, and progress reports. The student clinician learns to talk in professional language to the clients and their family. The clinician acquires the skills of counseling the clients and their family members about the treatment procedures and the progress they can expect. The clinician also learns to inform clients and their families about services offered by such other professionals as audiologists, physicians, psychologists, physical therapists, special education specialists, and social workers. Student clinicians learn how to keep clinic records and maintain confidentiality about the records they keep and the services they render. All clinicians, including the student clinicians, are expected to honor the confidentiality of persons who receive services from them. The clinicians should not discuss the identity of their clients in nonprofessional contexts and should not discuss their clients in social situations. In essence, the student clinician learns to practice the profession ethically and effectively.

Through supervised clinical practice, the student clinician fulfills the clinical requirements for the license, certification, or other credentials needed to work in various professional settings. A clinical supervisor plays a major role in teaching the professional skills to the student clinician. Lena said,

> I start with student clinicians with no experience in treating people with communicative disorders. By the time the clinicians leave us, they are professionals. I see how a student, who is unsure but eager to learn, becomes a confident and capable clinician. I become a part of that remarkable change, which happens right before my eyes, and that is very gratifying for me.

The code of ethics of the American Speech-Language-Hearing Association that clinicians adhere to is described in **Chapter 12.**

Joseph Smiley, PhD, CCC-SLP

Professor of Communicative Disorders, Hanson State University

In addition to clinical supervisors, departments of communicative disorders in universities have speech–language pathologists and audiologists who are members of the teaching faculty. In some cases, the same individuals may handle academic teaching and clinical supervision. In others, different people may be responsible for the two sets of duties.

Joseph Smiley got his bachelor's degree in speech and hearing sciences and his master's degree in speech–language pathology. Then he worked for 3 years as a clinician in a major hospital. He was a member of a team of specialists who treated patients with aphasia, which is an adult language disorder. His work at the hospital stimulated his interest in aphasia to the extent that he wanted to specialize in it. Therefore, Joseph decided to go on for his doctoral degree in speech and language pathology. Most doctoral degrees are research degrees. The doctoral students take more advanced courses to specialize in selected areas and do research on a significant problem. The doctoral candidates write a dissertation based on their research.

The doctoral degree is essential to teach in most colleges and universities. Joseph did his doctoral research on the treatment of aphasia. When he accepted a faculty position, he began to teach such courses as anatomy and physiology of the speech and hearing mechanism, aphasia, and speech disorders of neurologic origin. He also supervises student clinicians who work with patients with aphasia.

Joseph said,

Aphasia and related communicative disorders are described in **Chapter 9.**

I love teaching. Aphasia is both an intriguing and challenging disorder of communication. In my teaching, I have not found a student who is not touched by the story of patients with aphasia who, having been competent communicators, suddenly lose their speech and language abilities. Aphasia and its varieties illuminate the normally obscure relation between the brain and speech–language functions. Students are fascinated by the basic and applied research on the relation between the brain and language.

Although Joseph spends a major portion of his time teaching academic courses, he is also involved in research. His main interest is the treatment of patients with aphasia. He said about research,

I want to develop an effective treatment program for patients with aphasia. The problem is that there are different kinds of aphasia. We do not know if the same treatment procedure works with all kinds of aphasia. For the last few years, I have been researching a single treatment program to see if it is effective across patients who are diagnosed to have different kinds of aphasia. The answers are not in yet. I have to test the procedure with a variety of patients before I can draw some conclusions.

Joseph hires several graduate students as his research assistants who help him collect data. Under his supervision, the research assistants treat patients with aphasia with the experimental treatment procedures he designs. "This gives my students a valuable experience. They learn the research process while treating their patients. The students understand better how treatment procedures are researched and evaluated because they actually do it," said Joseph.

In addition to teaching, research, and clinical supervision, Joseph also advises students in the department of communicative disorders about their educational and clinical program. Joseph said,

> Advising is an important part of my duties in the department. The student who has decided to major in communicative disorders has a lot of questions about the required courses, the sequence in which they must be taken, the clinical practicum, and many other topics and issues. It is my job to provide them with answers, help them plan their educational program, and make sure they stay on the right course. I like this aspect of my job very much because it gives me a chance to take my students through a complex process of course work and clinical practicum and thus help them meet their educational and professional goals.

 ## Jennifer Johnson, PhD, CCC-SLP

Research Scientist, Western Research Laboratory

As already noted, most speech–language pathologists are clinicians in various settings. Some teach and supervise students at colleges and universities. However, a smaller number of individuals are full-time researchers. Full-time research scientists work in universities and specialized research laboratories.

Like clinicians, Jennifer also wished to help people who have disorders of communication, but not necessarily by directly working with them. She wanted to help by generating new knowledge through research. During her graduate study, she worked as a research assistant on a large federally funded program on the treatment of stuttering. She learned much about research methods and approaches in speech–language pathology. She was fascinated by the research process and realized that research eventually helps many people, even those the researcher did not work with. For example, a research scientist who develops a new method of treatment for stuttering will help, through the work of other clinicians who use that technique, many stutterers across the country. Therefore, treatment research is a powerful tool for helping a large number of people.

Research is needed to generate basic scientific information as well. What speech and language are, how speech and voice are produced, how language is acquired, and how the process of speech or language acquisition is disrupted are all questions for research. The causes, as well as the nature of communicative disorders, should be understood. Aspects of normal as well as disordered communication should be described. All this and more are the tasks of research scientists.

Some scientists who research communication and its disorders may not have clinical training at all. These scientists do not treat clients; they do research to find answers to questions that might help treat clients. Other scientists have clinical training and thus can treat and do research at the same time. Jennifer is one of those scientists who has both clinical and research training. She was trained as a clinician at the master's level and as a researcher at the doctoral level.

Jennifer has a government grant to research the relation between the family history of stuttering and the duration of stuttering treatment. She wants to know if stutterers who have stuttering relatives need longer treatment time than those who do not have such relatives. She said, "We know that some stutterers take more time to show improvement than others. But we are not sure what causes this variability in response to treatment. I thought that a starting point is to investigate the relation between family history of stuttering and the response to treatment."

Jennifer is very much involved in her research. She said,

> Research is a 24-hour obsession with me. A piece of research evidence is the most exciting thing I can see. I have four research scientists working under my direction. We work well as a team and we design studies together. We recruit stuttering persons who do and do not have family history of stuttering. We treat them with the same method of treatment. It is a long-term research project. It will take years of careful data gathering to find some answers.

Speech–Language Pathologists in Other Professional Settings

Besides public schools, hospitals and clinics, state hospitals for individuals with mental illness, private clinics, universities and colleges, and research laboratories, speech–language pathologists work in several other settings. These include Veterans Administration hospitals, rehabilitation institutes, and institutes for individuals with developmental disabilities. At the Veterans Administration hospitals, speech–language pathologists are likely to work with communicative disorders more commonly seen in older persons. These disorders include aphasia and speech disorders due to neurological damage and diseases.

The speech–language pathologist working in rehabilitation institutes works mostly with people with various kinds of physical disabilities that affect speech and language. For example, patients with head injury and children with cerebral palsy are among those served in such facilities. The speech–language pathologists working in institutes for people with developmental disabilities develop and implement speech–language treatment programs for those residents.

Finally, speech–language pathologists who have private practice may have contracts to serve people in nursing homes, extended care facilities, and senior citizen homes. They also may have contracts with home health care agencies, in which case the speech–language pathologist visits the homes of patients who, for many reasons, cannot travel to a clinic.

Audiologists

 Dianne Harris, MA, CCC-A

Clinical Audiologist, Children's Hospital, Speech and Hearing Clinic

Dianne is an audiologist who specializes in hearing and its disorders. She has a master's degree in audiology. She holds the American Speech-Language-

Hearing Association's **Certificate of Clinical Competence in Audiology (CCC-A).** She also is licensed by the state government to practice audiology. Dianne has been working in the speech and hearing clinic of a children's hospital for the last 2 years.

When she graduated from the university, Dianne had several job options. Like some audiologists, she could have worked out of a physician's office. An ear, nose, and throat specialist in town was looking for an audiologist to work for her. A private speech and hearing clinic in town also had an opening for an audiologist. But she decided to take a position at the children's hospital because she could work exclusively with children, which is what she liked most. She said, "I like testing hearing in young children and babies. The younger the child, the harder it is to give a hearing test. I like that challenge."

Read **Chapter 10** to learn more about hearing, its disorders, and the work of audiologists.

Dianne spends most of her time assessing hearing in children. The clinic sees children from birth to 21 years of age. Because of her special interest in testing the very young, Dianne tends to see most of the younger children and infants. The clinic employs two other audiologists who mostly work with older children. She also works with five speech–language pathologists. A speech–language pathologist directs the clinic.

Dianne spends much time counseling parents of children with hearing impairments. She said,

> I take time to discuss fully what it means to have a child with a hearing impairment. I enjoy this aspect of my work. It is also a difficult aspect of my work. I know I have to handle it in a sensitive and professional manner. Parents of very young children often suspect a hearing loss in their child but are not yet ready to accept that the child has a hearing impairment.

Once the parents accept that fact, Dianne talks about various means of rehabilitation. She discusses hearing aids, speech and language treatment, sign language and other means of communication, educational needs of the child, and related issues.

Dianne does a complete hearing-aid evaluation on children who might benefit from amplification through hearing aids. She is responsible for the fitting of the aid. (Figure 2.4 shows how an audiologist typically fits a hearing aid on a child.) Dianne closely monitors the child's use of it. She counsels the classroom teachers on the special needs of the child with a hearing loss. For example, Dianne might suggest to the teacher that the child must be seated in front of the class and that the teacher should face the child while talking. This helps the child understand the speech by lipreading, which is understanding speech by watching the movements of the mouth.

"Since my audiological work is with children, I am very involved with the family members and the educational system. I enjoy dealing with different people to make sure the hearing impaired child's special needs are met," said Dianne.

Cheryl Logan, MA, CCC-A

Audiologist, Logan Hearing Center

Cheryl Logan is an audiologist who owns her own private practice. After she graduated with a master's degree in audiology, Cheryl worked in an ear, nose,

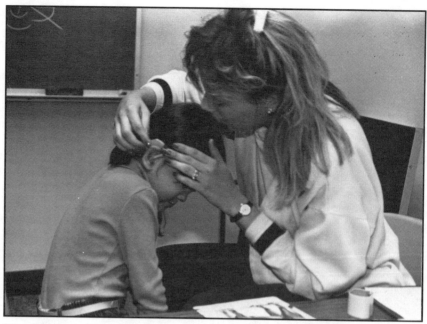

Figure 2.4. An audiologist fits a hearing aid on a child.

and throat specialist's office for about 5 years. Her primary responsibility there was to assess the hearing of patients referred to her by the ear, nose, and throat specialist. She assessed hearing in both children and adults. She also did hearing-aid evaluations, which is a procedure to determine the type of hearing aid best suited for a particular patient.

Cheryl said,

> I always wanted to have my own professional practice. But I needed some experience in my profession before I ventured on my own. After having worked for 5 years in a physician's office, I thought I could handle it, and so I opened my office. It has been a challenge, but I have enjoyed it tremendously.

Cheryl knew that getting established in a professional practice takes time, patience, and hard work. To succeed in private practice, she should know the business aspect of it. She should manage her accounts, taxes, and professional and secretarial employees. Above all, to succeed in private practice, she must build a referral base. This means that Cheryl should have physicians and other specialists who refer patients to her. "I have quite a few clients who just look up my name in the phone book and call for an appointment. But a majority of clients are referred to me by other physicians, especially ear, nose, and throat specialists," said Cheryl. She should be in touch with the professionals who send her clients. She keeps them informed of her hearing assessment results and her recommendations. Cheryl tests her clients in a specially constructed soundproof booth as shown in Figure 2.5.

Audiologists in private practice also may dispense hearing aids to individuals with hearing impairments. They need a special state license to do this. Cheryl has the license to dispense hearing aids. Her work, therefore, involves hearing-aid evaluations and fitting hearing aids to her clients. She buys different models of hearing aids directly from manufacturers. This helps her select

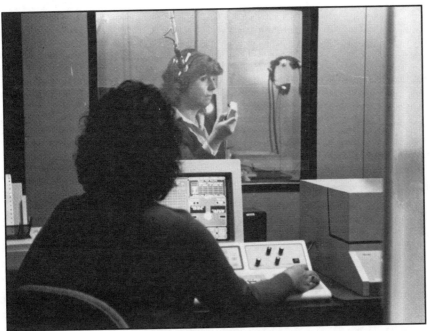

Figure 2.5. An audiologist tests the hearing of an adult.

the aid that is most suitable for a given client. She tries different aids on a client and determines which aid improves the client's ability to detect sounds and understand speech.

For about 2 years, Cheryl was the only audiologist in her practice. Then Cheryl's practice expanded. She developed two contracts with the area hospitals to provide audiological services to their patients. To serve those contracts, Cheryl hired an audiologist. Their clients who need speech–language services are referred to the area speech and language clinics.

Audiologists in Other Professional Settings

In addition to hospitals and private practice, audiologists work in several other settings. They work in college or university departments as instructors, clinical supervisors, and research scientists. In this respect, their work is similar to that of speech–language pathologists who work in colleges and universities.

Audiologists also may work for the armed forces to monitor the hearing of military personnel. Most, if not all, Veterans Administration hospitals hire audiologists to conduct hearing and hearing-aid evaluations. Military audiologists also may do various kinds of research on hearing and speech perception.

Another professional setting for audiologists is industry. Workers in many industries are exposed to a high level of dangerous noise. Constant exposure to high intensity noise can damage the hearing of workers. Noise also tends to induce fatigue and reduce efficiency. Workers in noisy places are prone to accidents. Therefore, there are both federal and state laws that require employers to take reasonable steps to protect the hearing of their employees. Under federal laws, workers who sustain hearing loss because of a noisy job environment can seek compensation. Therefore, employers need to periodically monitor the hearing of their workers and implement procedures to reduce the risk of noise-induced hearing impairment in their employees. It is the industrial audiologist who periodically monitors the hearing of employees and suggests steps to protect the hearing of individuals exposed to noise. Such steps are a part of a hearing conservation program.

Most industrial audiologists work on contracts with specific industries. Industrial audiologists usually have a mobile unit with all the equipment needed to evaluate the hearing of workers. The audiologists drive their unit to the industrial setting to administer hearing tests. Whenever possible, such tests are administered at the time new employees are hired and then periodically to monitor their hearing. Industrial audiologists may suggest earplugs and other devices that reduce the risk of hearing impairment.

Summary

- Speech–language pathologists, audiologists, and speech and hearing scientists are people who specialize in the study and treatment of human communication disorders.

- The speech–language and hearing scientists work in research laboratories and university departments.

- Speech–language pathologists and audiologists work in a variety of professional settings which are illustrated in Figure 2.6.

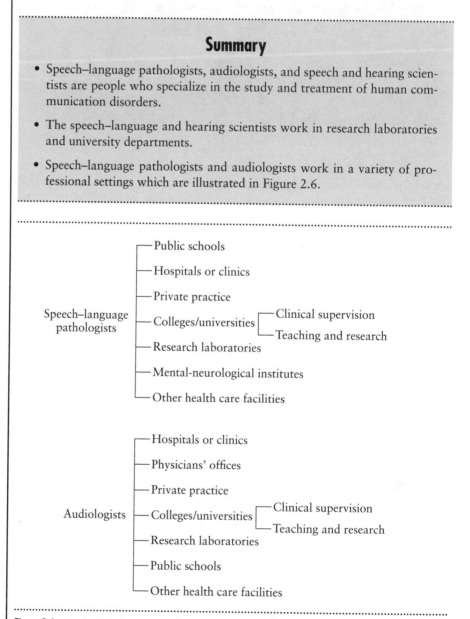

Figure 2.6. Professional settings of speech–language pathologists and audiologists.

An Overview of Anatomy and Physiology of Speech and Hearing

- Structural Mechanisms of Speech Production
- Anatomy and Physiology of Hearing
- The Nervous System
- Dialogue
- Study Questions
- References

Tammy Speeks owns a private speech and language clinic in Los Angeles. She holds a master's degree in speech–language pathology and the Certificate of Clinical Competence from the American Speech-Language-Hearing Association. She also is licensed to practice her profession by the state of California. Two other clinicians work in her clinic.

It is Monday afternoon. Tammy is sitting in her clinic office and reading her mail. Most adults and children who come to her clinic for services are referred by physicians. In their letters of referral, the physicians mention a disorder of communication, a medical problem that may be a cause of a certain disorder of communication, or both. Today, Tammy received several referral letters that told her brief stories of people with problems.

A Referral from a Neurologist

I am referring Mr. Ben Tilley, a 65-year-old man, to you for a speech–language evaluation to determine the usefulness of speech–language therapy. Ben has been diagnosed with parkinsonism. The results of neurological examinations show marked hypokinesia. Damage to the extrapyramidal system is indicated. His articulation is indistinct. He talks too softly, and his phrases are too short. His speech is monotonous, and his voice is breathy. Apparently, parkinsonism has affected his articulatory, respiratory, and phonatory mechanism. Please let me know the results of your evaluation, and thank you for helping Mr. Tilley.

A **neurologist** is a medical specialist who diagnoses and treats disorders of the nervous system.

Parkinsonism is a degenerative disease of the nervous system.

Hypokinesia is reduced range and force of muscle movements.

The **extrapyramidal system** is a part of the nervous system involved in movement control.

See **Chapter 9** for more information on neurological problems.

A **laryngologist** is a medical specialist who diagnoses and treats throat problems.

An **endoscope** is an instrument used to examine vocal folds.

Vocal **nodules** are small nodes that develop on vocal folds.

An **oral surgeon** performs surgery on oral structures.

Clefts are openings in the roof of the mouth, repaired by surgical methods.

In **cineradiography,** moving X-ray pictures are taken.

See **Chapter 9** for details on communication problems associated with neurological problems or diseases.

A **stroke** is a cause of brain damage due to interrupted blood supply.

Aphasia is a language problem due to stroke and other causes.

Hemiplegia is paralysis of one half of the body.

An **audiologist** is an expert in hearing and its disorders.

In **sensorineural hearing loss,** portions of the inner ear or auditory nerve are damaged.

An **audiogram** is a graph showing hearing thresholds.

See **Chapter 10** for details on hearing disorders and audiologists.

A Referral from a Laryngologist

I am referring Mrs. Melinda Baily, a 32-year-old woman, for a voice evaluation and consideration for voice therapy. She is a lead singer with a musical group in town. She came to me with a hoarse voice. She has a long history of hoarseness, which has become progressively worse during the last few weeks. My endoscopic examination has revealed bilateral vocal nodules. I believe Mrs. Baily can benefit from voice therapy. After a few weeks of voice therapy, I would like to repeat the endoscopic examination of her vocal folds.

A Referral from an Oral Surgeon

I am referring James Redding, a 4-year-old boy, for a speech evaluation. Jimmy had bilateral cleft of the hard and soft palate. His palatal clefts have been closed with the Veau–Wardill–Kilner surgical procedure. Our cineradiographic procedure indicates a reasonably mobile velopharyngeal mechanism. Nonetheless, Jimmy's speech is hypernasal. We believe that a speech training program may be helpful in increasing the efficiency of the velopharyngeal mechanism and in reducing hypernasality. Let me please have your recommendations.

A Referral from a Family Physician

I am referring Mr. Thomas Tanner, age 62 years, for a language evaluation. Mr. Tanner suffered a stroke about 3 weeks ago; he has right hemiplegia. He has great difficulty in expressing himself. Neurological evaluation suggests damage to motor speech areas of the brain. His physical condition has improved markedly. I believe he is now a good candidate for speech and language rehabilitation. I would appreciate your report and recommendations for speech and language therapy.

A Referral from an Audiologist

I am referring Timothy Noll, a 10-year-old boy, for a speech and language evaluation. My audiological findings suggest a sensorineural hearing loss. I have enclosed a copy of his audiogram. Timothy has been fitted with binaural hearing aids, which improve his hearing thresholds; aided and unaided thresholds also are indicated on his audiogram. I think that Timothy needs an intensive speech training program. Your assessment and recommendations will be greatly appreciated.

As you found out, these referral letters are full of technical terms that I do not expect you to fully understand now. The purpose of introducing these referral letters to you at this stage of your knowledge is to emphasize the need to learn certain technical matters, especially the anatomy and physiology of speech and hearing. Because of their knowledge of anatomy, physiology, and related technical matters, the referral letters mean much more to speech–language pathologists or audiologists than they do to you at this stage of your training. In the subsequent chapters, you will learn more about the disorders and diseases mentioned in the letters.

In this chapter, we shall take a brief and simplified look at the physical mechanism that makes hearing and speech production possible. More detailed discussion of anatomy and physiology, and neurology of speech, language, and hearing can be found in several sources including Bhatnagar and Andy (1995), Seikel, King, and Drumright (2000), Kent (1997), Perkins and Kent (1986), Calvin and Ojemann (1980), Ornstein and Thompson (1984), Smith (1984), Webster (1999), and Zemlin (1998). Students majoring in communicative sciences and disorders will have additional courses on anatomy, physiology, and neurology of speech, language, and hearing.

At a gross level, talking is like walking. For both, one needs a physical mechanism. Several bodily structures that are parts of different neuroanatomic systems provide these physical mechanisms. Various bones, muscles, membranes, tendons, cartilage, and nerves are involved in speech production.

Structural Mechanisms of Speech Production

The major structures of speech include the respiratory, phonatory, and articulatory systems. The central nervous system (the brain) is responsible for integrating all the activities of other structures into a more abstract activity called language. A related but important system is that of hearing. Figure 3.1 illustrates the major systems of speech, language, and hearing. For the sake of simplicity, nerves involved in speech production are not included in Figure 3.1.

When a person begins to speak, the various structures in the chest, abdomen, throat, and mouth are activated. The brain regulates this complex action. The hearing mechanism helps the speaker become aware of speech others produce. The same mechanism also helps the speaker self-monitor what he or she says or has just said. The speaker uses the airstream (especially the breathing-out) to set the vocal cords into vibration. This vibration produces the vocal sound. Then, for the most part, the tongue, teeth, and soft and hard palates help shape the vocal sound into recognizable speech sounds. The cavities of throat, mouth, and nose also help modify the qualities of the sound produced by the larynx. This modification results in a voice that is pleasant and appropriate for age, sex, and the kind of communication attempted.

Vocal folds are a pair of thin muscles in the throat used to produce sound.

Palate is the roof of the mouth; its front portion is hard; its back portion is soft.

A **cavity** is a space containing certain structures.

The Respiratory System

That a speaker needs air to speak is common knowledge. A person who is out of breath finds it difficult to speak. The amateur opera singer who runs out of air and interrupts singing at unexpected junctures dramatically illustrates this fact. The air used for speaking comes from the lungs. We breathe in (**inhale**)

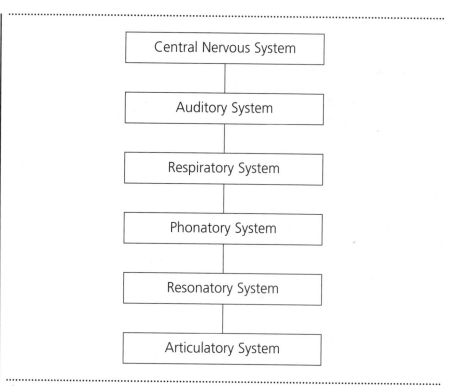

Figure 3.1. Schematic of the major systems (structures) of hearing, speech, and language. *Note.* From *Assessment and Treatment of Articulation and Phonological Disorders in Children* (p. 3), by A. Peña-Brooks and M. N. Hegde, 2000, Austin, TX: PRO-ED. Copyright 2000 by PRO-ED, Inc. Reprinted with permission.

and breathe out (**exhale**), and we normally speak on exhalation. Inhalation and exhalation and the act of speaking are related in a complex manner. Several structures including the rib cage, the diaphragm, and the lungs make this action possible. Many muscles under the control of the nervous system implement the action of breathing and talking.

The rib cage provides the main structural frame for respiration. Also known as the thoracic cage and commonly called the chest, the **rib cage** consists of 12 pairs of **ribs** that form a cylinder-like structure. All ribs are attached at the back to the vertebral column. The upper 7 ribs are directly and independently attached to the sternum (the breast bone) in front. The 3 false ribs also are attached to the sternum but with a common cartilaginous band. The lowest 2 ribs are not attached to the sternum, and hence are called the false ribs. The rib cage houses such vital organs as the heart and the lungs. Figure 3.2 illustrates the rib cage.

The floor of the thoracic (chest) cavity is the **diaphragm,** which is a thick muscle, shaped like a dome. It separates the stomach from the thorax. The diaphragm plays a major role in breathing because the lungs rest on it. Figure 3.3 illustrates the lungs and the diaphragm.

The cone-shaped lungs are a part of the **pulmonary system,** which includes the lower and upper airways. The upper airway includes the mouth, nose, and upper portions of throat. The **trachea,** which is a tube formed by about 20 rings of cartilage, is the starting point of the lower airway.

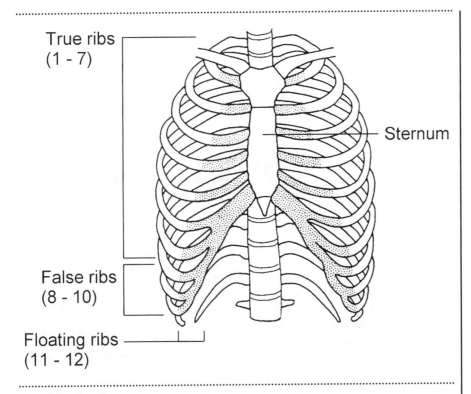

Figure 3.2. The rib cage.

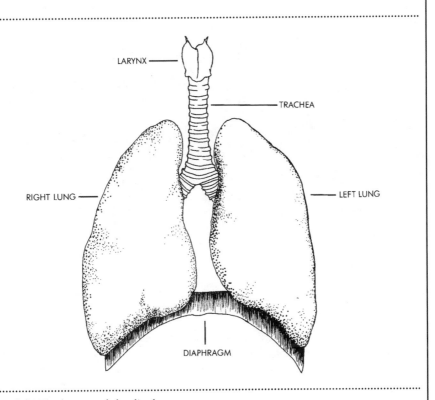

Figure 3.3. The lungs and the diaphragm.

Besides the diaphragm, several other muscles move during breathing. These include muscles in between the ribs (**intercostal muscles**), and several muscles in the neck, chest, and stomach.

When we breathe in, we bring in oxygen to the blood, and when we breathe out, we get rid of the accumulated carbon dioxide. When an excessive amount of carbon dioxide creates a need for oxygen, a structure in the brain stem called the **medulla oblongata** fires impulses to the muscles of respiration. Adults normally breathe about 12 times a minute, although this rate can be reduced by special exercises. Young children's rate of breathing is typically higher, and infants breathe at rates of 60 times per minute or higher.

Inhalation and exhalation create the rhythmic cycle of respiration. Inhalation brings the air into the lungs where oxygen and carbon dioxide are exchanged. Through the actions of the diaphragm and other muscles of respiration, we expand the chest cavity and with it the lungs. When the lungs expand, the pressure within the lungs, compared to that outside, is reduced. Through the open laryngeal valve, the air then moves into the lungs and equalizes the pressure inside and outside the lungs. Soon the muscles contract to reduce the volume of the chest cavity. This creates a positive pressure within the lungs. As a result, the air moves out (exhalation). In this manner, the cycle of inhalation and exhalation keeps going automatically.

The production of speech needs a supply of moving air that can set the vocal folds into vibration. Respiration provides such an air supply. However, speech modifies the breathing cycle. Because speech is typically produced on exhalation, the duration of exhalations during speech tends to be longer than that during silent periods or inhalation. A longer or louder utterance may require deeper inspiration than the usual. Compared to quiet breathing, breathing during speech is more consciously monitored and adjusted to meet the demands of speech. Such adjustments are rapid and continuous.

Respiratory problems most frequently found in speech and voice disorders result from an improper use of breathing for the purposes of speaking. Persons who stutter, for example, may try to speak while inhaling air. They also may continue to speak on the rapidly dwindling air supply, instead of stopping to breathe in. Some speakers with voice disorders are known to waste the air by improper modifications of exhalation.

Neurological diseases and brain damage may cause respiratory problems. In the case of Mr. Tilley, who was referred for a speech–language evaluation by a neurologist, the respiratory problems were caused by brain damage due to parkinsonism. Patients who have this neurological disorder talk in a soft voice and with short phrases, because they cannot sustain a strong breath supply for louder and more continuous speech.

The Phonatory Mechanism

With the lungs providing the necessary air supply for speech, the **larynx**, popularly known as the voice box, makes it possible to *phonate*. To **phonate** is to produce voice.

The larynx, whose major structures are illustrated in Figure 3.4, is a valve; it opens and closes. Like all other structures of speech, the laryngeal valve has its primary biological functions. Essentially, it closes the entry into the trachea so that food and other substances that do not belong in the lungs do not enter them. The laryngeal valve also is involved in the cough reflex that expels for-

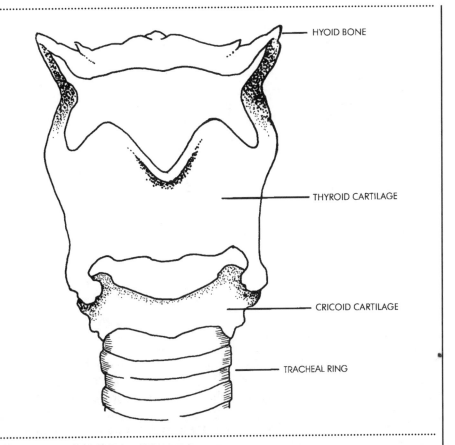

Figure 3.4. The major laryngeal structures.

eign substances that accidentally enter the trachea. Finally, the valve can be closed to build up air pressure below it. This pressure, described as the **subglottal pressure,** is essential for such biological functions as excretion and child delivery and for such actions as lifting heavy objects.

The larynx includes muscles, membranes, and cartilages. The larynx lies at the top of the trachea, in the front portion of the neck. The larynx is suspended by the U-shaped **hyoid** bone, which floats under the jaw but is not an integral part of the larynx. The muscles of the tongue and various muscles of the skull, larynx, and jaw are attached to this bone.

Several cartilages provide the framework for the larynx. The relatively large, butterfly-shaped **thyroid cartilage** forms the frontal and side walls of the larynx. Of the laryngeal cartilages, the **cricoid** is the most important. The cricoid is the top ring of the trachea. It is linked with the thyroid cartilage and a pair of **arytenoid cartilages,** which are two small, pyramid-shaped cartilages. The arytenoids are connected to the cricoid through the **cricoarytenoid joint,** which permits circular and sliding movements. Because the vocal folds are attached to the arytenoid cartilages, their movements cause the folds to open or close. The cricoarytenoid joint is shown in Figure 3.5.

Various muscles are found in the laryngeal area, but we will be concerned with only a few of them here. Because of these muscles, we can make the necessary movements and adjustments needed to phonate (produce voice). The

Subglottal pressure is air pressure below the vocal cords.

Cartilages are tough connective tissue.

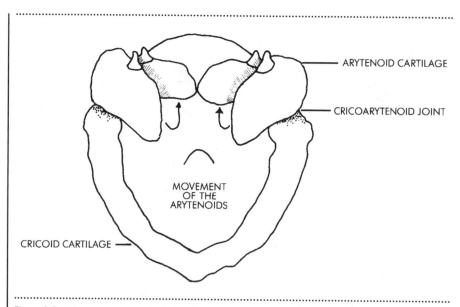

Figure 3.5. The cricoarytenoid joint.

muscles are capable of shortening, lengthening, tensing, and relaxing the vocal folds. Muscular movements also bring the folds together or pull them apart. All of these movements are important in the production of speech and variations in voice.

An important point to remember is that the basic structure that vibrates and produces sound is a pair of muscles known as the **thyroarytenoid muscle.** As the name suggests, the thyroarytenoids are attached to the thyroid and the arytenoid cartilages. The thyroarytenoid muscles are divided into two muscle masses: the internal thyroarytenoids and the external thyroarytenoids. The internal thyroarytenoids are the primary portions of the thyroarytenoid muscle that vibrate and produce sound. Therefore, they also are known as the **vocal folds, vocal cords,** or the **vocalis muscle.** The vocal folds are illustrated in Figure 3.6.

The muscles that bring the vocal folds together and those that pull them apart work in **antagonism** (in opposition to each other). Folds that are closed or nearly closed are **adducted,** and those that are drawn apart are **abducted.** The muscles that achieve these results are either adductors (those that pull together) or abductors (those that pull apart).

Two pairs of muscles that bring the vocal folds together (the adductors) are the **lateral cricoarytenoid** and the **interarytenoid muscles.** These two muscles act in harmony and in opposition to the major vocal folds abductor called the **posterior cricoarytenoid muscle.**

The muscle that lengthens and tenses the vocal folds is the **cricothyroid.** It is attached to the cricoid and the thyroid cartilages. Of course, the vocal folds themselves (the thyroarytenoid muscle) can be lengthened and tensed. Lengthening and tensing of the vocal folds result in thinning and thickening of the folds.

When the vocal folds are abducted (pulled apart), a small opening results. This opening has a name: **glottis.** The anatomist's insistence that a space between the vocal folds be given a name can create some awkward phrases: *the opening is closed when the glottis is closed,* and *the opening is open when the glottis is open.* The point is that the glottis should not be confused with an

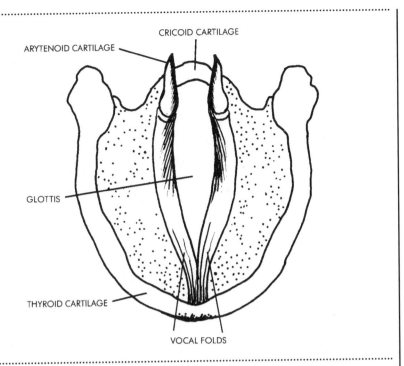

ARYTENOID CARTILAGE

CRICOID CARTILAGE

GLOTTIS

THYROID CARTILAGE

VOCAL FOLDS

Figure 3.6. The vocal folds.

anatomical structure; it is space that varies with the varied behavior of the vocal folds.

The muscles described so far (the thyroarytenoid, the cricothyroid, the posterior cricoarytenoid, the lateral cricoarytenoid, and the interarytenoid) are known as the **intrinsic muscles** of the larynx because their attachments are within the larynx. They are more directly associated with phonation. However, there are **extrinsic laryngeal muscles,** which have at least one attachment to structures other than the larynx. These muscles help keep the laryngeal structures in place. Their actions can lower or raise the larynx and thus indirectly influence sound production.

Phonation

The vocal folds are capable of fast and rapidly changing actions necessary to produce speech, especially conversational speech. Such fast action is possible because the folds are richly supplied by the nerves, and their anatomy is highly flexible. The folds can vibrate at a faster or slower rate. They can open and close quickly or slowly, and with greater or lesser force. They can close fully or partially, or they can just approximate. They can assume any intermediate positions resulting in various shapes of the space between them (glottis). The folds can be thickened by shortening and thinned by elongation. They can be tensed or relaxed. In essence, their actions range from one extreme to the other. This flexibility of the vocal folds is primarily responsible for both the beauty and the range of human vocal response, including such superb and unique human accomplishments as vocal music. Figure 3.7 shows the shape of the vocal folds during quiet breathing, forced inhalation, normal phonation, and whisper.

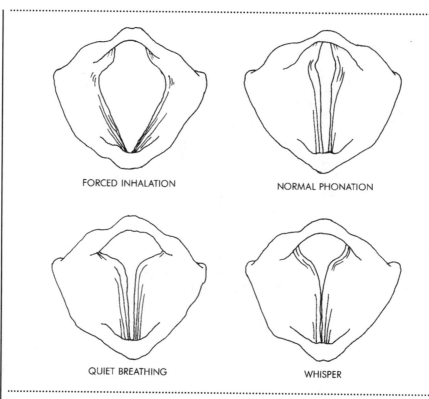

FORCED INHALATION

NORMAL PHONATION

QUIET BREATHING

WHISPER

Figure 3.7. The shape of the vocal folds during various functions.

During silence, the folds are open (abducted) and the glottis is V-shaped. To produce voice, the vocal folds must vibrate, and they cannot vibrate unless they come together (adducted). The vocal folds are primarily adducted by the action of the interarytenoid muscle, which moves the two arytenoid cartilages together.

When the vocal folds are closed, the airflow stops. This results in a buildup of air pressure below the folds. This subglottal air pressure is higher than the pressure above the glottis. Consequently, the vocal folds begin to vibrate and open. The opening begins at the bottom and moves toward the top. This is the opening phase. As the opening phase reaches the top of the folds, the bottom portion begins to close. The closing process also moves from the bottom to the top of the folds. The folds may remain closed for a brief duration (the closed phase). This closure once again causes a buildup of subglottal air pressure, which restarts the cycle of opening and closing.

Whereas the opening of the vocal folds is explained on the basis of the subglottal air pressure, their closing is explained partly on the basis of the **Bernoulli effect.** The theory says, among other things, that when gasses or liquids move through a constricted passage, **velocity** increases and **pressure** decreases. In the case of phonation, as the air moves from the lungs to the laryngeal area, it passes through the open but constricted vocal folds, which results in increased velocity of the air and decreased pressure between the edges of the folds. This lowered pressure between the folds draws them together. Thus, whereas an increased pressure below the folds blows them apart, a drop in pressure between the edges of the folds pulls them together.

Bernoulli was a Swiss scientist who developed the kinetic theory of gases and liquids.

Velocity is quickness of motion.

Pressure is force distributed over a certain area.

Another factor responsible for the opening and closing of the folds is their elasticity. The folds are strong enough to resist and thus help build air pressure under them, but they also are elastic enough to move back to their earlier position, and thus close again. Therefore, the full explanation of the vocal fold movements includes the buildup of air pressure, the pressure differences (positive and negative), and the elasticity of the muscles. This explanation of phonation is called the **myoelastic–aerodynamic theory.**

The sound the larynx produces is not the same sound that is eventually heard. This is because the structures or cavities (upper throat and mouth) that lie beyond the glottis modify the laryngeal sound. The laryngeal sound is then articulated into speech sounds of the language.

The Pitch and Loudness of Voice

The two important characteristics of voice are pitch and loudness. Both refer to how we perceive voice. Pitch and loudness are often described as *perceptual* or *psychological;* they are sensations. These sensations depend on certain physical and physiological factors.

The vocal folds normally move in a regular manner. The patterns of movement repeat themselves. Among other factors, the amount of subglottal air pressure, the degree of muscular effort, and the velocity of the moving air determine these patterns of vibrations. Variations in these patterns, in turn, create differences in pitch and loudness.

The pitch of a speaker's voice is determined primarily by the frequency with which the vocal folds vibrate. The frequency of vibration is measured in terms of hertz (abbreviated Hz); 100 Hz means 100 vibrations per second. The greater the frequency of vocal fold vibrations, the higher the pitch. The rate at which given vocal folds vibrate is called the **fundamental frequency,** a physical variable that is different from person to person. The differences in the fundamental frequency of vocal fold vibrations are perceived as differences in **pitch,** a psychological variable.

It is a common knowledge that men tend to have lower vocal pitches than women. This is because the fundamental frequency of male vocal fold vibration is about 125 Hz, whereas the fundamental frequency of female vocal fold vibration is about 225 Hz. Young children of either sex tend to have higher pitches because their fundamental frequency may be as high as 400 Hz. The fundamental frequency changes with age and the change is dramatic for the male. These changes are associated with the growth of the laryngeal musculature and cartilages.

The **elasticity, tension,** and **mass** of the vocal folds determine the fundamental frequency of vocal fold vibration. Longer and thicker vocal folds vibrate at lower frequency; hence, the vocal pitch of a male speaker is generally lower than that of a female. Thinner and shorter folds vibrate at higher frequency; hence, the vocal pitch of a female speaker is higher than that of a male. However, a speaker who has longer and thicker folds can stretch and lengthen the folds and thereby increase his or her fundamental frequency. This is because stretched folds are tense, and tensed folds vibrate at higher frequency, resulting in higher pitch.

Loudness, another perceived characteristic of voice, also has physical and physiological bases. The main physical factor that determines perceived loudness of voice is the degree of subglottal (below the vocal folds) air pressure. To build greater air pressure, however, the two vocal folds must compress

Pitch is determined by the rate of vocal fold vibration (physical factor) and the mass, tension, and elasticity of the vocal folds (physiological factors).

harder. Therefore, the degree of vocal fold compression also is a factor in loudness. When a person is called on to speak louder, he or she tends to inhale more air and exhale somewhat more forcefully. To achieve forceful exhalation, the vocal folds need to compress more than usual to build up extra subglottal pressure.

The two main interrelated physiological factors that determine loudness are the intensity and amplitude of vocal fold vibrations. The greater the subglottal air pressure, the higher the **intensity** of phonation; it is the force or vigor with which the folds open and close. Higher intensity of phonation is associated with increased amplitude of vibration. **Amplitude** is the extent of vocal fold movements; the greater the extent of movement, the higher the amplitude. This occurs when the folds swing apart wider. Thus, loudness is caused by increased subglottal air pressure, intensity, and amplitude of vocal fold vibration.

> Just as the "membrane" of a loudspeaker bulges out to produce louder sound, the vocal folds bulge more and move with greater force to produce louder sound.

Voice Quality

As mentioned before, the tone produced at the larynx does not sound anything like the sound of speech (and song) that people produce. The structures and cavities above the larynx modify the laryngeal tone to a great extent, resulting in the ultimately heard speech with all its deep, rich, and varied characteristics. These cavities of the throat and mouth resonate the sound and change its quality. **Resonance** is modification of a sound by structures through which the sound passes. Resonating bodies do not produce sound; they only affect its quality. The manner of vocal fold vibration also influences perceived vocal quality. Compared to frequency and intensity of voice, vocal quality is a more subjective aspect of voice production.

Vocal quality is affected by many of the factors we have discussed so far: the mass, length, and tension of the vocal folds; the degree of compression between the folds; subglottal air pressure; and frequency, intensity, and amplitude of vocal fold vibrations. Another factor that affects vocal quality is the physical symmetry of the two folds. If the paired vocal muscles are not symmetrical, they do not vibrate in harmony. For example, if one of the folds is thicker than the other, then the rate at which they vibrate will differ. This will affect the vocal quality.

The commonly described vocal qualities include breathiness, harshness, and hoarseness. Excessive nasality is a related quality, but it often is described as a resonance problem. A **breathy voice** results when the vocal folds do not completely close. Vocal nodules, for example, can prevent the two folds from achieving closure. Lack of such closure causes air leakage during phonation and adds frictional noise to the voice. This kind of voice is perceived as breathy.

Harshness, or roughness of voice, is a vocal quality due mainly to the irregular vibration of vocal folds. In irregular and aperiodic vibrations, the duration of vibrations, the intensity, or both may change abruptly. Also, the vocal folds may have excessive tension and they may compress too hard.

When both breathiness and harshness are present, the vocal quality is described as **hoarse.** Therefore, hoarseness results from excessive air leakage through the glottis and irregular vocal fold vibrations. However, the predominant quality of the hoarse voice may be breathiness or harshness.

Nasality refers to the added nasal resonance to voice. Nasal resonance is the quality added to the sound when the sound passes through the nose. Nasal speech sounds (the *m, n,* and *ng* in the English language) require nasality. Nonnasal or oral speech sounds (all of the other sounds of English) should not have perceivable nasal resonance. Note that nasal resonance is not abnormal in itself. It is abnormal when misplaced; then it is called **hypernasality.**

Nasality is not a vocal quality but a resonance quality, because it is not related to the behaviors of the vocal folds. It is a matter of what happens to the laryngeally phonated sound when it passes through the cavities of the throat and mouth.

Deviant voice qualities may signal laryngeal pathology. Therefore, they should be taken seriously. Mrs. Baily, who was referred to Tammy, the speech–language pathologist, had developed vocal nodules. Nodules result in hoarse voice.

Vocal nodules and many other kinds of vocal pathologies and the resulting voice problems are described in **Chapter 7.**

Summary

- The breathing mechanism provides the power needed for phonation.

- The laryngeal mechanism with its vocal folds is the voice-producing mechanism.

- The airflow from the lungs passing through the closed or nearly closed vocal folds sets them into vibration.

- The vibrations create laryngeal tones.

- The structures above the larynx (resonators), including the mouth and the nose, modify the laryngeal tone.

Even the modified laryngeal tones, however, are not yet speech. Additional modifications are needed to turn the laryngeal and subsequently modified tones into recognizable speech sounds. These modifications are called *articulation* and the structures that accomplish it are *articulators*.

Articulatory System

The word *articulation* has different meanings. In anatomy, it means connection of movable parts. In speech, it means movements of structures to produce speech sounds. In speech science and pathology, as well as in everyday language, articulation also means the act of saying something clearly. In this section, **articulation** means the movement of joined anatomic parts as well as the production of speech sounds by such movements.

The tone the larynx produces and gets modified as described is shaped into speech sounds by several structures including the tongue and the lips. This shaping of the speech sounds is articulation.

The sound the larynx produces travels through the cavities of the throat and mouth, collectively known as the **pharynx** or the vocal tract. The pharynx is divided into three segments: the laryngopharynx, the oropharynx, and the nasopharynx.

The **laryngopharynx** starts just above the larynx and ends at the base of the tongue. The laryngopharynx is connected to the **oropharynx,** which extends up to the soft palate. The oropharynx is connected to the **nasopharynx.** The nasopharynx ends where the two nasal cavities begin. These cavities of speech are illustrated in Figure 3.8.

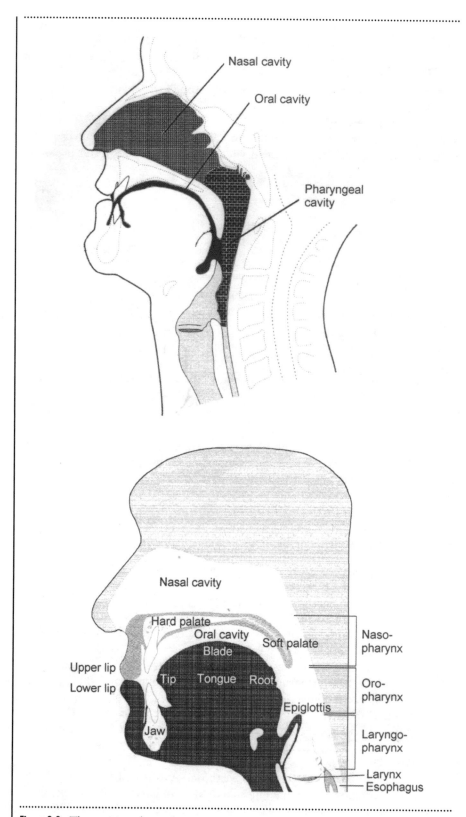

Figure 3.8. The cavities of speech.

The laryngopharynx and the oropharynx add resonance to the sounds the larynx produces. However, as noted before, the nasopharynx adds noticeable resonance to only the nasal sounds (*n, m,* and *ng*). The nasal cavity is normally closed during the production of the non-nasal sounds of speech. The soft palate and the surrounding muscles of the throat help achieve this closure. Movable parts, including the soft palate, tongue, and lips play a major role in articulating the speech sounds.

The Soft Palate

Also known as the **velum,** the **soft palate** is a flexible muscular structure at the juncture of the oropharynx and the nasopharynx. Located at the back of the mouth, it hangs from the hard palate, which is the roof of the mouth. The small, cone-shaped tip of the velum is called the **uvula.** Figure 3.9 shows the major structures of the oral cavity, including the soft palate.

The soft palate is a dynamic structure of muscles that can be lowered or raised. When it is lowered, the nasal cavities are opened and breathing through the nose is possible. When it is raised, it helps close the nasal cavities from the oral cavity. In this process, the muscles of the pharynx also move inward to meet the muscles of the soft palate. Like a sphincter, the nasal port is then closed. The phonated sound exits only through the mouth, and the nasal speech sounds do not have the desirable nasal resonance.

If the muscular bulk of the soft palate is inadequate, then the nasal cavity may always remain open to some extent. When this happens, the speech of the speaker will sound excessively nasal because sound energy passes through the nasal cavities when it should not. The person sounds as though he or she is speaking through the nose. This condition often is seen in patients with cleft palate. Jimmy Redding's problem described at the beginning of this chapter is of this kind.

Read more about cleft palate in **Chapter 8.**

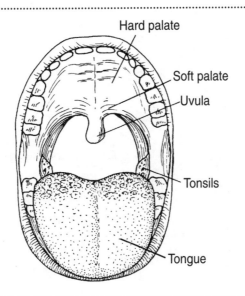

Hard palate

Soft palate

Uvula

Tonsils

Tongue

Figure 3.9. The major structures of the oral cavity.

The Hard Palate

The bony roof of the mouth and the floor of the nose is called the **hard palate.** The major portion of the hard palate is made up of a pair of bones called **maxillae** (singular, maxilla). The hard palate is illustrated in Figure 3.10.

The front portion of the maxillary bone is called the **premaxilla,** and it houses the four upper front teeth known as the **incisors.** In the fetal stage, the premaxilla grows as a separate structure which eventually fuses with the maxillary bone.

The portion of the maxillary bone that forms most of the hard palate is called the **palatine process.** The palatine process consists of two pieces of bone that grow and fuse at the midline during the fetal stage. The outer edges of the maxillary bone are called the **alveolar process,** which houses the molar, bicuspid, and cuspid teeth.

Due to genetic and toxic environmental reasons, the premaxilla may fail to fuse with the maxillary bone. Similarly, the palatine processes may fail to fuse at the midline. Such failures cause **clefts of the palate.**

At the back, the maxillary bone joins with the **palatine bone** (not the palatine process, which is part of the maxillary bone). The soft palate attaches to the palatine bone.

The Jaw

The jaw is an important bone of the face. Its anatomic name is the **mandible.** It houses the lower set of teeth and forms the floor of the mouth. In adults, it is considered a single bone, although it is the result of the fusion of two bones. The line of fusion is in the midpoint of the chin.

The part of the mandible that houses the teeth is called the **alveolar arch.** The two arches of the mandible are hinged to the skull with a set of muscles and tendon. The mandible is attached to the temporal bone, which is a part of the skull. Therefore, the joint is known as the **temporomandibular joint (TMJ).**

A group of muscles helps open and close the jaw. Other kinds of movements needed to chew food also are made possible by muscles. Though its major task is to chew food, the mandible is important for speech because it houses the lower teeth, serves as a framework for the tongue and lower lip, and is a part of the oral cavity.

Clefts of the palate and lips are described in **Chapter 8.**

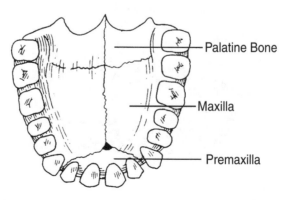

Figure 3.10. The hard palate.

The Teeth

As noted earlier, the upper dental arch is part of the maxillary bone and the lower arch is part of the mandible. Although their major function is **mastication** (chewing), the teeth help make some speech sounds. For example, in producing the *f* and the *v* sounds, the teeth and the lips come in contact. Therefore, the teeth also are articulators.

As you know, each tooth has an anatomic name. Figure 3.11 illustrates the teeth. The temporary teeth, whose appearance in a baby is joyfully celebrated in the family, are known as the **deciduous** teeth. Babies normally have 20 deciduous teeth, 10 in each arch. Of the 10, 4 are incisors, 2 are canines, and 4 are molars. Adults have 32 teeth, 16 in each arch. Of the 16, 4 are incisors, 2 are canines, 4 are premolars, and 6 are molars. The deciduous dental arch does not have premolars or the third molar.

The way the two dental arches meet each other is described by the term **occlusion.** If the individual teeth in the two arches are properly aligned and the upper and lower dental arches meet each other in a fairly symmetrical manner, the occlusion is normal. Deviations in the shape and the dimensions of the upper and lower jaw bones and the positioning of individual teeth, among other factors, will create **malocclusions,** which are classified as Class I, II, or III. The normal occlusion and Class II and III malocclusions are illustrated in Figure 3.12.

In **Class I malocclusion,** only some individual teeth are misaligned, but the two arches are normally aligned. In **Class II malocclusion,** the upper jaw is protruded and the lower jaw is retracted or receded. In **Class III malocclusion,** the upper jaw is receded and the lower jaw is protruded. In individual cases, each type of malocclusion may vary considerably in the degree of abnormality.

The dental specialty of **orthodontics** is concerned with the study and treatment of dental deviations.

The Tongue

The biological function of the tongue is to sense taste and to move food around in the mouth for better chewing and swallowing. A nonbiological function of the tongue is to help produce speech sounds.

Anatomically, the tongue is divided into its tip, blade, dorsum, and root. The tip, being the thinnest and most flexible part of the tongue, plays an important

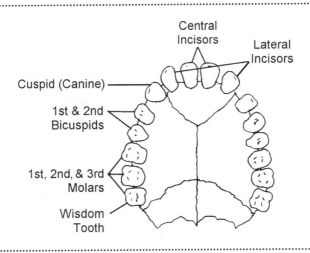

Central
Incisors

Lateral
Incisors

Cuspid (Canine)

1st & 2nd
Bicuspids

1st, 2nd, & 3rd
Molars

Wisdom
Tooth

Figure 3.11. The teeth.

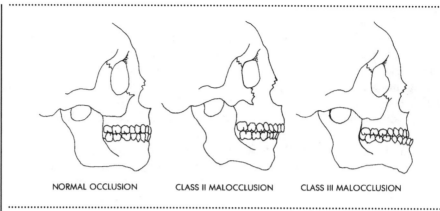

NORMAL OCCLUSION   CLASS II MALOCCLUSION   CLASS III MALOCCLUSION

Figure 3.12. The normal and deviant forms of dental occlusions.

role in articulation. The tip is a narrow structure (and it can be proverbially sharp in the nonanatomic sense). The blade is a small region next to the tip. In a resting position, the blade is the portion of the tongue that lies just below the alveolar ridge. The dorsum is the larger area of the tongue that lies in contact with both the hard and soft palates. The very back of the tongue contains its root.

Because of a rich supply of nerves, the longitudinal, vertical, and transverse muscle fibers of the tongue can move swiftly. Due to the action of these muscles, the tongue can be lengthened, shortened, curled up, pulled down, and flattened. Such actions change the dimensions of the oral cavity and modify the resonant characteristics of the voice.

In everyday speech, the importance of the tongue is very much recognized because it often is equated with language or speech. Recall such expressions as "mother tongue," "sharp tongue," and so forth. The tongue is a major articulator. It can stop the airflow and release it in a plosive manner. The voiceless sounds *t* or *k* and the voiced sounds *d* or *g*, for example, are produced in this manner. The tongue can constrict the air passage and thus create hissing or friction noises. The voiceless *s* and the voiced *z* are made this way. The tongue can stop the airflow and then release with a fricative noise. The *ch* (as in *chalk*) and the *j* as in (*job*) are produced in this manner. Such noises and sounds are made with the help of other oral structures as well.

Lips and Cheeks

The muscles of the lips and cheeks are a part of the facial musculature. Anatomically, smiles and laughter are different kinds of contractions of the lip and other facial muscles. Expressions of anger, resentment, disapproval, contentment, joy, frustration, and many other complex emotions also are different contractions of various muscles of the face.

The lips are made up of the **orbicularis oris** muscle of the mouth. Several muscles of the chin and the cheeks are connected to the orbicularis oris. Together, they make a variety of lip movements possible.

A large flat muscle that makes up most of the cheeks is called the **buccinator**. Its inner surface is covered with mucous membrane. Along with other muscles of the face and lips, the buccinator helps articulate several speech sounds.

With practice, speech sounds can be articulated with minimal movement of lips, just like a ventriloquist does. However, under most normal circum-

Not all speech sounds need vocal fold vibrations. Those that do are **voiced** sounds.

Sounds that are made without vocal fold vibrations are **voiceless.**

See **Chapter 4** for a discussion of speech sounds and how they are produced.

stances, lips are important in producing a group of sounds called the **labial sounds.** For example, in producing a *p* or *b,* both lips are used. The lips are closed for a short duration, which stops the airflow, and are then opened to release the air. Lip closure builds intraoral (within-the-mouth) air pressure, which is then released in a plosive manner. The orbicularis oris muscle of the mouth, the buccinator, and other facial muscles are involved in such productions. All these structures are under the control of the central nervous system. A later section offers a brief look at this system.

Summary

- Articulation is movement of such structures as tongue, lips, soft palate, and jaw to produce speech sounds.

- The modified laryngeal tone is articulated into speech sounds.

- The soft palate, hard palate, tongue, teeth, lips, lower jaw, and cheek muscles are primary articulators.

Anatomy and Physiology of Hearing

Speaking and hearing are closely related. The spoken form of speech and language requires normal hearing. The child learns the language he or she hears and becomes aware of. The hearing mechanism also helps regulate the production of speech. Because speakers hear themselves speak, they can change various aspects of their speech. For example, speakers who hear themselves speak softly or less clearly may restate more loudly or more clearly. More important, speakers can make such changes as they speak. The speech, language, and voice problems of deaf children and adults show that normal hearing is essential to effortlessly acquire, maintain, and monitor oral speech and language skills.

Hearing also is of biological importance. The hearing mechanism alerts the organism to dangers in the environment. Noises made by a careless predator in the wild may serve as lifesaving signals for the potential prey who, on hearing them, runs for its life. Although humans may loathe the sounds associated with danger, those sounds are a signal of impending danger that, when heeded, enhances the survival of individuals and their species.

The Ear

The ear is complex and what it does is amazing. The human ear is divided into the outer ear, the middle ear, and the inner ear. The gross anatomy of the ear is illustrated in Figure 3.13.

The Outer Ear

The most visible part of the outer ear, and biologically the least useful, is called the **auricle** or **pinna.** Its role in hearing is limited to funneling some sounds to

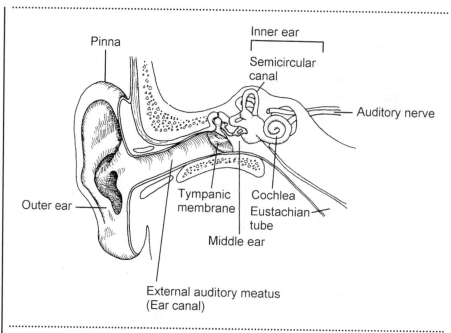

Figure 3.13. The gross anatomy of the human ear.

the ear canal. However, it does have some cosmetic value. This is the part that serves as a hanger for jewelry and eyeglasses.

The **ear canal,** also known as the **external auditory meatus,** is the more useful part of the outer ear. The canal is a muscular tube that resonates the sound that enters it. On average, the canal is about 2.5 cm (1 in.) long, slightly curved, and ends at the point where the eardrum is located. Most of the canal is made up of cartilage. Therefore, it is flexible and prone to injury. When people insert things that do not belong in the ear, they run the risk of damaging their eardrum.

The Middle Ear

The middle ear structures include the eardrum (the tympanic membrane), a chain of three small bones (the ossicular chain), and the Eustachian tube, which connects the middle ear cavity to the nasopharynx. These structures are housed in a cavity of the **temporal bone,** which is a part of the skull.

The **tympanic membrane** is thin, semitransparent, cone-shaped, and relatively tough, although flexible enough to vibrate. It vibrates very much like the membrane of a loudspeaker. The tympanic membrane is sensitive to different sound frequencies. Although all portions of the membrane can respond to low frequency sounds, particular portions respond to specific high frequencies. Through its vibrations, the tympanic membrane transmits the sound to the auditory ossicles (the small bones). The tympanic membrane and the ossicular chain of the middle ear are illustrated in Figure 3.14.

The **ossicular chain** is suspended in the middle ear by ligaments. The first bone of this chain is called the **malleus** (Latin for *hammer*), because it resembles a hammer. It is attached to the tympanic membrane. The second and middle bone of the chain is called the **incus** because it resembles an anvil. It is connected to the malleus in a tight joint that permits very little movement. The third and last bone is called the **stapes,** which resembles the stirrup on an Eng-

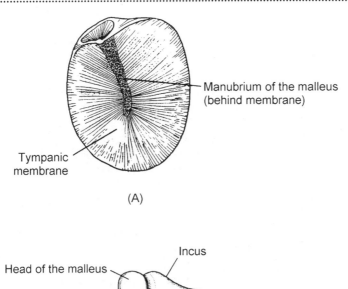

Manubrium of the malleus
(behind membrane)

Tympanic
membrane

(A)

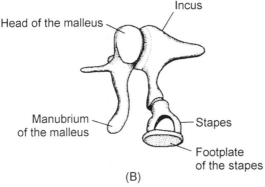

Incus

Head of the malleus

Manubrium
of the malleus

Stapes

Footplate
of the stapes

(B)

Figure 3.14. (A) The tympanic membrane and (B) the ossicular chain of the middle ear.

lish saddle. Therefore, the three bones also are known as the *hammer*, the *anvil*, and the *stirrup*.

The incus is attached to the stapes. The vibrations of the malleus and the incus are transmitted to the stapes. The stapes then conducts the sound to an opening called the **oval window** of the inner ear.

There are two small muscles in the middle ear that dampen the vibrations of the eardrum and the ossicular chain: the tensor tympani and the stapedius. The **tensor tympani** tenses the eardrum so that its vibrations are reduced. The **stapedius muscle** stiffens the ossicular chain so that its vibrations also are reduced. These reactions are reflexive and are known as the **acoustic reflex.** This reflex protects the ear from very loud sounds and noises that could damage the ear.

The Inner Ear

The **oval window**, the point where the inner ear begins, is a small opening in the bone of the inner ear. The foot of the stapes is positioned at this opening. The oval window receives sound vibrations from the foot of the stapes, which also acts like a door of the inner ear.

The inner ear is a complex system of interconnecting canals and passages called the **labyrinth** within the temporal bone. These canals, filled with a fluid called **perilymph,** house the sensitive inner ear organs of hearing and the organ that helps maintain balance (equilibrium) and body movement. The structures responsible for equilibrium are the three **semicircular canals.**

The **cochlea** is the main inner ear structure of hearing. The cochlea (and the semicircular canals) is illustrated in Figure 3.15. The cochlea appears like the shell of a snail or a coiled hose filled with a fluid called **endolymph.** When stretched, the human cochlea measures about 3.8 cm (1.5 in.). The floor of the cochlea is called the **basilar membrane.** When the stapes pushes into the inner ear, what gets really pushed around is the endolymph (fluid) in the inner ear.

The basilar membrane contains the inner ear's most important structure of hearing, called the **organ of Corti,** which bathes in the endolymph. This organ contains the **hair cells** that respond to sound. These cells, the **cilia,** which are anatomically hairlike structures, respond to sound vibrations.

The vibrations delivered by the foot plate of the stapes into the inner ear's oval window create wavelike movements in the perilymph. Through **Reissner's membrane,** these movements are transmitted to the endolymph, which then transmits them to the basilar membrane.

The hair cells of the organ of Corti respond to the vibrations of the basilar membrane. The vibrations create a shearing force on those cells. At this point, the mechanical forces of vibrations (wavelike movements of the fluids and membranes) are transformed into electrical energy, which can stimulate the nerve endings. This energy transformation within the organ of Corti is essential because the nerve fibers that carry the sound can respond only to electrical impulses, not to mechanical vibrations.

The nerve that picks up the neural impulses created by the movement of the hair cells of the cochlea is called the **acoustic nerve,** also known as the **cranial nerve VIII.** It has two divisions. The **vestibular division** is concerned with body equilibrium or balance. The **auditory division** is concerned with hearing.

The auditory division of the acoustic nerve has many endings in the cochlea. These nerve endings are in contact with the hair cells to pick up the sound vibrations transformed into neural impulses. Some 30,000 nerve fibers of the auditory nerve can be found in the cochlea. The auditory nerve exits the inner ear through the **internal auditory meatus.**

Diseases of the inner ear and of the auditory nerve cause a type of hearing loss known as **sensorineural hearing loss.** The cochlear hair cells may be dam-

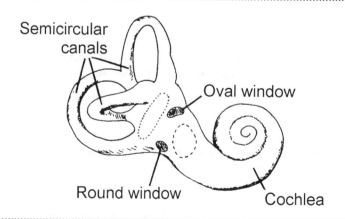

Figure 3.15. The cochlea and the semicircular canals.

aged due to prolonged exposure to noise. The hair cells then do not respond to the sound stimuli. Or the auditory nerve may be damaged, perhaps due to a tumor. In this case, the sound stimuli are not efficiently transmitted to the brain. Timothy Noll, who was referred to Tammy Speeks by an audiologist, had sensorineural hearing loss. It means that Timothy's middle ears are normal, but his hearing loss is due to problems in the cochlea, auditory nerve, or both.

The nerve impulses carried by the left and the right auditory pathways enter the brain stem. Also, the auditory pathways up to this point are considered peripheral (related to structures outside the brain), and those beyond this point are considered central (related to the brain).

At the brain stem, many auditory nerve fibers that come from one ear cross over (**decussate**) to the opposite side, forming **contralateral** pathways. Some continue on the same side, forming **ipsilateral** pathways. Because of this crossover of signals, the brain can compare sounds sent to it from each of the two ears. It helps the brain localize and integrate the sounds. The two sides of the temporal cortex are connected, so additional integration of sounds is possible because of this reason as well.

Summary

- In the absence of hearing, it is difficult to acquire and produce speech.

- The ear is divided into the outer ear, middle ear, and inner ear.

- The auricle and the external ear canal are the two major structures of the outer ear.

- The tympanic membrane, the Eustachian tube, and a chain of three small bones called the malleus, incus, and stapes are the major structures of the middle ear.

- The inner ear is filled with fluids and contains the organs of hearing and balance; the cochlea with its basilar membrane and hair cells is the most important structure of hearing.

- The acoustic branch of the cranial nerve VIII carries sound in the form of neural impulses from the hair cells to the brain.

- Sound waves, striking the tympanic membrane, set vibrations in the ossicular chain. These vibrations are transmitted to the inner ear in the form of waves in its fluid and the basilar membrane; the hair cells on the membrane react to these vibrations; and the mechanical vibrations are transformed into electrical (neural) impulses, which are carried to the brain by the acoustic nerve.

The Nervous System

The finely coordinated and complex activity we call speech is made possible by the respiratory, phonatory, and articulatory mechanisms. However, these structures need neural impulses to make them work. These impulses are generated in the nervous system.

The nervous system is a two-way street. It carries impulses to the peripheral systems and organs from the brain, and it carries impulses from these systems and organs back to that central regulator. The brain also regulates, integrates, and formulates communicative messages. In this sense, the brain executes many complex activities that make it all happen.

The Neuron

The central nervous system is made up of billions of nerve cells called **neurons.** A neuron, illustrated in Figure 3.16, has three parts: a cell body, dendrites, and an axon. The core of the cell body is called the **nucleus.** The body is covered with a membrane. The **dendrites** and **axons** are more like projections of the cell body, which specialize in receiving and conducting stimuli.

Dendrites receive neural impulses generated elsewhere, and axons send out impulses generated within the neuron. Neural impulses flow either *toward* the cell body or *away* from the cell body. The flow of information toward the cell body is described as **afferent.** Information flowing out of the cell body is known as **efferent.** A nerve carrying information to the brain also is described as afferent, and the one that carries information away from the brain is called efferent. A nerve carries information by conducting electrical impulses known as **action potentials.**

Many nerve fibers (axons), especially those in the peripheral nervous system and the larger axons of the central nervous system, have a white sheath

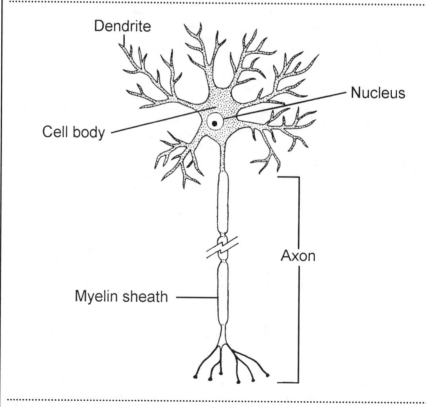

Figure 3.16. The neuron.

around them. This insulating sheath, called the *myelin,* has breaks at the junction between cells to facilitate the impulse transfer. The brain cells do not have this sheath, and hence they appear gray. Myelinated neurons can transfer information at a faster rate than the nonmyelinated.

Whereas nerves are neurons arranged in the form of fibers, a **nervous system** is an organization of nerves according to some structural, spatial, and functional principles. The peripheral, central, and autonomic systems often are collectively known as the nervous system.

Peripheral Nervous System

A collection of nerves that are outside the skull and the spinal column forms the **peripheral nervous system.** These nerves carry **sensory** impulses originating in the peripheral sense organs to the brain. They carry **motor** impulses originating in the brain to the muscles and glands in the body.

The peripheral nervous system is a collection of three kinds of nerves: the cranial, the spinal, and the peripheral autonomic. The cranial nerves are more directly involved in speech, language, and hearing than the other two kinds.

Cranial Nerves

The **cranial** nerves are so called because they enter or exit the same structural space that is occupied by the brain—the skull. Cranial nerves exit through holes, called **foramina,** in the base of the skull. The nerves exit at different levels of the brain stem and the top portion of the spinal cord. Some exit at a higher level than others. Consequently, the cranial nerves are numbered according to the vertical order in which they exit from the skull. They go out to connect to various sense organs and muscles of the head and neck. Table 3.1 lists the cranial nerves by their numbers, names, and functions.

Table 3.1
Cranial Nerves and Their Functions

Nerve No.	Name	Function
I	Olfactory	Sense of smell (sensory)
II	Optic	Vision (motor)
III	Oculomotor	Eye movement (motor)
IV	Trochlear	Eye movement (motor)
V	Trigeminal	Face (sensory); jaw (motor)
VI	Abducens	Eye movement (motor)
VII	Facial	Tongue (sensory); face (motor)
VIII	Vestibular acoustic	Hearing and balance (sensory)
IX	Glossopharyngeal	Tongue and pharynx (sensory); pharynx only (motor)
X	Vagus	Larynx, respiratory, cardiac, and gastrointestinal systems (sensory and motor)
XI	Accessory	Shoulder, arm, throat movements (motor)
XII	Hypoglossal	Mostly tongue movements (motor)

Some cranial nerves carry sensory information from a sense organ to the brain. Therefore, they are called **sensory nerves.** Other nerves carry impulses from the brain to the muscles to make those muscles move. Therefore, they are called **motor** (movement-related) **nerves.** A few cranial nerves do both: they carry sensory as well as motor impulses. They often are described as **mixed nerves.**

There are 12 pairs of cranial nerves, designated with Roman numbers. As shown in Table 3.1, five pairs of cranial nerves are not concerned with speech or hearing. Cranial nerve I is concerned with smell, whereas nerves II, III, IV, and VI are related to vision and the movements of the eyes.

Cranial nerves V, VII, VIII, IX, X, XI, and XII—seven in all—are important for speech or hearing, most of them for speech.

- **Trigeminal Nerve V.** Both a sensory and a motor nerve, the trigeminal is the largest of the cranial nerves, with three branches that serve many structures of the face, including the forehead, eyes, nose, and upper lip; the jaw; the tongue; and the cheeks.
- **Facial Nerve VII.** This also is a sensory and motor nerve. As a sensory nerve, the facial nerve is partly responsible for taste. As a motor nerve, it controls a variety of facial movements and expressions, including wrinkling of the forehead, tight closure of the mouth, retraction of the corners of the mouth, and cheek movements. Damage to this nerve usually gives the face a masklike appearance with minimal or no expression.
- **Vestibular Acoustic Nerve VIII.** This nerve has two branches, the **vestibular,** which is concerned with the sense of balance, and the **acoustic,** which carries sensory information (sound impulses) to the brain.
- **Glossopharyngeal Nerve IX.** This is a mixed nerve, containing sensory, motor, and autonomic fibers. It supplies the tongue (sensory) and the pharynx (motor). The motor portion helps regulate the movements of the muscles in the pharynx. Such movements are involved in speech production.
- **Vagus Nerve X.** This is called a wandering ("vagus") nerve because it wanders into the chest and stomach as well. It also is a mixed nerve with sensory, motor, and autonomic fibers. It is motor to the heart, lungs, and digestive system. It also is sensory to those structures along with the larynx, throat (including the base of the tongue), and external ear. A branch of the vagus nerve, the **recurrent laryngeal nerve** is important for speech. Its right and left branches regulate the intrinsic muscles of the larynx, excluding the cricothyroid. The recurrent nerve can be damaged during thyroid surgery. This usually results in total or partial paralysis of the vocal folds. Depending on the extent of paralysis, the speaker may not be able to produce voice, or if able, the voice may be hoarse.
- **Accessory Nerve XI.** This is a motor nerve, but it is unlike other cranial nerves. It is both a cranial nerve and a spinal nerve because it has a cranial and a spinal origin. Its major function is to regulate some of the muscles of the pharynx and the soft palate. It also is involved in head and shoulder movements.
- **Hypoglossal Nerve XII.** This is a motor nerve to the tongue. Running under it, the nerve controls most of the tongue movements.

Spinal Nerves

The spinal nerves of the peripheral nervous system are closely related to the autonomic nervous system. Together, they control various bodily activities, which are executed without much conscious knowledge or effort.

There are 31 pairs of spinal nerves. They are attached to the spinal cord through two roots: one afferent (dorsal, toward the back) and the other efferent (ventral, toward the front). The spinal nerves can be sensory, motor, or mixed; they supply the various small and large muscles throughout the body. They also control such automatic functions as breathing. Hence, some of them are indirectly involved with speech.

Autonomic Nervous System

The physical environment we live in is full of sensory stimuli. To survive, to adapt, to change, and to enjoy, we must be in touch with this environment. The nervous system, for the most part, is the means by which we change and adapt to the environment. However, our bodies also have a busy internal environment, which needs control and regulation. The **autonomic nervous system** controls this internal environment. This system, with **sympathetic** and **parasympathetic** divisions, supplies the smooth muscles within the body and the various glands that secrete hormones.

The sympathetic and the parasympathetic branches act in an opposing manner. The sympathetic branch generally mobilizes the body so that we can cope with emergencies. It helps us run from a dangerous situation or fight our enemy. The sympathetic branch accelerates the heart rate, raises the blood pressure, dilates the pupils, and increases the blood flow to the peripheral body structures (such as the legs that run). The action of the sympathetic division makes us feel emotionally aroused.

> The sympathetic branch mobilizes the body, and the parasympathetic branch calms the body.

The parasympathetic action helps bring the mobilized body back to its relatively relaxed state. The parasympathetic branch goes to work after we run or win (or lose) a fight. It slows the heart rate, lowers the blood pressure, increases the activity within the stomach, and generally relaxes the body. The action of the parasympathetic division makes us feel calm and relaxed.

The autonomic nervous system does not directly control the muscles of speech. However, emotionally aroused and relaxed states have contrasting effects on speech fluency, speech rate, voice quality, and other not well-understood aspects of communication. Relaxation of muscles of the body, especially of the speech-related muscles, sometimes is included in the treatment of fluency and voice problems. Think of the differences in one's speech, language, and voice under excited versus relaxed conditions. When excited, speech may be louder and faster than usual. When relaxed, speech may be softer and slower than usual. By mediating such states of excitement and relaxation, the autonomic nervous system may exert an indirect effect on speech.

Central Nervous System

The complex and highly evolved central nervous system has made it possible for humans to think, talk, write, paint, sing, and dance. It also has made it possible to create a human world and environment that differ from the animal world and environment. More important, the brain has made it possible to create a unique world of imagination, curiosity, creativity, music, art, architecture, poetry, mathematics, and science. Many neuroscientists believe that it is because of the brain that we study ourselves and try to understand our body as well as behavior (Calvin & Ojemann, 1980). All of these add up to a beautiful and enlightened human world.

The brain probably needed some help from the environment to do all that. After all, the nervous system, including the brain, is an instrument that allows organisms to live and work as efficiently and as successfully as possible in their environment. As a result, the organisms survive, and in the case of humans, enjoy life, too.

The peripheral nervous system is the means by which the brain gathers information about the environment. The brain then sends various impulses that lead to various appropriate actions. The peripheral systems and organs receive and send a variety of information and possibly demand directions for action. Therefore, there needs to be a centrally coordinating instrument that integrates information and issues commands. The brain is such an instrument.

The central nervous system includes the **brain** and the **spinal cord**, depicted in a general diagram in Figure 3.17. The spinal cord is an elongated structure within the spinal canal of the vertebral column. As noted before, pairs of spinal nerves branch out on either side of the vertebral column and reach most parts of the body. The upper portion of the spinal cord is continuous with the lower portion of the brain, known as the brain stem.

The Brain

The brain is the most important structure for speech, language, hearing, and all "higher" activities found in humans. The brain is housed within the cranial cavity of the skull. Its three major divisions are the brain stem, the cerebellum, and the cerebrum.

Chapter 9 describes the speech disorders that result when the brain does not properly control motor speech production.

The Brain Stem. The primary structures of the brain stem are the medulla, the pons, the midbrain (mesencephalon), the diencephalon, and the reticular formation. (Some neuroanatomists consider only the medulla and the pons as the structures of the brain stem.) The medulla is the uppermost portion of the spinal cord, which enters the cranial cavity. The pons and the midbrain are above the medulla. The brain stem (minus the reticular activating system) is illustrated in Figure 3.18.

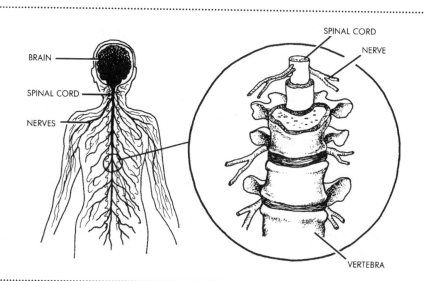

Figure 3.17. The brain and the spinal cord.

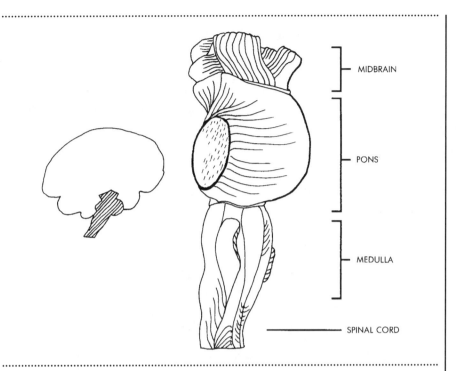

MIDBRAIN

PONS

MEDULLA

SPINAL CORD

Figure 3.18. The brain stem structures.

The **medulla** controls breathing and other vital functions of the body. The medulla contains nerves that carry commands from the motor center in the brain to various muscles. These pathways are known as the **pyramidal tracts.** Some of the muscles supplied by the pyramidal tracts are involved in speech. The pyramidal tract is a major structure that controls all kinds of movements. Therefore, it is important for speech production.

At the level of the medulla, the pyramidal tracts from the left and the right side of the brain cross over to the other side. Therefore, the left side of the body is primarily controlled by the right side of the brain and vice versa.

Although it means bridge, the **pons** is roundish and bulging. It bridges the two halves of the cerebellum (not cerebrum). It also projects fibers to other parts of the brain.

The **midbrain** is a narrow structure, also known as the **mesencephalon.** It lies above the pons. As its name implies, it is in the middle of other brain structures. The midbrain links the higher centers of the brain with the lower centers. Certain auditory and visual relay stations (way stations) also can be found in the midbrain.

The **reticular activating system** is a structure within the midbrain, brain stem, and upper portion of the spinal cord. This system integrates sensory impulses flowing into the brain with motor impulses flowing out of it. Therefore, it plays a role in the execution of motor activity. The system is the primary mechanism of attention and consciousness. It sends diffuse impulses to various regions of the cortex and alerts it about the incoming impulses.

The **diencephalon** includes the thalamus and the hypothalamus. The **thalamus** integrates the sensory information that flows into the brain and relays the sensory impulses to various parts of the cerebral cortex. The **hypothalamus,** which lies below the thalamus, helps integrate the actions of the autonomic nervous system. It controls emotional experiences.

Basal Ganglia. The structures deep within the brain that help to integrate motor impulses are called **basal ganglia,** illustrated in Figure 3.19. Basal ganglia are a part of the **extrapyramidal system,** which controls motor movements indirectly. (The pyramidal system controls movements more directly.) Both the systems control various voluntary movements of the body. As such, both are involved in speech production as well. Mr. Ben Tilley, who was referred to Tammy Speeks, suffered from damage to the extrapyramidal motor system, mostly to the basal ganglia. This damage is frequently seen in patients with parkinsonism, a progressive neurological disorder.

The Cerebellum. The cerebellum ("little brain") is a major structure of the central nervous system. As illustrated in Figure 3.20, the cerebellum lies just behind the brain stem and below the cerebrum. The portion of the brain that lies above the cerebellum is known as the occipital lobe of the cerebral hemispheres.

The cerebellum is a major structure of movement. Therefore, its function affects speech. The cerebellum regulates equilibrium (balance), body posture, and coordinated fine motor movements. Because such movements are essential for rapid speech, the activities of the cerebellum are important for speech. It is not a primary motor integration center, however. It receives impulses from other centers in the brain and helps coordinate those impulses.

See **Chapter 9** to find out more about ataxic dysarthria.

Damage to the cerebellum causes a neurological condition called **ataxia,** which is found in some children with cerebral palsy and adults who have suffered cerebellar damage. Disturbed balance and abnormal gait are major neurological symptoms. Patients are likely to show a speech disorder called **ataxic dysarthria.**

The Cerebrum. For speech, language, and hearing, the **cerebrum** (cerebral cortex) is the most important of the central nervous system structures. Its complex, intricate, and multitudinous neural connections distinguish the human brain from the subhuman brain. It is the biggest of the central nervous system structures.

The cerebrum has gray cells on top, unlike the spinal cord and the brain stem, which have such cells on the inside. This is the reason why the brain is popularly known as the gray matter. The cortex includes the topmost portion of the brain, but it is actually arranged in a series of six layers. Each layer consists of a different type of cell. The surface looks wrinkled because it is folded

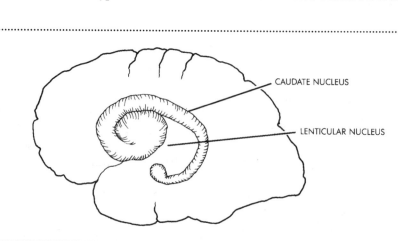

CAUDATE NUCLEUS

LENTICULAR NUCLEUS

Figure 3.19. The location of the basal ganglia within the brain.

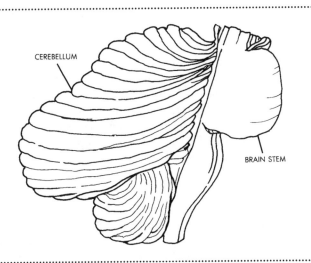

Figure 3.20. The cerebellum.

to accommodate more tissue in a somewhat small space. Billions of neural cells are packed into this structure and folded into numerous ridges and valleys. A ridge on the cortex is called a **gyrus,** and the cortex has many **gyri** (plural). Some of its valleys are shallow, but others are deeper. A shallow valley is a **sulcus,** and there are many **sulci** on the brain surface. The deeper valleys are fewer than sulci and are called **fissures.**

The fissures also are the boundaries of broad divisions of the cerebrum. The **longitudinal** fissure divides the cerebrum into the left and right hemispheres. The **fissure of Rolando** creates the frontal portion of the brain. The **lateral fissure,** or the **fissure of Sylvius,** creates a smaller area that lies under the frontal portion of the brain and is a part of the temporal lobe. The lobes of the cerebral cortex are illustrated in Figure 3.21.

There are four lobes in each hemisphere: the frontal, parietal, temporal, and occipital. For the most part, these names are based on the cranial bones with

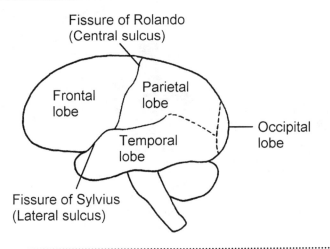

Figure 3.21. The lobes of the cerebral cortex.

which they are in contact. Hence, those divisions are not necessarily based on function. Nevertheless, each lobe has a major function, although the brain is an integrated structure and most of its activities are interconnected.

The **occipital** lobe is at the lower back portion of the head, just above the cerebellum. It is primarily concerned with vision and hence is of little direct relevance to speech and hearing. The **parietal lobe** is the primary somatic sensory area. It integrates such body sensations as pain, touch, temperature, and pressure. Such sensations are called **somesthetic.** Two specific areas of the parietal lobe, the areas including and surrounding the supramarginal gyrus and the angular gyrus, are involved in speech and language. For example, reading, writing, and word-finding problems have been found in persons who have suffered damage to the angular gyrus.

The remaining two lobes of the cerebrum, the frontal and the temporal, are of greater relevance to speech and hearing. The **frontal lobe** contains areas that are especially important for speech production. These include the **motor cortex** and **Broca's area.** The major speech–language and hearing areas of the brain are illustrated in Figure 3.22.

The **motor cortex** has specific representations for most of the muscles of the body. With the help of the pyramidal tract, this center controls movements. When specific areas of the primary motor cortex are stimulated, particular motor responses, such as a hand or lip movement, result. Neurosurgeons have studied the effects of direct brain stimulation before conducting brain surgery (Calvin & Ojemann, 1980). To find out what areas are directly related to what actions, neurologists electrically stimulate exposed areas of epileptic patients prior to surgery. Such "mapping" techniques have shown that compared to the control center for legs and other body structures, a large brain area controls lips, jaw, tongue, and larynx, suggesting the importance of cortical control of structures involved in speech. The hand also is controlled by a relatively large area.

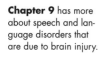

Chapter 9 has more about speech and language disorders that are due to brain injury.

Broca's area, named after the 19th-century French neurosurgeon and anthropologist Paul Broca who "discovered" it, is an important **motor speech center.** After a brain autopsy of a former patient with aphasia, Broca reported that an area in the frontal cortex was damaged. That area, located in the third

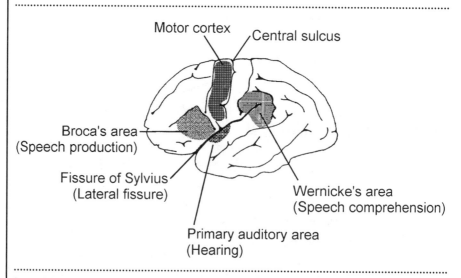

Figure 3.22. The major speech, language, and hearing areas of the brain.

convolution of the left cerebral hemisphere, came to be known as Broca's area. Although strict localization of functions in specific areas of the brain is now considered oversimplified neurology, specialists generally agree that in a majority of people, the left hemisphere controls speech production.

The **temporal lobe** contains two structures that are important for speech and hearing. First, the temporal lobe is the seat of the **primary auditory cortex,** which receives the sound stimuli from the acoustic nerve. It is believed that the auditory cortex processes what the ear hears and determines the meaning of sound stimuli, including heard speech.

Another important structure within the temporal lobe is named after Carl Wernicke, a famous German neurologist of 19th century. Wernicke found that an area in the first convolution of the left temporal lobe was responsible for understanding speech. It is now believed that **Wernicke's area** is responsible for both understanding and formulating speech.

Most structural landmarks and divisions of the brain are arbitrary. The lobes and other structures of the brain are an interconnected, integrated unit. The interconnected pathways of the brain help integrate sensory input and achieve coordinated execution of motor actions. In fact, there are specialized fibers that connect different parts of the brain to integrate its work. For instance, **association fibers** connect areas *within* a hemisphere. **Commissural fibers** connect the corresponding areas of the two hemispheres. At their base, the two hemispheres also are connected by a thick band of fibers known as **corpus callosum.** Finally, there are **projection fibers** that form pathways to and from the brain stem and spinal cord and from the sensory and motor areas of the cortex.

The brain is housed in, and protected by, the strong bony structure called the **skull.** The skull is not a single structure. It is made up of different pieces of bone, which eventually fuse into a unified structure. The brain has many small spaces called **ventricles** that are filled with the **cerebrospinal fluid,** which flows over the brain. Along with the bones of the skull, the fluid-filled cavities help protect the brain from external shocks.

The brain is covered with layers of membrane called **meninges.** Infectious diseases (**meningitis**) that destroy these meninges also can cause brain damage.

The brain is richly supplied with blood by four blood vessels. They are the two **vertebral** and two **carotid** arteries. Each has an internal and an external branch. The internal carotid artery divides into two arteries. One of them, the middle carotid artery, moves into the inner portions of the brain and, dividing again into branches, supplies most of the brain cells. The middle carotid artery supplies brain structures involved in speech and language. Therefore, damage to this artery can cause aphasia, a profound language problem.

Chapter 9 has more about aphasia and related disorders.

Summary

- The actions of the speech muscles and organs are initiated and regulated by the nervous system.

- The nervous system carries impulses from the sensory organs to the brain and from the brain to the muscles.

- The nervous system consists of the peripheral, central, and autonomic divisions.

(continues)

- Several cranial nerves of the peripheral nervous system are directly involved with speech.

- The spinal and the autonomic nerves are not directly involved with speech, although they have certain indirect effects.

- The central nervous system includes the spinal cord and the brain.

- The cerebrum contains various areas that specialize in speech, language, and hearing functions.

Dialogue

In the beginning, Ms. Noledge-Hungry was not thrilled about the anatomy and physiology of speech and hearing. Professor Speech-Wisely's simple descriptions and his efforts to make them as clinical as possible were helpful. On occasion, it was even interesting. At the least, she understood why she should study anatomy and physiology.

N-H: Dr. Speech-Wisely, we normally do not think about all the muscles, bones, nerves, and membranes that are involved in speech.

S-W: Yes, but it is true of eating or walking. Normally, we have no compelling reason to think of the structure. It often is a disorder that forces our attention to the anatomy and physiology.

N-H: I understand that speech is social, but it needs a biological system.

S-W: Exactly. Respiration, phonation, articulation, and higher neural integration are the four biologically based functional systems of speech. Can you summarize the respiratory system?

N-H: Yes. **Respiration** supplies power for speech production. Respiration is a function of the lungs which is housed in the rib cage. An important muscle of respiration is the **diaphragm** below the rib cage. Other muscles, especially the intercostal muscles, also are important for respiration.

S-W: That is correct. We talk mostly on exhalation. The exhaled air sets the vocal folds into motion. Can you describe the vocal folds?

N-H: The **vocal folds** are a part of the larynx, which includes muscles, cartilages, and membranes. The larynx is suspended from the hyoid bone. The **vocalis muscle** forms the vocal folds.

S-W: Good. Remember that vocal folds are attached to **arytenoid cartilages,** which permit various kinds of movement.

N-H: Yes, and the arytenoids are attached to the **cricoid.** But I am not sure of how vocal folds vibrate.

S-W: OK. The **myoelastic–aerodynamic theory** explains how the vocal folds vibrate and produce sound. When the vocal folds are closed, the air pressure below is higher than that above the folds. Consequently, the folds begin to burst open, and they vibrate as a result. However, when the air escapes through the opened folds, the pressure between the folds decreases. This draws the folds together;

thus, they close. The elasticity of the folds also makes this happen. How is the frequency of vocal fold vibrations measured?

N-H: The frequency of vocal fold vibrations is measured in cycles per second and called **hertz.** The pitch of the voice depends on the frequency and the loudness on the amount of subglottal air pressure. But I find the descriptions of vocal qualities subjective.

S-W: You are correct. Vocal quality is **breathy** when the folds are not closed and there is air leakage. The quality is **harsh** when it is rough; this is due to irregular fold vibration. The quality is **hoarse** when it is both breathy and harsh. Can you define resonance?

N-H: I will try. **Resonance** is the modification of the laryngeal tone by the structures above it. The **laryngopharynx,** the **oropharynx,** and the **nasopharynx** dampen or enhance certain tones. That is why the eventual sound we hear is different from the laryngeal tone.

S-W: Good. Now, **articulation.** The sound of the vocal folds, modified by the oral and nasal cavities, are shaped into sounds of speech. The articulators that accomplish this task include the soft palate, the hard palate, the jaw, the tongue, the lips, and the cheeks. You must be able to describe the basic parts of these structures.

N-H: I figured that! I found the ear more complex than I could ever imagine.

S-W: You are right. But it does a lot. Just imagine all the complex sounds and noises you can hear and distinguish. Besides, the ear also is concerned with balance and body position. Can you give a brief description of the ear?

N-H: OK. It is divided into three parts: the outer ear, the middle ear, and the inner ear. The **outer ear** includes the pinna and the external ear canal and ends with the **eardrum,** which is a thin membrane. It vibrates when the sound waves hit it. The most important parts of the **middle ear** are the three small bones forming a chain: the **malleus,** the **incus,** and the **stapedius.** The malleus is attached to the eardrum, and the stapedius is attached to the oval window of the inner ear. The **inner ear** is filled with fluids and contains the **cochlea,** the most important structure for hearing. On its **basilar membrane,** the cochlea has the sensory hair cells that are connected to the auditory nerve fibers. The **auditory nerve** carries the sound to the brain.

S-W: Excellent! I might just add that the sound that strikes the eardrum is transmitted to the **ossicular chain.** The **stapedius bone** transmits the energy into the fluids of the inner ear. The movement of the fluids stimulates the hair cells of the cochlea. The stimulation of the hair cells is transformed into neural impulses, which are carried to the temporal lobe of the brain by the auditory nerve.

N-H: The brain is the controlling center for speech production and for hearing, too, right?

S-W: A more accurate description is that the brain *controls* speech production and *interprets* hearing and spoken language. You should be able to describe the neuron and the **peripheral** and the **central nervous systems.** Of the peripheral nerves, the **cranial nerves** are more important for speech and hearing than the spinal nerves. You should remember the major cranial nerves involved in speech and hearing. Now, tell me about the brain stem.

N-H: The **brain stem** contains the **medulla,** the **pons,** the **midbrain,** and the **reticular formation.** I was confused by cerebellum and cerebrum. But I think I got them straightened out. The **cerebellum** looks like a little cerebrum, and it lies behind the brain stem and below the cerebrum. It coordinates motor impulses.

S-W: Yes, the **cerebrum** is roughly the cerebral cortex. It has ridges called **gyri** and valleys called **sulcus,** or fissures. The cortex is divided into four lobes. The **frontal lobe** is concerned with movement, including speech articulation; it has the primary motor area and Broca's speech production area. The **temporal lobe** contains the primary auditory area and Wernicke's speech comprehension area. The **occipital lobe** is concerned with vision, and the **parietal lobe** is concerned with somesthetic sensations.

N-H: As we study more about various disorders of communication, I suppose we will learn more about the significance of the structures we studied.

S-W: Certainly. And also, as we go along, we will review the basic anatomy and physiology needed to understand a particular topic or disorder of communication.

N-H: I think that will be very helpful, Dr. Speech-Wisely. Thank you for your time, and I will see you in class.

S-W: OK!

Study Questions

1. Why should we study the anatomy and physiology of speech to understand disorders of communication?

2. What are the major structural mechanisms of speech?

3. We normally speak while we are _____ the air.

4. The rib cage contains _____ pairs of ribs.

5. Give a brief description of diaphragm.

6. Define trachea.

7. Which brain stem structure fires impulses to the muscles of respiration?

8. What are some of the biological functions of the larynx?

9. Describe the major laryngeal structures.

10. Describe the cricoarytenoid joint. Why is it important for phonation?

11. The vocal folds also are known as internal _____.

12. The term *adducted* means that the vocal folds are _____.

13. The term *abducted* means that the vocal folds are _____.

14. Glottis is a small _____ between the folds.

15. What is electromyography? What can we accomplish with it?

16. Give a brief description of the myoelastic–aerodynamic theory of phonation.

17. Differences in the frequency of vocal fold vibration are perceived as differences in _____.

18. Compared to thinner and shorter vocal folds, longer and thicker vocal folds vibrate at _____ frequency.

19. What two factors determine the loudness of voice?

20. Define resonance.

21. What are the three commonly described vocal qualities?

22. What is nasality? What is hypernasality?

23. What are the different meanings of the word *articulation?*

24. Give a brief description of the cavities of speech.

25. Define soft palate. Describe its functions.

26. The major portion of the hard palate is made up of bones called _____.

27. Define alveolar process.

28. The anatomic name of the jaw is the _____.

29. Give a brief description of the three types of malocclusion.

30. What are the anatomic names of the four parts of the tongue?

31. The ear canal also is known as the _____.

32. Give a brief description of the ossicular chain of the middle ear.

33. What is the acoustic reflex?

34. What is otitis media?

35. What is a disease of the ossicular chain?

36. Give a brief description of the cochlea.

37. What are the two branches of the acoustic nerve? What are their functions?

38. Distinguish the meaning of the terms *afferent* and *efferent*.

39. What are cranial nerves? What is their significance to speech?

40. Give a brief description of the sympathetic and the parasympathetic branches of the autonomic nervous system.

41. The central nervous system includes the _____ and the _____.

42. Describe the primary structures of the brain stem and their functions.

43. What is the function of basal ganglia?

44. What is the function of the cerebellum?

45. Briefly describe the four lobes of the brain.

46. The primary auditory area is found in the _____ lobe.

47. Broca's area is found in the _____ lobe.

48. What are the functions of Broca's and Wernicke's areas?

References

Bhatnagar, S. C., & Andy, O. J. (1995). *Neuroscience for the study of communicative disorders.* Baltimore: Williams & Wilkins.

Calvin, W. H., & Ojemann, G. A. (1980). *Inside the brain.* New York: New American Library.

Kent, R. (1997). *The speech sciences.* San Diego: Singular.

Ornstein, R., & Thompson, R. F. (1984). *The amazing brain.* Boston: Houghton Mifflin.

Peña-Brooks, A., & Hegde, M. N. (2000). *Assessment and treatment of articulation and phonological disorders in children.* Austin, TX: PRO-ED.

Perkins, W. H., & Kent, R. D. (1986). *Functional anatomy of speech, language, and hearing: A primer.* Boston: Little, Brown.

Seikel, J. A., King, D. W., & Drumright, D. G. (2000). *Anatomy and physiology for speech, language, and hearing* (2nd ed.). San Diego: Singular.

Smith, A. (1984). *The mind.* New York: Viking Penguin.

Webster, D. B. (1999). *Neuroscience of communication* (2nd ed.). San Diego: Singular.

Zemlin, W. R. (1998). *Speech and hearing science* (4th ed.). Needham Heights, MA: Allyn & Bacon.

Articulation and Phonological Disorders

The basic unit of oral language, the organized system of verbal communication, is speech. Speech, in turn, can be broken down into its basic units: speech sounds. Speech sounds are used in forming syllables, which are necessary to form words. When spoken words are organized into sentences, the organized system of oral language is formed.

This chapter is about speech sounds. The basics of the sound system of the English language, the classification of English sounds, how children learn to produce the sounds, and what problems arise in this learning process are covered in this chapter. The problems children have in learning and producing the sounds of their language are known as **articulation** or **phonological disorders**. The chapter concludes with a brief description of the methods speech–language pathologists use in treating articulation and phonological disorders.

Experiments in Infant Speech Perception

Lisa and John Larson and their son Timmy live in a Midwestern university town. One day they saw an announcement in the local newspaper that solicited infants for a research project. Both Lisa and John appreciate the need for research because, as undergraduate psychology students, both had served as subjects in several experiments. Therefore, they decided to let the scientists study 7-month-old Timmy in an experiment on speech perception.

A speech scientist at the university, Dr. Jean Simon was working hard to produce answers to some fascinating questions about young babies' perception of speech. Do 4- or 6-month-old babies understand the difference between speech sounds? Can a 4-month-old hear the difference between *p* and *b* or *s* and *z?* Do babies learn to understand the difference between speech sounds in a certain sequence? Questions like these have always fascinated speech scientists and clinicians who want to know how we come to understand differences between speech sounds we hear and how we learn to produce them. The first question concerns the **perception** of speech and the second concerns the **production** of speech sounds. Dr. Simon's research involved speech perception.

On the appointed day, Lisa took Timmy to the speech research laboratory at the university. Both Lisa and John had met Dr. Simon before. Dr. Simon had observed Timmy and considered him suitable for the experiment. Timmy did not have a hearing problem and he was physically healthy. He was growing normally. Dr. Simon had fully described the experiment to the Larsons. According to the federal law and the university policy, human subjects (or parents of child subjects) must understand what an experiment would involve and give informed consent to voluntarily participate in it. The Larsons had earlier signed a form to that effect. They were also guaranteed the right to withdraw their son from the experiment at any time and without any negative consequences.

At the laboratory, Dr. Simon introduced her research assistant, Steve, a doctoral student, to Lisa. To take advantage of Timmy's cheerful mood, Dr. Simon wanted to start the experiment right away. Lisa and Timmy were taken to a suite of two rooms divided by a one-way mirror. As shown in Figure 4.1, one of the rooms (the experimental room) was furnished with two chairs, a round table, a video camera (C), a loudspeaker, and a smoked Plexiglas box in front of the loudspeaker (VR). Steve was carrying a bag in which he had some toys. Lisa was asked to sit in one of the chairs (P) and hold Timmy on her lap (I) so that he looked straight ahead. She was made to wear a pair of headphones through which she would hear soft music during the experiment. Steve, also wearing a pair of headphones which fed music to his ears, sat to Lisa's right (A); the speaker and the Plexiglas box were to her left. Dr. Simon went to the adjoining room (the control room) from which she could see through the one-way mirror. She sat in front of her electronic equipment (E) that controlled much of the experiment.

A logic device can be programmed to control various parts of an experiment.

Steve pulled out a puppet from his bag and began to manipulate it in front of Timmy. Timmy liked to watch Steve's actions. During the experiment, Steve manipulated other toys to hold Timmy's attention. Soon Dr. Simon pushed a button to start the experiment. A tape deck began to play. Various syllables were taped on two channels of the tape recorder. The electronic equipment, known as a **logic device,** began to present various speech stimuli through the loudspeaker in the experimental room.

Timmy began to hear *va* through the speaker. The syllable repeated once every second (*va-va*). But Timmy was more interested in the puppet than in the meaningless *va-va*. When Timmy was still looking at the toys, the logic device changed the stimulus to *sa* (*sa-sa*) for 4 seconds. Timmy then *turned his head* to the left and looked in the direction of the speaker. Immediately, both Steve and Dr. Simon pushed a button to tell the logic device that the child made a correct response. Instantaneously, the device lit up the Plexiglas box in front of the speaker; to his delight, Timmy saw a monkey in the box dancing and striking cymbals. The box remained lit for about 2 seconds, and then it went dark again. The device changed the stimulus to *va* and Timmy renewed his interest

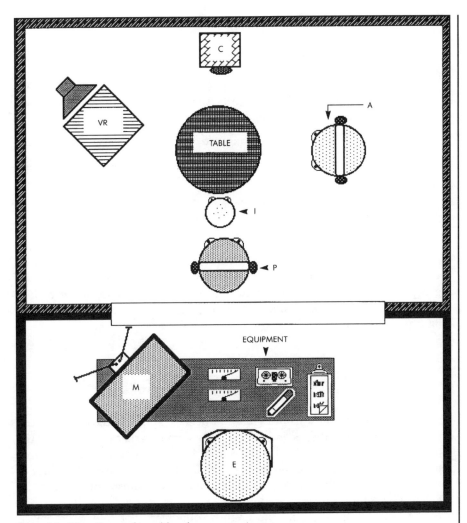

Figure 4.1. Visually reinforced head turn experiment.

in Steve's actions. Again, after a while, the device changed the stimulus to *sa;* Timmy turned toward the box which reinforced the response as before.

The presentations of *va* were the **control trials** (presentation of the same syllable) and the presentations of *sa* were the **change trials** (presentation of a new syllable). Several control and change trials were run to make sure that Timmy *reliably responded to a change in the speech stimulus.* To conclude that Timmy discriminated between *va* and *sa,* he had to turn his head only during the change trials and not during the control trials. The experiment continued in this fashion. Dr. Simon presented such syllable pairs as *sa–za* and *sa–sha* before concluding the experiment. Timmy's mother and the two scientists were pleased with his cooperative mood and good discrimination between speech syllable pairs.

The experimental procedure Dr. Simon used is the **visually reinforced head turn paradigm.** In fact, my description of the procedure is based on experiments conducted by several scientists (Kuhl, 1987). With the help of this and a few other methods, we have learned that infants and young babies can be taught to discriminate between a variety of speech stimuli and also that it is hard to teach discrimination between certain other stimulus pairs.

- Four- to 17-week-old infants can be taught to discriminate between vowels [u] and [i] and between [a] and [i].

- Two- to 3-month-old infants can be taught to discriminate between [ra] and [la].

- One- to 4-month-old infants can be taught to discriminate between [va] and [sa] and between [sa] and [sha], but *not* between [sa] and [za].

- Two-month-old infants can be taught to discriminate between [ba] and [ga].

- One- to 4-month-old infants can be taught to discriminate between [pa] and [ba].

- Six- to 8-month-olds can be taught to discriminate between [sa] and [za], but *not* between [fi] and [ti] or [fa] and [ta].

An interesting finding is that infants under 1 year of age can be conditioned (taught) to discriminate sounds that are *not* used in their language. However, this teachability begins to decline around 12 months of age. With increasing experience with the sounds of their own language, babies begin to lose their ability to learn to discriminate between sounds that are not used in their language.

The Inadequate Alpha, Beta

The term **alphabet** comes from *alpha* and *beta*. The first letter of the Greek alphabet is alpha and the second is beta. It is supposed that each letter of the alphabet stands for a sound. This is more or less true of languages. It is only minimally true of English because the spoken English sounds are not faithful to the written alphabet that represents them. Sounds of Spanish and some Asian languages are more true to their alphabets.

The English alphabet and the English sounds are not fully harmonized because the alphabet did not keep pace with the changes in the spoken sounds. As new sounds emerged in speech, new letters were not created. In Europe, the alphabet was standardized around the time when printing became more common. Printing presses could not handle an ever-changing alphabet or spelling of words. If the spelling had to be fixed, the alphabet also had to be fixed. Obviously, a fixed alphabet is insensitive to changes in speech sounds. As time passed the discrepancy between the alphabet and the sounds of English became wider (Tizard, 1980). Centuries later, we still have the same 26 letters but there are 46 or so sounds. Nevertheless, we may still be lucky. Centuries from now the discrepancy between the alphabet and the sounds may be even greater. The sounds are still changing.

The problems of an inadequate alphabet first becomes evident when the child begins to read aloud. In oral reading, the sounds must be matched with the letters of the alphabet used to spell the words. Trouble begins here because the same sound is spelled in many different ways. Table 4.1 shows a few examples of varied spellings for the same sound or phoneme. At this point, recall from Chapter 1 that a sound is also called a phoneme and that it is placed within two slash marks.

The problem is not limited to different spellings for the same sound. There are simply not enough letters to represent the sounds of the language. Adding

Table 4.1

Examples of Alternate Spellings for the Same Sounds of English

....

The /i/ sound may be spelled with e as in even, but also as:

ee (seen)
ea (read)
ei (deceive)
ie (field)
i (ravine)
eo (people)
oe (amoeba)
ae (Caesar)
ey (key)

The vowel /u/ has at least 13 spellings. Consider how different they are:

u (rule)
oo (boot)
o (move)
ew (knew)
ue (due)
ou (group)
ui (fruit)
ough (through)
ous (rendezvous)
wo (two)
ieu (lieu)
oe (shoe)
eu (maneuver)

The consonantal sounds are also spelled in different ways. Take just one example, the /s/:

s (six)
ss (miss)
sc (scene)
c (circle)
ps (psalm)
st (listen)
x (fox)
z (quartz)

....

insult to injury, the inadequate alphabet contains some useless letters. Both *c* and *q* are redundant and useless. The *c* often masquerades as /k/ or /s/ and the *q* as /k/. As though the three letters *k, c,* and *q* were not enough to represent the single /k/ (sound), it also is spelled with both *c* and *k* (*luck*), double *c* (*account*), *c* and *h* (*echo*), and *k* and *h* (*khaki*).

Most languages have similar problems. Therefore, specialists have developed a different set of phonetic symbols that could represent most of the sounds adequately. The system is called the **International Phonetic Alphabet (IPA)**. It is presented in Table 4.2. In IPA, each symbol stands for only one sound. Note that it does not contain the *c* or the *q*. Diphthongs are expressed with two symbols because they are a combination of two vowels. In the following sections of this chapter, the IPA symbols are used to represent the sounds.

Table 4.2
The International Phonetic Alphabet (IPA)

IPA Symbol	Examples	IPA Symbol	Examples
/p/	pot	/ʃ/	shine
/b/	bat	/ʒ/	vision
/m/	mat	/θ/	thin
/n/	net	/ð/	then
/ŋ/	sing	/ʧ/	chin
/d/	dime	/ʤ/	Jane
/t/	time	/v/	van
/g/	gum	/w/	wine
/k/	Kim	/l/	lean
/f/	fun	/j/	yawn
/s/	sun	/h/	hen
/z/	Zen	/r/	run
/ɑ/	fall	/ɛ/	bet
/æ/	fat	/e/	late
/ɔ/	fought	/o/	overcoat
/ə/	atop	/ʊ/	put
/ʌ/	upset	/u/	boot
/ɪ/	infect	/ɝ/	shirt
/i/	eat	/ɚ/	later
/eɪ/	main		
/aɪ/	lime		
/oʊ/	dome		
/aʊ/	how		
/ɔɪ/	boy		
/ɪʊ/	fuse		

Sounds, Phonemes, and Allophones

As described in Chapter 1, specialists make a distinction between speech and language. **Language** is an abstract system of symbols used to communicate; it is a system larger than speech. It includes rules of meaning, grammar, and social use. Narrowly defined, **speech** is the production of speech sounds. More broadly defined, speech is the actual production of oral language. In studying speech, we analyze the sounds, their relationship to one another, and the way they are combined to form syllables and words. These rules are studied in phonology, which is the scientific study of the sound system and patterns used to create words of a language.

Although speech and language can be analyzed separately, the two are a part of the same event we call verbal communication. Speech is the building block of language. Sounds or the phonemes are the individual elements of speech.

A **phoneme** is a class of speech sounds; it is an abstract name given to variations of a speech sound. Phonemes make a difference in meaning. Therefore, a phoneme often is described as the smallest unit of sound that can affect meaning. For example, /p/ and /b/ are different phonemes because at the word level,

Review descriptions of speech and language in **Chapter 1.**

when one is changed to the other, the meaning changes. The words *pat* and *bat* have different meanings because of different initial phonemes. The final consonant and the middle vowel of the two words are the same.

A phoneme is not a single, invariable entity. That is why it is defined as a *group* or *family* of sounds. The individual sound /k/ is a phoneme, but, when different speakers produce it in different linguistic contexts, the sound is not the same. Such variations of a phoneme are called **allophones.** But, in spite of its variations, a phone is always perceived as the same, just as a /k/ is always perceived as a /k/, regardless of the subtle variations in its individual productions. For example, the /k/ in *key* is produced more toward the front of the mouth than the same sound in *cool*, which is produced more toward the back of the mouth. To a trained ear, the two productions of /k/ sound different. Nonetheless, most listeners do not distinguish between those variations of /k/. In essence, a phoneme varies depending upon contexts, speakers, and occasions of production, but, nonetheless, most listeners may not even be aware of such variations.

The term *phonemic* is distinguished from *phonetic*. **Phonemic** refers to the abstract system of sounds, whereas **phonetic** refers to concrete productions of specific sounds. For example, the idealized and abstract description of /g/ is phonemic. Phonemic representations, or phonemes, are enclosed within slash marks, as, for example, /g/. The description of an actual production of /g/ in a word by a specific speaker is phonetic. Phonetic productions are enclosed in brackets [ ]. Thus, sounds within slash marks suggest a general and abstract class of sounds (phonemic representation); those within brackets suggest specific sound productions by given speakers (phonetic representation).

Some languages have more phonemes than others. English has 46 phonemes, which is considered a larger number. In contrast, Spanish contains only 26 phonemes. Certain phonemes can be found in most languages, but some phonemes may be unique to certain languages.

The term *phonemes* is a more technical term than speech sounds. Nonetheless, they mean the same. Therefore, in this chapter, the terms *speech sounds* and *phonemes* will be used interchangeably.

Classifications of Speech Sounds

The speech sounds are classified in various ways. Only a few classifications are described here. A traditional classification of speech sounds includes vowels, consonants, manner of sound production, and place of articulation. A nontraditional classification is based on distinctive features of sounds.

Traditional Classifications

Vowels

Vocal fold vibrations are involved in the production of all vowels. The differences in vowels are created largely by differences in the shape of the oral tract. The oral tract (roughly the mouth) is more open in the production of vowels than in the production of consonants. However, one vowel sounds different from another because of differing shape of the vocal tract.

The tongue and the jaw are the major structures that change the shape of the vocal tract. The tongue moves back and forth. It lifts its tip or stays low. It bulges its body or flattens out. Different movements of the jaw create wider or narrower mouth opening. These and other movements continuously change the shape of the oral cavity. The sound produced by the larynx passes through the oral cavity. The different shapes of the cavity modify the laryngeal tone in different ways. Therefore, the vowels sound different.

The vowels are classified according to the tongue positions needed to produce them. The *front, central, back, high, mid,* and *low vowels* describe the relative positions of the tongue in the oral cavity. These positions combine with each other. For example, some vowels are produced with a *high* and *front* tongue position, whereas some others are produced with a *low* and *back* tongue position. Figure 4.2 illustrates the various tongue positions with which different vowels are typically produced.

Lips also contribute to the articulation of vowels. The lips are rounded in the production of some vowels. Vowels /u/ and /o/ are examples. Other vowels are produced without rounding the lips.

When two vowels are combined, they form **diphthongs.** A diphthong is produced by a continuous change in the vocal tract shape. The *ai* sound in such words as *buy* and *why* and the *ei* in *day* and *stay* are diphthongs.

Consonants

Whereas the vowels are produced by opening the oral cavity, the consonants are produced by constricting it. A combination of a consonant and a vowel is a **syllable** (e.g., *sa* or *si*).

Manner, place, and voicing are the three factors traditionally used to classify consonants. The **manner** of articulation describes the degree or type of constriction. The **place** of articulation describes the location of constriction. **Voicing** describes the presence or absence of vocal fold vibrations in the pro-

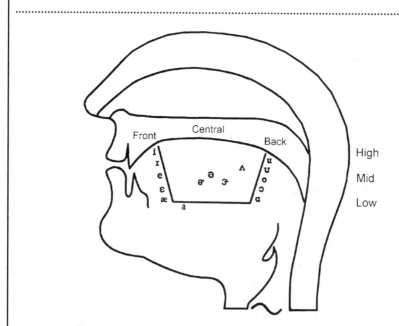

Figure 4.2. The vowel chart.

duction of consonants. Table 4.3 shows the classification of English consonants according to the manner, place, and voicing factors.

The Manner of Articulation

Classification based on the manner of articulation (production) results in six major categories of consonants: stops, fricatives, affricates, glides, liquids, and nasals.

Stops are produced by completely stopping the airflow. The air pressure is built up within the oral cavity. The pressure is then released in a manner resembling a small explosion. This is typically described as the **plosive** manner. Therefore, stops are also known as **stop-plosives.** Produce an exaggerated /p/ and you know what a stop-plosive is. The /p/, /b/, /t/, /d/, /k/, and /g/ are stop plosives.

Fricatives are produced by severely constricting the oral cavity and then forcing the air through it. This creates a **hissing** or **friction** type of noise. Hence, the name fricatives. A prolonged /s/ or /f/ gives you a good idea of a fricative. The /f/, /v/, /θ/ (as in *th*ink), /ð/ (as in *th*em), /s/, /z/, /ʃ/ (as in *sh*oe), /ʒ/ (as in bei*g*e), and /h/ are fricatives.

Affricates are a combination of stops and fricatives. Only two sounds, /tʃ/ (as in *ch*air) and /dʒ/ (as in *j*ump), are affricates. Make the *ch* sound and note that you first stop the air and then force it through a narrow constriction.

Glides are produced by gradually changing the shape of the articulators. Only two sounds, /w/ (as in *w*ine) and /j/ (as in *y*es), are glides.

Liquids are produced with the least restriction of the oral cavity. Therefore, they are more like vowels. Two sounds, /r/ and /l/, are liquids. Liquids are also called **semivowels.** Of the two liquids, the /l/ also is called a **lateral** because in producing this sound, air escapes around the sides of the tongue.

Nasals are produced while keeping the velopharyngeal port open so that the sound produced by the larynx passes through the nose. As a result, nasal resonance is added to these sounds. The /n/, /m/, and /ŋ/ (*ng* as in comi*ng*) are the three nasal sounds of English.

Table 4.3

Classification of English Consonants

	Manner of Production						
Place of Articulation	**Nasals**	**Stops**	**Fricatives**	**Affricates**	**Liquids**	**Glides**	**Laterals**
Bilabial	ⓜ	p ⓑ				ⓦ	
Labiodental			f ⓥ				
Linguadental			θ ⓓ̵				
Lingua-alveolar	ⓝ	t ⓓ	s ⓩ		ⓛ		ⓛ
Linguapalatal			ʃ ③	tʃ ⓓ͡ʒ	ⓡ	ⓙ	
Linguavelar	ⓝ̇	k ⓖ					
Glottal			h				

Note. Voiced sounds are circled.

The Place of Articulation

Classification of consonants also is based on the primary articulators that shape the sounds. Therefore, the same sounds grouped under the six categories of manner of articulation are reclassified on the basis of place of production. Seven categories are described: bilabial, labiodental, dental, alveolar, palatal, velar, and glottal. The different places where these sounds in the oral cavity are produced are shown in Figure 4.3.

Bilabial sounds are produced primarily by the two lips. Four sounds, /p/, /b/, /m/, and /w/, are bilabials. Of these, the first two are stops, the third is a nasal, and the fourth is a glide.

Labiodental sounds are produced by the lips and teeth. Only two sounds, /f/ and /v/, are labiodentals. Both are fricatives.

Dental sounds, also known as **linguadentals** are produced by the tongue, which makes contact with the upper teeth. Only two sounds, /θ/ (*th*ink) and /ð/ (*th*em), are dentals. Both are fricatives.

Alveolars, also known as **lingua-alveolar** sounds, are produced by raising the tip of the tongue to make contact with the alveolar ridge, which is the place immediately behind the front teeth. Six sounds, /t/, /d/, /s/, /z/, /n/, and /l/, fall into this category. Of these, the first two are stops, the next two are fricatives, the fifth is a nasal, and the sixth is a liquid.

Palatals, also known as **linguapalatal** sounds, are produced by the tongue, which comes in contact with the hard palate. The tongue contact is at the back of the alveolar ridge. Six sounds, /ʃ/ (*sh*ip), /ʒ/ (rou*ge*), /tʃ/ (*ch*alk), /dʒ/ (oran*ge*), /r/, and /j/ (as in *y*ou), are palatals. Of these, the first two are fricatives, the next two are affricates, the fifth is a liquid, and the sixth is a glide.

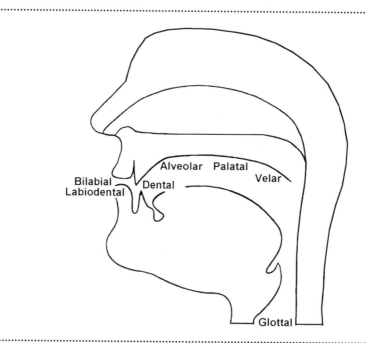

Figure 4.3. The place of articulation of English consonants.

Velars, also known as **linguavelar** sounds, are produced by the back of the tongue, which raises to make contact with the velum (soft palate). Three sounds, /k/, /g/, and /ŋ/, are velars. The first two are stops and the third is a nasal.

Glottal sounds are produced by keeping the vocal folds open and letting the air pass through; the result is friction noise. Therefore, glottals are also fricatives. Normally, only the /h/ is classified as a glottal. However, when the air is stopped by an abrupt closure of the vocal folds and then released in a plosive, another glottal, which is represented by /ʔ/, is produced. The glottal /ʔ/ is most frequently heard in such exclamations as "oh oh!" and "huh huh."

Voicing

The category of speech sounds based on the behavior of the vocal folds is called **voicing.** Not all sounds require vocal fold vibration. Noise created by forcing the air through a narrow constriction can be shaped into speech sounds. In this case, the vocal fold vibrations are absent. Therefore, sounds are either voiced or voiceless. The source of sound is the vocal fold vibration in voiced sounds; it is noise in voiceless sounds. Most voiced and voiceless sounds form a pair. In the following consonant pairs, the first is voiced and the second is voiceless: /z/ and /s/; /d/ and /t/; /b/ and /p/; /g/ and /k/; /v/ and /f/; /ð/ and /θ/; and /ʤ/ and /ʧ/. As you can see, consonants can be voiced or voiceless. However, all vowels are voiced (except when they are whispered).

Nontraditional Classification

A nontraditional method of classifying speech sounds is based on distinctive features. Linguists who proposed distinctive features believe that the phoneme is not the basic unit of speech. They proposed that a **phoneme** is a **collection of independent features.** A **distinctive feature** is a unique characteristic of a phoneme that distinguishes one phoneme from the other (Chomsky & Halle, 1968; Jakobson, Fant, & Halle, 1952).

According to the distinctive features theory, a feature is either present or absent in a phoneme. Therefore, the system is called **binary;** a phoneme can be assigned either a plus value if a feature is present or a minus value if the feature is absent. For example, voicing is a distinctive feature. A sound is either voiced or unvoiced. So a phoneme is assigned a plus value if it is voiced or a minus value if it is unvoiced. A speech sound is either a consonant or a vowel. Therefore, on the distinctive feature **consonantal,** a sound is assigned a plus value if it is a consonant or a minus value if it is not a consonant. On the distinctive feature **vocalic,** a sound is either a plus value because it is a vowel or vowel-like, or a minus value because it is a consonant. The distinctive features of English consonants described by Chomsky and Halle (1968) are presented in Table 4.4.

The distinctive features approach has influenced the treatment of articulation disorders. As discussed later in this chapter, clinicians have sometimes taught missing distinctive features to children with articulation disorders.

The distinctive features approach is not too different from the traditional analysis of manner, place, and voice. Most distinctive features listed in Table 4.4 have their counterparts in the traditional analysis, although the binary notion and the method of applying a feature across all the phonemes make the approach different.

Table 4.4

The Chomsky–Halle Distinctive Features of English Consonants

	w	f	v	θ	ð	t	d	s	z	n	l	ʃ	ʒ	j	r	tʃ	dʒ	k	g	ŋ	h	p	b	m
Voiced	+	−	+	−	+	−	+	−	+	+	+	−	+	+	+	−	+	−	+	+	−	−	+	+
Consonantal	−	+	+	+	+	+	+	+	+	+	+	+	+	−	+	+	+	+	+	+	−	+	+	+
Anterior	+	+	+	+	+	+	+	+	+	+	+	−	−	−	−	−	−	−	−	−	−	+	+	+
Coronal	−	−	−	+	+	+	+	+	+	+	+	+	+	−	+	+	+	−	−	−	−	−	−	−
Continuant	+	+	+	+	+	−	−	+	+	−	+	+	+	+	+	−	−	−	−	−	+	−	−	−
High	−	−	−	−	−	−	−	−	−	−	−	+	+	+	−	+	+	+	+	+	−	−	−	−
Low	−	−	−	−	−	−	−	−	−	−	−	−	−	−	−	−	−	−	−	−	+	−	−	−
Back	−	−	−	−	−	−	−	−	−	−	−	−	−	−	−	−	−	+	+	+	−	−	−	−
Nasal	−	−	−	−	−	−	−	−	−	+	−	−	−	−	−	−	−	−	−	+	−	−	−	+
Strident	−	+	+	−	−	−	−	+	+	−	−	+	+	−	−	+	+	−	−	−	−	−	−	−
Vocalic	−	−	−	−	−	−	−	−	−	−	+	−	−	−	+	−	−	−	−	−	−	−	−	−

Summary

- Speech sounds are classified on the basis of

  Place of articulation
  Manner of articulation
  The presence or absence of voicing
  Distinctive features

- The methods cross-classify sounds; the same sound is classified and reclassified with different methods.

Acquisition of Speech Sound Productions and Sound Patterns

As the experiments on speech perception have shown, infants are good at learning to discriminate between speech sounds they hear. But what about learning to *produce* speech sounds? Can we find a pattern in the normal acquisition of speech sounds? Are some sounds easier than others to learn? Answers to questions such as these help us understand speech and language learning and treat disorders of communication.

Acquisition of Speech Sounds

Though a newborn baby's crying means something, speech communication begins months later. Three-month-old infants make various vowel sounds called **cooing**. However, researchers have paid more attention to a later behavior called **babbling** because of its presumed relation to speech production. Infants in the age range of 5 to 7 months begin to babble. A well-fed, dry, and cheerful baby lying on his or her back makes plenty of vocal noises. The baby begins to produce more vowels, and some vowels are repeated. Such syllables as "ba-ba," "ma-ma," and "ga-ga" may frequently be heard. Infant babbling consists of recognizable speech sounds. The sounds that are present in the surrounding language are babbled more frequently than those that are not. For these and other reasons, it is now generally believed that babbling and speech sound acquisition are related.

There are two types of studies on the acquisition of speech sounds. The goal of the first type of study is to establish norms of articulation. **Norms** are the typical behaviors of a representative group of children. The main question researched is this: At what age do children master different speech sounds? In answering this question, the **cross-sectional method** is used. A certain number of children are selected from each age level targeted for the study. The children's speech production is sampled by various test stimuli and spontaneous conversation. At each age level, the specific sounds a majority of children will have mastered are determined. The different sets of sounds children of different ages have mastered are the norms. In a variation of this method, some researchers focus on the acquisition of a class of speech sounds. For example, the researcher may study the acquisition of fricatives in children.

The goal of the second type of study is to observe the process of learning. These studies use the **longitudinal method,** in which only one or a few children are observed for an extended period of time. Speech samples are recorded frequently to trace the development of speech sound learning. One or a few studies of this kind will not produce norms because norms are established by testing many children. Nevertheless, this kind of research can also help us understand various stages and processes of sound acquisition. The results of the two kinds of studies on the acquisition of speech sounds can be summarized as follows (Peña-Brooks & Hegde, 2000):

- Vowels are acquired before consonants. Before age 3, children use most if not all the vowels.

- Among the consonants, the nasals (/m/, /n/, and /ŋ/) are acquired the earliest. They are generally mastered between 3 and 4 years of age.

- Stop sounds are mastered earlier than fricatives. Most stops are mastered between 3 and 4.5 years of age. Among the stops, /p/ may be mastered the earliest.

- Glides (/w/, /j/) are also mastered earlier than fricatives. Glides are mastered between 2 and 4 years.

- The liquids (/r/, /l/) are mastered relatively late (between 3 and 5 years).

- Fricatives and affricates are mastered later than stops and nasals. The fricative /f/ is mastered earlier than other fricatives (around age 3). Fricatives /θ/, /ð/, /dʒ/, /s/, and /z/ are mastered last (between 3 and 6 years).

- Consonant clusters (e.g., *tr* in the word *train*) are acquired later than most other sounds.

The norms clinicians use are mostly based on the cross-sectional studies. Studies by Wellman, Case, Mengurt, and Bradbury (1931); Poole (1934); Templin (1957); Sander (1972); and Prather, Hedrick, and Kern (1975) have provided widely used norms. Sander's is a reanalysis of some published studies. Subsequent studies that have provided norms include those of Art and Goodban (1976); Stoel-Gammon (1985); Preisser, Hodson, and Paden (1988); and Smit, Hand, Freilinger, Bernthal, and Bird (1990). Frequently used norms are presented in Table 4.5.

The studies do not agree entirely on the age at which children master speech sounds because of differences in methods of study. For example, some researchers consider a sound mastered at a particular age level when 90% of children produce it correctly, whereas others so consider a sound when only 75% produce it correctly. Compared to older studies, some recent studies have reported earlier ages at which children acquire speech sounds.

Norms are based on statistical averages, which apply to large groups of children. Therefore, norms are useful only as broad guidelines. Norms are of little help in predicting the performance of an individual child. Studies have shown that individual children vary tremendously in their articulatory skills. Some children produce most speech sounds correctly by age 2 or 3. Others continue to master various sounds even at age 6 or 7. Generally speaking, however, the sounds that are acquired the last—the fricatives and the affricates—also are the most frequently misarticulated.

Table 4.5

Ages (Years-Months) at Which Children
Mastered the Phonemes in Five Studies

Phonemes	Wellman et al. (1931)	Poole (1934)	Templin (1957)	Sander (1972)	Prather et al. (1975)
m	3-0	3-6	3-0	before 2	2-0
n	3-0	4-6	3-0	before 2	2-0
h	3-0	3-6	3-0	before 2	2-0
p	4-0	3-6	3-0	before 2	2-0
f	3-0	5-6	3-0	3-0	2-4
w	3-0	3-6	3-0	before 2	2-8
b	3-0	3-6	4-0	before 2	2-8
ŋ		4-6	3-0	2-0	2-0
j	4-0	4-6	3-6	3-0	2-4
k	4-0	4-6	4-0	2-0	2-4
g	4-0	4-6	4-0	2-0	2-4
l	4-0	6-6	6-0	2-0	2-4
d	5-0	4-6	4-0	2-0	2-4
t	5-0	4-6	6-0	2-0	2-8
s	5-0	7-6	4-6	3-0	3-0
r	5-0	7-6	4-0	3-0	3-4
ʧ	5-0		4-6	4-0	3-8
v	5-0	6-6	6-0	4-0	4-0
z	5-0	7-6	7-0	4-0	4-0
ʒ	6-0	6-6	7-0	6-0	4-0
θ		7-6	6-0	5-0	4-0
ʤ			7-0	4-0	4-0
ʃ		6-6	4-6	4-0	3-8
ð		6-6	7-0	5-0	4-0

Speech Sound Patterns

In recent years, the attention has shifted from the acquisition of single phonemes to the acquisition of sound patterns and processes underlying such patterns. Researchers believe that the misarticulations of a normally developing
child are not random mistakes but mistakes that show certain patterns. Children's errors are a way of simplifying the adult model of correct articulation.
Such attempts children make at simplifying adult production of speech sounds
are called **phonological processes.** For example, a normally developing child
may omit a syllable not stressed by adults. A child may say "jama" instead of
pajama because the *pa* syllable is usually not stressed in adult speech. This is an
example of an **unstressed syllable deletion process.** The child simplified the
adult production of the word by deleting an unstressed syllable, presumably
because unstressed syllables are harder to learn.

Researchers have discovered many phonological processes by analyzing
normal as well as disordered speech. However, the different age levels at which
the processes appear have not been clearly identified. The phonological processes
are currently most generally used in the analysis of misarticulations. Therefore,
we will return to this topic later in the chapter.

Articulation and Phonological Disorders

The Nelsons lived in a small town in southern Minnesota. David was the 5-year-old son of Kathy and Ron Nelson. David had an older brother and a younger sister. He spent much of his time playing in his backyard; his dog kept him company while keeping away unwanted company. The moment he saw one of us in our backyard, David would start talking.

One cool and colorful autumn afternoon, while I was reluctantly trying to start my even more reluctant lawn mower, David shouted from his backyard:

"Hi Giwi, how aw you?" (*Hi Giri, how are you?*)

"I am fine David, how about you?" I said.

"Goo. You know wha?" asked David. (*Good. You know what?*)

"What?"

"My Mom ga me a new gogy."

"Oh! Your Mom got you a new dog?"

"Ya. You know hi<u>sl</u> name?" quizzed David, knowing well that I did not.

"No, tell me," I said.

"Hi<u>sl</u> name i<u>sl</u> Dumpy." (*His name is Gumpy.*)

"Is it Dumpy?" I asked.

"No!" David protested in an annoyed tone. "Not Dumpy (pausing for a moment and slowing down his speech), Dumpy."

"Oh! You call him Gumpy!"

"Ya!" he said, with a proud smile on his face.

"I like the name. When did you get him?" I asked David.

"Yeterday."

"Where did you find Gumpy?" I asked.

"In Tommy hou." (*In Tommy's house.*)

"He didn't want to keep Gumpy any more?"

"They ha to moo sa pe." (*They had to move some place.*)

"So they gave the dog to you?"

"Yu." (*Yup.*)

"Do you feed Gumpy?"

"Yeah. I gave him a cu a goggy foo." (*Yeah. I gave him a cup of doggie food.*)

"Does he like you?"

"Yeah. He ike me." (*Yeah. He likes me.*)

"Is Gumpy a good dog?"

"He is goo, ba you know wha? He tied to wun away dis monin." (*He is good, but you know what? He tried to run away this morning.*)

"Is that right? I bet he likes you and your home now. He is not going to run away."

"I tink so!" said David. (*I think so.*)

Then he went on with another story. We talked long enough to decide that it was too late to mow the lawn.

David had an articulation disorder. And so did Jason, another child from our neighborhood in Clovis, California.

Jason Johns, a 4-year-old boy, lived across the street with his parents Jennifer and Kevin and his 6-year-old sister Amanda. He liked to visit us often as he was a special friend of my wife Prema. He loved to talk and usually (certainly not accidentally) ended up at the dining table with some cookies and a glass of milk.

One warm summer evening, when we were taking care of typical household chores, we heard the gentle and unmistakable knock on the door. Of course, it was Jason.

"Hi Pwema. Hi Giwi. Hi Manu." he said. (*Hi Prema. Hi Giri. Hi Manu.*)

The three of us said, "Hi Jason."

Our son Manu asked, "How are you doing today?"

"Pine" (*Fine*), he said. He directly went to the dining room where Prema was going through her paperwork at the dining table. He settled himself on a chair and began his delightful conversation.

"What aa you doowin, Pwema?" he asked. (*What are you doing, Prema?*)

"I am going through these bills that I have to pay."

"Oh. My mom d da, too." (*Oh, my mom does that, too.*)

"Oh yeah?" said Prema.

"Yup. My mom say a lot of es word, you know da, wigh, when si look e da bill." (*My mom says a lot of es word, you know that, right, when she looks at the bills.*) Prema just smiled at him.

"You know wha?" asked Jason.

"What?"

"I awedy ee my dinnew." (*I already ate my dinner.*)

"Oh you did? That's a good boy."

"I ee all a ii." (*I ate all of it.*)

"Very good."

"I ee vetab, too."

"What kind of vegetables did you eat?"

"I ee cawa and bee."

"Carrots and beans. Good for you. What else did you eat?"

"I ha su mea." (*I had some meat.*)

"What kind of meat?"

"I foga." (*I forgot.*)

"You forget so soon!"

"Yeah. I ha su tato, too." (*Yeah. I had some potatoes, too.*)

"Potatoes, too? Looks like you had a good dinner!"

"Yeah. I kween u da pwe." (*Yeah. I cleaned up the plate.*)

"You cleaned up the plate? I bet your mom was happy about that!"

"Yeah. I dwan aa da mi, too." (*Yeah. I drank all the milk, too.*)

"Milk is good for you."

"I know. Ee da a baee gu." (*I know. It does a body good.*)

"What is that? It does a body good?"

"Yeah. You know wha de say on TE." (*Yeah. You know what they say on TV.*)

"Yes, I know."

"I kween u da pwe, kween u da gwa." (*I cleaned up the plate, cleaned up the glass.*)

"I am so proud of you, Jason."

"My mom say OK to ea cooee when you pini you dinnew."

"Your mom says it is OK to eat cookies when you finish your dinner?"

"Yeah. Se say OK to ea ieem, too!" (*She says OK to eat ice cream, too!*) Jason's enthusiasm was on the rise.

"Manu sometimes eats ice cream after he finishes his dinner."

"Yeah. Su cany ee OK, too!"

"Some candy is OK, too! Looks like you can eat anything after you have cleaned up your dinner plate."

"Aa you goin to gee su cooee to Manu now?" (*Are you going to give some cookies to Manu now?*)

"I will ask him. If he wants, both of you can have some. If he doesn't, you can still have some."

"I kween u d pwe!" (*I cleaned up the plate!*)

Soon Jason was eating his cookies and drinking a glass of milk.

David and Jason were healthy, cheerful, playful, and talkative children. They were like most other children of their age. They were not mentally retarded. There was no evidence of brain injury. There was no weakness or paralysis of the muscles of speech; their speech mechanism had no structural problems. The two children's language was not deficient. They talked in grammatically complete sentences like other young children. Their parents' speech and language were within the limits of typical variation. The two children's home environment was that of a typical suburban middle-class family. Each child had at least one sibling who spoke normally. Except for the difficulty they had in producing certain speech sounds, the two children were not unusual.

Healthy and normal children's difficulty in producing certain speech sounds is called a **functional articulation disorder.** A functional disorder (sometimes also described as **idiopathic disorder**), as described in previous chapters, cannot

It is assumed that a disorder is functional when no organic factor explains it.

be explained on the basis of some neurological damage, muscle weakness or paralysis, or structural problem such as a cleft palate. The term *functional* does not explain the disorder; it implies only that an organic cause was not found. Some clinicians assume that functional articulation disorders are learned behaviors; others, who do not make that assumption, think that the origin is unknown.

Descriptions of Articulation and Phonological Disorders

There are several methods of describing errors of articulation. Some are simpler than others. A few methods are relatively new. We shall take a brief look at some of the major methods of describing errors of articulation.

Description of Individual Errors

In determining individual sound errors, the clinician listens to the production of each phoneme and judges whether it was correct or not. The errors are then grouped according to types. Within this approach, four types of errors are described: omissions, substitutions, distortions, and additions. The first three types of errors are more common than the last one.

An **omission** is an absence of a required sound in a word position. For example, a child who says "ka" for *car* or "boo" for *boot* omits the /r/ and the /t/. In this case, the omitted sounds are in the final position within the words. Both David and Jason had several omissions. For example, David said "goo" for *good* and "ga" for *got,* omitting the /d/ and /t/ in word final positions. David said "yeterday" for *yesterday.* Therefore, he omitted /s/ in the medial word position (actually, in the *st* cluster). Jason's "ee" for *eat* and "ha" for *had,* among many others, illustrate omissions of word final consonants.

A sound **substitution** involves the production of a wrong sound in place of a right one. A person who says "wadio" for *radio* or "toup" for *soup* is substituting /w/ for /r/ and /t/ for /s/. David and Jason had several substitutions. For example, David said "tink" for *think* and "goggy" for *doggie.* Therefore, he substituted /t/ for /θ/ and /g/ for /d/ in word final positions. Similarly, Jason said "pine" for *fine* and "kween" for *clean.* Therefore, among others, he substituted /p/ for /f/ (initial position) and /w/ for /l/ (medial position).

A **distortion** is an imprecise sound production that does not match its normal production. The listener typically knows what the distorted sound stands for. A "slushy" production of /s/ in *soup,* for example, is a distortion. In one of the more frequently observed variety of /s/ distortion, the air escapes from the sides of the tongue. In this case, the /s/ begins to sound somewhat like an /l/. David distorted his /s/ sounds. He said "hisl" for *his.* Besides /s/, the most frequently distorted sounds include the /r/, /l/, /z/, /ʃ/, and /ʧ/.

An **addition** occurs when a sound that does not belong in a word is added. For example, the child who says "cupa" for *cup* is adding an extra sound at the end of the word. An addition also can be observed within a word as in "salow" for *slow.*

The approach of describing individual errors involves a sound-by-sound analysis of misarticulations (Elbert & Gierut, 1986). The production of each sound is judged as either correct, distorted, substituted, or omitted. Whether a sound is added to a word is also noted. Finally, the misarticulated sound's position within a word is determined (initial, medial, or final). A clinician using this method would summarize the misarticulations of David and Jason in the following way:

Summary of David's Errors of Articulation

Omissions: /d/, /t/, /p/, /s/, /v/, /m/ in word final positions.
Substitutions: /w/ for /r/ in word final positions; /g/ for /d/ in word initial positions; and /t/ for /θ/ in word initial positions.
Distortion: /s/ in word final positions.

Summary of Jason's Errors of Articulation

Omissions: /r/, /t/, /s/, /m/, /p/, /l/, /k/, /d/, /ʃ/, and /v/ in word final positions; and /r/, /v/, and /k/ in word medial positions.
Substitutions: /w/ for /r/, /p/ for /f/, /d/ for /ð/, /w/ for /l/, and /s/ for /ʃ/ in word initial positions; /w/ for /r/ and /w/ for /l/ in word medial positions; and /w/ for /r/ in word final positions.

In the sound-by-sound method of describing individual errors, the clinician does not look at the overall pattern of misarticulations. There is no effort to see if sounds that are misarticulated share certain common characteristics such as voicing or stridency. Most clinicians think that the sound-by-sound analysis is better suited to those clients who show only a few errors of articulation. For clients who misarticulate many sounds, an analysis of the overall pattern of misarticulations may be more appropriate. The clinician then uses one of the methods of determining the pattern of errors.

Patterns Based on Methods of Sound Production

An older method of finding a pattern in errors of articulation is based on how the sounds are produced. As described in an earlier section, speech sounds are classified on the basis of place of articulation, manner of articulation, and the presence or absence of voicing. This place–manner–voice approach can be used to identify patterns of errors.

Take, for instance, a child who shows errors of the following kind:

"ban" for *fan,* "bive" for *five,* "bun" for *fun*
"bad" for *pad,* "baid" for *paid,* "banda" for *panda*
"dime" for *time,* "dell" for *tell,* "dable" for *table*
"gan" for *can,* "gum" for *come,* "gid" for *kid*

These errors have a pattern. The clinician can find a common principle that can describe all of these errors. The child uses /b/ instead of /f/ and /p/, /d/ instead of /t/, and /g/ instead of /k/. While the /f/, /p/, /t/, and /k/ are voiceless sounds, /b/, /d/, and /g/ are voiced sounds. Therefore, the pattern in this case is that the child *substitutes a voiced sound for voiceless sounds.* Obviously, this pattern is based on the voicing feature of speech sounds.

Suppose the child also makes the following two categories of errors:

1. "wadio" for *radio,* "wamp" for *lamp,* "yewo" for *yellow*
2. "base" for *vase,* "balue" for *value,* "bote" for *vote*

"tink" for *think,* "tum" for *thumb,* "tanks" for *thanks*
"toup" for *soup,* "tay" for *say,* "tome" for *some*
"pine" for *fine,* "peel" for *feel,* "pour" for *four*

Two patterns can be noted in these errors. The errors of the first category suggest that the child *substitutes glides for liquids.* While /r/ and /l/ are liquids, /w/ and /j/ (the *y* sound in *yellow*) are glides. The errors of the second category suggest that the child *substitutes stops for fricatives.* While /b/, /t/, and /p/ are stops, /v/, /θ/, /s/, and /f/ are fricatives. The two patterns are based on the manner of speech sound productions.

Should the child make additional errors of the following kind, other patterns based on place of articulation may also be identified:

"dem" for *them,* "dis" for *this,* "dere" for *there*

Such errors suggest that the child *substitutes alveolars for linguadentals* because /ð/ (as in *them*) is a linguadental but /d/ is an alveolar. Other substitutions, listed earlier, can also be used to identify patterns based on place of articulation. For example, the substitutions of /p/ for /f/ and /b/ for /v/ suggest that bilabials (/p/ and /b/) are substituted for labiodentals (/f/ and /v/).

Patterns Based on Distinctive Features

Distinctive features of speech sounds provide yet another method of finding patterns in an array of misarticulations. As described in an earlier section, distinctive features are critical elements that distinguish one sound from another. Clinicians typically use Chomsky and Halle's (1968) distinctive features to find patterns based on elements that contrast speech sounds (see Table 4.4).

Suppose a child makes the following kinds of errors:

"pine" for *fine,* "pool" for *fool,* "pollow" for *follow*
"base" for *vase,* "beal" for *veal,* "bain" for *vain*
"toap" for *soap,* "tun" for *sun,* "tale" for *sale*
omits /s/, /ʃ/ (sh), /tʃ/ (ch), /ʒ/, and /dʒ/

The child substitutes /p/ for /f/, /b/ for /v/, and /t/ for /s/. The target sounds for which the child substituted other sounds all share a common feature: stridency. Therefore, after having listed three kinds of substitutions and five omissions, the clinician summarizes the results by stating the pattern: *The child has not mastered the distinctive feature stridency.*

Consider another example:

"tum" for *come,* "tup" for *cup,* "tate" for *cake*
"dum" for *gum,* "dame" for *game,* "das" for *gas*
"san" for *sang,* "ban" for *bang,* "lon" for *long*

The child in this case substitutes /t/ for /k/, /d/ for /g/, and /n/ for /ŋ/ (ng). According to the Chomsky–Halle system, the target sounds are all back sounds (produced at the back of the mouth); the sounds the child uses instead of them are all front sounds (produced in the front of the mouth). The pattern here is that the child *has not learned the back sounds.* Another way of saying it is that the child *has not learned the contrasting features of front and back.*

The following gives a final example of a child with a different feature problem:

"dice" for *nice,* "dote" for *note,* "dap" for *nap*

"buther" for *mother,* "bice" for *mice,* "bake" for *make*

"hug" for *hung,* "lug" for *lung,* "wrog" for *wrong*

The child in this case substitutes /d/ for /n/, /b/ for /m/, and /g/ for /ŋ/ (ng). The target sounds are nasals, which are substituted with non-nasal sounds. In this case, the clinician concludes that the child *has not mastered nasals* or *has not mastered the contrast between nasal and non-nasal sounds.*

The distinctive feature approach helps us group sounds according to shared characteristics. It also helps us contrast sounds on the basis of unique features. When sounds are grouped, they form a class. Sounds within a class are similar because of their shared features; sounds across classes contrast because of lack of common features.

Some clinical research suggests that when a child misarticulates several sounds that share a common feature, it may not be necessary to teach all of the sounds. When some of the sounds are taught, other sounds that are in the same class may be produced without additional training. In one of our earlier examples, the child did not correctly produce /f/, /v/, /s/, /ʃ/ (sh), /tʃ/ (ch), /ʒ/, and /dʒ/ (all *strident* sounds). In this case, the clinician using the traditional analysis identifies seven target sounds to be taught. On the other hand, the clinician using the distinctive feature analysis thinks that it is sufficient to teach only a few of the seven sounds. A child who masters, for example, /f/, /v/, and /ʃ/ may produce the remaining four strident sounds without further training.

Production of untrained behaviors following training of similar behaviors is called **generalization** or **generalized production.** Research has shown generalized production of some untrained sounds (Bernthal & Bankson, 1998; Peña-Brooks & Hegde, 2000). However, there is need for more research. All distinctive feature contrasts have not been experimentally tested to see if generalized productions occur within the feature classes.

Phonological Patterns

More recently researched patterns of misarticulations are based on phonological analysis. In this analysis, different patterns of errors are explained on the basis of different processes or the lack of phonological knowledge on the part of the child.

Analysis of phonological processes tries to find logic and patterns in children's misarticulations.

As noted before, in the phonological process analysis, errors are thought to be simplifications of more complex adult articulatory responses. For example, the omission of a sound in a word makes that word simpler to say. The many ways (or patterns) of simplifying difficult sound productions are identified as different **phonological processes.** For example, a child who omits several final or initial consonants is said to exhibit the **consonant deletion process.**

Many phonologists and speech–language clinicians assume that phonological processes also are rules that children use in simplifying difficult articulatory responses. In the case of the final consonant deletion process, for example, the child is supposed to use the following rule: simplify the response by deleting the final consonants. There is very little evidence to make this assumption, however. It is a rule the phonologist or the clinician extracts from the child's pattern of responses. The fact that the child's misarticulations show patterns may not necessarily mean that the child is "using a rule."

Many phonological processes that help organize multiple errors of articulation have been described and summarized in many sources devoted to articulation and phonological disorders (Hodson, 1986; Ingram, 1981; Peña-Brooks & Hegde, 2000; Shriberg & Kwiatkowski, 1980; Stoel-Gammon & Dunn, 1985; Weiner, 1984). The following are a few examples:

Final Consonant Deletion. Final consonants are omitted: "bo" for *boat*, "bee" for *beep*, "hi" for *hide*, "hau" for *house*, "bu" for *book*.

Initial Consonant Deletion. Initial consonants are omitted: "ot" for *pot*, "us" for *bus*, "eep" for *deep*, "ink" for *sink*, "op" for *top*.

Cluster Reduction. One or more consonants of a cluster are omitted: "kate" for *skate*, "bu" for *blue*, "tong" for *strong*, "teep" for *steep*.

Fronting. Sounds produced in the front of the mouth are substituted for those produced at the back of the mouth; alveolars are used in place of palatal and velar sounds: "tak" for *chalk*, "seep" for *sheep*, "tum" for *come*.

Denasalization. An oral sound is substituted for a nasal sound: "mad" for *man*, "bother" for *mother*.

Reduplication or Doubling. A syllable of a target word is repeated: "baba" for *bottle*, "dada" for *dog*, "tata" for *television*.

Unstressed Syllable Deletion. "medo" for *tomato*, "tephone" for *telephone*, "ephent" for *elephant*.

Epenthesis. An unstressed vowel, typically the schwa /ə/, is inserted inappropriately: "sapoon" for *spoon*, "looka" for *look*, "cupa" for *cup*.

There are several other phonological processes (Peña-Brooks & Hegde, 2000). Different authors have used somewhat different names for the same or similar processes. The clinician selects a system of classifying errors according to phonological processes and determines the kinds of processes presumably used by a given client. The treatment is then directed toward eliminating a faulty phonological process instead of individual sound errors. For example, if the child is missing many final consonants, the errors are classified under the final consonant deletion process. The clinician's aim then is to eliminate this phonological process. It is assumed that teaching a few of the missing consonants in the final position will result in generalized production of other final consonants. This assumption has not been fully tested in clinical treatment studies.

It is possible that some of the phonological processes are new names for the same behaviors described differently in other methods of analysis. For example, *omissions* in older terminology becomes a *deletion process*. One kind of *substitution* in the older terminology becomes the *fronting process*. It must also be noted that no phonological process can be eliminated without training some individual sounds. The main clinical question is whether treatment of some individual sounds has an effect on other, untreated sounds grouped according to some concept or theory. We need more research to fully answer this important question.

A variation of the phonological approach to finding patterns in misarticulations is to determine a child's **knowledge of the phonological system.** It is assumed that a normal speaker has full knowledge of the sound system used in his or her language and that the children who misarticulate have varying levels of knowledge of the adult phonological system (Elbert & Gierut, 1986). For example, the child who correctly articulates all except a few sounds that are omitted in the word final position has one level or type of knowledge, whereas another child who misarticulates a variety of sounds all the time in all of the word positions has another type of knowledge.

In the phonological knowledge approach, the sounds that are always misarticulated are treated first, and those that are misarticulated only some of the time in only one or two positions are treated last. This unusual sequence is supported by some evidence that when the most consistent errors are corrected, the less consistent errors may be eliminated without further training (Elbert & Gierut, 1986).

Summary

- Multiple sound errors are not isolated occurrences.

- Sounds belong to classes or categories. Therefore, errors also may belong to similar classes and categories.

- When errors are classified according to some system of classes or categories, we have patterns of errors.

- Except in cases of clients who misarticulate just one or two sounds, it is necessary to find patterns of correct and incorrect productions.

- When a pattern is found, treatment may be more efficient and economical because correction of some sounds within a pattern may be sufficient to generate correct production of other sounds within that pattern.

- To find patterns, the clinician first identifies individual sounds that are in error. After that, the clinician may use one of the patterns that group those errors.

- Patterns are alternative methods of describing errors of articulation. For example, after having noted individual errors, the clinician might point out that the client (a) does not use fricatives; (b) does not use one of the distinctive features such as stridency; (c) shows a phonological process such as consonant deletion; and (d) shows limited knowledge of the adult phonological system.

Potential Causes of Articulation and Phonological Disorders

Describing articulation and phonological disorders is easier than specifying their causes. Decades of research has not found factors that are reliably associated with problems of sound production in a majority of cases. Nevertheless, the studies have served a purpose. We know now that many variables that may appear to be related to defective articulation may not be related at all.

The potential causal variables investigated by researchers fall into two main categories. One category of variables includes such personal characteristics as intelligence, gender, or birth order of people who misarticulate. The other set of variables includes such organic factors as hearing loss, dental problems, and neuropathologies.

Personal Characteristics

Intelligence

It was once thought that low intelligence might be a cause of articulation problems. However, several studies have shown that children with normal intelligence can also have difficulty learning the speech sounds. Indeed, many children who are treated for problems of articulation in speech and hearing clinics have normal intelligence.

Intelligence is associated with defective articulation only when it is significantly below normal. A majority of institutionalized children with mental retardation have problems of articulation.

Gender

There is some evidence that female children generally have slightly superior articulatory skills than male children. However, the evidence is weak, and the reported sex differences are small or negligible (Bernthal & Bankson, 1998; Peña-Brooks & Hegde, 2000). Nonetheless, more boys than girls tend to have articulation and phonological disorders. A majority of children treated for these disorders in speech clinics are boys.

Socioeconomic Status

Research has shown that socioeconomic status is not a strong factor in the etiology of articulation disorders (Bernthal & Bankson, 1998; Peña-Brooks & Hegde, 2000). Nevertheless, more children in the lower socioeconomic levels than in the upper levels have errors of articulation. Other studies have reported that children from lower levels make more errors of articulation than those in the upper classes.

Birth Order and Sibling Status

There is some evidence that firstborn and only children have better articulation skills than those who have older siblings (Bernthal & Bankson, 1998; Peña-Brooks & Hegde, 2000). The age difference between the siblings is also a factor. The greater the difference, the better the articulation of the younger child. It is suggested that when the siblings are too close to each other in age, the slightly older sibling may provide a model of defective articulation for the younger children.

Language Development

Because speech is a part of language, the relationship between language development and misarticulations has been researched. Studies have shown that the language development of children with severe misarticulations is somewhat delayed. The children may be less proficient in using complex sentence structures. However, children with less severe disorders of articulation may not show language delay or disorders.

Motor Skills

Because the production of speech is a motor task, defective speech suggests deficiency in general or speech-specific motor skills. Research into general motor skills (gait, coordinated fine or gross movements, etc.) has not shown anything of significance. Studies of speech-related motor skills also have not produced anything significant except that the children who misarticulate may be slower in repeating syllables.

The speed at which a speaker can repeat selected syllables (*pa-ta-ka,* for example) is called the diadochokinetic rate. Most clinicians use a diadochokinetic test in assessing articulation disorders. However, the significance of the slower rate in the etiology of articulation disorders is not clear. It may be an effect of the disorder, not its cause.

Auditory Discrimination

Clearly hearing and understanding differences between speech sounds is known as **auditory discrimination.** Many researchers in the past were concerned with the possibility that a child misarticulates because he or she cannot hear the difference between speech sounds others produce. If the child cannot hear the difference between /s/ and /z/, then that child's substitution of /s/ for /z/ may be due to this lack of auditory discrimination.

Studies on the auditory discrimination abilities of children with misarticulations have produced inconsistent results. Some children have scored poorly on auditory discrimination tests, whereas others have scored within the normal range. In general, the relationship between auditory discrimination and articulation does not appear very strong.

Organic Variables

Oral Structures

Lips, teeth, tongue, and hard and soft palates are all involved in speech production. The traditional classification of speech sounds (bilabials, labiodentals, lingua-alveolars) suggests the importance of those structures. However, most children who misarticulate have normal lips, teeth, tongue, and palates. Therefore, in a majority of cases, misarticulations cannot be explained on the basis of significant structural anomalies.

In a few cases, **tongue-tie,** also known as **ankyloglossia,** may be an organic cause of misarticulations. Normally, the free tip of the tongue is mobile. This mobility is needed to make sounds such as /t/ and /d/. However, if the **lingual frenum,** which attaches the tongue to the base of the mouth, is too short, the range of the tongue-tip movement is reduced. The frenum is then attached too close to the tip of the tongue. This is diagnosed as tongue-tie. In the past, clipping of the frenum to free the tongue tip was more common than it is now. However, research has shown that tongue-tie is not a frequent cause of misarticulations. Only an extreme case of tongue-tie can affect articulation. Such cases are rare.

Although most children who misarticulate do not show gross organic defects, such defects, when present, are associated with misarticulations. For example, children with unrepaired clefts of the palate and lips show various kinds of misarticulations. Oral-structural deviations and dental anomalies are common in such children.

Clefts occur because certain bones of the face do not fuse together during the fetal and embryonic periods. Cleft palate and associated disorders of communication are described in **Chapter 8.**

Some children may have dental abnormalities with no clefts. The teeth may be missing, or the two dental arches may be misaligned. The upper incisors are important in the production of some speech sounds (/f/, /v/, /s/, /z/, and others). Nevertheless, missing incisors may or may not cause defective articulation of the target phonemes. Whereas some children misarticulate the target sounds, others do not.

The effects of malocclusion of the dental arches on articulation has been a topic of several studies. **Malocclusion** is a problem of misaligned upper and lower dental arches. In Class I malocclusion, only some individual teeth are misaligned, but the arches themselves are generally aligned. In Class II malocclusion, the upper jaw is protruded and the lower jaw is receded. In Class III malocclusion, the upper jaw is receded and the lower jaw is protruded. The degree of deviation, of course, varies within the classes.

See **Chapter 8** for more information and illustrations of malocclusions.

Studies do not suggest that articulation and dental malocclusions are strongly related. Individuals with an extreme degree of malocclusions are likely to show some problems. Many people with diagnosed malocclusions do not exhibit problems of articulation.

When an organic problem that could affect articulation exists, but its effects are not observed, the clinician usually concludes that the child has learned a **compensatory response.** In essence, the child will have learned unusual ways of producing the target sounds. People who do not learn compensatory responses show problems of articulation. This seems to be true of missing teeth, malocclusions, and variations in lip mobility and tongue size. Among individuals who are left with a stiff upper lip because of the surgical repair of the cleft lip, some may have articulation problems, whereas others may not. Due to diseases of various kinds, portions of the tongue may be surgically removed. Only a few individuals who have had this kind of surgery may show problems of articulation.

Hearing Loss

Hearing loss causes a variety of oral speech and verbal language problems. Various kinds of articulation problems are frequently seen in children and adults with moderate to severe hearing loss. Individuals who are born with deafness have the greatest difficulty in articulating speech sounds. Severe hearing loss makes it difficult not only to hear other people's speech but also to monitor one's own speech production. Even when the hearing loss is mild, what the person hears may be distorted.

Hearing impairment and its effects on communication are described in **Chapter 10.**

Individuals with hearing impairment are likely to omit consonants in the final and initial positions. Omissions of /s/ and /z/ are common. They tend to substitute voiced for voiceless and nasal for oral consonants. They distort many speech sounds, especially the fricatives.

Neuropathologies

Although most children with errors of articulation do not show gross neurological problems, neural damage of various kinds tends to cause articulation and other communicative problems. These problems are found more frequently in adults than in children. However, communicative problems resulting from neural damage are different from functional misarticulations.

Various diseases and accidents can damage portions of the central nervous system concerned with speech production. When certain parts of the brain or

Dysarthrias and other disorders of communication that have a neurological basis are described in **Chapter 9.**

various nerves that control speech muscles are damaged, speech production is affected. In such cases, the speech muscles are not able to execute the complex and rapid movements necessary to produce speech. Central or peripheral nerve damage causes a group of speech disorders called **dysarthrias.** The damage to the nervous system causes paralysis, weakness, or incoordination of the muscles of speech. The patient is not able to articulate speech sounds properly. The speech is hard to understand. Besides problems of articulation, dysarthrias are also associated with deviant voice quality, monotonous pitch, variable rate of speech, hypernasality, and other problems.

See **Chapter 9** for more information on apraxia of speech.

Another speech disorder of neurological origin that includes errors of articulation is called **apraxia of speech.** Damage to the central nervous system causes apraxia of speech. However, there is no paralysis or weakness of the muscles of speech because the peripheral nerves that supply them are not damaged. It is believed that the brain damage makes it difficult to program the precise movements necessary for smoothly articulated running speech. Therefore, apraxia is described as a *motor programming disorder.* The apraxic person makes highly inconsistent errors of articulation. At times, the person is able to speak without errors of articulation. The person has difficulty positioning the articulators correctly and appears unsure of the movements necessary to produce a word. Therefore, the articulatory efforts are described as **groping.** Every time the speaker tries to say a word, he or she produces a different kind of error. Based on these and other characteristics, functional articulation in children is easily distinguished from apraxia of speech, seen more frequently in adults with neurological problems.

In recent years, some researchers have suggested that a small group of children who show errors of articulation may have apraxia of speech. That is, disorders of articulation in some children may be due to brain damage which makes it difficult to program the movements of speech. This variety of articulation disorder is called **developmental apraxia of speech (DAS).** Like the apraxic adults, the children with DAS may show signs of trial-and-error groping while trying to say certain words. The children can produce the movements necessary to make a speech sound but have difficulty making them in the context of speech production. Therefore, some clinicians diagnose DAS in a small number of children who are then presumed to have central neural problems (Hall, Jordan, & Robin, 1993).

Tongue Thrust

In recent years, the relationship between swallowing and articulation has received much attention. A pattern of abnormal swallow is called **tongue thrust.**

Orthodontists, specialists who treat people with misaligned teeth and upper and lower dental arches, are concerned with tongue thrust because of the belief that tongue thrust works against orthodontic treatment. While the orthodontist tries to move the upper dental arches back, tongue thrust is supposed to move it forward. Some speech–language pathologists are concerned with tongue thrust because of its potential association with articulation disorders, especially the frontal lisp (distortion of /s/ and /z/).

In the normal swallow, the tip of the tongue is placed against the alveolar ridge, which is that portion of the inner gum ridge behind the upper central incisors. The body of the tongue then pushes the fluid or the solid into the back of the mouth and the upper throat. From then on, swallowing is mostly reflexive. During deviant swallow, the tip of the tongue is supposed to push the front teeth, often the upper central incisors. The tongue tip may protrude between the upper and lower teeth and thus come in contact with the lower lip. During speech production, the tongue also may exert some force against the front teeth. Even at rest, the tongue may be carried more toward the frontal portion of the mouth. There is no satisfactory explanation for tongue thrust, though both bottle-feeding and thumb-sucking have been blamed for it.

There is controversy about whether deviant swallow causes articulation problems and whether correcting deviant swallow is the work of speech–language pathologists. Orthodontists often refer children with deviant swallow to speech–language pathologists for **myofunctional therapy,** which is treatment aimed at correcting tongue thrust. Some speech–language pathologists provide myofunctional therapy. However, there also are myofunctional therapists who are not speech–language pathologists. Many speech–language pathologists accept a referral from an orthodontist only when the client has an articulation disorder, which they treat. Other speech–language pathologists may treat articulation disorder as well as tongue thrust. More research is needed to determine the exact relationship between deviant swallow and speech disorders.

Summary

- Most personal characteristics that are within the range of normal variation are not significantly related to defective articulation.

- Unusually low intelligence and low socioeconomic levels are associated with defective articulation.

- More males than females exhibit disorders of articulation.

- Firstborn children, only children, and those with siblings who are much older have better articulatory skills.

- A child may show mild to moderate articulation problems while exhibiting normal language skills.

- Within the normal limits, general and speech-related motor skills do not play a significant role in articulation skills.

- Auditory discrimination problems do not seem to be causally related to articulation problems.

- Significant organic deviations are not associated with articulation disorders in a majority of children.

- Dental malocclusions do not explain articulation disorders of many children.

- Hearing loss is a major physical cause of articulation disorders.

- Although children with articulation disorders do not exhibit neuropathologies, those who do tend to have articulation disorders.

- Tongue thrust may or may not be associated with articulation disorders.

Assessment of Articulation and Phonological Disorders

When a child is referred for articulation treatment, the clinician's first job is to determine whether or not there is a clinical problem, and if there is, what its characteristics are. This process of identifying and describing a clinical problem is **assessment**.

A thorough assessment of articulation takes time. Therefore, the clinician often screens clients to determine who has normal articulation and who, because they seem to have a problem, must be assessed.

Articulation Screening

A **screening** is a brief procedure that helps determine whether or not a person should be assessed at length. Those who pass a screening procedure are judged to have age-appropriate articulation. Those who fail it are scheduled for a complete assessment. In the public schools, speech–language clinicians routinely screen children in kindergarten and the lower elementary grades. Besides articulation, the clinician also screens language, voice, and fluency.

There are different procedures to screen articulation skills. If the child is talkative at all, a brief conversational speech sample is tape-recorded for later analysis. Or, with the help of pictures, clinicians test the production of speech sounds. Clinicians make sure that /s/, /z/, /ʃ/ (sh), /tʃ/ (ch), /dʒ/, /r/, /l/, /θ/, /f/, /v/, /t/, /k/, and /g/, which are frequently misarticulated, are tested in all word positions. The clinician also may use standardized screening tests or the screening portions of full-length assessment tests of articulation.

The sounds that are misarticulated are often compared to the developmental norms. If the clinician determines that the sounds a child misarticulates should have been produced correctly, then that child is considered a candidate for a complete evaluation. It is possible that some misarticulations would not be considered serious because of the age of the child. Also, in the case of children who speak a different dialect, or speak English that is influenced by a primary language other than English (e.g., Spanish), the clinician may decide that the child speaks a different form of English and does not exhibit a disorder of articulation.

Procedures of Evaluation

A child who fails the screening test is thoroughly evaluated to find out the number and types of errors and their patterns. In addition, the presence of any gross organic deviations in the oral structures and any signs of neurological damage also are noted. A case history is taken to get a larger picture of the client's behavior, health, and development. The clinician is especially interested in speech and language development. Finally, the client's hearing is screened. Table 4.6 shows the articulation assessment module.

Case History

The first step in the evaluation of any communicative disorder is to take a case history, through which the clinician finds out when the problem was first noted,

Table 4.6

Assessment of Communicative Disorders: Articulation Disorders

1. History of the client, the family, and the disorder

2. Interview of the client, the family members, or both

3. Orofacial examination

4. Hearing screening

5. Speech and language sampling

6. **Measurement/assessment of articulation:**
   a. **sampling conversational speech**
   b. **administration of standardized tests of articulation**
   c. **analysis of individual errors, their types, and their word positions**
   d. **analysis of patterns of misarticulations**

7. Recommendations

8. Report writing

Note. Procedures unique to assessment of articulation are in bold print.

what the client and the family think the problem is, whether the problem is stable or changing, and whether the client previously received treatment. In addition, the clinician seeks information on the child's general health and his or her family. Information on language, physical, social, and behavioral development also is obtained.

Although a history rarely reveals the causes of an articulation disorder, the clinician is alert to such factors as potential accidents, injuries, and diseases that could cause brain damage. The child's academic performance and the effects of the speech disorder on the child's academic and social life also are investigated. Family members provide much of the information. The clinician typically has the parent or the client fill out a case history form and then interviews him or her to get more detailed information.

Orofacial Examination

The clinician examines the client's facial and oral structures to rule out gross organic problems. The clinician notes the general symmetry of the facial structures. The shape and the mobility of the lips and the tongue are examined by having the client perform various tasks. Missing teeth and dental malocclusion, if any, are noted and described. The hard and soft palates are viewed for signs of structural abnormality. This examination may reveal a submucous cleft of the palate, which is an opening in the palate covered by the mucous membrane. This type of cleft can go unnoticed. The mobility of the soft palate is evaluated to make sure that it can move back and up to close the velopharyngeal port during the production of non-nasal sounds. These and other procedures constitute an **orofacial examination**, also known as an **oral-peripheral examination**.

Hearing Screening

The client's hearing is screened by a brief audiological screening procedure. Like any other screening test, a hearing screening does not determine the actual

Hearing screening and assessment procedures are described in **Chapter 10**.

thresholds of hearing but only suggests either that the hearing is within the normal limits or that the client needs to be evaluated with a complete audiological test battery. A client who fails a hearing screening is referred to an audiologist for a complete hearing evaluation.

Assessment of Sound Production

Conversational speech samples, standardized tests that evaluate the production of individual sounds, and assessment tools that help evaluate phonological processes are the major sources of information on articulation and its disorders. The clinician talks to the child and tape-records the conversation, which is directed to make sure that the child produces most of the sounds of the language. Conversational speech provides a natural means of assessing speech sound productions.

Several commercially available standardized tests help assess the production of individual sounds. Of these tests, the *Templin–Darley Tests of Articulation* (Templin & Darley, 1969), the *Goldman–Fristoe Test of Articulation* (Goldman & Fristoe, 1986), the *Fisher–Logemann Test of Articulation Competence* (Fisher & Logemann, 1971), the *Deep Test of Articulation* (McDonald, 1964b), the *Arizona Articulation Proficiency Scale–Second Edition* (Fudala & Reynolds, 1986), and the *Photo Articulation Test–Second Edition* (Pendergast, Dickey, Selmar, & Soder, 1997) are among the better known and frequently used tests.

Most tests of articulation contain pictures the clients are asked to name. The words that are evoked in this manner are selected to test all or most of the sounds of English in the word initial, medial, and final positions. In addition, consonant clusters (*stop, strike, bread, sleek*) are also tested. To assess sound production in continuous speech, some tests require the clients to retell a brief story that has been read to them.

Distinctive features, phonological processes, and phonological knowledge are often assessed by a sample of conversational speech. Several tests or assessment protocols to analyze phonological processes also are available. Among these, *The Assessment of Phonological Processes–Revised* (Hodson, 1986a, 1986b) is available in both English and Spanish versions. Other tests or protocols for analyzing phonological processes include the *Bankson–Bernthal Test of Phonology* (Bankson & Bernthal, 1990), the *Khan–Lewis Phonological Analysis* (Khan & Lewis, 1986), *Phonological Process Analysis* (Weiner, 1979), and *Natural Process Analysis* (Shriberg & Kwiatkowski, 1980). Computer programs that analyze phonological process when a speech sample is typed into the program also are available (Hodson, 1986c; Weiner, 1984).

Test of Stimulability

In testing for stimulability, the clinician produces the child's misarticulated sounds correctly and asks the child to imitate. The child is said to be **stimulable** if he or she imitates the correctly modeled productions. Most clinicians think that stimulable sounds are easier to teach and, therefore, provide a starting point for treatment.

Writing an Assessment Report

After the assessment, the clinician must evaluate information obtained from all sources and make recommendations for treatment. The clinician considers the case history and interview data, the results of the orofacial examination, and the client's performance on standardized tests and conversational speech. The production of each sound is classified as correct or incorrect. If incorrect, the types of errors in terms of omissions, distortions, substitutions, and additions are determined. Finally, if the child has multiple misarticulations, an analysis of the pattern of errors based on phonological approaches or distinctive features is made.

An assessment report is then prepared that summarizes the history and the results of tests and other observations. The report is typically concluded with a statement regarding the presence of an articulation disorder and recommendations for treatment.

Assessment of Articulation in Relation to Ethnocultural Factors

Assessment of articulation disorders, especially disorders of articulation, requires a careful consideration of a client's ethnocultural background. Cultural and ethnic factors greatly influence speech and language behaviors. What appears to be a deviation from the norms of one group may be an accepted part of cultural practice in another group. In the realm of communication, too, what appears to be a disorder from the standpoint of one cultural group's norms may not be a disorder from the standpoint of another group.

In assessing articulation in children (or adults) who speak a different dialect, variety, or form of English, the clinician needs to consider the accepted patterns of speech sound production in that dialect, form, or variety. For example, compared to standard English production of speech sounds, a child who speaks African American English may produce certain speech sounds differently. However, this difference alone is not a cause for diagnosing an articulation disorder. It is because the difference is a part of African American English rules of speech sound production. The child has an articulation disorder only when his or her speech sound productions are not consistent with the accepted rules of African American English.

Similarly, a child (or an adult) whose primary language is not English may produce English speech sounds differently. Such a speaker's English speech sound production is influenced by his or her primary language. For example, a bilingual child whose primary language is Spanish may produce certain English speech sounds in a manner that is different from a monolingual English speaking child's. This, too, is not a cause for diagnosing an articulation disorder. The correct assessment of such a child is that he or she speaks a variety of English that is influenced by the primary language. A bilingual child has an articulation disorder only when his or her patterns of speech sound production are consistent neither with English phonological rules nor with those of the primary language.

See **Chapter 11** for details on how culture, ethnic factors, and bilingualism affect communication and communicative disorders.

Treatment of Articulation and Phonological Disorders

There are many approaches to treating disorders of articulation. Within the scope of this chapter, it is not possible to describe even all of the major approaches.

Therefore, an overview of the treatment process and some details about selected aspects of treatment are provided. A few variations and specific approaches also are mentioned.

The major components of most treatment programs include the selection of target responses, the development of stimulus materials, the implementation of treatment procedures, and the use of procedures to assess generalization and to ensure maintenance of correct sound productions outside of the clinic and over time.

Selection of Target Behaviors

The final goal of articulation treatment is the correct production of misarticulated phonemes in conversational speech in all situations. In most treatment programs, this goal is stated as a **criterion of performance.** For example, clinicians may specify a criterion of 90% accuracy in the production of the target phonemes in conversational speech produced at home and other nonclinical situations.

When a client has only a few misarticulations, the targets are the correct productions of those sounds in conversational speech at 90% accuracy. In cases of clients with multiple misarticulations, one or more of the patterns we discussed earlier may be the treatment targets. For example, when the pattern is based on methods of sound production, the target behavior may be the correct production of voiced sounds. In the case of distinctive features, the treatment targets are the features that are missing or not used frequently. When patterns of errors are based on phonological processes, the goal of treatment is the elimination of faulty processes. For example, the treatment goal for a child who does not produce many consonants in the final position is the elimination of the final consonant deletion process. Of course, this is the same as saying that the goal is to teach the production of final consonants.

> A client who meets a criterion of performance has mastered a **treatment target.**

Antecedent Stimulus Events

Once the target behaviors are selected, the clinician finds appropriate stimulus materials to be used in treatment sessions. The stimulus materials include pictures or objects, clinician's modeling of target sound productions, instructions on how to produce them, and manual guidance to help the articulators make appropriate movements. Stimulus events are antecedent events because the clinician presents them *before* the client produces, or makes an attempt to produce, the target sounds.

> Anything a clinician does to trigger a target response is an **antecedent event.**

In the initial treatment sessions, the clinician asks the client to name pictures selected to evoke words with target sounds in them. For example, in teaching the target sound /s/ in the initial word position, the clinician might select 15 to 20 pictures that represent such words as *soup, sink, soap,* and *sock.* When practical, objects may be used instead of pictures.

The child who does not produce a sound at all often needs additional help in producing it. In such cases, **modeling** the correct response is a frequently used additional antecedent. The clinician asks the child to name a picture and immediately names it so the child can imitate the correct response. For example, the clinician asks, "What is this?" and immediately adds, "Say *soap.*"

In producing the word, the clinician might place an extra emphasis on the target sound.

A traditional approach to articulation treatment that emphasizes the role of instructions and demonstrations is called the **phonetic placement method.** In this method, the clinician describes how a target sound is produced correctly. In front of a mirror, the clinician may demonstrate the placement of the tongue, the shape of the lips, the movement of the soft palate, the extent of mouth opening (jaw movement), and the relation between the teeth and the lips. In addition, the clinician also may use charts, diagrams, and plastic models to show the kinds of contacts the tongue, palate, teeth, and lips make in producing certain sounds.

In some extreme cases, the clinician may have to use manual guidance to facilitate the correct production of a target sound. In **manual guidance,** the clinician uses his or her fingers to shape the articulators. For example, in teaching the production of /f/, the clinician might gently push the lower lip under the upper dental arch and hold it there when the child softly bites on the lip and pushes the air out. A treatment approach based on manual guidance of the articulators is called the **moto-kinesthetic method.** When the clinician manually moves the articulators, the client receives motor and kinesthetic feedback. Kinesthetic feedback makes the child aware of the position and movement of the speech articulators.

Treatment Procedures

After the clinician develops pictures, words, and other stimulus materials for a client, the treatment is started. However, the actual starting point and the way the treatment process is organized differ from clinician to clinician. Three variations are described.

Auditory Discrimination or Production?

Some clinicians start training not by asking the child to produce or imitate the correct production of the target sound, but by asking the child to listen to the differences between the target sound and the error sound. As noted before, this is done on the assumption that a child who says "wadio" for *radio* may not auditorily discriminate between /w/ and /r/.

In auditory discrimination training, the child is asked to listen to the clinician's paired word productions. For example, the clinician says "radio" or "wadio," "run" or "wun," "road" or "woad," and so on. The child may be asked to raise his or her left hand when the word with the /r/ sound is heard and the right hand when the word with /w/ sound is heard. In this manner, the child learns to auditorily discriminate between /r/ and /w/. The important point is that the child is not asked to *produce* the target sound correctly until he or she discriminates between the error sound and the correct target sound. Some specialists recommend exclusive auditory discrimination training done over many treatment sessions (Van Riper & Emerick, 1984; Winitz, 1984).

Clinicians who do not think that the auditory discrimination training is necessary begin training with production. The child is asked to produce or imitate the target sound from the very beginning. To evoke target responses, clinicians may initially use modeling, instructions, demonstrations, and manual guidance, when found necessary. There is some evidence that production training is sufficient to teach both production and auditory discrimination, whereas discrimination training teaches only discrimination, not production (Williams & McReynolds, 1975).

Sound, Syllable, or the Word?

Almost all communicative behaviors are taught first by teaching their simpler forms and then by progressing to more complex forms.

Whether discrimination training is done or not, the first stage of production training may be started at the sound, syllable, or word level. Most clinicians simplify the target response in some manner. The most obvious simplification is to teach the sound in isolation, although stop-plosive sounds (/p/, /b/) cannot be taught in isolation. (When a stop-plosive is released, a short *a* sound is added to it.)

Most traditional approaches to articulation therapy start production treatment at the sound level. In other approaches, treatment is started at the syllable level because the syllable is a more natural unit of speech. In a treatment program known as the **sensory-motor approach** (McDonald, 1964a), the treatment is *always* started at the syllable level. In this approach, the clinician must first find a context in which the client can produce the target sound correctly. For example, a child who generally misarticulates /s/ may correctly produce it in the context of "watchsun" (two words, *watch* and *sun* are produced as though they were one word). The target sounds are trained in such newly created syllabic contexts.

Still other clinicians start training at the word level. In a treatment program known as the **paired-stimuli approach,** the clinician first finds a *key word* in which the error sound is produced correctly (Weston & Irwin, 1985). If one cannot be found, the correct production of the sound is taught in a single word, thus creating a key word. The key word is then paired with 10 other training words. The child is asked to produce the key word first and a training word next. For example, in teaching the target /f/, the key word may be *fan,* which the child produces correctly. The child is then asked to say *fight.* Initially, the child is likely to omit the /f/. Next, the child says *fan* again, followed by another training word such as *four.* In this manner, the key word is paired with each of the selected training words. Soon, the child begins to produce the target sound in training words.

Most clinicians use a more simplified level only when a given client needs it. Some clients need to start at the sound level; others can handle the syllable level. If a client can respond at the word level as in the paired-stimuli approach, it is even better because the target sounds must eventually be produced correctly in words and conversational speech.

Single or Multiple Sound Targets?

A child who misarticulates many sounds has multiple treatment targets, even when the sounds are grouped into classes. However, in the beginning, the clinician may focus either on one sound or on multiple sounds. To begin with, some clinicians prefer to focus on a single sound because of the possibility that multiple sounds may confuse the client.

Believing that it is less monotonous and may lead to more rapid improvement, some clinicians train more than one sound at a time. Such an approach, called the **multiple-phoneme approach,** may be useful (Bradley, 1989; McCabe & Bradley, 1975). In this method, the clinician works on several sounds in any given session. All sounds are initially trained in isolation. Then in successive stages, the sounds are trained at the level of syllables, words, phrases, or sentences; reading; and conversational speech. The multiple-phoneme approach is attractive in cases of children with numerous misarticulations.

Sequence of Treatment

Treatment of articulation follows a general sequence, which is individualized to suit specific children. Most target sounds are treated in the order of sounds, syllables, words, phrases, and sentences. As the child gains mastery of the sound, the task during treatment becomes increasingly more complex and more natural. It starts with imitation of single sounds, syllables, or words, and ends with conversational speech.

At each level of training, a certain performance criterion may be required. For example, 90% accuracy at the word level may suggest that it is time to move on to the next level of training, the phrase level. Note that to adhere to such criteria, the client's correct and incorrect productions must be measured in each session. Such measurements demonstrate the clinician **accountability.** The measures indicate whether the treatment is working or not.

Management of Treatment Contingencies

Treatment programs differ in one or more respects, but many use behavioral principles to teach correct responses (Baker & Ryan, 1971; Bernthal & Bankson, 1998; Blache, 1989; Bradley, 1989; Elbert & Gierut, 1986; McCabe & Bradley, 1975; McLean, 1970; Mowrer, 1989; Sommers, 1983; Weston & Irwin, 1985). Such behavioral principles as modeling and positive reinforcement have been proven effective in modifying articulation disorders.

The clinician instantaneously evaluates every attempt to produce the target sound and gives immediate and appropriate feedback to the child. The feedback given to correct responses to increase their frequency is called **positive reinforcement.** Verbal praise is a frequently used **positive reinforcer.** Such verbal statements as "Excellent!" "Good job!" and "I like that!" can be powerful reinforcers. In some cases, however, tangible reinforcers may be necessary. The child may earn tokens for correct responses, which are exchanged for small gifts such as stars or other kinds of stickers. The amount of reinforcers given a child is gradually reduced.

The clinician gives a different kind of feedback for incorrect responses. Such feedback is called **corrective feedback,** which tends to decrease the rate of incorrect responses (Hegde, 1998). The clinician might say "No" or "Wrong" every time an incorrect response is made. Time-out and response cost are two other frequently used procedures that decrease the frequency of error responses. In **time-out,** immediately following an incorrect response, the clinician says "Stop," and looks away from the client for 5 to 10 seconds. Eye contact is then reestablished and the training is continued. In **response cost,** a wrong response costs a reinforcer that the child had earned for correct responses. These and other response reduction procedures (Hegde, 1998) help decrease the rate of incorrect sound productions. As long as the clinician also positively reinforces correct productions, the response reduction procedures do not produce negative or undesirable effects.

Generalization and Maintenance

The final treatment goal is the correct production of sounds in sentences in everyday situations when no systematic feedback is given. Throughout the treatment, the clinician periodically asks the child to produce the target sounds in new, untrained words. Brief conversational speech may also be recorded in the absence of any feedback. Known as **probes,** such a procedure helps assess whether a trained sound is produced in untrained words and sentences and while speaking in such natural settings as home and school.

As the treatment progresses, correct responses become stable in the presence of the clinician because the clinician has reinforced them. If the parents, siblings, friends, and others reinforce the correct responses at home and in other nonclinical situations, the correct responses are more likely to be produced and maintained there. Therefore, one of the **response maintenance strategies** is to train the family members to reinforce correct productions of target sounds at home and in other situations.

Another maintenance strategy is to teach the client self-monitoring skills. Teaching a client to count his or her own correct and incorrect productions of a target sound is an excellent technique of promoting self-monitoring skills. The client who can monitor his or her own productions is more likely to maintain the gains of treatment.

Dismissed clients are **followed up** to assess maintenance of correct articulation. The first follow-up is recommended 3 months after the dismissal. Additional follow-ups are scheduled less frequently. In all follow-up sessions, a conversational speech sample is recorded and the correct production of previously taught sounds is analyzed. Standardized tests also may be administered. If the client has maintained correct articulation for a year or more, further follow-ups may be unnecessary. If any of the follow-ups show an increase in the frequency of incorrect responses, a few treatment sessions are necessary. This is called the **booster treatment.** Often, the same procedure that has been effectively used before is applied in booster treatment.

Summary

- Treatment of articulation disorders includes a variety of procedures in which individual or a group of phonemes are trained with the help of modeling, multiple cues for correct production, and appropriate feedback.

- Treatment begins at the syllable or word level and ends with correct production of target sounds in conversational speech exhibited in natural settings.

- To promote maintenance, family members and others are trained to reinforce correct articulation at home and in other settings.

Dialogue

Ms. Noledge-Hungry, one of the students in Professor Speech-Wisely's class on introduction to communicative disorders, is not sure of her major. She thinks she might enjoy working with people with speech, language, or hearing problems. She came to the professor's office to discuss articulation and its disorders. The professor always summarized and highlighted the information during these visits. The professor also answered his inquisitive student's questions about the science and the profession.

N-H: Professor Speech-Wisely, I was fascinated by the experiments on speech perception. I thought that the experimenters conditioned the infants to discriminate between speech sounds. We do not know if the infants "perceive" the differences between phonemes.

S-W: You are absolutely correct.

N-H: You know, Dr. Speech-Wisely, at one time I was teaching the alphabet to my niece, and when I began to describe to her what letter sounded like what, both she and I were confused. Often you wonder how we sort this out at all!

S-W: You are correct. The alphabet is inadequate, redundant, and confusing. Therefore the specialists have devised the **International Phonetic Alphabet.** It can be used to describe the sounds of English and sounds in other languages. In the IPA, each symbol stands for a specific sound. Can you define phonology?

N-H: Yes. **Phonology** is the study of the sound system of a language. The sounds are the building blocks of a language. Technically, speech sounds are phonemes.

S-W: Very good. A **phoneme** is a class of speech sounds. Phonemes make a difference in meaning.

N-H: But phonemes are abstracts. When they are actually produced, they vary from one production to another. Those variations are called **allophones.**

S-W: Very good. Now tell me about speech sound classifications.

N-H: Well, one way of classifying speech sounds is to make a distinction between **vowels** and **consonants.** The vowels are produced by keeping the vocal tract relatively open and by vibrating the vocal folds.

S-W: Correct. You must remember the front, central, mid, back, high, and low vowels. A combination of two vowels is called a **diphthong.** All consonants are produced with some constriction of the vocal tract. Consonants are classified on the basis of place–manner–voicing characteristics. What are the consonantal types based on this classification?

N-H: The **place of articulation** yields seven categories: bilabials, labiodentals, linguadentals, lingua-alveolar, linguapalatal, linguavelar, and glottal. The **manner of articulation** yields six categories: stops, fricatives, affricates, glides, liquids, and nasals. The **voicing feature** yields the voiced and unvoiced consonants.

S-W: You should be able to describe each category and give examples. Now, what are distinctive features?

N-H: **Distinctive features** are unique characteristics of sounds that help differentiate one sound from the other.

S-W: Good. Now can you summarize the research on speech sound acquisition?

N-H: I will try. **Babbling** is the beginning of the acquisition of speech sound and language. Vowels and back consonants are frequently heard in babbling. Later acquisition of speech sounds is studied by either the **cross-sectional** or the **longitudinal method.** Both can find patterns of acquisition. By and large, vowels are acquired before consonants, nasals before other consonants, stops and glides before fricatives. Fricatives and liquids are mastered relatively late.

S-W: Excellent! Also, remember that the late developing phonemes, especially the fricatives and affricates, are also most frequently misarticulated.

N-H: Yes, I remember that. Dr. Speech-Wisely, how do you describe disorders of articulation?

S-W: There are different descriptions. Basically, a person does not produce certain speech sounds correctly. The errors themselves may be described individually or by identifying certain patterns in them. An error may be in the initial, medial, or final position of words. What are the four traditional categories of errors?

N-H: **Omissions, substitutions, distortions,** and **additions.**

S-W: Good. You should be able to describe each category and give examples. Now, what do you know about the pattern analysis of misarticulations?

N-H: Patterns may be found on the basis of the **place–manner–voice characteristics of phonemes, distinctive features,** and **phonological processes or phonological knowledge.**

S-W: You should be able to describe a few phonological processes.

N-H: You mean processes such as consonant deletions?

S-W: Yes. Now, tell me what factors have been researched to find the causes of articulation disorders.

N-H: Research has shown that disorders of articulation are more prevalent among children of lower **socioeconomic status** and among those who have lower than normal **intelligence. Oral structures,** unless grossly deformed as in some cases of cleft palate, do not seem to be related to articulation problems. **Hearing loss** causes speech and language problems, but many children with articulation problems have normal hearing. Various **diseases of the nervous system** can cause disorders of speech, but again, children with functional articulation disorders do not have neurological problems. It looks like in individual cases, it is often not possible to detect a cause of the disorder.

S-W: Good summary. Treatment of articulation disorders typically involves correcting the faulty articulations and teaching the production of target sounds. What do you have to do before you start the treatment?

N-H: You must **assess** the disorder. Case history, an orofacial examination, hearing screening, recording conversational speech samples, administering standardized tests of articulation, and determining stimulability are all parts of assessment.

S-W: The assessment data are analyzed for the number and kinds of errors. Omissions, substitutions, distortions, and additions are noted. What is done next?

N-H: Some clinicians find **patterns** in the errors. This is done only when the client has multiple misarticulations. The patterns may be based on an analysis of place–manner–voice, distinctive features, or phonological processes.

S-W: Excellent. What is an important factor to be considered in assessing articulation disorders?

N-H: Ethnocultural factors. The essence of the argument is that a difference is not necessarily a disorder. We need to consider if the speaker speaks a different variety of English, such as African American English or English that is influenced by a primary language in a bilingual speaker.

S-W: Very good. The treatment of articulation disorders starts with the selection of individual target sounds or specific patterns. The clinician then selects **antecedent stimulus events** including pictures, objects, modeling, manual guidance, phonetic placement, and moto-kinesthetic cues. What is the actual starting point of treatment?

N-H: Well, three variations were discussed. First, some clinicians train **auditory discrimination training** followed by **production training**. Others train only production. Second, some clinicians start training at the **sound level**. Others start it at the **syllable** or **word level**. Third, some clinicians start training on **multiple sounds,** whereas others train only one sound at a time.

S-W: Good. Most clinicians, however, simplify the target response in some way. For this and other reasons, treatment follows a general sequence of training at the sound, syllable, word, phrase, and conversational speech levels.

N-H: In most treatment programs, the clinician reinforces correct responses and gives corrective feedback for incorrect responses.

S-W: That is correct. Throughout the training, the clinician probes the correct production of sounds in untrained words to assess generalization. To help clients maintain their target responses in natural settings, members of the family may be trained to reinforce correct productions at home and other places. The clients dismissed from therapy are followed up and, if necessary, booster treatment is given.

The Outlook

N-H: Dr. Speech-Wisely, I am not sure I want to major in communicative disorders. I am hoping that this course will help me make a decision. What does a non-major gain from learning about articulation disorders?

S-W: You gain a lot even if you do not major in communicative disorders. This kind of knowledge can be useful to any person, in any profession. You know now that a child who mispronounces words may have an articulation disorder in need of treatment. If you become a teacher, a physician, a psychologist, or a counselor, you can identify problems of articulation in children or adults you work with and refer them to speech–language clinicians at the right time. Even people going into careers in business, broadcasting, and journalism must have a basic knowledge of communicative disorders.

N-H: You are right! I never thought of it. I think everyone needs to know something about disorders of communication. If I do decide on majoring in communicative disorders, what more will I learn about disorders of articulation?

S-W: You will learn more about phonetics, the science of speech production. You will learn more about the anatomy and physiology of the articulatory mechanisms. You will have advanced courses in articulation and phonological disorders. You will learn more about treatment and specific methods of treatment.

N-H: Can students observe how disorders of articulation are treated?

S-W: Of course! You can observe treatment of articulation or any other form of communicative disorder in our own speech and hearing clinic.

N-H: When do students get practical experience in treating articulation disorders?

S-W: In some programs, undergraduate students who have taken all the preclinic courses can start their clinical practicum in their senior year. Most students start their clinical practicum at the graduate level.

N-H: How much time does it take to treat a child or an adult?

S-W: It depends on the severity of the articulation disorder, the intelligence of the client, the amount of time the family members spend on assigned tasks, the frequency of treatment sessions in a week, and the duration of each session. Some need just a few weeks of treatment. Others need months of treatment.

N-H: Where can people get treatment for problems of articulation?

S-W: Most children who misarticulate get treatment in public schools. Federal laws mandate speech, language, and hearing services to children with communicative disabilities in public schools. Treatment is also available in speech and hearing departments at major hospitals, many university campuses, and private speech and hearing clinics.

N-H: Is it possible to specialize in articulation disorders?

S-W: Yes. Disorders of articulation is one of the areas in which clinicians specialize. You can get a doctoral degree with specialization in articulation disorders and do research.

N-H: Well, I think I have taken a lot of your time. Thank you.

S-W: You are welcome.

Study Questions

1. Distinguish between speech perception and speech production.

2. Describe the visually reinforced head turn procedure.

3. Four- to 17-week-old infants can discriminate between vowels ____ and ____, and between ____ and ____.

4. One- to 4-month-old infants cannot discriminate between ____ and ____ or between ____ and ____.

5. At what age are infants able to discriminate between sounds not used in their language?

6. Define articulation or phonological disorders.

7. Why is there a discrepancy between the sounds of English and the English alphabet?

8. Why was the International Phonetic Alphabet created? What are its advantages?

9. Define phonology.

10. Define a phoneme. Give an example.

11. What are allophones?

12. What is common to all vowels?

13. What is a diphthong?

14. How are consonants produced?

15. The manner of articulation yields _____ major categories.

16. Stops are also known as _____.

17. What are fricatives? Give an example.

18. What is a common characteristic of all nasal sounds?

19. Describe at least two categories of sounds identified under the "manner of articulation."

20. What are glides? How are they produced?

21. What are linguadentals? How are they produced?

22. Define distinctive features. Give at least two examples.

23. What is meant by the statement that the distinctive features are binary?

24. Distinguish between the cross-sectional and longitudinal methods of studying the acquisition of speech sounds.

25. Before age 3, children use most if not all of the _____.

26. Among the consonants, the _____ are acquired the earliest.

27. What class of sounds are mastered the last?

28. What are phonological processes? Give two examples.

29. What are functional articulation disorders?

30. Define omissions, substitutions, and distortions.

31. Summarize the research on the etiology of articulation disorders.

32. What is ankyloglossia?

33. What is malocclusion?

34. What is dysarthria? What are its characteristics?

35. What is a tongue thrust?

36. Distinguish between articulation screening and assessment.

37. List the steps involved in making as assessment of articulation disorders.

38. Give a brief description of articulation assessment.

39. Defend the statement that a difference in the production of speech sounds does not necessarily suggest an articulation disorder.

40. Why is it that a child speaking African American English, though producing certain speech sounds differently, does not necessarily exhibit an articulation disorder?

41. What are antecedent stimulus events?

42. Define the phonetic placement method.

43. Define the moto-kinesthetic method.

44. In the sensory-motor method, at what level is treatment started?

45. Give a brief description of the paired-stimuli method.

46. In treatment sessions, what are the two kinds of feedback given by the clinician to the client?

47. Distinguish between time-out and response cost.

48. What are probes?

References

Art, P. B., & Goodban, M. J. (1976). A comparative study of articulation acquisition as based on a study of 240 normals, age three to six. *Language, Speech, and Hearing Services in Schools, 7*, 173–180.

Baker, R. D., & Ryan, B. P. (1971). *Programmed conditioning for articulation.* Monterey, CA: Monterey Learning Systems.

Bankson, N. W., & Bernthal, J. B. (1990). *Bankson–Bernthal Test of Phonology.* Chicago: Riverside Press.

Bernthal, J. E., & Bankson, N. W. (1998). *Articulation and phonological disorders* (4th ed.). Needham Heights, MA: Allyn & Bacon.

Blache, S. E. (1989). A distinctive feature approach. In N. A. Creaghead, P. W. Newman, & W. Secord (Eds.), *Assessment and remediation of articulatory and phonological disorders* (2nd ed., pp. 361–382). Columbus, OH: Merrill.

Bradley, D. P. (1989). A systematic multiple-phoneme approach. In N. A. Craighead, P. W. Newman, & W. Secord (Eds.), *Assessment and remediation of articulatory and phonological disorders* (2nd ed., pp. 305–322). Columbus, OH: Merrill.

Chomsky, N., & Halle, M. (1968). *The sound pattern of English.* New York: Harper & Row.

Creaghead, N. A., Newman, P. W., & Secord, W. (Eds.). (1989). *Assessment and remediation of articulatory and phonological disorders* (2nd ed.). Columbus, OH: Merrill.

Elbert, M., & Gierut, J. (1986). *Handbook of clinical phonology.* San Diego: College-Hill Press.

Fisher, H. B., & Logemann, J. A. (1971). *The Fisher–Logemann Test of Articulation Competence.* Boston: Houghton Mifflin.

Fudala, J., & Reynolds, W. (1986). *The Arizona Articulation Proficiency Scale–Second Edition.* Los Angeles: Western Psychological Services.

Goldman, R., & Fristoe, M. (1986). *Goldman–Fristoe Test of Articulation.* Circle Pines, MN: American Guidance Service.

Hall, P. K., Jordan, L. S., & Robin, D. A. (1993). *Developmental apraxia of speech.* Austin, TX: PRO-ED.

Hegde, M. N. (1998). *Treatment procedures in communicative disorders* (3rd ed.). Austin, TX: PRO-ED.

Hodson, B. W. (1986a). *The Assessment of Phonological Processes–Revised.* Austin, TX: PRO-ED.

Hodson, B. W. (1986b). *Assessment of Phonological Processes–Spanish.* San Diego: Los Amigos Associates.

Hodson, B. W. (1986c). *Computer analysis of phonological processes.* Stonington, IL: Phono-Comp.

Ingram, D. (1981). *Procedures for the phonological analysis of children's language.* Baltimore: University Park Press.

Jakobson, R., Fant, G., & Halle, M. (1952). *Preliminaries to speech analysis* (2nd ed.). Cambridge, MA: MIT Press.

Khan, L., & Lewis, N. (1986). *Khan–Lewis Phonological Analysis.* Circle Pines, MN: American Guidance Service.

Kuhl, P. (1987). Perception of speech and sound in early infancy. In P. Salapatek & L. Cohen (Eds.), *Handbook of infant perception: From perception to cognition* (Vol. 2). New York: Academic Press.

McCabe, R. B., & Bradley, D. P. (1975). Systematic multiple phonemic approach to articulation therapy. *Acta Symbolica, 6,* 2–18.

McDonald, E. T. (1964a). *Articulation testing and treatment: A sensory-motor approach.* Pittsburgh: Stanwix House.

McDonald, E. T. (1964b). *A Deep Test of Articulation.* Pittsburgh: Stanwix House.

McLean, J. E. (1970). Extending stimulus control of phoneme articulation by operant techniques. *Asha Monographs, 14,* 24–47.

Mowrer, D. (1989). The behavioral approach to treatment. In N. A. Creaghead, P. W. Newman, & W. Secord (Eds.), *Assessment and remediation of articulatory and phonological disorders* (2nd ed., pp. 159–192). Columbus, OH: Merrill.

Peña-Brooks, A., & Hegde, M. N. (2000). *Assessment and treatment of articulation and phonological disorders in children.* Austin, TX: PRO-ED.

Pendergast, K., Dickey, S., Selmar, J., & Soder, A. (1997). *Photo Articulation Test–Second Edition.* Austin, TX: PRO-ED.

Poole, I. (1934). Genetic development of articulation of consonant sounds in speech. *Elementary English Review, 11,* 159–161.

Prather, E. M., Hedrick, D. L., & Kern, C. (1975). Articulation development in children aged two to four years. *Journal of Speech and Hearing Disorders, 40,* 179–191.

Preisser, D. A., Hodson, B. W., & Paden, E. (1988). The developmental phonology: 18–24 months. *Journal of Speech and Hearing Disorders, 53,* 125–130.

Sander, E. (1972). When are speech sounds learned? *Journal of Speech and Hearing Disorders, 37,* 55–63.

Shriberg, L., & Kwiatkowski, J. (1980). *Natural Process Analysis.* New York: Wiley.

Smit, A. B., Hand, J. J., Freilinger, J. J., Bernthal, J. E., & Bird, A. (1990). The Iowa articulation norms project and its Nebraska replication. *Journal of Speech and Hearing Research, 26,* 486–500.

Sommers, R. K. (1983). *Articulation disorders.* Englewood Cliffs, NJ: Prentice Hall.

Stoel-Gammon, C. (1985). Phonetic inventories, 15–24 months: A longitudinal study. *Journal of Speech and Hearing Research, 28,* 505–512.

Stoel-Gammon, C., & Dunn, C. (1985). *Normal and disordered phonology in children.* Austin, TX: PRO-ED.

Templin, M. (1957). *Certain language skills in children: Their development and interrelationships* (Institute of Child Welfare Monograph No. 26). Minneapolis: University of Minnesota Press.

Templin, M., & Darley, F. L. (1969). *The Templin–Darley Tests of Articulation.* Iowa City: Bureau of Educational Research and Services, University of Iowa.

Tizard, W. (1980). *Webster's new world dictionary of the American language.* New York: IDG Books Worldwide.

Van Riper, C., & Emerick, L. (1984). *Speech correction: An introduction to speech pathology and audiology.* Englewood Cliffs, NJ: Prentice Hall.

Weiner, F. (1979). *Phonological process analysis.* Baltimore: University Park Press.

Weiner, F. (1984). *Process analysis by computer* [Computer program]. State College, PA: Parrot Software.

Wellman, B., Case, I., Mengurt, I., & Bradbury, D. (1931). *Speech sounds of young children.* University of Iowa studies in child welfare. Iowa City: University of Iowa.

Weston, A. J., & Irwin, J. V. (1985). Paired-stimuli treatment. In P. W. Newman, N. A. Creaghead, & W. Secord (Eds.), *Assessment and remediation of articulatory and phonological disorders* (pp. 337–368). Columbus, OH: Merrill.

Williams, G., & McReynolds, L. V. (1975). The relationship between discrimination and articulation training in children with misarticulations. *Journal of Speech and Hearing Research, 18,* 401–412.

Winitz, H. (1984). Auditory considerations in articulation training. In H. Winitz (Ed.), *Treating articulation disorders: For clinicians by clinicians.* Baltimore: University Park Press.

Language Acquisition and Disorders in Preschool Children

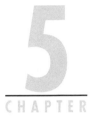

As noted in the previous chapter, the speech sounds are used to form spoken words and sentences, which are the basic structures of oral language. Competency in oral communication requires mastery in the complex and organized system called language. The questions of how most children easily acquire mastery in using this system and how some children find it an extremely difficult task to accomplish have been fascinating to investigate but challenging to provide answers for. Consider the stories told by two children presented in the next section to demonstrate the difference between children in the two groups: those with normal and those with deficient language skills.

Tales of Two Children

While being shown pictures, the two children were told a story called "There Is No Such Thing as a Dragon." The children were then asked to retell the story while looking at the same pictures. (Note the ages of the two children.)

 Erika, Age 5

Billy woke up one morning and found a small dragon in his room. He told his mother about it. But the mother said, "There is no such thing as a dragon." When Billy began to eat breakfast, the dragon sat on the table. The dragon ate all the pancakes. The mother did not say anything because she did not believe in dragons. The dragon became bigger. Soon, the dragon filled the house. When the dragon got hungry, he just ran after a bakery truck. See, the dragon is carrying the house! When Billy's dad came home for lunch, the house was not there! Daddy went looking for the house. Here he finds it! Billy and his mom wave from the upstairs window. They came down, stepping on the dragon's head and neck. Daddy asked "What happened?" Billy said, "It was the dragon." He patted it on the head. The dragon then became small like a kitten. The mother said dragons this size are OK!

 Erick, Age 9

Billy see dragon in room. Mother say no dragon. Dragon ate pancake. Dragon big. Dragon carry house. He hungry. Daddy say, "Where is house?" Daddy look for house. He find it here. Daddy say, "What happen?" Billy say, "Dragon." Dragon small.

By the time they are 5 or 6 years of age, most children, like Erika, will have mastered the basic structure of their language. By this time, the children have a vocabulary that serves them well and startles adults on occasion. Although they continue to learn and refine certain aspects of language, a majority of 6-year-old children speak in grammatically complete sentences. They can take part in conversations and use language appropriately in most social situations. These are the children with normal or better than normal language skills. These children are the subjects of this chapter.

At the same time there are children, like Erick, who do not fully acquire the language spoken around them. Some children are silent companions of those who talk incessantly. Others say a few words but do not combine words into phrases and sentences. Some children use simpler or broken sentences. These children omit various grammatical elements of language. The children are not sure of word meanings and do not always understand what they hear. They are often not sure of what to say or when to say it. They cannot take part in conversations. These are the children with language disorders. These children also are the subjects of this chapter.

The Study of Language Acquisition

Susan was delighted when her professor Dr. Sol Logos asked if she would be interested in a research assistantship. Dr. Logos said that he was studying language acquisition in young children and was looking for a research assistant. Susan thought that the research assistantship would help pay some bills and allow her to gain valuable experience. So she agreed to help.

Once every 2 weeks, Susan and Dr. Logos went to the homes of 4 young children. They carried portable video recording equipment, a high-quality audiotape recorder, and a separate notebook for each child. They spent about 45 minutes in each home.

Dr. Logos had been collecting data on alternate Tuesdays for the past 3 months. The research would be continued for the next 2 years or so. He had selected 4 children who were, at the beginning of the study, ages 16, 22, 24, and 26 months. But all of them were using mostly single-word utterances at the beginning of the study. Both parents of all 4 children were college graduates and the mothers worked at home.

On this Tuesday morning, Susan and Dr. Logos loaded the equipment into his minivan and drove off to Matt's home. At 29 months, Matt was their oldest subject. Matt's mother, Mrs. Tanner, had set up the living room the way Dr. Logos wanted it. There were several of Matt's toys. There were some children's books with many big pictures in them. Susan and Dr. Logos quickly set up the video and audio recording equipment. Susan and Matt's mother sat on the floor with Matt and began their conversation with him. Their job was to stimulate Matt to talk. They used pictures and toys to strike a conversation. They also performed various actions to evoke speech from him. They asked many questions and answered Matt's questions. For example, today Susan made one of the puppets walk and asked Matt what the puppet was doing. "Walking," said Matt. Mrs. Tanner took a cup and pretended to drink out of it. "What is Mommy doing?" asked Susan. "Mommy drinking," replied Matt. When shown a picture of two boots, Matt said, "Boots." When he saw something in the book that he did not understand, he asked, "What dat?" The mother made a male toy run and, after a few seconds, stopped the action. When she asked Matt, "What did he do?" Matt said, "He runned."

While Susan and Mrs. Tanner evoked various kinds of speech from Matt, Dr. Logos wrote down in the notebook everything Matt said. Sometimes he wrote down what Matt was looking at or the question asked of Matt. He made sure that the video camera remained focused on the three people. Occasionally, he would ask Matt a question.

The session lasted about 40 minutes. Matt was talkative. He named things and actions, answered questions, and asked about many things and events Susan and Mrs. Tanner manipulated. Dr. Logos thought that they had a good language sample from Matt.

The next home Susan and Dr. Logos visited was Jenny's. At 19 months, Jenny Thomas was the youngest and the most advanced child. When the familiar research team arrived, Jenny was ready for them. As soon as the team stepped in, Jenny asked "Like some coffee?" to which Dr. Logos replied, "Yes, please." Jenny asked Susan, "What about you?" Susan said, "No, thanks." Jenny then told Mrs. Thomas, "Only one cup, Mom."

Jenny could say many more words than most children her age. She was already talking in simple sentences. Susan placed a small toy truck in a box and asked Jenny, "Where is the truck?" Jenny replied, "It's in the box." When she was playing with some blocks, Jenny's mother asked, "What are you doing?" Jenny said, "Can't you see? I am playing with blocks. I am building a house."

Jenny could use pronouns (*I, me, you*), prepositions (*in, on, under*), regular plurals (*blocks*), present progressive *ing* (play*ing*), auxiliaries (*is* as in "The boy *is* walking"), articles (*a, the*), and many other grammatical features. She had begun to use most of these features in the last month or so.

After about 30 minutes of recording Jenny's speech, Susan and Dr. Logos took a lunch break. At 1 P.M., they visited their third subject, Nate, and at 2 P.M. they visited their last subject, Kathy.

The next morning, at 9 A.M., Susan came to Dr. Logos's laboratory. Viewing both the tapes and the notes taken by Dr. Logos, Susan entered everything each child said into a computer on which the data were stored. With Susan's help, Dr. Logos would later analyze the data.

Dr. Logos and Susan were studying language acquisition in 4 young children. Once every 2 weeks, each child's language was sampled and stored on a computer disk. Dr. Logos had planned on observing the same children for a period of 2 years or more. The researchers did not do anything to speed up language

The more expensive and time-consuming **longitudinal** method gives detailed, child-specific information.

acquisition; they simply observed and recorded what the children said. This is the **longitudinal method** of studying language acquisition. In the longitudinal method a small number of children are repeatedly observed over a long period of time. Sometimes, a single child may be observed for months or years. Recorded language samples are analyzed to see when (at what age) children begin to produce new language responses, the sequence in which they produce different language responses, and the overall pattern of language acquisition.

Dr. Logos had earlier studied language acquisition in a different way. He had studied 60 children who were in the age range from 2 years to 3 years 6 months. He had four subgroups of 20 children each. The age of the children in the first through the fourth group was 2 years, 2 years 6 months, 3 years, and 3 years 6 months. He visited each child only once and recorded a 10-minute conversational sample from each child. He also administered a standardized test of language development. The conversational speech samples and the test results were used to analyze language acquisition in the age range from 2 years to 3 years 6 months. Dr. Logos did not wait to see the same 24-month-old child to show changes in language as he or she grew older. He had different children at different age levels. This is the **cross-sectional method** in which many subjects are selected from different age levels and are studied simultaneously for a relatively brief duration.

Using the longitudinal and cross-sectional methods, researchers have studied ages at which specific language behaviors are acquired and the sequence in which they are acquired. The term language acquisition, however, is too broad. What exactly is acquired? There are different answers to this question because language acquisition researchers have studied different aspects of language. However, most researchers have generally studied the various linguistic components of language including preverbal behaviors, semantic features, grammatical structures, and pragmatic aspects.

Acquisition of Preverbal Behaviors

The **preverbal behaviors** are those that precede the production of words and phrases. An infant, even a newborn, is highly vocal. The infant's cry is a powerful communicator. Older children who have not acquired language often cry and whine to express themselves. However, an infant's cry is a reflexive response to pain, hunger, and discomfort. Its communicative effects are limited.

Most researchers have focused on babbling as the most significant preverbal behavior. When well fed, happy, dry, and lying on his or her back, a 4-month-old baby typically spends much time making various kinds of vocal sounds. This is called **babbling.** The baby typically produces strings of consonant–vowel combinations such as "babababa" or "nananana." A parent–child response-loop is commonly observed during this stage. For example, the mother says "bababababa" and the baby imitates it; in turn, the mother imitates the baby's production, which the baby repeats (McLaughlin, 1998; Owens, 1996).

Experimental research has shown that babbling can be increased by social reinforcement. For example, a mother who gently tickles, smiles, or picks up the baby as soon as the baby babbles often sees an increase in babbling (Schumaker & Sherman, 1978).

Babbling increases between 4 and 10 months. Also, it becomes more complex and varied. New sounds are heard in babbling. Many speechlike sounds appear in late babbling. Babies first produce the labial stop sounds (/p/, /b/) and

---

*The faster and less expensive **cross-sectional** method is not suitable to study changes over time in individual children.*

*A **linguistic definition** of language is that it is a mental or cognitive system of rules. The system consists of codes or symbols that help represent objects, events, and relations.*

*A **behavioral definition** of language is that it is verbal behavior shaped and maintained by a verbal community.*

*Review **Chapter 1** for definition and description of language.*

eventually fricative consonants (/f/, /s/). Research data suggest that babbling and early speech–language production are closely related (McLaughlin, 1998; Owens, 1996; Sachs, 2001).

By the end of the first year, most babies are communicating with a variety of means. The baby's gestures, noises, sounds, and eye contact are full of messages for the parents. The baby points to things wanted. A child who can walk begins to physically move the parents to indicate the needs. For example, a child takes the mother's hand and leads her to the toy chest to get something out of it.

The First Words

On the average, children produce their first words around 12 months, although there are significant individual differences. The first few words are related to children's world of things and events. These words tend to be names of toys, animals, and food items (McLaughlin, 1998; Owens, 1996). The words "mama" and "dada" are likely to be among the first few words. Verbs, or action words (*give, do*), although fewer, also are part of the first 50 words. Children are quick to learn words that are easily pronounced and those that name objects or animals that move. For example, children learn such words as *dog, cat, car,* and *choo choo* earlier than *kitchen* or *sofa*. Most children produce about 50 words by the age of 18 months, although individual children differ.

Two-Word Utterances

Around the age of 18 months, most children begin to produce two-word phrases by combining words they already know. The two-word utterances signal the beginning of **syntax,** which is arranging words in proper order to form meaningful sentences.

The word order in the two-word utterances of young children may differ from that in adult speech. A child may produce expressions that are uncommon in adult speech. Generally, single-word utterances lack certain grammatical features. For example, "Mommy hat" and "Daddy shoe" lack the possessive inflection ('s). Because they lack one or more grammatical features, two-word phrases are not grammatically complete sentences. However, it often is not possible to determine the missing feature because the child's phrases can be translated into different sentences. For example, "Mommy eat" may be translated into "Mommy eat*s*" or "Mommy *is* eat*ing*" or some other sentence.

Experts depend on the **context of an utterance** to determine the meaning of children's ambiguous productions. For example, if the mother is eating and the child is asked the question "What is Mommy doing?" the child's reply "Mommy eat" may mean "Mommy *is* eating." The situation in which an utterance is produced usually provides a clue to the meaning.

Speech that does not include required grammatical features is called **telegraphic speech.** The speech is like telegrams, in which words that are not essential for communication are omitted. In a child's telegraphic speech, various grammatical features are missing. The child may use nouns, adjectives, and verbs but omit articles (*a, the*), conjunctions (*and, but*), and inflections (possessive 's, past tense *ed*). As children acquire various grammatical features of language, their speech becomes less telegraphic. Their utterances become

Examples of **two-word utterances:**
"more high"
"Daddy shoe"
"all gone"
"Mommy come"
"no wet"
"there kitty"
"see doggie"

grammatically more correct. The length of their utterances increases. More complex grammatical features become part of their sentences.

Acquisition of Grammatic Morphemes

Morphemes, as defined in Chapter 1, are the smallest meaningful units of language. All words are morphemes. Most words also are single morphemes. Single morphemes of language that can stand alone and convey meaning are called free morphemes. For example, the word *cat* is a single morpheme; its isolated production can be meaningful. It cannot be broken down into a smaller element without destroying its meaning.

Grammatic morphemes, though important in producing meaningful sentences, are not meaningful when produced alone. For example, the **present progressive** *ing* is a grammatic morpheme. Isolated production of *ing* makes no sense, but a similar production of *cat* makes some sense. Other grammatic morphemes include inflections of English language: adding /s/ to a word to make it a plural (*cup* vs. cups); adding /ed/ to a word to indicate past tense (*walk* vs. walk*ed*); adding /s/ to a word to indicate possession (*Mommy* vs. Mommy's); articles *a* and *the;* and prepositions (*in, on, under*). These grammatic morphemes are usually not produced by themselves. They are added to other morphemes (words). Therefore, they are called **bound morphemes.** A word is *inflected* by adding a bound morpheme to a free morpheme. This action changes or modifies the meaning. For example, when you add /ed/ to the word *walk,* the tense and, hence, the meaning changes.

Brown (1973) conducted a well-known study of the acquisition of selected grammatic morphemes. The research of Sol Logos described earlier is modeled after Brown's research, although many others have used similar methods. Brown selected 3 children, Adam, Eve, and Sarah, and studied them for approximately 3 years to trace the development of 14 grammatic morphemes. When the study was started, the children were of different ages. Eve was the youngest at 18 months, and Adam and Sarah were older at 27 months. But all 3 were at the same level of language production, highlighting the hazards of describing language development strictly in terms of the age of children. Visiting the children in their home once every 2 weeks, Brown recorded language samples and analyzed the stages of development.

In measuring the changes in language produced by the children, Brown used a concept called the **mean length of utterance (MLU).** The MLU is the average length of a child's multiple utterances; the length is measured in terms of morphemes, both bound and free. For example, the utterance "Mommy come!" has two free morphemes, both individual words; but the utterance "Mommy's hat" has three (*Mommy* and *hat,* two free morphemes, both individual words, plus the possessive *'s,* a bound morpheme, not an independent word). MLU is widely used to measure language acquisition and language behaviors in children. Two children exhibiting the same MLU are at the same level of language acquisition.

According to Brown's analysis, the children acquired the morphemes in roughly the same sequence. For example, all 3 mastered the production of the present progressive *ing* before the other morphemes. The children next mastered the prepositions *in* and *on.* Then they mastered the regular plural inflection, followed by irregular past tense and other morphemes. The contractible copula and the contractible auxiliary were the last morphemes the children mastered. The average order of acquisition of the 14 morphemes and examples are given in Table 5.1.

A cross-sectional study by de Villiers and de Villiers (1973) showed similar (but not the same) sequence of acquisition of the 14 morphemes Brown studied. Most researchers have concluded that the order of acquisition of grammatic morphemes Brown described is fairly typical of most normally developing children. Nonetheless, this order of acquisition is not invariable across children nor is it insensitive to environmental input as Brown and others often claimed in the 1970s and 1980s. Much subsequent research has shown that the order of acquisition can be changed by explicitly teaching more advanced grammatical features to young children (Hegde, 1993) and that parents normally implicitly teach language to their children in various ways (Moerk, 1983, 1992).

Acquisition of Complex Forms of Language

Generally, the morphemes acquired earlier are grammatically and semantically simpler than those acquired later. As the child acquires more complex grammatic morphemes, including articles, copulas, and auxiliary verbs, the child's utterances become longer and more complex.

The morphemes learned later are used in more complex utterances. For example, the auxiliary *is* cannot typically be used in combination with just

Table 5.1

Average Order of Acquisition of 14 Grammatical
Morphemes in Three Children

Order of Acquisition	Morphemes	Examples	Age of Mastery (Months)
1	Present progressive *ing*	Daddy com*ing*	19–28
2/3	Prepositions (*in, on*)	Car *in* box Book *on* table	27–30
4	Regular plural inflection	My book*s*	24–33
5	Irregular past	Came, went, sat, broke	25–46
6	Possessive	Daddy*'s* hat	26–40
7	Uncontractible copula	It is!	27–39
8	Articles	I want *a* cookie. Give me *the* ball.	28–46
9	Regular past *ed*	I pour*ed* the milk.	26–48
10	Regular third-person *s*	Daddy cook*s*.	26–46
11	Irregular third person	Does, has	28–50
12	Uncontractible auxiliary	He *was* painting.	29–48
13	Contractible copula	He *is* nice. or He*'s* nice.	29–49
14	Contractible auxiliary	Mommy *is* coming. or Mommy*'s* coming.	30–50

Note. Adapted from *A First Language: Early Stages,* by R. Brown, 1973, Cambridge, MA: Harvard University Press.

another word (unless it is an emphatic assertion as in *"He is!"*). It typically is a part of a grammatically complete sentence: *"The boy is running."* Unless the child already produces nouns (*girl, boy, dog*) and verbs (*running, walking*), the auxiliary *is* is useless. Therefore, a child who produces auxiliaries correctly is already using simple sentence forms.

The articles, auxiliaries, copulas, present progressive *ing*, prepositions, and regular past tense morphemes, among others, make it possible for the child to produce a variety of sentences. In subsequent stages of language acquisition, the child begins to produce other sentence forms, including the **negative sentences** and **questions**.

Note that the use of double or multiple negatives is accepted adult usage in African American English.

Negative sentences involve a semantic notion called **negation**. Even before a negative sentence is produced, the child will express this semantic notion by saying, "No!" The negative sentence forms emerge in several stages. In the beginning, the child is more likely to add *no* to other words (*No car, Not Mommy, No go*). In the next stage of development, the child begins to insert the negative within a phrase or sentence. The child produces such utterances as "He no like it" and "I no want milk." After having mastered the auxiliary, the child begins to produce grammatically correct negative sentences like "Boy is not running" or "Kitty is not eating." Whereas most of these negative forms are mastered during the preschool years, more complex forms are not acquired by the time a child enters school. These include the indefinite negative forms (*nobody, no one, none,* and *nothing*). Many elementary school-age children continue to say, "I don't want none" and "Nobody don't like me."

Grammatically, there are many kinds of questions, and one kind is grammatically not a question at all but used as such by a change in intonation. For example, you can change the affirmative sentence *you are smart* into a question by saying it with a rising intonation (the pitch of the voice is raised at the end of the sentence). Children often ask this type of question (*"No cookie?" "Mommy gone?"*). The most frequently used questions are called the *wh*-questions: *what, why, when, who, whose, which, where,* and *how*. These questions require the use of the auxiliary and the placement of the *wh*-word at the beginning of sentences.

The first questions of young children do not contain the auxiliary. Such expressions as "What dat?" for "What *is* that" are frequently heard. In the next stage, the child is likely to ask a question by simply starting an otherwise affirmative phrase or sentence with a *why*. Therefore, a child is likely to ask, "Why she is crying?" and "Where we are going?" Children generally acquire *what, where,* and *who* earlier than *when, how,* and *why*. It has been hypothesized that *what, where,* and *who* questions are semantically simpler than *when, how,* and *why* questions.

By the time they enter the first grade, most children will have learned the major grammatic morphemes and sentence structures. They also will have begun to understand and produce more complex forms of sentences. However, many complex or unusual forms of sentences may not be fully mastered by the age of 6 or 7 years. Children continue to learn new forms of more advanced sentence forms throughout the early school years.

Acquisition of Pragmatic Aspects of Language

Recall that **pragmatics** is the study of social use of language.

It is not enough for a child to learn words, phrases, grammatical features, and various forms of sentences. The child also should learn to use language in social situations. Chapter 1 contains a description of the pragmatic component of language. The pragmatic view is concerned with how children learn to use language in social situations to communicate effectively.

Initially, a baby's communication may be **unintentional.** That is, the baby may not do something to affect a caregiver's behavior. For example, a baby who cries because he or she is wet is not doing so to make the caregiver change the diaper, though the caregiver might do just that. The same cry, however, may be **intentional** when it is exhibited to get attention. Generally, social communication is intentional; its simpler forms, which often are nonverbal, may be found early in life. By 3 weeks of age, the infant begins to show signs of social smile. Such smiles, gestures, and other nonverbal behaviors are among the early attempts at intentional communication.

Babies 8 to 10 months of age show more definitive evidence of intentional communication. Around this age, the child's speech begins to serve specific **functions.** In the pragmatic view, functions are roughly the same as purposes or intentions. For example, speech serves the purpose of getting various kinds of help from others. This is called the **instrumental function** of language ("I want it"). Through speech, children come to control other people's behavior. This is the **regulatory function** ("Stop it!"). Research has shown that instrumental and regulatory functions develop early (McLaughlin, 1998; Owens, 1996). Through speech, children quickly learn to regulate and control events and people.

Experts have studied the development of many complex pragmatic language behaviors, including **dialogue** or **discourse.** An aspect of dialogue is **turn-taking,** which is a conversational skill that develops over several years. Turn-taking implies that there is a time to express verbally or nonverbally, and there is a time to listen and watch. Communication consists of a sequence of behaviors. Two or more people involved in this sequence know when to express and when to watch and listen. Many children in the age range of 18 to 24 months are able to take turns in conversation. However, more refined turn-taking behavior may not develop until the child is 5 or 6 years old.

Extended dialogue not only requires turn-taking but also **topic maintenance,** which is continued conversation on the same topic for socially acceptable durations. The child who has not yet learned this pragmatic skill may shift the topic of conversation abruptly or interject unrelated comments. Most 3-year-old children are able to maintain the topic of conversation for at least some time, although frequent shifts are common. Children 4 to 5 years of age can maintain the topic of conversation for longer periods of time.

Many other pragmatic skills continue to be acquired over the school years. All skills improve as the child gains more experience in the social use of language (Gleason, 2001; Hulit & Howard, 1993; McLaughlin, 1998).

Individual Differences in Language Acquisition

Although researchers have identified broad stages and patterns of language acquisition across children, a major characteristic of language acquisition is that children differ from each other. Each child has a characteristic pattern of language acquisition, which may be different from those of other children.

Individual differences are evident in the rate of acquisition as well as in the acquisition of specific aspects of language. Within normal limits, some children are slower than others. Some children's words are more intelligible than the words of other children. A number of children use gestures more often than others. A few children persist with single words longer than others who quickly begin to combine words into sentences. Some children make more word order mistakes than others.

Compared to other children, some talk more readily, talk more, or talk more often. Depending on the individual child, speech may be characteristically brief or elaborate. In essence, the kinds of differences adults show in their use of language also are seen in children.

The major milestones of language acquisition are presented in Table 5.2. The summary must be understood in light of the individual differences in language acquisition. Therefore, the milestones generally apply to groups of children, not necessarily to an individual child.

Table 5.2

The Major Milestones of Language Acquisition in Children

Age Range	Typical Language Behaviors
0–1 months	Startle response to sound; quieted by human voice
2–3 months	Cooing, production of some vowel sounds; response to speech; babbling
4–6 months	Babbling strings of syllables; imitation of sounds; variations in pitch and loudness
7–9 months	Comprehension of some words and simple requests; increased imitation of speech sounds; may say or imitate "mama" or "dada"
10–12 months	Understanding of "No"; response to requests; response to own name; production of one or more words
13–15 months	Production of 5 to 10 words, mostly nouns; appropriate pointing responses
16–18 months	Following simple directions; production of two-word phrases; production of 20 or more words
19–22 months	Response to two-step directions; production of 50 single words; production of *I* and *mine*
2–2.6 years	Response to some yes/no questions; naming of everyday objects; production of phrases and incomplete sentences; production of the present progressive, prepositions, regular plural, and negation "no" or "not"
3–3.6 years	Production of 3- to 4-word sentences; production of the possessive morpheme, several forms of questions, negatives *can't* and *don't*; comprehension of *why, who, whose,* and *how many*; and initial productions of most grammatic morphemes
3.6–5 years	Greater mastery of articles, different tense forms, copula auxiliary, third-person singular, and other grammatic morphemes; production of grammatically complete sentences

Summary

- Through the cross-sectional and longitudinal methods, researchers have noted broad patterns of language acquisition.

- Certain language skills are learned earlier than other skills. Generally, simpler forms are learned before more complex forms are learned.

- Many times, the child learns several aspects of the language simultaneously. While the vocabulary is expanding rapidly, new sentence forms are learned and certain pragmatic aspects also are mastered. The child's language becomes more complex as he or she grows older.

- By age 5 or 6, a majority of children will have acquired the basic forms and functions of language.

- Children continue to acquire more complex forms of language and advanced pragmatic skills throughout their school years.

Theories of Language Acquisition

Though much needs to be known, scientists have a fairly clear understanding of *what* is learned in the language acquisition process. What is not so clear is *how* language is acquired, though there is no dearth of theories of language acquisition. Because a comprehensive review of theories will not be attempted here, the reader is referred to other sources for further information (Gleason, 2001; Hulit & Howard, 1993; McLaughlin, 1998; Moerk, 1983, 1992; Owens, 1996). A few differing viewpoints are sketched below.

The Nativist Viewpoint

Everyone knows that only humans speak languages. Through their language, people communicate socially. Animals, too, communicate with each other, but this communication is limited. Animals communicate through movements, postures, and limited vocal responses. Although animals, especially chimpanzees, have been taught some surprising forms of communication, the most complex form of oral, manual, and other symbolic communication for which the word *language* is used is found only in humans. Although each language is unique in certain respects, all languages share many universal characteristics. Rules of word formation and word combination, for example, are common to all languages.

It also is known that children normally acquire language rapidly. Within the first 5 to 6 years, children acquire the basic structures and functions of a very complex and abstract system of communication. Most children seem to go through similar sequences of language acquisition, although there are individual differences in the rate of acquisition. It also appears that children do not seem to need or receive systematic and extended instruction in learning to speak. Arguments of this kind have led to a well-known theory of language acquisition: the nativist theory.

The modern nativist theory of language acquisition is based on some ancient ideas because **nativism** is an ancient philosophy. Early Greek thinkers,

See **Chapter 1** for Chomsky's theory of language.

for example, explained human knowledge on the basis of nativism. They suggested that much of human knowledge is **innate,** which means that it is already given when the child is born. Nativism assumes that certain forms of knowledge are not learned.

Chomsky, the linguist who proposed the transformational generative grammar, revived nativism in the study of language. Chomsky (1968) suggested that language is not learned through environmental stimulation, reinforcement, or teaching. The basic knowledge necessary to acquire language is already present at the time a child is born. As already described, Chomsky made a distinction between competence and performance. He said that competence, which includes the knowledge of the rules of universal grammar, is innate. Because of this competence, the child can learn language without much help from the parents, siblings, or other caregivers.

Chomsky's ideas quickly became popular and many other experts who studied language acquisition proposed variations of the basic nativist theory. One such variation states that children are born with an **innate mechanism** of language acquisition, called the **Language Acquisition Device (LAD).** It is a part of all children's biological makeup. The LAD knows much about languages in general because it contains the universal rules of language. The environment provides information about the unique rules of the language the child is exposed to. The LAD then integrates the universal and the unique aspects of the language and thus helps the child learn the language in a relatively short period of time (Bohannon & Bonvillian, 2001; Owens, 1996).

Another variant of the nativist theory is the **cognitive theory. Cognition** includes knowledge and such mental processes as memory and auditory and visual perception. The cognitive theory states that language acquisition is made possible by cognition and general intellectual processes. Unless the child first develops nonlinguistic knowledge of things and events, words to describe them may not be learned. In other words, a child must first acquire concepts before producing words. For example, the child who does not know about a *dog* or a *triangle* is not likely to say those words. According to this view, knowledge comes first and language later.

The cognitive theory also has its variations. Some scientists believe that language is the cause of cognition, not the other way around. According to this viewpoint, concepts are learned through language. Therefore, language comes first and knowledge later. Others think that language and cognition influence each other. Accordingly, concepts may be learned through language, and language learning may be enhanced by nonlinguistic concepts. In essence, scientists have suggested every possible relation between language and cognition (McLaughlin, 1998; Owens, 1996). No single viewpoint has been fully supported by scientific evidence.

The Behavioral Viewpoint

Recall that **mands, tacts,** and so forth are functional units of verbal behavior.

The behavioral viewpoint does not explain the acquisition of *language* because language often is described by linguists and others as a mental system. Scientists who use Skinner's behavioral analysis explain the acquisition of *verbal behavior.* As described in Chapter 1, verbal behavior is categorized not on the basis of structure, but on the basis of function. The different kinds of verbal behaviors are acquired under appropriate conditions of stimulation and social consequences (McLaughlin, 1998; Skinner, 1957; Winokur, 1976).

The behavioral scientists have not been especially interested in the developmental sequence through which verbal behaviors are acquired. These experts believe that it is more important to find out the causes of behaviors than the sequence in which the behaviors are acquired. Instead of studying the ages at which different kinds of verbal behaviors are mastered, the behavior scientists try to determine under what conditions those behaviors are learned.

Behavioral scientists suggest that **learning**, not an innate mechanism, plays a major role in the acquisition of verbal behaviors. They find it difficult to believe that the child has a knowledge of the rules of the universal grammar when neither the child nor the average adult can describe that knowledge. A person acquires the knowledge of the rules of grammar by special study; it is not naturally "given" as innate mechanisms are. Behavior scientists assert that just because a child speaks in grammatically correct sentences does not mean that the child knows the rules of grammar.

The events in the child's environment are more important in the behavioral theory than in the nativist theory. Children learn only the language they are exposed to; severe social deprivation results in language deprivation as well. Practically all forms of verbal behaviors can be increased or decreased experimentally. Social reinforcement, for example, can increase babbling, word and phrase responses, and the production of grammatical features. One of the commonly used methods of teaching language to children with language disorders is to model the correct responses and reinforce the child's correct productions.

Recent research on language acquisition has questioned the nativistic assumption that the environment does not offer much assistance to the child in language acquisition. For example, research on mother–child interactions has suggested the possibility that mothers, fathers, older children, and adults in general may do much to help the child learn language (Moerk, 1983, 1992). It has been shown that mothers (and other caregivers) speak differently when they are addressing younger children than when they are addressing older children or adults. Because of its distinct characteristics, the speech addressed to young children is called *motherese*. While addressing young children, mothers use

- Simple and concrete words
- Greater pitch variations
- Higher pitched voice
- Shorter, simpler sentences
- Slower rate of speech
- Greater fluency of speech
- Clearer enunciation (articulation) of speech

As the child grows older, the mother's speech changes. The speech rate increases, the pitch variations decrease, the words become more complex, the sentences get longer, and the speech is less carefully enunciated and not as conspicuously fluent as before. The mothers also begin to talk more about abstract concepts and relations.

Research on motherese has also shown that mothers are more likely to expand or correct a child's ungrammatical utterances than grammatically correct utterances. Also, children are more likely to imitate mothers' expanded or correct utterances (Bohannon & Bonvillian, 2001). Furthermore, infants and young children attend more to motherese than to adult speech. Possibly, an infant reinforces certain kinds of responses from the mother. If the infant more readily responds to certain kinds of speech from the mother, the mother then is more likely to exhibit those kinds of speech. Research on motherese, therefore, shows the power of interactional patterns that shape the behavior of children as well as their caregivers.

Disorders of Language

When Mrs. Bateson brought her son Todd to the University Speech and Hearing Clinic, he was 2 years 6 months old. The following conversation between a speech–language pathologist (SLP) and Mrs. Bateson (Mrs. B) highlights not only Todd's problem of communication but also the problems of many other children who exhibit language disorders.

SLP: How would you describe Todd's language problem?

MRS. B: Todd is slow in speaking the language. Compared to my daughter Lani at his age, Todd has very little language. When he wants something, Todd makes noises, points to things, or just whines and cries. When he wants to eat or drink something, he may take my hand and lead me to the kitchen or the refrigerator. When I don't understand what he wants, he just fusses. He and I both get frustrated.

SLP: Are there some words he can say?

MRS. B: Only a few. He can say "Mommy" clearly. He also can say "Dada" for *daddy,* "Aani" for *Lani,* "mi" for *milk,* "wawa" for *water,* "ba" for *ball,* and "aggie" for *doggie.* There are a few other words he can say, but not very consistently.

SLP: Does Todd combine words into phrases? For example, has he ever used phrases like "Mommy here" or "Daddy come"?

MRS. B: No, he doesn't. He says only single words.

SLP: Do people understand Todd when he says something?

MRS. B: Not many people can understand him. But I can!

SLP: At what age did he begin to babble? You know the "baba" and "dada" types of sounds babies make?

MRS. B: Yes, I know what babbling is. I once took a course on child development. We discussed the stages of language acquisition in the class. I don't think Todd babbled much before he was 11 months. My daughter babbled a lot when she was only 5 months.

SLP: How old was Todd when he could sit, stand, and walk without support?

MRS. B: I think he did those like any other child. He may have been 7 months old when he sat, 10 or 11 months when he stood up, and a little over a year when he began to walk. At least I didn't think he was much delayed in this respect.

SLP: What about Todd's health? Did he have any major illnesses?

MRS. B: Todd has been a healthy child. He has not had any illnesses. An occasional cold and runny nose, maybe. But nothing serious.

SLP: Do you think Todd can hear well?

MRS. B: I think so. He turns when I call his name. We don't have to speak louder to him. He responds to the sounds and noises around the house.

SLP: Does he understand what you say to him?

MRS. B: He can understand more than he can talk. He understands "Come here," "Let's go," "Dinner is ready," "Where is Daddy?" "Give this to Lani," and things like that. He does what I ask him to do, so I figure he understands the words I speak to him even though he cannot say the same words.

SLP: OK. I will probably ask you more questions later. Now let us spend some time with Todd. I need to observe his speech and record a sample of his language. You and I will use these pictures, objects, and toys to encourage Todd to talk. I also will screen his hearing, look into his mouth, and administer a few tests. We will talk again after all that.

Todd had a language problem. He did not talk like other children of his age. At 2½ years of age, he spoke only a few words. He did not combine words to form phrases or sentences. He often communicated nonverbally; he pointed to things he wanted and used gestures. When people did not understand him, he whined or cried. Some of his words were not fully articulated; only the family members could understand them. However, Todd enjoyed good physical health. He had no significant motor delay.

The clinician found that Todd's oral structures (lips, tongue, teeth, hard and soft palates) appeared normal. Todd passed the hearing screening test, which indicated normal hearing. There were no signs of mental retardation or neurological damage. Physically, Todd was growing as expected. Nonetheless, his language was extremely limited.

A Description of Language Disorders in Children

Limited language skills are described as language delay, language disorder, language impairment, or language problem. Language disorders vary in severity; they are more severe in some children than in others. As we shall see shortly, language disorders in some children may be associated with such physical and sensory disabilities as cerebral palsy and deafness. Other children, like Todd, may be essentially normal in most, if not all, respects and yet exhibit a language problem. Language disorder in children who are otherwise essentially normal is called **specific language disorder** or **disability**. In other cases, the language disorder typically is described in terms of the associated disability or clinical condition: language disorder associated with mental retardation, language disorder associated with hearing impairment, and so forth. A school-age child who has limited language skills is likely to be considered as having a **language learning disability** or simply a **learning disability**.

Children who show language problems are a diverse group. Many potential causes could lead to language disorders. Even within a diagnostic category, such as specific language disability or language disorder associated with mental retardation, individual differences are notable.

Although some technical distinctions can be made between them, we use the terms *language delay, disorders, impairment,* and *problems* to mean the same.

Keeping all such variations and individual differences in perspective, we might say that, among other symptoms, children with language disorders show the following major problems (Hegde, 1996):

- Limited skills in understanding spoken language
- Poor listening skills
- Limited understanding of word meanings and meanings in general
- Limited expressive language skills
- Limited use or lack of use of morphologic elements of language
- Limited use of sentence structures (limited syntactic performance)
- Inappropriate use of language
- Deficient use of language that has been learned
- Limited conversational skills
- Limited skills in narrating experiences

In addition, certain children with language disorders also may experience

- Limited cognitive skills
- Later academic problems (reading and writing problems)
- Some abnormal patterns of language

Aspects of Children's Language Disorders

Phonological disorders are described in **Chapter 4.**

The language problems just listed are typically classified under semantic, syntactic, morphological, and pragmatic aspects of language. In a given child, a language disorder may affect any or all aspects of language. Typically, multiple aspects or skills are affected. Therefore, to gain a better understanding of language disorders, we must look at some of the specific kinds of problems the child shows in semantic, morphological, syntactic, and pragmatic skills of language (Hegde, 1996; Johnston, 1988; McCormick & Schiefelbusch, 1990; Nelson, 1993; Paul, 1995; Reed, 1994; Van Kleek & Richardson, 1988).

Semantic Problems

A slow acquisition of words and word meanings is an early sign of language disorder. The child may not learn to say the first few words until he or she is 2 or even 3 years old. After learning to say words like *Mama, doggie, kitty,* or *nighty-night,* the rate of acquisition of new words may be extremely slow. In other words, the child's vocabulary does not grow at a normal rate. Words that are learned may not be readily used. The child may have difficulty remembering the words.

The semantic problems also are evident in the kinds of words a child with language disability tends to learn. At his or her own slow rate, the child tends to learn simpler and frequently used words faster than more complex and less frequently used words. Concrete words are more readily learned than abstract words. The child's vocabulary may be limited to the names of a few objects (*ball, kitty, truck*) and people (*Mommy, Daddy*), but abstract words (*good, bad, nice, yesterday, holiday*) may be missing.

The child with a language disorder may not understand the meanings of spoken words. Many theorists believe that semantic problems are due to cognitive problems. That is, the child may have difficulty in learning the *concepts* that underlie word meanings.

Morphological Problems

The morphological aspect refers to various ways in which words are formed and modified to change meaning. This aspect also includes grammatic morphemes such as the plural and possessive inflection, articles *the* and *a,* regular past tense (*ed* as in walk*ed*), and many others.

Review **Chapter 1** which describes the structure of language, including the morphological aspects of language.

Difficulty in the acquisition of morphological aspects of language is a dominant aspect of childhood language disorders. The child continues to use words and phrases without adding grammatic morphemes. Consider the following utterances of a 5-year-old child:

- Give me two block. (Plural inflection *s* is missing.)

- Daddy coming home. (Auxiliary *is* is missing.)

- Book on table. (Article *the* is missing.)

- Mommy hat. (Possessive inflection *'s* is missing.)

- Yesterday I walk home. (Past tense *ed* is missing.)

- He goed. (Inappropriate use of regular past tense *ed* in place of the irregular verb *went*.)

- He happy. (Copula *is* is missing.)

- Me going. (Inappropriate pronoun is used.)

When the morphological elements are missing, the utterances become grammatically incomplete. The utterances are more like telegrams; only the most essential words are used and certain grammatical elements are omitted. Therefore, this kind of speech often is described as *telegraphic.*

Syntactic Problems

Syntax is the arrangement of words into meaningful sentences. **Syntactic problems** are difficulties in sentence construction, as expressed in grammatically inappropriate forms. The child with language disorders speaks in short or incomplete sentences. The word order may be incorrect. The child's sentences may lack variety; only simple, active, declarative sentences may be produced. Complex or unusual forms of sentences (such as the passive sentence) may be acquired very late or not at all.

Syntactic problems may be more pronounced in the comprehension of spoken language. The child may be unable to understand longer, complex, or unusual types of sentences.

Pragmatic Problems

Pragmatic aspects of language refer to appropriate use of language in social contexts. Therefore, **pragmatic problems** are those of language use. The child with language disorders may have acquired some language structures but may not appropriately use them in social situations. The limited language the child has acquired may not be used at all or may be used inappropriately.

The child with language disorders is more likely to just respond to questions than to initiate conversation. If another person somehow initiates conversation, the child with language disorders is likely to show poor discourse skills. For example, the child may not maintain a topic of discussion, may interrupt a speaker with irrelevant utterances, and may not take turns in conversation. The child may not appreciate that the listener did not understand what he or she said. Or, the child may not know how to modify statements when they are not understood. As a result, the child may simply repeat the defective utterance. Problems of this kind are described as *pragmatic* problems. Consider the following exchange between a speech–language clinician and a 7-year-old boy with a language disorder:

CLINICIAN: Did you go to school today?

CHILD: Yes.

CLINICIAN: What did you do there?

CHILD: (Merely shrugs his shoulders)

CLINICIAN: Did you do anything special?

CHILD: We play.

CLINICIAN: Don't you play there every day during recess time?

CHILD: Yeah.

CLINICIAN: Did you learn anything new?

CHILD: (Merely shrugs his shoulders)

CLINICIAN: Did the teacher . . .

CHILD: You know what? I got new shoe.

CLINICIAN: When did you buy them?

CHILD: Buy what?

As you can see, the child did not use certain morphological features. The past tense /ed/ (*play* for play*ed*) and the plural inflections (*shoe* for sho*es*) were missing. From a pragmatic standpoint, the child was unable to answer two questions. He probably did not understand the phrase "anything special." The child did not maintain the topic of conversation; he introduced a new topic (concerning his shoes) in the middle of another by interrupting the clinician. But he soon forgot the new topic he had just introduced.

Research has identified many other kinds of pragmatic problems. The child with language disorders has difficulty narrating a story. Contrast the story retold by Erick and Erika, reproduced at the beginning of this chapter. Compared to the sequential and logically consistent story of the 5-year-old Erika, the 9-year-old Erick's story lacked details and sequenced events. The unduly brief story is told in limited words with no progression of events. These also are pragmatic problems.

Summary

Children with language disorders show deficiencies in many aspects of language, including:

- An overall slowness in the acquisition of language

(continues)

- Limited vocabulary

- Omission of many grammatical features and misuse of other grammatical features

- Shorter and simpler word arrangements, limited varieties of sentences

- Inadequate or inappropriate use of the learned language skills

- Problems in comprehending spoken language

Potential Causes and Associated Problems

Like Todd, described earlier in this chapter, many children with language disorders are otherwise normal, while other children have language problems along with other kinds of problems. A growing body of research evidence suggests that language disorders may be a part of inherited conditions. Many genetic syndromes are associated with language disorders. Although a child with language disorders can be of normal intelligence, a child with mental retardation almost always exhibits some deficiency in language. Although a child with language disorders may have normal hearing, children with severe hearing impairments almost always have language problems. Likewise, many children with language disorders may not show severe emotional, behavioral, or psychological problems of the kind seen in autistic children. However, autistic children always have language problems. Finally, although the environment of many children with language disorders may be normal, severe environmental deprivations may be associated with language problems.

It is tempting to conclude that mental retardation, hearing loss, autism, and similar conditions are *causes* of language disorders. They may be causes in a rough sense; had there been no mental retardation, hearing loss, or autism, the child may have acquired language normally. However, we cannot be sure. More important, a child has mental retardation, hearing impairment, or autism *in addition* to language disorder. These conditions and language disorders exist together. It is difficult to separate the cause from the effect, especially in cases of associated congenital organic or genetic problems. Theoretically, causes and effects can be more easily separated when the causes are environmental than when they are genetic or congenital. For example, clinicians can better defend the conclusion that brain injury caused language problems in a child who had normal language skills prior to the injury than the conclusion that mental retardation caused the language problem. Therefore, it is better to describe mental retardation and similar problems as *associated conditions* and not as causes of the language disorder.

Hereditary Factors and Genetic Syndromes

Some research evidence suggests that hereditary (genetic) factors may be involved in language disorders. If a child in a family has a language disorder, other children in the family, especially the brothers of the child with the language disorder, have a higher risk of developing language problems (Tomblin, 1989). Some experts have suggested that language disorders in otherwise

normal children reflect the lower point in the normal range of language variation. Like all skills, language skills vary in the population; some people have
higher skills than others (Leonard, 1991). This suggestion also implies that
some portion of limited language performance in some children may be due to
normal genetic variations in the population.

There are, however, specific genetic syndromes that are associated with varying degrees of language disorders. In several syndromes, the language disorders
may be of extreme severity. New information on speech–language performance
of children born with various genetic conditions is constantly emerging.

In addition to those listed below, many other genetic syndromes that cause
mental retardation and behavioral problems also are associated with language
delay. The reader is referred to other sources for more information on genetic
syndromes and associated communicative disorders (Hegde, 2001a; Jung, 1989;
Schopmeyer & Lowe, 1992; Shprintzen, 2000).

Down Syndrome

Down syndrome is a well-known genetic syndrome associated with certain
physical characteristics and mental retardation all traced to genetic abnormality. An extra chromosome is the most frequently reported genetic abnormality
associated with Down syndrome. Whereas normal children have 46 chromo-
somes (23 pairs), those with Down syndrome have 47. However, children with
Down syndrome have shown varied genetic abnormalities. Some children have
dislocated chromosomal materials, and others have a mixture of some normal
and some abnormal cell structures. Depending on the degree of mental retardation, children with Down syndrome show varied levels of language skills,
although a generally slow development of language is typical. Hearing loss is a
common sensory deficit in children with Down syndrome.

Fragile X Syndrome

Fragile X syndrome is another genetic syndrome associated with mental retardation and speech and language delay. Fragile X syndrome is thought to cause
the most common form of mental retardation in males. The syndrome is so
named because in the affected person, the long arm of the X chromosome has
a fragile site. Therefore, it is one of the X-linked syndromes of mental retardation. The defective gene is carried by the mothers, but only one third of the carrier females may show signs of mild mental retardation or subtle learning problems (Schopmeyer & Lowe, 1992). The syndrome tends to appear in multiple
male members of affected families. The affected children show significant language delay, attention deficit, hyperactivity, and autistic-like behaviors, including hand-flapping, hand-biting, perseveration, and poor eye contact.

Prader-Willi Syndrome

Another genetic syndrome thought to cause mental retardation in a majority of
affected children, Prader-Willi syndrome, is associated with significant speech
and language delay. Children with this syndrome are likely to show difficulties
in executing oral movements necessary to produce speech. Although some

children may show near-normal language skills, others may show up to 4 years of delay.

Environmental Syndromes

Even inherited, genetic syndromes may have environmental causes. For example, pesticides and other toxic agents can cause genetic damage. Defective genes may then be transmitted. However, there also are syndromes that may be noticeable at the time of birth and are caused by maternal exposure to drugs, including alcohol.

Fetal Alcohol Syndrome

Fetal alcohol syndrome is observed in children of chronic alcoholic mothers. The fetus is especially vulnerable to maternal alcohol consumption during the first 3 months of pregnancy. Growth in the facial region often is negatively affected. The children may show near-normal intelligence to profound mental retardation. Over 80% of children with fetal alcohol syndrome may show speech, language, voice, and fluency problems. All aspects of language, including phonological, semantic, morphological, and pragmatic aspects, may be deficient. The children also show behavioral signs of brain injury, including hyperactivity, attention deficit, and academic learning problems.

Fetal Exposure to Crack Cocaine

In recent years, fetal exposure to crack cocaine has received much attention. In the mid-1980s, many cases of infants born to cocaine-addicted mothers were documented and widely reported. Often referred to as *crack babies,* these infants are prenatally exposed to a smokable form of cocaine (crack). Because crack cocaine is somewhat inexpensive, its use has been widespread in people of lower socioeconomic levels. Consequently, the number of babies born each year with prenatal exposure to crack has been variously estimated at 100,000 to 375,000 a year. Such exposure is likely to cause low birth weight, prematurity, and smaller head circumference, suggesting that fetal growth is retarded. Children born to cocaine-addicted women tend to show hyperactivity, impulsivity, learning and memory problems, and a difficulty in understanding cause–effect relationships. These children are at high risk for brain damage, neurological problems, and associated disorders of communication.

Brain Injury

Brain injury often is associated with speech and language problems. It is a frequent cause of mental retardation. The brain injury, in turn, has many causes. Excessively premature children with low birth weight are especially vulnerable to brain injury. Difficult and prolonged labor and delivery also can injure the baby's brain. Various kinds of accidents, especially auto accidents, are a major cause of brain injury in children. Many kinds of toxic (poisonous) chemicals cause brain injury. For example, children who accidentally or otherwise swallow lead suffer serious brain damage.

Mental Retardation and Genetic Syndromes

Children with mental retardation are a diverse group mostly because of the diverse causes of mental retardation. As noted, such diverse factors as inherited genetic syndromes, environmentally induced genetic abnormalities, and such external trauma as brain injury cause mental retardation. Consequently, children with mental retardation show a variety of communicative problems. The severity of these problems, however, varies with the extent of retardation. The greater the degree of retardation, the more severe the communicative problems. Children with retardation are generally slow in learning the speech sounds of the language. Once learned, they are likely to show many errors of articulation.

The language of children with mental retardation is deficient in all aspects of language: vocabulary, meaning, morphological features, syntax, and social use. Compared with children without retardation, children with retardation are slow in saying their first words. These children continue to produce fewer words than children without retardation, and the meaning of the words they have learned may be limited. Children with retardation are slower than those without retardation in combining words into phrases and sentences. These children tend to omit many grammatical features. Their sentence structure may be limited to simpler forms. The limited language they acquire may not be freely used. For these reasons, their conversational skills are extremely limited.

Research has shown that children with retardation generally do not show abnormal or unique types of language; their language resembles that of younger children. Although progress is slow, the children with retardation follow the same sequence of language development as normally developing children. However, a few children with profound retardation who are institutionalized may show **echolalia** (repetition of heard speech) and **jargon** (utterance of meaningless string of words). Some children with retardation, especially those with Down syndrome, do not show language skills that match their general intellectual level. On certain nonverbal tasks, some children with retardation exhibit intellectual level that would presumably support higher language skills than they actually exhibit.

The child with retardation can benefit greatly from language training programs. Much of the research on language training has been done with children with mental retardation.

Autism

Psychiatrists are medical specialists who treat mental and behavioral disorders.

Leo Kanner, a child psychiatrist, originally described autism as a profound emotional disorder of childhood. Consequently, and for many years, it was believed that autism was an emotional and psychiatric disorder. It was often suggested that a profound disturbance in the mother–child relationship might have been the cause of autism. As a psychiatric disorder, autism was considered a form of childhood psychosis, which is a severe form of mental or behavioral disorder, characterized by disorientation to time, place, and person; strange sensations (hallucinations); and beliefs that have no basis in reality (delusions).

In recent years, there has been some new thinking on the nature and etiology of autism, although the causes still are not understood. It is now believed that autism is a *pervasive developmental disorder*, not a psychiatric or emotional disorder (American Psychiatric Association, 1994). Therefore, autism is more like mental retardation than childhood schizophrenia. Most experts now believe that because autism is present at birth, a failure to form an emotional bond between the mother and the child is a consequence, not the cause, of autism. There is some evidence that, at least in some cases, autism may have a genetic basis. In some cases autism has a higher familial incidence (more than one case among blood relatives), and in other cases families with a history of autism also have a history of mental retardation and language disorders. Also, some specialists believe that various portions of the brain that control communication, social interaction, and motor skills may not develop normally.

> **Schizophrenia,** the most devastating of the mental illnesses, is a form of psychosis.

Autism may be present at birth in a child, but it is typically noticed sometime during the first 3 years of age. The dominant feature of many peculiar nonverbal and verbal behaviors of the infant with autism is a disconcerting lack of desire to relate to people, including the parents. Whereas a normal infant enjoys looking at the mother's face or her smile, the infant with autism fixes its gaze on the mother's ear ring or key bunch. When held by the mother, the infant is distressed; when hugged by others, the infant stiffens. When left alone, the infant is generally happy. Soon the baby begins to show precise and decisive movement away from people and toward objects.

The child with autism prefers solitude to social contacts. As written by one mother, her daughter Elly

> sought enclosed places; every time she saw a playpen, she tried to get in; if there was no physical fence between her and the world, she erected one. She looked through human beings as if they were glass. She created solitude in the midst of company, silence in the midst of chatter. (Park, 1982, pp. 4–5)

The disturbing uniqueness of the autistic child soon becomes apparent in many respects. The child wants to be left alone with some objects he or she finds endlessly fascinating. The child may not point to things or ask for help; there is very little he or she wants from people. The child is typically self-absorbed or lost in some apparently meaningless physical activity. The autistic child may spend hours in a corner, arranging and rearranging blocks in the same routine a hundred times. The child may hold his or her hands in front of his or her face and make snakelike movements for hours on end. An entire morning may be spent sitting on the floor and rocking back and forth.

A few autistic children are prone to hurt themselves constantly. They bang their heads against walls, pull their hair, chew on their fingers, bite their own arms, and scratch their faces. Those who hurt themselves are often institutionalized and placed in padded cells. Such children may be made to wear thick gloves they cannot remove; some may be physically restrained to prevent serious self-injury.

The autistic child is deeply disturbed by a change in routine. Everything must be the same, day after day. If the chest in the bedroom is moved only a foot from its original place, the child may become very upset and remain so until the chest is moved back to its place. Park (1982) has given many vivid examples of her daughter Elly's desire for "arbitrary order." When her older sister Sara was not home one evening, Elly became upset that only five people, instead of the usual six, were going to eat dinner. The family could eat dinner in peace only after Elly placed a doll in Sara's dining chair.

Profound language disturbances are a major characteristic of autism. In the beginning, the parents are likely to suspect deafness because the infant may not respond to voice or speech. The autistic child may take no notice of speech but promptly respond to nonhuman sounds. A child who pays no attention when his or her name is called in a loud voice may quickly turn toward a toy car that makes a soft buzz. Soon the parents realize that the child is not deaf but prefers nonhuman sounds and noises to human speech.

On their own, most autistic children do not learn language at the usual rate. Nor do they use whatever they have learned to communicate with others. They learn words at a painfully slow rate. A 5-year-old autistic child may produce only 25 words; that is fewer than what some 24-month-old children can say. The autistic child is more likely to learn words that refer to objects than those that refer to concepts, people, or human relations. Nouns are preferred to verbs. One of the curious aspects of the autistic language is that some apparently difficult words are more easily acquired than those that are easier to learn. For example, the child may correctly use words like *oak, maple, square,* or *triangle* but not *love, hate, home, sister,* or *mommy* (Park, 1982). The child who can say *hexagon* may be unable to ask, "What's that?"—a question a young normal child is rarely tired of asking.

The autistic child is especially slow in learning words that express emotion. Having shunned human relationships, the child finds no use for words like *love, hate,* or even *want.* The child's use of words like *good* or *bad* are devoid of emotional tone (Park, 1982).

The words learned are used in a restricted sense and context. The child may use the word *ball* to refer only to his or her own red ball of medium size. A smaller, a bigger, or a blue ball is not at all a ball for the child. Therefore, the autistic learning is described as **context-bound.** In other words, the autistic child does not generalize what has been learned to other, appropriate contexts, situations, or stimuli.

One of the early language problems the autistic child shows is echolalia. **Echolalia** is parrotlike repetition of what is heard. It was originally thought that autistic echolalia was not intended communication, and therefore it was meaningless. Experts now believe that although some echolalic responses may be automatic parroting of what is heard, other responses may be the autistic child's attempts at communication (Prizant, 1983). This is evident when the echoed response includes the child's words that may be the actual answer. For example, when asked, "What do you want?" the child may reply, "What do you want candy."

A notable aspect of autistic language is **pronoun reversal.** Autistic children typically refer to themselves as "you," "he," or "she." They may refer to other people as "I." Some autistic children do not learn to use the pronoun "I" correctly until after age 6. There is much speculation about the reasons for pronoun reversal. Most experts think that it may be due to the autistic child's persistent echolalia. The child is always addressed as "you" and not as "I"; people refer to themselves as "I" and not "you." Therefore, for the autistic child who echoes other people, "you" stands for "I" and "I" stands for "you." Experts have noted that when echolalia decreases, the correct usage of pronouns increases (Schiff-Myers, 1983).

Autistic children generally speak in shorter, simpler sentences. They tend to omit various grammatical features such as conjunctions and prepositions. The auxiliary *is* (as in *the boy is running*) and the present progressive *ing* are especially difficult for the autistic child to learn. Equally difficult are the morphological inflections, including the regular plural *s* or the past tense *ed*. Probably because the autistic child often learns whole phrases, word boundaries are often not understood. For example, the child who has acquired "Going to the store" may rigidly repeat that phrase when it is time to go anywhere.

The child's sentences may have wrong word order. A child may say, "Table on hat," "Is running boy," or "Put toy it in" (Park, 1982; Wing, 1972). The child also may include words that do not make syntactic sense. A child may say, "Good girls don't wet your pants" or "I want a water" (Wing, 1972). Such mistakes are rare in the language of normal children or those with retardation.

Teaching language to autistic children has received much attention in recent years. Many autistic children have been taught various kinds of language behaviors. Behavioral methods of controlling unwanted activities and teaching language have generally been fruitful. Nonetheless, attempts at rehabilitating autistic children have not always been successful. Some are permanently institutionalized. Others show varying degrees of progress. Some grow to be near-normal individuals who may continue to exhibit a few odd and autistic-like behaviors.

Hearing Impairment

Oral language development and hearing are closely related. In fact, normal hearing is essential for spoken (oral) language development. Children who do not hear the language spoken around them have difficulty learning that language. Therefore, among children with language disorders, some have associated hearing impairment.

Hearing loss and hearing impairment are general terms that mean a person's hearing ability is deficient or below normal. Hearing loss is measured in terms of a unit called a decibel, abbreviated dB. It is a relative unit that helps determine how much louder a sound must be before a person can detect it. People with −10 to 15 dB hearing levels are considered to have normal hearing. Any person for whom the sound must be louder than 15 dB before he or she can detect it has a hearing problem. Earlier, hearing was considered normal if it fell in the range between −10 to 25 dB (this still is the medical and legal definition of hearing loss). More recent research has shown that even a 15 dB hearing loss may be significant in children because of its potential impact on language acquisition (Bess, 1988; Martin & Clark, 2000; Kelly, Davis, & Hegde, 1994; Northern & Downs, 1991; Wallace, Gravel, McCarton, & Ruben, 1988). Therefore, most experts now consider the range of normal hearing, especially for children, to be within −10 to 15 dB.

The term **hearing impairment** includes two groups of people: those who are hard of hearing and those with deafness. The hearing loss in individuals who are **hard of hearing** typically ranges between 16 dB and 70 dB. This range is so wide that it is hard to make general statements about the group as a whole. People at the two ends of that range have extremely different hearing sensitivity. Although children with a hearing loss that ranges between 16 and 25 dB may run the risk of language delay, adults who acquire a similar loss after the acquisition of language may manage to function normally in most communicative situations. Generally, a person who is hard of hearing is aware of normal conversation. Depending on the degree of loss, a hearing aid may or may not be required.

Read more about hearing and its measurement in **Chapter 10.**

However, the hard of hearing child can acquire oral language. The more severe the loss, the greater the amount of difficulty the child will have in learning the language. Although both may be considered to have a hearing impairment, a child with a 30 dB hearing loss is not the same as one with a 70 dB loss.

Hearing loss in people who are deaf typically exceeds 70 dB. Without hearing aids, a person who is deaf cannot hear normal conversation. Therefore, he or she has the greatest amount of difficulty in understanding and learning the spoken language. Unless special methods are used to teach the spoken language, a child who is deaf may never acquire it.

The greatest amount of difficulty in learning the oral (spoken) language is experienced by the child who is born deaf. Such a child who is **congenitally deaf** is deprived of the sound stimulation from the beginning. The child may show a more natural tendency to learn signs and gestures than the spoken language.

In the absence of extensive early training, the oral language of people who are deaf may be severely impaired. The child who is deaf usually is slow in the acquisition of spoken words, phrases, and sentence structures. A great deal of difficulty is experienced in learning such grammatic morphemes as the plural and the possessive *s* inflections, past tense forms, conjunctions (*and, but*), and prepositions (*of, on*). Many of these morphemes do not receive enough stress in normal conversation. Therefore, the child who is deaf, even with amplification, may not be aware of them. Additional difficulties are experienced in learning complex forms of sentences. The child is more likely to use simple, active, declarative sentences instead of complex sentences.

> Rehabilitation of persons with hearing impairment is described in **Chapter 10.**

Some children are born with normal hearing but become deaf later. This type of deafness is described as **acquired** or **adventitious.** The amount of oral language or the extent of oral language disorder a child with acquired deafness shows depends on the time of onset of the hearing loss. The earlier the onset, the greater the adverse effects on language acquisition.

Neurological Impairment

> Communicative disorders of neurological origin are described in **Chapter 9.**

Some experts believe that language disorders of certain children may be a form of **aphasia,** variously called childhood aphasia, developmental aphasia, or congenital aphasia (Eisenson, 1986). Aphasia is a language disorder caused by brain damage. It is more typically observed in adults who have had normal language until a stroke, a neurological disease, or a head trauma damages certain portions of the brain, and consequently the person loses some or most of his or her language.

Developmental aphasia, in which the child does not acquire language as usual, is different from adult aphasia. Due to demonstrable brain damage, normally acquired and used language is lost in adult aphasia. But the child with developmental aphasia may not show such clear signs of neurological damage as muscle weakness or paralysis. These children may show hyperactivity, distractibility, and frequent mood changes. When the signs of neurological damage are subtle or even nonexistent, some experts use the term *minimal brain damage.* The term is questionable because the brain damage is mostly presumed.

An important characteristic of children with developmental aphasia is their marked difficulty in listening and understanding spoken language. They seem to understand the nonhuman sounds of the environment more readily than the meaning of speech stimuli. Therefore, some experts believe that these children have difficulties in auditory processing of verbal stimuli. In addition, the children also may have problems of memory and speech sound discrimination (difficulty in distinguishing similar-sounding phonemes).

The concept of childhood or congenital aphasia is controversial. Many experts believe that the concept is based on questionable evidence. The critics point out that the obvious difference between the loss of language in the adult with aphasia and the inability to learn language in childhood language disorders and the practice of inferring brain damage in the absence of neurological evidence make it difficult to believe that language disorders of many children can be explained on the basis of aphasia.

Isolation, Abuse, and Neglect

Among the many other factors that are either associated with or suspected to cause language disorders in children, isolation, abuse, and neglect have received attention in recent years. Because language is a form of social behavior, it is reasonable to think that a child must experience affectionate, loving, close, and supportive family, social, and personal relations to acquire language. **Physical or social isolation** reduces the human contacts that are needed to acquire language. A completely socially isolated child who does not hear human language is unlikely to acquire it. Discovery of nonverbal "closet children" or those who were reared by wolves or lions is sometimes reported. Unfortunately, because many such children have not been studied by scientists, credible data on the effects of reported isolation on language and social development are limited.

Children who are not totally isolated but experience reduced social contacts also may show a slower than normal rate of language acquisition. Such children may be described as **socially deprived.** Children who are frequently hospitalized for prolonged illness may be somewhat slow in the acquisition of language. Some research has raised the possibility that children who are abused and neglected, especially the latter, may be prone to language delay (Fox, Long, & Langlois, 1988).

Summary

- Language disorders are associated with many conditions and possibly have many causes.

- Many genetic syndromes that are associated with mental retardation, autism, brain damage, hearing impairment, and possibly physical isolation, neglect, and abuse are among the associated conditions.

- Much research needs to be done to isolate causes of language disorders.

- In many individual cases, it is not possible to specify a cause or causes of the language disorder.

Assessment of Language Disorders

When a parent seeks help for the child who does not talk much, the clinician must make an assessment of the child's language behaviors. Essentially, **language**

assessment is a process of observation and measurement of a client's language behaviors to determine (1) whether or not a clinical problem exists; (2) the nature and extent of the problem; and (3) a course of action to help the child.

The assessment of language disorders is outlined in Table 5.3. Accordingly, the case history, hearing screening, and orofacial examination are done in assessing any form of communicative disorder. The specific procedures are designed to get as much information as possible on the language of the child (Nelson, 1993; Reed, 1994).

The Case History and Interview

A pediatrician, a teacher, a psychologist, or any other professional may refer a child to a speech and hearing clinic. Concerned parents also may bring a child directly to the clinic.

Through the case history and the interview, the clinician learns about the child's birth; physical, social, and behavioral development; education; and communication. The clinician is especially interested in the child's speech and language development and the coexistence of such complicating conditions as neurological problems, autism, mental retardation, or hearing loss.

The interview also serves the purpose of getting acquainted with the parents and understanding how they view the problem and how they react to the child's communicative difficulties. For example, the clinician may wish to know how the child and the parents communicate with each other. Do they use speech or gestures and signs? Does the child understand what is spoken? What do the parents do when they do not understand the child's productions? The clinician seeks answers to questions such as these.

Observation and Measurement of Language

Following the interview, the clinician might observe the child from an adjacent room, which contains a one-way mirror through which the child can be seen.

Table 5.3

Assessment of Communicative Disorders: Language Disorders

....

1. The history of the client, the family, and the disorder

2. Interview of the client, the family members, or both

3. Orofacial examination

4. Hearing screening

5. **Measurement of language behaviors:**
   a. **Language and speech sampling**
   b. **Administration of standardized language tests**
   c. **Obtaining home language samples**
   d. **Administration of client-specific language measurement procedures**

6. Recommendations

7. Report writing

....

Note. Procedures unique to language assessment are in bold print.

Through an audio system, the clinician also can hear the conversation between the child and his or her family. The clinician may hear mostly single-word productions, phrases, or utterances that are not grammatically complete. The child may be silent most of the time. The child and the parents may use signs and gestures to communicate with each other. A sibling might constantly answer questions asked of the child. Even before the child makes any attempt at communication, the parents might anticipate what is wanted and supply it. The clinician uses information of this kind to plan for more formal assessment with the help of standardized tests and other procedures.

Standardized tests are frequently administered to determine whether or not the child lags behind children of his or her age in the use of language. These tests sample various aspects of language performance, including expressive and receptive language skills. **Expressive language skills** refer to a person's talking (language production), whereas **receptive language skills** refer to an understanding of what is said (spoken language).

Some tests focus on the child's use of such grammatic morphemes as the regular plural inflection and the present progressive *ing* (*coming, going*). One such test, the *Test for Examining Expressive Morphology* (Shipley, Stone, & Sue, 1983), contains pictured test items that are used to evoke morphological productions. For example, pointing to the picture of one book, the examiner says, "Here is one book," and then immediately points to the picture of two books and says, "Here are two . . . ." The child is expected to say, "books."

Several other tests are available to assess various aspects of language. For example, the *Northwestern Syntax Screening Test* (Lee, 1969) samples grammatic morphemes as well as certain syntactic features including word order and specific sentence types. The *Carrow Elicited Languages Inventory* (Carrow-Woolfolk, 1974) tests how well children can imitate different sentence types (such as the passive and active forms) and various grammatic morphemes. Another test, the *Test for Auditory Comprehension of Language* (TACL–3) (Carrow-Woolfolk, 1999), measures how well children understand selected morphologic and syntactic structures. The *Test of Early Language Development* (Hresko, Reid, & Hammill, 1999) yields an overall score for spoken language along with separate scores for receptive and expressive languages.

A frequently used test to assess children's comprehension of word meanings is the *Peabody Picture Vocabulary Test–Revised* (Dunn & Dunn, 1981). The typical test items consist of four pictures printed on a single card. The child who points to a specific picture when asked indicates comprehension of the spoken word. Another test of receptive and expressive vocabulary is the *Comprehensive Receptive and Expressive Vocabulary Test* (Wallace & Hammill, 1994).

Standardized tests, though convenient to use, have their limitations. Often, children who do not produce grammatical features in a test situation may produce them in normal conversation at home. Also, children who imitate certain sentence types may not be able to produce them in conversational speech. Furthermore, most tests give only one or two opportunities for the child to produce or imitate a given language structure (Paul, 1995). Because of these and other limitations, clinicians also use other procedures, including language samples.

Language Sampling

A measure of language vital to a diagnosis of language disorders in children is called **language sampling,** which is the procedure of recording a person's language productions under relatively normal conditions and, whenever possible, with the help of conversational speech. In this procedure, the clinician and the family members spend time talking with and listening to the child.

The clinician's main task in obtaining a language sample is to stimulate the child to speak as freely and naturally as possible. To accomplish this, the clinician may use toys, books, pictures, and objects. The parents or siblings also may participate in this interaction. During the sampling, the child is encouraged to look at the books and pictures, play with the toys, manipulate objects, and talk. The clinician may tell a story to the child and ask the child to answer questions about it or retell the story.

When the child talks more in the presence of the clinician, the two may engage in conversational speech. The clinician may ask about the child's school, pets at home, friends, cartoon shows, birthday parties, and favorite play activities. The clinician also can listen to the conversation between the parents and the child.

The language sample is tape- or video-recorded so that the clinician can make a thorough analysis of the child's responses later. The clinician takes notes on what the child was doing before, during, and after an utterance was made. The meaning of most utterances are clear only when we know the context or situation in which they were produced. For example, a child who says "Blocks" may mean, among other things, "Give me those blocks," "Look at these blocks," or even "I am playing with the blocks." A mere tape recording of this utterance may not help in understanding the meaning of it. If it is recorded that the child was reaching for the blocks while saying the word and that, when the clinician handed them to the child, the child said, "Thank you," then the single-word response "Blocks" was indeed a request.

Other Procedures

A hearing screening is a quick test done to find out if the client needs to be assessed fully.

A complete language assessment includes several other procedures designed to rule out various problems that can cause language or other problems of communication (Hegde, 2001a). For example, an orofacial examination is made to make sure that the child's oral structures are not deformed or deficient. To rule out hearing loss, the child's hearing is screened. A child who fails this screening is referred to an audiologist for a complete hearing assessment.

More about hearing and its disorders is discussed in **Chapter 10.**

Several other conditions that may be associated with language disorders must also be assessed either by the speech–language pathologist or by other professionals. For example, a psychologist may evaluate a child with mental retardation or autism. A medical professional will evaluate a child with physical and neurological disabilities.

The Assessment Report

After having gathered as much information as possible, the clinician makes an analysis of the information and writes an assessment report. This report states whether the child has a problem, and, if so, the nature or extent of the problem and what should be done to remediate it.

The information obtained through the case history, standardized tests, language samples, hearing screening, oral-peripheral examination, and reports from other specialists is integrated to obtain a total picture of the child's performance and potential. The clinician makes a diagnostic statement only after considering all sources of information.

The child's performance on a standardized language test is typically evaluated in relation to the range of age-based norms for that test. If the child's performance falls below this range, then that child's language behaviors are considered below normal.

The language sample is analyzed to determine what language structures the child has learned and what structures the child has not learned but should have. The child's production of grammatic morphemes, word order, sentence types, and related aspects also are described. Missing structural elements that might be targeted for treatment are identified. How well the child comprehends spoken language also is determined.

The pragmatic analysis determines how the child uses the amount of language that he or she has learned. A child may have some language, but may be unwilling to talk. A child who talks may be unable to stay on a topic, take turns in conversation, or maintain eye contact. The language used may be inappropriate for the situation, time, or persons involved in conversation. Such observations are summarized in an assessment report.

Finally, the report offers recommendations for treatment and includes a statement of prognosis for improvement. The **prognosis** is a statement about the future course of the disorder when certain steps are taken or when nothing is done. For example, in the case of a child who might be held back from the first grade because of a language disorder, the clinician might suggest that if the child received systematic language treatment over the next 9 months, the child might be able to attend the first grade or that without treatment the child might repeat the grade.

Treatment of Language Disorders

For three major reasons, the treatment of language disorders in children is a diverse venture. First, different approaches have suggested different targets for language treatment. Clinicians have variously emphasized the importance of teaching grammatical rules, semantic concepts, production of language behaviors, pragmatic rules, and cognitive processes.

Second, different approaches advocate different treatment procedures. Should the treatment sessions be highly structured or loosely organized? Should the clinician control the stimuli or let the child control them? Should the clinician systematically reinforce the child for correct responses or should there be no such consequence? Different experts have given different answers to these and other questions. Consequently, there are a variety of approaches to language treatment.

Third, the children who exhibit language disorders are themselves a diverse group. Disorders vary in severity across children. In some respects, the treatment of a mild language disorder is different from that of a severe disorder. Children with language disorders who have such associated conditions as hearing impairment need additional procedures.

In spite of all the diversity of target behaviors and treatment approaches, generally applicable principles and procedures of treatment have emerged (Hegde, 2001b). Although many procedures have been advocated, only a few have been experimentally tested and found to be effective. Therefore, an overview of these general treatment procedures and principles that have received some research support is presented.

Selection of Treatment Targets

To the extent possible, the final target of treatment is normal conversation in everyday situations. The child should understand and take part in conversation. Therefore, the child should have an adequate vocabulary, good sentence structure, and correct production of morphological features. The child should gain an understanding of word and sentence meanings. Finally, the child should appropriately use the learned language in diverse social situations (Hegde, 1998).

Even with extensive training, some children with language disorders may not achieve normal language functions. Nonetheless, the clinician never loses sight of such a final target. The goal is to help the child realize his or her maximum communicative potential.

The **usefulness** of the language behaviors is a major consideration in their selection. Although all language behaviors are useful, some are more useful or of more immediate value than other language behaviors. For example, it is more useful for a young child to be able to say *milk* or *Mommy* than *blue* or *ceiling*. Children are more likely to use names of siblings and friends, pets, toys, clothing items, and foods. Teaching such targets, therefore, is meaningful to the child and his or her family. Useful language behaviors are more likely to be produced at home and maintained over time.

Sequence of Treatment

The final goal is realized through a sequence of treatment. The treatment for a child who has not learned words at all must be started, obviously, at the word level. In the case of a nonverbal child, any vocalization (such as an *a* or *m* sound) may be the initial treatment target. Once vocalization is established, the production of certain meaningful words may be the treatment target. In the next stage, the clinician might combine already taught words into simple phrases. For example, a child who learns to say *mommy, hat, car, big,* and *come* may be taught many phrases created out of these words: "Mommy hat," "Mommy come," "big car," and so forth.

Once the phrases are learned, the clinician targets simple sentences. This requires that the child learn various grammatical features. For example, the phrase "Mommy hat" must be expanded to "Mommy's hat" to make it grammatically more correct; this requires the teaching of the possessive *s* inflection. The phrase "big car" may be expanded to different forms such as "This is a big car," "It is a big car" or "That's my big car." Such expansions require the teaching of additional grammatic morphemes and word order.

Once the child learns simple sentences, more complex sentences may be taught. The child who has mastered simple, active, declarative sentences (e.g., "This is a car" or "He is a man") may be taught question forms (e.g., "What is this?" or "Who is that?"). Other, more complex forms of sentences are taught in subsequent stages of treatment.

The language the child learns in the treatment sessions may or may not be used in spontaneous conversational speech. Therefore, in the final stages of treatment, the target is almost always conversational speech. In this stage, the child is encouraged to use specific language structures learned in the earlier treatment sessions in conversational speech. Certain pragmatic language skills, including staying on a conversational topic, taking turns in talking and listening, and narrating events and experiences, also are taught at this stage. Unless this complex stage of treatment is managed appropriately, the pragmatic use of language may not emerge.

Some Basic Treatment Procedures

After selecting the target behaviors, the clinician prepares a set of stimulus materials, which may be pictures, objects, and toys, that help evoke the target responses from the child. Suppose the target is to teach selected words to a 3-year-old child who does not produce words at all. The clinician starts treatment in a small therapy room, which is typically equipped with children's furniture. The child and the clinician may sit across a small table or next to each other. The clinician then shows a picture, perhaps that of a car, and begins to establish the production of the single-word response, *car*.

Many children with language disorders who cannot produce words or phrases can imitate when others produce them. To exploit this tendency to imitate, the clinician **models** a desired response, which the child imitates. In teaching the word *car*, for example, the clinician places a picture of a car in front of the child and asks, "What is this?" and immediately models the correct response by saying, "Say *car*." If the child says "Car," the clinician immediately praises him or her by saying, "Excellent!" or "I like that!" or "Very good." This kind of immediate praise is known as **verbal reinforcement**. A given opportunity to produce a correct target response also is called a **trial**. Most language target responses can be established only by many repeated trials (Hegde, 1998).

Modeling is a common procedure in the treatment of articulation, language, voice, fluency, and other disorders of communication.

If the child did not say anything when the correct response is modeled, the clinician simply proceeds to the next trial. As before, the picture is placed in front of the child again, the same question is asked, and the correct response is modeled. If the child produced a totally wrong response, such as "truck" or "train" for *car*, most clinicians say "No" or "That is not a truck (train)." This kind of verbal disapproval, when it reduces the production of wrong responses, is called **corrective feedback** or verbal punishment. The term *punishment* does not mean the same as it does in everyday speech. **Punishment** is a procedure designed to decrease the frequency of selected behaviors by arranging an immediate consequence for those behaviors (Hegde, 1998).

When the child begins to imitate the modeled response consistently on a certain number of trials, the clinician stops modeling. The child is shown the stimulus, asked a question, and given a few seconds to respond. Target responses that are not imitated but produced in relation to more natural stimuli, such as a question or some event, are known as **evoked responses**. As before, the correct evoked responses are reinforced and the incorrect responses are given corrective feedback.

When the child begins to produce evoked responses of a given word with a certain degree of accuracy—usually 90% correct—the clinician introduces other words selected for training. When a certain number of words are taught, the training is shifted to two-word phrases and eventually to sentences and conversational speech.

Treatment in the advanced stage is usually less structured. Being more informal, it better approximates the natural conversation between individuals.

Also, by this time, the clinician will have reduced the amount of reinforcement given to the child. Only periodic praise will be given. This is done because children normally, and in everyday situations, are not explicitly reinforced for producing specific structures of language. It is thought that making the final stages of the treatment situation resemble natural communicative exchanges promotes pragmatic use of language.

The Role of the Family and Others

Successful treatment of language disorders in children requires the cooperation of many individuals who normally interact with them. Under the controlled condition of the clinic and in the reassuring presence of the clinician, most children begin to produce what has been taught. Unfortunately, the same children may be speechless in other situations, including the home and the school. To encourage the child to use in natural social contexts what has been taught in the clinic, the clinician must implement additional procedures known as **generalization** and **maintenance procedures** (Hegde, 1998).

The logic behind generalization and maintenance procedures is rather simple. The clinician and the clinical situation are helping the child to produce the behaviors; however, the home, the school, and other situations are not, because the child has not learned the new responses in those situations. Also, unlike the clinician, people at home and in other situations may not be supporting (reinforcing) the child's newly acquired skills. Therefore, to achieve response generalization to the everyday situations, the clinician must somehow make those situations part of the treatment. In addition, people in the life of the child must somehow be a part of the teaching process. If these two goals are accomplished, then the child is likely to produce the newly learned language behaviors in home and in other situations. If the parents and others learn to reinforce the child's correct productions, then those productions also may last (Hegde, 1998).

The clinician takes several steps to make the responses generalize and last. The most important of these steps is to get the family, friends, teachers, and others involved in the teaching process. Parents are especially encouraged to observe the treatment sessions. At appropriate times, the clinician may ask the parents to present stimuli, ask questions designed to evoke the target responses, and reinforce correct productions. The parents are encouraged to engage the child in conversation. The parents are told what target behaviors are being trained and how to reinforce the child when those behaviors are produced at home.

The siblings, friends, and teachers of the child also may be similarly trained. Many times, an older sibling can be effective in strengthening newly taught language behaviors. When teachers know how to get the child to say what he or she has learned, the child will begin to talk in the school. When steps such as these are implemented, the child does not see the clinic as the only special place where the newly learned language responses may be produced.

Another important step the clinician takes is to systematically change the setting in which the treatment is carried out. When the child begins to converse with the clinician, the treatment sessions may be moved out of the small and formal room and into more naturalistic settings. The child may be taken to a restaurant or a store where he or she will order food or talk to salespeople. The clinician may visit the child at home and engage in conversation. The interaction between the family and the child may be observed and suggestions for improvement offered. Steps such as these are usually successful in encouraging the child to use the newly learned language in social situations.

Some Procedural Variations

The general outline of the treatment procedure given so far may be described as the behavioral approach to the treatment of language disorders. The behavioral approach has been researched extensively and shown to be effective in generating various aspects of language in children with language disorders. The approach uses such procedures as modeling, reinforcement, corrective feedback, and systematic shaping of nonexistent behaviors (Hegde, 1996, 1998, 2001b).

Generally speaking, the behavioral approach is more structured than some of the nonbehavioral approaches. An exception is known as the incidental teaching procedure. It is a behavioral approach that uses a loose structure. **Incidental teaching** is a procedure in which the naturally occurring opportunities for communication are used to teach language (Hart & Risley, 1982). Instead of using systematically arranged trials in which the target responses are evoked, the clinician using the incidental teaching procedure waits until the child brings up a topic of interest. Thus, it is a method of teaching language through talking. When the child says something, the clinician shows interest and asks for more information. This request usually leads the child to elaborate on the language he or she typically uses. The clinician also elaborates on the child's production. Such elaborations may be repeated by the child, although there is no insistence on such imitations.

Children present many opportunities to elaborate language. In fact, research has shown that parents often repeat and elaborate what the child says. Such elaborations are called **expansions.** For example, a child points to her shoes and says, "Mommy, shoe." The mother then might expand the child's utterance by saying, "Yes, they are your new shoes. Can you say 'My new shoes?'" The child might imitate "My new shoes," which is a more elaborate, longer, and grammatically more correct utterance than the original. It is believed that expansions of this kind help normally developing children, as well as those with language disorders, learn complex forms of language.

Other variations of language treatment include an emphasis not on what the child says but on what the child *knows* about things and events. This approach, generally known as the **cognitive** or **semantic approach,** relies heavily on teaching concepts that underlie the production of language. The focus within this approach is the mental or cognitive processes thought to be basic to language acquisition. At least in the initial stages of language training, the child is not required to imitate or produce words, phrases, or sentences. Instead, the child is encouraged to explore objects and engage in physical activities with a view to teach the child information about those objects and activities. For example, instead of teaching the word *car* to a child, the clinician may allow the child to play with a toy car and to manipulate it. The clinician may demonstrate all kinds of actions with the car and describe its color and shape. It is thought that the child will find out from this experience what a toy car is. The knowledge the child gains about the car is considered a prerequisite to the verbal production of the word *car,* which may need additional training.

Some Special Considerations

The general treatment procedure sketched so far is modified to suit the needs of particular children. In addition, the children who have associated problems need special considerations.

For children who have language disorders but have no other associated problems, language treatment is the primary, if not the only, concern. However, for children who have associated problems that need special considerations, the clinician keeps all of their needs in perspective. Many of these children need the services of other professionals. It is the responsibility of the speech–language pathologist to see that the child's multiple needs are met.

The child who has **mental retardation,** for example, needs the services of a psychologist who evaluates the mental, behavioral, and cognitive skills of the child. The child often is enrolled in various special educational programs. The child who is profoundly retarded tends to be institutionalized and is in need of constant care. The speech–language pathologist typically serves on the interdisciplinary team that manages such children. In teaching language to children with mental retardation, the clinician takes into consideration their behavioral potential. However, without prejudging their potential, most clinicians prefer to teach increasingly complex language until it becomes evident that further progress is not possible.

The child who is **autistic** also needs the help of an interdisciplinary team, which includes a psychologist or psychiatrist, nurse, social worker, and special educators. Serving on such a treatment team, speech–language pathologists are mainly responsible for teaching communicative skills. However, teaching speech and language to children with autism poses special challenges. Powerful reinforcers, such as food and drink, are often needed to motivate the generally withdrawn autistic children to perform in language treatment sessions. Research has shown that generalization of clinically taught language behaviors to natural settings is one of the most troublesome issues. The child who is autistic is extremely **stimulus-bound,** which means that a behavior learned in a particular situation is bound to that situation only. In other situations, the child may not exhibit that behavior. Therefore, the treatment must be implemented in many different settings, so that the child produces language in a variety of situations.

The rehabilitation of children with hearing impairment is covered in more detail in **Chapter 10.**

Children who have **hearing impairment** compose another group that requires special considerations. Most children with a significant hearing impairment can benefit from sound amplification. Individual hearing aids children wear can help them to understand spoken speech and to improve speech production by making it possible to self-monitor their speech. In group treatment sessions, clinicians may use **desktop auditory trainers** that consist of an amplifier, to which multiple earphones are attached. The clinician's speech is fed to the amplifier, which in turn feeds the amplified speech to the children's ear through the headphones.

Methods of nonverbal communication are described in **Chapters 9 and 10.**

Finally, children with **physical disabilities** who have language disorders also need special considerations. Along with speech and language treatment, these children need the services of medical specialists, physical therapists, occupational therapists, and others involved with rehabilitation. Individuals with severe physical disabilities, including some with cerebral palsy, may not be able to learn oral language. For example, paralysis of the vocal cords and the speech muscles may make it impossible to talk. In such cases, nonverbal means of communication must be taught. American Sign Language is one of the better known nonverbal means of communication taught to children who are deaf and profoundly retarded. Other means of nonverbal communication include communication boards on which the speaker arranges words or points to standard messages. Sophisticated computer programs are becoming available for nonverbal individuals to communicate with others.

Summary

- The goal of language treatment is to remediate the specific kinds of language deficiency in a given child.

- The clinician selects useful and relevant language targets to teach.

- The final goal of conversational speech in naturalistic environment is realized through carefully planned sequence of treatment, starting with the simpler and advancing to the more complex language structures.

- The clinician uses various stimuli to evoke the target responses.

- When necessary, the clinician models the correct responses for the child to imitate.

- The child is praised for correct productions.

- Members of the family, teachers, and other significant people may be trained to evoke and reinforce language in nonclinical settings.

- Children who have language problems along with sensory or physical disabilities need additional services.

Dialogue

The student Ms. Noledge-Hungry found the topic of language acquisition and disorders in treatment very interesting. She was beginning to get a better appreciation for the profession of speech–language pathology, especially through her discussions with Dr. Speech-Wisely.

N-H: Dr. Speech-Wisely, it seems that how children acquire language and why some do not are both difficult to answer.

S-W: True. Nonetheless, we know enough to help those who do not acquire language on their own.

N-H: That is the most encouraging part. Well, we have to start with the methods of studying language acquisition. I learned that in the **longitudinal method,** one or a few children are observed repeatedly over months and years. In the **cross-sectional method,** many children of different ages are selected and observed only one time. The results are used to trace the development of language across time or across age groups.

S-W: That is right. Experts have looked at the acquisition of preverbal behaviors, vocabulary, morphological features, grammatical structures, meaning, and pragmatic aspects. An early sign of language development in a child is **babbling,** which appears around age 4 months. First words appear around 12 months of age. The first words the child learns are about the objects the child can manipulate. Around age 18 months, most children begin to combine words into phrases. Soon the child begins to learn various **grammatic morphemes,** which are grammatical features that affect meaning. Among others, Brown has described a sequence of the acquisition of selected grammatic morphemes. You should have a general idea of his findings.

N-H: But children differ, don't they?

S-W: Most certainly. A given grammatical feature may be acquired at different ages by two healthy and normal children, although the rough sequence is more stable across children.

N-H: I understand that the child is more likely to produce simple, active, declarative sentences before producing more complex or passive or negative forms of sentences. The acquisition of each type of sentence has a certain rough sequence to it.

S-W: Yes, we took a look at a few sentence types such as the negative or interrogative (questions). You should be able to describe at least one such sequence.

N-H: It appears that by the time they enter the first grade, most children will have acquired the basic structure of their language.

S-W: That is true to a large extent, although children continue to learn complex words and meanings beyond the first grade.

N-H: The pragmatic aspect of language acquisition seems to begin very early in life, right?

S-W: That is right. From the very beginning, the mother and the child are special partners in communication. Babies 8 to 10 months of age show various kinds of language **functions** or intentions. Children begin to indicate what they want by using gestures and words. The **instrumental** function of language helps children get what they want, and the **regulatory** function helps them control the behavior of others.

N-H: Eventually the children learn strategies of normal conversation and social use of language.

S-W: What about the theories of language acquisition?

N-H: The nativistic and the behavioral are the two major and contrasting theories of language acquisition. The **nativistic theory** argues that language acquisition is made possible largely by innate mechanisms, whereas the **behavioral theory** argues that it is largely due to the influence of a verbal community.

S-W: Can you summarize disorders of language in children?

N-H: Each component of language may be disordered. **Semantic deficiencies** include a slow acquisition of words and word meanings. **Morphologic deficiencies** include slow acquisition of grammatic morphemes. **Syntactic deficiencies** include inappropriate sentences and wrong word orders. **Pragmatic deficiencies** include problems in the social use of language. Other problems include poor **language comprehension.**

S-W: Very good. Are language disorders associated with other kinds of problems?

N-H: Many children with language disorders are otherwise normal. But some children with language disorders have other associated problems. These include various **genetic syndromes** that are associated with mental retardation; **autism,** which is a pervasive developmental disorder; **hearing impairment,** which includes people who are hard of hearing or deaf; **neurological impairment,** which includes childhood aphasia; and **social deprivation** and **social isolation.**

S-W: That is right. Now tell me about the assessment of language disorders.

N-H: In making an **assessment,** the clinician observes and measures the language of a child to find out whether a problem exists, and, if it does, the clinician determines the extent of the problem and what can be done about it. The clinician takes a case history, interviews the parents, observes the child's language, records a language sample, administers standardized tests of language behaviors, screens the hearing, and examines the child's oral speech mechanism. An assessment report is then written, which summarizes the child's language behaviors and the problems noted and offers recommendations.

S-W: Excellent! Then the clinician plans for treatment. How does a clinician select target behaviors for treatment?

N-H: The clinician selects target behaviors that are useful to the child. Many clinicians also consider the age-based norms in selecting appropriate targets. Dr. Speech-Wisely, can you summarize the treatment procedures for me?

S-W: Of course. The clinician first selects stimulus materials that help evoke the target responses from the child. The training is started at a level that the child can respond to. Initially, the child is reinforced for imitating the clinician's correct production of target responses. Eventually, the child is encouraged to produce more natural, nonimitative responses; the training focuses on conversational speech. Behavioral techniques, including reinforcement and corrective feedback, are used by many clinicians to teach the selected target responses. Incidental teaching and expansion of the child's utterances also are frequently used.

N-H: I liked the idea of getting the family members, teachers, and friends of the child involved in treatment. I realize how important it is in the generalization and maintenance of treated language behaviors in the child.

S-W: Then there is the question of special needs of children who have associated problems such as autism or hearing impairment.

The Outlook

N-H: Dr. Speech-Wisely, if I decide to major in speech–language pathology, what kinds of courses will I take in the area of language and language disorders?

S-W: You will take a full course on language acquisition in children. There is so much more to learn there. You will probably take a full course on the language disorders of children. You will make a more detailed study of the characteristics, assessment, and treatment of language disorders in a variety of children. In many universities, you also may be offered a course on linguistics. At the graduate level, you may take additional seminars on language, its disorders, and treatment. Remember, we talked only about the language disorders in children. There are language disorders in adults, which we will study later. Additional graduate courses are offered on that topic as well.

N-H: Sounds very interesting! I wonder in what settings the children with language disorders are typically treated.

S-W: Most school-age children with language disorders are treated at public schools by the speech–language pathologist who works for the school district. Younger children are often seen at private, college, and hospital-based speech and hearing clinics. Language disorders are now a major part of the speech–language pathologist's caseload in many settings.

N-H: Being able to give children a skill like language must be very satisfying.

S-W: That is really the whole point of the profession of speech–language pathology. Successful treatment in our profession means the gift of communication. The proud smile on the face of the mother who, for the first time in her life, hears the word *Mommy* from her child may be your biggest reward.

N-H: I can imagine that. I find that information on language and its disorders useful even for people who do not specialize in speech–language pathology.

S-W: That is true. A general awareness of language acquisition and what can go wrong in that process is very useful to parents of young children. They can recognize the signs of delay in their children and consult a speech–language pathologist at an early time.

N-H: Dr. Speech-Wisely, thank you for your time. I will see you in class.

S-W: OK, have fun and hit the books!

Study Questions

1. Describe the two methods of studying language acquisition.

2. What is babbling? At what age do babies typically begin to babble?

3. What are some of the characteristics of children's first words?

4. What are overextensions and underextensions? Give examples.

5. Roughly, at what age do most children begin to combine words into phrases?

6. Describe the characteristics of telegraphic speech.

7. How many morphemes are in the words *hat* and *books?*

8. What are grammatical morphemes? Give two examples.

9. Give a brief description of the results of Brown's study of language acquisition in three children.

10. Through what stages does a child acquire the negative sentence forms?

11. Distinguish between simple, compound, and complex sentence forms. What is the order of acquisition of these types of sentences?

12. What are communicative functions? Give two examples.

13. Describe at least two pragmatic skills associated with conversational speech.

14. Compare and contrast the nativist and the behavioral viewpoints of language acquisition.

15. What is motherese? What are its characteristics?

16. How do some clinicians distinguish language delay from language disorders?

17. Describe the semantic problems of a child with language disorders.

18. Describe four utterances of a child with language disorders that illustrate morphological problems.

19. Define pragmatics.

20. What are syntactic problems?

21. Describe the pragmatic problems of a child with language disorders.

22. Is mental retardation a cause of the language disorder or an associated condition? Explain.

23. What are some of the causes of mental retardation?

24. Describe the language of children with mental retardation.

25. Summarize the language problems of a child with autism.

26. What is echolalia? What is a possible cause of it in people with autism?

27. Distinguish between hard of hearing and deaf. Summarize the language problems of people who are deaf.

28. What is assessment of language disorders?

29. Give an outline of the language assessment procedures.

30. What is an oral-peripheral examination?

31. What principles are followed in selecting the target behaviors for language treatment?

32. What are generalization and maintenance?

33. Give a brief description of a language treatment procedure.

34. Define reinforcement and corrective feedback (punishment). How are they used in language treatment?

35. Why is it important to get the child's family and other people involved in the child's language treatment?

36. What is incidental teaching?

37. Give an example of expansion used in language treatment.

38. What is the basic assumption of the cognitive or semantic approach to the treatment of language disorders in children?

39. What special considerations are required in the treatment of language disorders in the group with hearing impairment?

40. What special considerations are required in the treatment of language disorders in children with physical disabilities?

References

American Psychiatric Association. (1994). *Diagnostic and statistical manual of mental disorders* (4th ed.). Washington, DC: Author.

Bess, F. (1988). Basic hearing measurement. In N. Lass, L. V. McReynolds, J. L. Northern, & D. E. Yoder (Eds.), *Handbook of speech–language pathology and audiology* (pp. 1094–1122). Philadelphia: Decker.

Bohannon, J. N., III., & Bonvillian, J. D. (1993). Theoretical approaches to language acquisition. In J. Gleason (Ed.), *The development of language* (5th ed., pp. 254–315). Needham Heights, MA: Allyn & Bacon.

Brown, R. (1973). *A first language: Early stages.* Cambridge, MA: Harvard University.

Carrow-Woolfolk, E. (1974). *The Carrow Elicited Language Inventory.* Hingham, MA: Teaching Resources.

Carrow-Woolfolk, E. (1999). *Test for Auditory Comprehension of Language–Third Edition.* Austin, TX: PRO-ED.

Chomsky, N. (1968). *Aspects of the theory of syntax.* Cambridge, MA: MIT Press.

de Villiers, J. G., & de Villiers, P. A. (1973). A cross sectional study of acquisition of grammatical morphemes in child speech. *Journal of Psycholinguistic Research, 2,* 267–278.

Dunn, L., & Dunn, L. (1981). *Peabody Picture Vocabulary Test–Revised.* Circle Pines, MN: American Guidance Service.

Eisenson, J. (1986). *Language and speech disorders in children.* New York: Pergamon.

Fox, L., Long, S. H., & Langlois, A. (1988). Patterns of language comprehension deficit in abused and neglected children. *Journal of Speech and Hearing Disorders, 53,* 239–244.

Gleason, J. B. (Ed.). (2001). *The development of language* (5th ed.). Needham Heights, MA: Allyn & Bacon.

Hart, B. M., & Risley, T. R. (1982). *How to use incidental teaching for elaborating language.* Lawrence, KS: H & H Enterprises.

Hegde, M. N. (1993). *Experimental manipulation of the sequence of morphologic acquisition.* A paper presented in a symposium on experimental analysis of language acquisition at the National Convention of Association for Behavior Analysis, Chicago.

Hegde, M. N. (1996). *A coursebook on language disorders in children.* San Diego, CA: Singular.

Hegde, M. N. (1998). *Treatment procedures in communicative disorders* (3rd ed.). Austin, TX: PRO-ED.

Hegde, M. N. (2001a). *Hegde's pocketguide to assessment in speech–language pathology* (2nd ed.). San Diego, CA: Singular.

Hegde, M. N. (2001b). *Hegde's pocketguide to treatment in speech–language pathology* (2nd ed.). San Diego, CA: Singular.

Hresko, W. P., Reid, D. K., & Hammill, D. D. (1999). *Test of Early Language Development–Third Edition.* Austin, TX: PRO-ED.

Hulit, L. M., & Howard, M. R. (1993). *Born to talk: An introduction to speech and language development.* New York: Macmillan.

Johnston, J. R. (1988). Specific language disorders in the child. In N. J. Lass, L. V. McReynolds, J. L. Northern, & D. E. Yoder (Eds.), *Handbook of speech–language pathology and audiology* (pp. 685–715). Philadelphia: Decker.

Jung, J. H. (1989). *Genetic syndromes in communication disorders.* Austin, TX: PRO-ED.

Kelly, B. R., Davis, D., & Hegde, M. N. (1994). *Clinical methods and practicum in audiology.* San Diego, CA: Singular.

Lee, L. (1969). *Northwestern Syntax Screening Test.* Evaston, IL: Northwestern University Press.

Leonard, L. L. (1991). Specific language impairment as a clinical category. *Language, Speech, and Hearing Services in Schools, 22,* 66–68.

Martin, F. N., & Clark, J. G. (2000). *Introduction to audiology* (7th ed.). Needham Heights, MA: Allyn & Bacon.

McCormick, L., & Schiefelbusch, R. L. (1990). *Early language intervention: An introduction* (2nd ed.). Columbus, OH: Merrill.

McLaughlin, S. (1998). *Introduction to language development.* San Diego, CA: Singular.

Moerk, E. (1983). *The mother of Eve—As a first language teacher.* Norwood, NJ: Ablex.

Moerk, E. (1992). *A first language taught and learned.* Baltimore: Brookes.

Nelson, N. W. (1993). *Childhood language disorders in context: Infancy through adolescence.* New York: Macmillan.

Northern, J. L., & Downs, M. P. (1991). *Hearing in children* (4th ed.). Baltimore: Williams & Wilkins.

Owens, R. E. (1996). *Language development: An introduction* (4th ed.). New York: Macmillan.

Park, C. C. (1982). *The siege: The first eight years of an autistic child.* Boston: Little, Brown.

Paul, R. (1995). *Language disorders from infancy through adolescence.* St. Louis, MO: Mosby.

Prizant, B. (1983). Language acquisition and communicative behavior in autism: Toward an understanding of the "whole" of it. *Journal of Speech and Hearing Disorders, 48,* 296–307.

Reed, V. (1994). *An introduction to children with language disorders* (2nd ed.). New York: Macmillan.

Sachs, J. (2001). The emergence of intentional communication. In J. Gleason (Ed.), *The development of language* (5th ed., pp. 40–69). Needham Heights, MA: Allyn & Bacon.

Schiff-Meyers, N. (1983). From pronoun reversal to correct pronoun usage. A case study of a normally developing child. *Journal of Speech and Hearing Disorders, 48,* 394–402.

Schopmeyer, B. B., & Lowe, F. (1992). *The fragile X child.* San Diego, CA: Singular.

Schumaker, J. B., & Sherman, J. A. (1978). Parent as intervention agent. In R. L. Schiefelbusch (Ed.), *Language intervention strategies* (pp. 237–316). Baltimore: University Park Press.

Shipley, K. G., Stone, T., & Sue, M. (1983). *Test for Examining Expressive Morphology.* Tucson, AZ: Communication Skill Builders.

Shprintzen, R. (2000). *Syndrome identification for speech–language pathologists.* San Diego, CA: Singular.

Skinner, B. F. (1957). *Verbal behavior.* New York: Appleton-Century-Crofts.

Tomblin, J. B. (1989). Familial concentration of developmental language impairment. *Journal of Speech and Hearing Disorders, 54,* 287–295.

Van Kleek, A., & Richardson, A. (1988). Language delay in the child. In N. J. Lass, L. V. McReynolds, J. L. Northern, & D. E. Yoder (Eds.), *Handbook of speech–language pathology and audiology* (pp. 655–684). Philadelphia: Decker.

Wallace, G., & Hammill, D. D. (1994). *Comprehensive and Receptive and Expressive Vocabulary Test.* Austin, TX: PRO-ED.

Wallace, I. F., Gravel, J. S., McCarton, C. M., & Ruben, R. J. (1988). Otitis media and language development at 1 year of age. *Journal of Speech and Hearing Disorders, 53,* 245–251.

Wing, L. (1972). *Autistic children.* New York: Bruner/Mazel.

Winokur, S. (1976). *A primer of verbal behavior: An operant view.* Englewood Cliffs, NJ: Prentice Hall.

Fluency and Its Disorders

Normal acquisition of speech sounds and language structures is necessary but not sufficient for competent social communication. Speakers also should acquire fluency in the use of language. If language is not used in a flowing, rhythmic, and fluent manner, communication suffers. Impediments to fluent communication create problems of fluency, of which the most common form is stuttering. Another form of fluency disorder is cluttering. Both create not only impediments to fluent and efficient communication but also many personal and social problems. These two disorders of fluency are the subjects of this chapter. Of the two, stuttering will receive most of our attention.

A Child's Story of Stuttering

Brian was a 5-year-old boy who stuttered. His parents, Mr. and Mrs. Thomas, took him to a speech and hearing clinic. As a disorder of fluency, **stuttering** is the speech of repetitions, prolongations, silent intervals, interjections, and excessive muscular effort. The following dialogue between the parents and the clinician summarizes some of the basic information about stuttering.

CLINICIAN: When did you first think that there may be something wrong with Brian's speech?

MRS. THOMAS: About a month ago, on a Sunday morning, I noticed that Brian was repeating a lot. I remember asking him what he wanted to eat for lunch that day. Brian started to say something like, "I want a hot dog for lunch," but he had a lot of trouble saying it.

CLINICIAN: What exactly did he do?

MRS. THOMAS: Well, he started like, "I-I-I-I-I wa-wa-wa-want a hot d-d-d-d-dog, Mom." He was trying too hard to say it. I could see a lot of struggle to get it out.

CLINICIAN: You had not heard that kind of problem in Brian's speech before?

MR. THOMAS: My wife had not heard it, but I had. About 2 months ago, when I was reading a story to him, he wanted to interrupt me to ask a question about the story. I don't remember what exactly he said at that time, but I remember him repeating a lot. Periodically, I have heard him repeat a bit too much, but I thought it may be a passing thing. I remember him asking me once, "What t-t-t-time is it, Dad?"

CLINICIAN: Have you seen an increase in repetitions?

MR. THOMAS: I think so. During the last month or so, his speech problems have increased. He is repeating more and getting stuck more often. Now it takes him longer to get out of a block, and only after some struggle.

CLINICIAN: What do you mean by a block?

MRS. THOMAS: His mouth and face look like he is trying hard to say something but nothing comes out. His lips are quivering, and his mouth is sometimes open, at other times tightly shut. You can see the struggle to say something, but he is not saying anything. This is what scares me the most.

CLINICIAN: Did anything unusual happen around the time you first noticed his repetitions or more recently when you noticed an increase in them?

MR. THOMAS: No, not really. Things have been pretty routine at home.

CLINICIAN: Has he been sick lately?

MRS. THOMAS: No, Brian has always been a healthy boy.

CLINICIAN: What about your health when you were carrying Brian?

MRS. THOMAS: I was fine during pregnancy, and the delivery was normal. The baby was healthy. We did not notice any problem until this stuttering came about.

CLINICIAN: What about his speech and language development? Was there any reason to be concerned?

MRS. THOMAS: No. In fact, Brian began to speak earlier than my other son Chad, who is 4 years older than him. We thought he was quite advanced in his speech. He usually talked a lot and learned new words fast.

CLINICIAN: So everything has been normal until you began to notice his stuttering.

MR. THOMAS: We may have missed something, but that is our impression.

CLINICIAN: I want to go back to Brian's stuttering. You said that he repeats a lot. Does he prolong a sound? Have you heard him say something like, "I want ssssome sssssoup, please?" I prolonged the *s* sound in both the words. Does he do that?

Take note of the different *types* of dysfluencies that Brian exhibited.

MRS. THOMAS: Oh, yes. He does it all the time. This morning, while eating a new kind of cereal, he said, "It is rad, Mom," but he prolonged the *a* sound. It was more like, "raaaad."

CLINICIAN: Does Brian repeat words and phrases? Does he say, "I-I-I want it," or "Let-let-let me do it," or "He-was he-was he-was coming," and things like that?

MR. THOMAS: Yes, we have heard him do that. Sometimes he repeats a word or a bunch of words many times before he moves on to the next word. Yesterday I heard him say to his brother, "Why are you-why are you-why are you-why are you do-do-doing it?"

CLINICIAN: Does he use what we call interjections like *uh* or *um* or *er*? As you know, most speakers have them, but I wonder how much Brian interjects.

MRS. THOMAS: I think he interjects a lot. In fact, Brian drives me up the wall with his *uhs* and *ums*. He starts a lot of sentences with *ums*. This morning he said, "Um-um-um what am I-I-I g-g-g-going to have um-um-um-um for breakfast, Mom." Sometimes he keeps going with *ums*.

CLINICIAN: What about interjected words like *well, OK,* and phrases like *you know, I mean,* and *you see?*

MRS. THOMAS: He uses them some of the time. We hear more *ums* and *uhs* than what you just described.

CLINICIAN: Does Brian show any facial grimaces when he stutters? Some people who stutter blink their eyes, wrinkle their noses and foreheads, purse their lips, wring their hands, swing their arms, and move their legs. Does Brian do any of these?

MRS. THOMAS: Yes, he does a few of those. I have seen him blink his eyes and wrinkle his nose and forehead. His hands and feet also move when he stutters. His mouth is distorted when he has a bad block. He also looks away from you when he stutters.

CLINICIAN: Does Brian stutter all the time or only some of the time?

MR. THOMAS: His stuttering varies. One day we may hear just a few problems, and the next day he may stutter on most of the words he speaks. He may be quite fluent in the morning but struggling to say his name in the afternoon. I find this puzzling. Is this true of other children who stutter, too?

CLINICIAN: Yes, it is. A basic characteristic of stuttering is that it varies across time and speaking situations. Stuttering may occur more when speaking on complex or unfamiliar topics. Dialogues in which people must take quick turns to talk and be silent also are difficult for people who stutter. They are more fluent while talking aloud to themselves or when they are speaking in monologue. Stuttering also varies depending on the conversational partner. People who stutter may be very fluent talking to pets and babies. Many adults who stutter talk to their subordinates with increased fluency, but when they confront their bosses, fluency may break down abruptly. Does Brian stutter more with some people and less with others?

MR. THOMAS: He is more fluent with his younger sister Michelle, who is 3. He has the most trouble with me, somewhat less with his mother. I would say his stuttering is about average when he talks to his older brother.

MRS. THOMAS: But his worst stuttering comes out when he talks to a stranger or in a new place. I took him to Chad's school the other day. One of the teachers there talked to Brian who blocked on every word he tried to say. The poor kid couldn't say his name. It was a heartbreaking scene for me. Also, his stuttering is worst when he talks to some of the kids in the neighborhood.

CLINICIAN: Many stutterers avoid certain words. Older children and adults use substitutes for difficult words. Do you know of any words that Brian avoids saying?

MRS. THOMAS: I think I do. The other day Brian wouldn't say *John,* who is a friend of Chad's. Brian kept saying, "Your friend called," but wouldn't say who it was. When Chad asked about four times, "Who was it?" Brian finally said, "J-J-J-John," and stuttered very badly on it. Of late, I have not heard him say "Hi" to people because he can't get it out. Another puzzling thing about his problem is that he can sing songs and not have a trace of trouble. Is this also typical?

CLINICIAN: Yes, it is! Most people who stutter have no trouble singing.

MR. THOMAS: It's amazing! Although Brian has certain words on which he stutters frequently, he can say those very same words fluently. I suppose this also is characteristic of stuttering.

CLINICIAN: That also is true. Stuttering on words is a matter of probability. Stuttering is more probable on some words than on other words. But even the words on which the stuttering probability is the highest may be, on occasion, spoken fluently. Therefore, it is not a question of not being able to say a word. As you know very well, Brian can, on occasion, say fluently every word that he stutters on. He knows exactly what to say, but on certain occasions he just cannot say it smoothly and easily.

MRS. THOMAS: That makes sense.

CLINICIAN: I want to talk a little bit about the family history. Is there a history of speech disorders in the family? Are you aware of a speech problem on either side of the family?

MR. THOMAS: When I was a kid, I used to stutter. I don't believe that my father ever stuttered but an uncle of mine did.

CLINICIAN: Do you know when you began to stutter and how severe it was?

MR. THOMAS: I am not sure, but I think I began to stutter when I was about 4. I think it was pretty bad because I still remember having a lot of trouble in grade school. I remember the painful teasing and the frustration of getting blocked in front of the class and things like that.

CLINICIAN: Did you receive treatment? Do you remember what it was?

MR. THOMAS: I did go to a speech therapist but not very regularly. I can't remember much about what she did with me.

CLINICIAN: When did your stuttering disappear, if it has. So far, you have not stuttered here.

MR. THOMAS: I do not stutter any more. I think my stuttering was at its peak during my years in intermediate school. High school was different. I began to experience more fluency, although I was not taking speech therapy at that time. The problem became less noticeable when I started college, and it disappeared in the subsequent years. Is this common?

CLINICIAN: To some degree. Some people who stutter may recover from it at any age, although recovery is more common in preschool children. During the early childhood years, girls who begin to stutter recover more often than boys of the same age. Roughly, some 30% of stutterers recover from it without much professional help, although some experts think this percentage is much higher. We call this **spontaneous recovery.** Mrs. Thomas, how about on your side of the family?

MRS. THOMAS: I do not believe there was a stutterer on my side of the family. I can't be sure, though. I did read in a newspaper article that stuttering runs in the family. Is this true?

CLINICIAN: To a certain extent, stuttering tends to run in the family. The blood relatives of a person who stutters have a greater chance of stuttering, compared with the blood relatives of nonstuttering people. We call this the **familial** incidence of stuttering. But the higher familial incidence also is related to the **gender ratio.** You know that there are more male stutterers than female stutterers.

MRS. THOMAS: Yes, I have wondered about that. I have seen only one female stutterer in my life but many male stutterers. But how does it relate to the familial incidence?

CLINICIAN: The familial incidence is related to the gender of one or more people found to stutter in the family. If a male in a family is found to stutter, the familial incidence for that family may be higher compared with the incidence in the general population. However, if a female in a family is found to stutter, the familial incidence may be the highest. This means that though females are less likely to stutter, a female who does stutter poses the maximum risk to the members of her family. In fact, the brothers and sons of a female who stutters run a very high risk of developing stuttering. Sisters and daughters of a male or female who stutters do not run that much of a risk. Of all the people, the sons of mothers who stutter run the greatest risk of developing stuttering.

MR. THOMAS: Does it mean that stuttering is hereditary?

CLINICIAN: Some experts believe that stuttering is **genetically transmitted,** at least in a certain number of cases, although we do not know of a defective gene and its method of transmission. However, we must remember that not all people who stutter have stuttering relatives. Therefore, we cannot conclude that stuttering is inherited in all cases. Most experts believe that both heredity and environment play a role in the development of stuttering.

MRS. THOMAS: If it is inherited, is it more difficult to treat?

CLINICIAN: No, there are no data that suggest that. Research has shown that almost all children and adults who stutter improve under treatment and many to a significant extent. Early treatment of stuttering is especially effective, and I am glad that you brought Brian this early.

MR. THOMAS: Well, that is good news for Brian and for us!

Some Basic Characteristics of Stuttering

The conversation between Mr. and Mrs. Thomas and the speech–language clinician points out many basic characteristics of stuttering. What follows is a summary of some of those characteristics.

Forms of Stuttering: Dysfluencies

Stuttering is a disorder of fluency characterized by certain types of dysfluencies, excessive amounts of dysfluencies in general, or excessive durations of dysfluencies. Of course, in some individuals, stuttering may be a combination of excessive duration and frequency of some or all types of dysfluencies. In addition, stuttering also may be characterized by **associated motor behaviors,** which include excessive muscular effort in speaking, facial grimaces, and hand and feet movements. Several other features, including the tendency to avoid certain words and speaking situations, are probably due to the initial difficulty in saying the words. Eventually, they also become a part of the stuttering problem.

The term **dysfluency** is also spelled **disfluency.**

The term **dysfluencies** refers to the many forms of interruptions that prevent the easy, effortless, and smooth flow of speech. In other words, dysfluencies are behaviors that disrupt fluency. Brian had several types of dysfluencies: part-word repetitions ("t-t-t-time," "g-g-g-going"); whole word repetitions ("I-I-I-I"); phrase repetitions ("why are you-why are you-why are you"); sound prolongations ("sssssoup"); and interjections of sounds, syllables, words, and phrases (*uh, um, well, you see*). People who stutter exhibit several other types of dysfluencies. Table 6.1 shows the major types of dysfluencies and examples.

Table 6.1
Major Types of Dysfluencies That Disrupt Fluent Speech

Dysfluency Types	Examples
Repetitions	
Part-word repetitions	"What t-t-t-time is it?"
Whole-word repetitions	"What-what-what are you doing?"
Phrase repetitions	"I want to-I want to-I want to do it."
Prolongations	
Sound/syllable prolongations	"Lllllllet me do it."
Silent prolongations	A struggling attempt to say a word when there is no sound.
Interjections	
Sound/syllable interjections	"um . . . um I had a problem this morning."
Whole-word interjections	"I had a well problem this morning."
Phrase interjections	"I had a you know problem this morning."
Silent pauses	A silent duration between words and sentences considered too long: "I was going to the (pause) store."
Broken words	A silent pause within words: "It was won(pause)derful."

The Loci of Stuttering

The **loci** of stuttering refers to the locations in the speech sequence where stutterings are typically observed. Stutterings or dysfluencies are not randomly distributed throughout an utterance. For example, stuttering is more likely on the initial word of a phrase or a sentence. The very first or the first few words are more likely to be repeated than the last few words of a sentence. For example, "Let-let-let-let me do it," is heard frequently, but not, "Let me do it-it-it." Similarly, the initial syllable is more likely to be repeated than the final syllables. For example, we often hear, "Pro-pro-probably it is true," but not, "Probably-bly-bly it is true."

Stuttering is more likely on consonants than on vowels, although some people stutter predominantly on vowels. People who stutter tend to have greater difficulty with longer than shorter words. Words that are used more frequently in the language are stuttered less often than those that are used less frequently. It has been hypothesized that the longer and the less frequently used words are more difficult to produce; therefore, they tend to be stuttered more often (Bloodstein, 1995).

Diagnosis of Stuttering

Even a casual observation will reveal that most forms of dysfluencies listed in Table 6.1 may be readily observed in normal speakers. The normally fluent speech is not perfectly fluent; probably no one is 100% fluent all the time. Such dysfluencies as *uh* and *um* and word and phrase repetitions are fairly common in the speech of most, if not all, people. Pauses of varying durations are equally common, especially in young children whose language skills are still developing. Even part-word repetitions and sound prolongations may be observed, though less frequently, in everyday speech of most speakers. How, then, is a person who stutters distinguished from normal speakers on the basis of dysfluencies? This has been a difficult question and there are several answers to it.

There are at least three well-established bases to distinguish a person who stutters from those who do not: (1) the frequency of all dysfluencies combined, (2) the presence of certain specific types of dysfluencies, and (3) the duration of dysfluencies. A clinician may consider one or more of these three bases. Figure 6.1 summarizes these criteria along with ways of combining them.

Frequency of All Dysfluencies Combined

Both normal speakers and those who stutter vary a great deal in the amount (frequency) of dysfluencies. A normal speaker may be more or less dysfluent depending on the speaking situation, the topic being discussed, the kind of listener involved, fatigue, the amount of knowledge about the topic, and many other factors. When talking about a familiar topic, under relaxing conditions, when the listeners are sympathetic and approving, a speaker may be more fluent. When talking about a topic he or she knows very little about, under threatening or stressful conditions, when the listeners are unsympathetic or hostile, and when tired, speakers may be more dysfluent.

The variability found in the amount of dysfluencies of normal speakers also is found in people who stutter. But over and beyond that, dysfluencies of people who stutter fluctuate from day to day and from one speaking situation to the

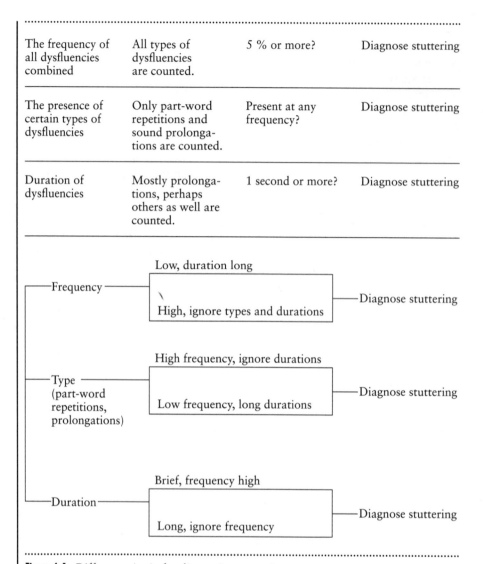

The frequency of all dysfluencies combined	All types of dysfluencies are counted.	5 % or more?	Diagnose stuttering
The presence of certain types of dysfluencies	Only part-word repetitions and sound prolonga-tions are counted.	Present at any frequency?	Diagnose stuttering
Duration of dysfluencies	Mostly prolonga-tions, perhaps others as well are counted.	1 second or more?	Diagnose stuttering

Frequency
Low, duration long
High, ignore types and durations
Diagnose stuttering

Type (part-word repetitions, prolongations)
High frequency, ignore durations
Low frequency, long durations
Diagnose stuttering

Duration
Brief, frequency high
Long, ignore frequency
Diagnose stuttering

Figure 6.1. Different criteria for diagnosing stuttering.

other. On the average, however, people who stutter do so on about 10% of the words they speak (Bloodstein, 1995). Therefore, a frequency of 10% of dysfluency is certainly abnormal, and the minimum frequency of dysfluency needed to diagnose stuttering is less than 10%.

Because it is difficult to precisely determine how dysfluent normal speakers are and what is the minimum (not the average) level of dysfluency needed to diagnose stuttering, experts have tried to determine how listeners respond to different amounts of dysfluencies. After all, if a society tolerates a certain amount of dysfluencies, then that amount may be judged normal. Ordinary people may be asked to listen to speech samples that contain varying amounts of dysfluencies and judge whether the speech is abnormal, stuttered, normal, or fluent, and so on. Results of these **listener judgment** studies have generally indicated that most dysfluencies are judged abnormal or stuttered when they reach or exceed 5% of the words spoken (Bloodstein, 1995; Van Riper, 1982). Therefore, some clinicians use the criterion of 5% or more dysfluencies to distinguish people who stutter from those who do not. In using this criterion, the clinician counts *all types* of dysfluencies because there is evidence that listeners judge a speech sample negatively if it includes an excessive amount of such fairly common types of dysfluencies as interjections and word repetitions (Hegde & Hartman, 1979a, 1979b). The clinician then counts the total number of words spoken or read. From these two measures, the clinician derives a percentage of dysfluency rate.

Presence of Certain Types of Dysfluencies

Some clinicians believe that normal and stuttered speech should be distinguished not by the amount of dysfluencies but by the **types of dysfluencies.** Although all kinds of dysfluencies are present in normal speakers, some types are infrequent. For example, part-word repetitions and speech-sound prolongations are not as frequent as interjections and word or phrase repetitions. However, these types of dysfluencies are heard quite frequently in the speech of people who stutter (Van Riper, 1982; Wingate, 1964). Therefore, some clinicians diagnose stuttering only on the basis of part-word repetitions and sound prolongations.

The diagnosis of stuttering based on the types of dysfluency may not have a quantitative criterion. The presence of part-word repetitions or prolongations may be sufficient to diagnose stuttering. The amount of these dysfluencies does not have to meet a quantitative (frequency) criterion such as 5%.

Most experts think that part-word repetitions and prolongations are more likely to be associated with muscular tension and struggle. Word repetitions or interjections often are produced without much struggle or muscular tension. In fact, some clinicians place a heavy emphasis on tension and struggle, along with abnormal breathing patterns (such as an attempt to speak while inhaling the air) associated with certain types of dysfluencies. Accordingly, *any* type of dysfluency is a stutter if it is produced with tension and struggle. For example, if a child said, "What-what-what are you doing?" and while repeating *what* the child showed facial grimaces, tension, and struggle, then that word repetition may be counted as a stutter.

Duration of Dysfluencies

Still other clinicians diagnose stuttering on the basis of **excessive durations** of dysfluencies. A dysfluency may be so brief that only an expert would notice it or it may be so long that none would miss it. Accordingly, a speaker may be considered a stutterer if his or her dysfluencies are of abnormal durations (Van Riper, 1982). Most clinicians diagnose stuttering if the duration of dysfluencies lasts a second (Van Riper, 1982).

The durational criterion may or may not use the frequency criterion as well. When the durations are very brief, the frequency may be important in the diagnosis of stuttering. When the durations are noticeably long, the frequency of dysfluencies may be ignored. In essence, stuttering is diagnosed when the durations are brief but the frequency of dysfluencies is high, or when the frequency is low but the durations are long.

Combined Use of the Three Criteria

A clinician may consider the three criteria as a set of rules to use in diagnosing stuttering. If one rule fails, the other rule may be applied to evaluate if a speaker stutters. For example, if a speaker's dysfluencies (all types counted and combined) exceed 5% of the words spoken, stuttering may be diagnosed. If a speaker's total dysfluency rate, when all types are counted and combined, does not meet the 5% criterion, then the presence of specific types of dysfluencies may be noted. If the speaker's dysfluencies are predominantly part-word repetitions and sound prolongations, stuttering may be diagnosed even if the rate is less than 5%. If neither of these rules apply, then the third rule may be applied. That is, if the speaker's dysfluencies are excessively long, then stuttering may be diagnosed.

Summary

- The diagnosis of stuttering is most certain when specific types of dysfluencies, notably part-word repetitions and prolongations, are both high in frequency and long in duration. The diagnosis depends on other factors such as tension, struggle, and breathing and other abnormalities when the frequency of these dysfluencies is low and the durations are short.

- When the frequency of all types of dysfluencies combined is high, their types and durations do not matter. Stuttering is diagnosed.

- When the duration of dysfluencies is very high, other factors do not matter; stuttering is diagnosed.

Associated Behaviors

In addition to dysfluencies of certain kinds and features, several associated behaviors also may characterize stuttering. As noted earlier, associated motor behaviors and avoidance of speech, speaking situations, and specific words may be parts of the stuttering problem.

Motor Behaviors

In some cases, associated motor behaviors may be the most attention-drawing deviations.

Stuttering-associated motor behaviors are many, and they vary across people who stutter, although a particular person is likely to have a characteristic pattern of behaviors. A majority of associated motor behaviors are observed in the face. Most adults who stutter tend to blink their eyes and wrinkle their noses and foreheads. Some tightly shut their eyes. Others purse their lips; their lips may quiver and tremble. Some keep their mouths wide open even while trying to say a word that starts with a /p/ or /b/, which requires the lips to be pressed together. Others repeatedly open and close their mouths while producing no speech sounds, although the flapping tongues and the forcefully closing and opening mouths may make various nonspeech sounds. Some people who stutter drop their jaws, and others so tightly close them that their heads begin to shake. One client I worked with ground her teeth and another clicked his tongue. A 10-year-old boy with severe stuttering slowly bent his torso until his face touched his own lap. A 35-year-old stuttering person jerked his neck every time he stuttered. Another person slowly moved his head toward his left shoulder during stuttering.

Movements of hands and feet also may be associated with stuttering. One person who stuttered swung his arms so widely, wildly, and suddenly that his wife had to keep a certain distance from him while he talked. Many just wring their hands. Some tap on the table or tap themselves, thinking that the rhythm of the taps makes them more fluent. Some clench their fist. An adult female person who stuttered violently rubbed the floor with the soles of her shoes. She said jokingly that her stuttering has a tendency to put holes in the carpet. Others may just wiggle their legs, move their feet, or tense their thighs.

Muscular tension associated with speech also is significant. Most people who stutter report a tightness in their throat, jaw, chest, shoulder, and stomach muscles while producing dysfluent speech. Most of the facial gestures described earlier are associated with excessive tension in the speech muscles. In some cases, tension may be felt in the entire body.

Certain breathing abnormalities also may be associated with stuttering. As noted before, a person who stutters may try to talk while inhaling air. Whereas normal speakers stop and breathe every so often during speech, a person who stutters may try to keep talking (and stuttering), although the air supply is exhausted. People whose stuttering is associated with this problem give the impression that they are trying to squeeze out the last bit of air from their lungs. In the middle of an utterance, some speakers who stutter stop and inhale unnecessarily. Breathing patterns of people who stutter may be jerky and arrhythmic during stuttered speech.

> Recall from **Chapter 3** that we speak on exhaled air.

Why do individuals who stutter exhibit these associated motor behaviors? Most likely because of accidental reinforcement of such behaviors. A man who says, "What t-t-t-t . . ." happens to swing his arm in frustration, and, just as he swings the arm, he happens to complete the word and the rest of the utterance: ". . . time are you coming?" The arm swing is accidentally reinforced by the release from an aversive stuttering. Next time when he stutters, he is more likely to swing the arm. At another time, a tight closing of the eyelids may be coincidental to the release from bad stuttering. Thus, initially, many associated motor behaviors may be coincidentally associated with the termination of stuttering. Eventually, they become a part of stuttering. At no time do the associated motor behaviors directly help stuttering people speak fluently.

The associated motor behaviors are not crucial for a diagnosis of stuttering. Not all speakers who stutter show marked associated behaviors. These behaviors are not necessarily related to age or the number of years of stuttering. A 5-year-old child with a history of only a few months of stuttering may show a complex set of bizarre motor behaviors. A 50-year-old adult with a 45-year history of stuttering may show only a few mild associated motor behaviors, if any at all. Typically, associated motor behaviors are exhibited only during the production of dysfluent and tensed speech. Therefore, associated motor behaviors are not a necessary minimum condition to diagnose stuttering. When they are present, however, the exaggerated associated movements and muscular tension make the diagnosis of stuttering virtually certain.

Negative Emotions and Avoidance Behaviors

A person who stutters is bound to experience certain emotional and behavioral effects of this profound speech difficulty. A 3-year-old boy who begins to repeat and prolong may not be aware of his speech difficulty. But this lack of awareness does not last too long. Soon the child is frustrated by his own struggle to express himself. The child gradually or even suddenly becomes aware of his unique struggles and tensions associated with speech. Some parents may "keep their cool" and not respond, at least for a while. But children whom the stuttering child plays with are more than likely to say something. To the boy who has not already figured that there is something wrong with his speech, a response from some person will certainly make it clear. The negative feelings and the eventual avoidance behaviors the person who stutters develops may have an origin in this awareness of being different in speech.

Parents and other adults cannot indefinitely withhold their reactions to the child's difficulties. To create a painful awareness in the child, the response need not be critical or negative. Polite, kind, and well-intentioned responses also can make the child aware of his or her difficulty or make the existing awareness more keen and painful. In an effort to help a child who is struggling to say something, some adults anticipate the child's words and say them. Other adults may politely look away from the child who is stuttering. Some may give such suggestions as "take a deep breath and say it" or "think of what you want to say before you say it," believing that such strategies will help the child. The effect of these and other adult reactions is an intensified unpleasant feeling that the child associates with his or her own speech problem.

The child who stutters is likely to confront impatient or outright rude responses from others. Some parents might criticize the child for being dysfluent and may urge the child to work harder to maintain fluency. Friends' teasing, strangers' occasional glances of surprise, or a sign of impatience can compound the situation for the child.

Repeated stutterings on certain words or in certain speaking situations eventually lead to the avoidance of those words and speaking situations. Each person who stutters may find some words more difficult to say than others. A client I treated had the greatest difficulty saying *pepperoni,* so he never ordered pepperoni pizza, which he loved, but ordered (and ate) mushroom pizza, which he hated. A 22-year-old female receptionist always said "Yes?" when she picked up the phone because if she tried to say "Hello" or the name of the company, a long silent pause resulted and caused some people to hang up on her. For a 10-year-old boy, his own last name was difficult to say. He gave a false name whenever he thought he could get away with it. A priest who counseled troubled couples to communicate better with each other could not say *communicate* or *communication* without stuttering badly. During his Sunday morning sermon, he could never say *communion* without hopelessly getting stuck on it; he simply avoided it. The priest substituted *talk* or *express* for *communication* and *the Lord's supper* for *communion.* But he was unhappy about his avoidance and word substitutions. He very much wanted to use the words he avoided.

Circumlocution also may be due to lack of knowledge of precise words to use or to a need to be indirect (diplomatic) in speech.

Circumlocution is another strategy that stuttering people use. They beat around the bush until the listener says the word they have been avoiding. Relieved, stuttering people then eagerly confirm it. A 15-year-old boy who stuttered surprised a student speech–language pathologist by saying, "My dad's wife is coming to pick me up soon." "She is your mother, isn't she?" asked the clinician. "Yes. You know it is an *em* word!" grinned the teenager. A mother of two daughters would not refer to them by their names; she always talked about "my younger daughter" or "my older daughter." Her listeners tended to ask, "You mean Jenny?" or "You mean Jeanne?" and the mother would say "Yes!" or "No." A client of mine stuttered severely on *June* and *July.* So in April he gave me advanced notice of his vacation by saying, "I will be spending the first and the second months that come after May in Europe." When I asked him where in Europe he would be spending his vacation, he fully taxed my knowledge of European geography: "First I go to Austria. Then I will visit the country that lies north of Austria. Then perhaps the country that is west of. . . ."

People who stutter carefully avoid many speaking situations. Apparently, this kind of avoidance is age-old. The legend has it that Moses was a stutterer who described himself as "slow of speech, and of a slow tongue." When he had to tell the people of Israel what God had told him, he recruited his brother Aaron to be his spokesman. Taking a clue from Moses, an executive of a large manufacturing company who did everything to avoid speaking on the telephone, hired an assistant just to talk on his behalf over the phone. The assistant, sitting next to the executive, relayed information back and forth like an interpreter of a foreign language. A 35-year-old woman would not order food at restaurants; she rarely went out alone to eat. A 23-year-old college student made sure that he never took a course in which oral presentations were mandatory. He met the instructor before registering for a class and made sure that there were no such assignments or that a written paper could be substituted. Another young man preferred to get lost in a city rather than to stop and ask someone for directions. Visiting Los Angeles for the first time, he found himself lost one evening while looking for a restaurant. After 2 hours of driving around, the restaurants he found were all closed. Needless to say, his avoidance behavior kept him hungry and awake that night.

Generally speaking, people who stutter tend to avoid strangers, formal audiences, counters where services or products are bought, telephones, restaurants, and self-introductions or other introductions. When such speaking situations cannot be avoided, people who stutter adopt other strategies, including word avoidance and circumlocution.

Like the associated motor behaviors, avoidance of words and speaking situations are not essential to the diagnosis of stuttering. They are the results of stuttering. The individuals would not have learned to avoid certain speaking situations if they did not stutter in those situations. Therefore, stuttering comes first and the avoidance responses next. However, avoidance of speaking situations, when combined with other evidence, strongly supports the diagnosis of stuttering.

Practically all people who stutter report the experience of painful emotions associated with stuttering. The emotional responses may get stronger as the stutterer gets older, especially when the stuttering severity increases. Consistent stuttering on certain words and in certain speaking situations creates apprehension and anxiety about speaking and speaking situations. Experts believe that these feelings of apprehension and anxiety are the causes of avoidance behaviors. These feelings are automatically reduced when a person avoids a word or a situation that causes them. Such reductions reinforce the avoidance reactions and thus perpetuate them.

Most adults who stutter can predict a certain amount of their stutterings before they occur. While reading aloud, people who stutter rapidly scan ahead to see if there are any difficult words. Tension mounts when some such words are spotted. In conversational speech, people who stutter constantly think about the inevitability of saying certain difficult words. An author whose lucidly written book on stuttering is based on his personal experience wrote, "Whenever I opened my mouth, I mentally glanced ahead at the sentence I wanted to say, to see if there was any word I was likely to stutter on" (Jonas, 1977, pp. 3–4). This phenomenon is known as **anticipation** or **expectancy** and is considered the basis of avoidance behaviors. If trouble in the form of stuttering is expected in a situation, the stuttering person tries to avoid it. In the past, if the person has had trouble speaking in that situation, then he or she expects the same trouble in that situation.

What Some Stuttering People Tell Us

Most people who stutter describe their stuttering as uncontrollable events. It is something that happens to them; they are not in charge of their speech mechanism when they stutter. Consider the following two dramatic descriptions, the first by the noted American author John Updike and the second by Jonas who was quoted earlier:

> I liked to imagine, all evidence to the contrary, that my stutter was unnoticeable, that only I was conscious of it. Conscious, that is, of a kind of window pane suddenly inserted in front of my face while I was talking, or of a barrier thrust into my throat. For there is no doubt that I have lots of words inside me; it's just that at moments, like rush-hour traffic at the mouth of a tunnel, they jam and I can't get them out. (Updike, 1987, p. 19)

> In the struggle to terminate a block, some stutterers became so agitated that they resemble an *epileptic having an attack:* cold sweat appears on their foreheads, they gasp for breath, their eyes bulge, their lips quiver, their arms jerk like a puppet's, they spray saliva in all directions; they seem to be literally trying to shake their words loose from their tongue. It is not hard to see why such people were once thought to be *possessed by demons;* when chronic stutterers talk about themselves, they often refer to their body as if it were under *alien control.* (Jonas, 1977, p. 70) [italics added]

A handyman who stuttered told me, "I feel like someone put a drop of crazy glue on the tip of my tongue. The tongue gets stuck to the roof of my mouth." People who stutter also say that the harder they try to get out of a block, the more difficult it becomes to get released. However, those individuals are puzzled as to why they suddenly get stuck on a word and then, just as suddenly, get released from it. For them, neither is their doing.

Many people who stutter believe that most listeners react unfavorably to their speech problem. Although very few people are outright rude to individuals who stutter, a single incidence of rudeness is always remembered and often generalized to other listeners, including those who do not react negatively. Occasionally, an impatient person on the phone hangs up on a speaker who has a long and silent prolongation. A gas station attendant tells a person who stutters to "come back when you know what you want." A teacher rolls her eyes when a child repeats endlessly. A tired and annoyed father asks a stuttering child to "spit it out." But such reactions are not as frequent as some people who stutter believe.

In fact, most people are polite. They want to help. However, people who stutter find the lay attempts to help them annoying and humiliating. If asked, many people who stutter will tell their conversational partners the following:

- Please do not finish sentences for us; instead, just be patient.

- Please do not politely turn your face away when we have a long dysfluency; keep looking at us as you normally would.

- Please do not tell us to "think what you want to say before you say it," for our stuttering is not due to confused or lack of thinking. We know precisely what we want to say; we just cannot say it at the moment.

- Please do not give us the perennial and useless suggestion "relax before you say something." Increased tension in speaking situations is part of our problem.

- Please do not ask us to "to take a deep breath before you speak," because only speech–language pathologists can teach us how to manage our airflow to sustain fluency.

Prevalence of Stuttering

Stuttering is found in almost all societies of the world. Some research suggests, however, that stuttering may be more prevalent in some societies than in others, but it is doubtful if stuttering is unheard of in any society (Bloodstein, 1995; Van Riper, 1982). In the United States, roughly 1% of the general population stutters. Assuming a population figure of about 280 million people, there are more than 2.8 million people in the United States who stutter.

Stuttering is more prevalent in school-age children than in the general population. Roughly 4% of school-age children may stutter at one time or another. The prevalence is probably still higher in preschool children. Stuttering in early childhood fluctuates across time. A child may stutter for a few days or weeks, and then the stuttering may suddenly disappear or gradually subside. In some cases, that is the end of it. In other cases, stuttering reappears gradually or with full force. One fourth of all children who stutter do so only for 6 months or less. As we noted before, depending on the age of onset, roughly one third recover from stuttering without professional help.

Stuttering can be found in all walks of life. It can be found in individuals with mental retardation as well as in those who are gifted. Philosophers, statesmen, kings, writers, and scientists have been among those who stutter. Besides Moses, Greek philosophers Aristotle and Demosthenes may have stuttered. In modern times, Sir Isaac Newton, Winston Churchill, and King George VI of England were stutterers. It was noted that the American writer John Updike stutters. Country singer Mel Tillis is a stutterer. Many other lesser known individuals who stutter have made significant contributions to government, science, education, and culture. Even more important is the fact that speech–language pathologists who were pioneers in researching and treating stuttering were attracted to this discipline because of their own stuttering. Wendell Johnson and Charles Van Riper are the two outstanding names in this category. Even today, many speech–language pathologists who are experts in stuttering stutter.

A well-established fact about the prevalence of stuttering is its gender ratio. Roughly four males stutter for every female who stutters (a 4:1 ratio). As noted before, more female than male children recover from stuttering. Still, many hypotheses have been advanced to explain this ratio. Both environmental and genetic factors have been suggested. An early environmental hypothesis was that parents expect the boys to excel in verbal skills and, therefore, put undue pressure on the boys. This pressure takes a toll on fluency. Currently, the hypothesis that the gender ratio is due to genetic factors is more attractive to many researchers. According to this hypothesis, stuttering may partly be an inherited disorder, at least in some individuals (Kidd, 1984).

The genetic hypothesis has received support from other kinds of data. As already noted, stuttering tends to run in families. This in itself is not a strong support for the genetic hypothesis; families may share similar environmental variables, which may account for the speech disorder. However, in combination with other kinds of evidence, it may support the genetic hypothesis.

Another kind of data on prevalence that supports the genetic hypothesis is what is called the concordance rate in **monozygotic** (identical) twins. If a disorder, disease, or trait is found in both the members of a monozygotic twin pair, then the twins are **concordant;** if only one of the twins is affected, then they are **discordant** for that disorder, disease, or trait. If a disorder shows a high concordance rate in monozygotic twins, then the disorder may have a genetic component. This is because the identical twins are formed out of a single fertilized ovum, which splits into two to form two embryos. The two individuals are genetically identical. **Dizygotic** or fraternal twins are formed out of two separate fertilized ova; genetically, they are no more similar than the ordinary siblings.

Stuttering was found to be concordant in several monozygotic twin pairs but not in all pairs studied. This suggests the importance of both heredity and environment in the etiology of stuttering. The presence of stuttering in some monozygotic twins, and its absence in their counterparts, points out the importance of environmental variables. More important, most of the concordant identical twins who stuttered were raised together. Therefore, the influence of environmental variables cannot be ruled out. Only concordant identical twins who were raised apart from the beginning provide strong support for the genetic hypothesis. Unfortunately, there are no such data.

Another factor that supports the role of environment is that even dizygotic twins who stutter show a higher concordance compared with ordinary siblings. There is no genetic reason why dizygotic twins should show greater concordance than brothers and sisters. The fact that they do suggests that twins, regardless of their genetic origin, may be reacted to more similarly than ordinary siblings and that they tend to learn behaviors—including stuttering—from each other.

In essence, the prevalence data suggest that both heredity and environment play a part in the etiology of stuttering. Most experts believe that genetic factors **predispose** an individual to stutter; under the right environmental circumstances, the individual is more likely to develop stuttering than the one not so genetically predisposed. Other kinds of data and theories are presented in the following sections.

Theories on Stuttering

Besides the genetic explanation discussed in the previous section, there are other theories that try to explain stuttering. A detailed discussion of many theories may be found in other sources (Bloodstein, 1995; Curlee & Siegel, 1997; Van Riper, 1982). In this section, two major sets of theories will be described briefly. One set of theories is related to neurophysiological variables and the other to environmental events.

Neurophysiological Aspects of Stuttering

From ancient times, philosophers, medical experts, and others have speculated about the **organic** or **neurophysiological** causes of stuttering. An idea central to these speculations is that one or more of the body structures or systems of people who stutter may be defective in some way. According to this view, stuttering may not be due to environmental factors but to faulty neurophysiological structures, functions, or both.

Historically, different organs or systems of the body, including those that have nothing to do with speech (e.g., the liver), have been blamed for stuttering (Van Riper, 1982). The Greek philosopher Aristotle thought that a too thick and sluggish tongue caused stuttering. The father of modern medicine, Hippocrates, thought that dry tongue was the cause. The ancient Roman physician Celsus suggested that a weak tongue was the culprit. Just when everyone thought that every kind of tongue had been blamed for stuttering, Galen, the great Greek physician of the 2nd century, suggested that cold and wet tongue was the real cause of stuttering. Then in the 17th century, the English philosopher Francis Bacon suggested that a frozen tongue was the cause. It is not known whether his treatment was welcome by the stuttering people of his time: he recommended hot wine to thaw the frigid tongue. We would not be surprised if some stutterers experienced temporary fluency soon after a session of hot wine treatment!

Not so old is the theory of the bad tongue, proposed by the Prussian surgeon Johann Friedrich Dieffenbach. He believed that stuttering was due to too large a tongue. The treatment was direct and swift: surgical removal of portions of the tongue. It is known that this treatment was carried out until the middle of the 19th century. Other organs of the body blamed for stuttering include the hyoid bone (a U-shaped bone in the upper throat), uvula, tonsils, hard palate, and brain.

The neurophysiological theories of modern day are based on extensive research on the speech mechanism and the brain that controls the movements of speech. Because speech is a finely regulated activity, the nerves, muscles, and brain must function properly to produce normal, fluent speech. Therefore, researchers have looked at all aspects of speech production and regulation to see if structures, functions, or both are abnormal.

Laryngeal Dysfunction

In recent years, researchers have looked at the larynx and its behaviors as a possible source of stuttering. Recall that the laryngeal mechanism in the throat is suspended by the hyoid bone at the base of the tongue and includes the vibrating vocal folds that produce voice. The larynx is a muscular structure controlled mostly by cranial nerve X. When a stuttering person suddenly stops talking, repeats syllables rapidly, or prolongs a sound, it is logical to assume that the vocal folds are behaving in an unusual manner.

In some studies, the laryngeal activity during stuttering and fluent speech was directly observed through a **fiberoptic scope,** which consists of a thin flexible tube inserted through the nose or mouth to the laryngeal area. It illuminates the larynx and allows the researcher to see it in action. In other studies, the electrical activity of laryngeal muscles was recorded through **electromyography.** Laryngeal activity also has been studied by **cineradiography,** in which moving X-ray pictures are taken. Unlike the conventional static X ray, cineradiography helps study the movement of structures.

Fiberoptic scopes, also known as **endoscopes,** are illustrated in **Chapter 7.**

Such studies have shown that during stuttering, the laryngeal muscles are too tense and excessively active. Pairs of muscles that oppose each other may be simultaneously active. For example, muscles that open and close the vocal folds may be active at the same time. This results in blocked or interrupted speech. The vocal folds normally vibrate in a regular and rhythmic manner, but in the production of stuttering, they vibrate irregularly and arrhythmically. People who stutter also tend to close their vocal folds very tightly, which blocks voicing and speech (Adams, Freeman, & Conture, 1984; Bloodstein, 1995).

The abnormal behaviors of the larynx just described are a part of stuttering, not its cause, because it is not possible to separate stuttering from those abnormal laryngeal behaviors. Clinically judged fluent speech is not associated with such abnormalities.

The Brain and the Speech Mechanism

Because it is the brain that controls the speech mechanism, it is thought that stuttering may be due to faulty structures or functions of the brain. Several lines of research have investigated the relation between brain functions and stuttering.

One line of investigation has suggested that in most stuttering individuals, one hemisphere of the brain may not be in full control of language or that language may be processed in the right side of the brain. In most normal speakers, regardless of handedness, the left side of the brain is dominant for speech. The right side of the brain is dominant for musical and other nonverbal activities. The two halves of the brain, known as the **cerebral hemispheres,** are identical in many respects, but the left hemisphere is slightly larger, and experts believe this is because of the importance and complexity of speech and language that this hemisphere controls. In a small percentage of individuals in the general population, the right hemisphere may be dominant for language. In any case, one hemisphere seems to take a leading role in controlling speech. However, if for some reason one of the hemispheres is not dominant for language, both may try to control a function in discoordinated fashion, causing stuttering (Bloodstein, 1995; Van Riper, 1982).

Such a theory was originally proposed by Orton and Travis in the 1920s. As summarized later by Travis (1931), the theory essentially stated that in the brain of a person who stutters neither hemisphere is dominant for speech. This theory was popular for many years in the United States and abroad. Later it was discarded in favor of other theories.

In recent years, researchers have developed new ways to study brain and speech production. For example, the **electroencephalographic method** by which the electrical activity of the brain is recorded has suggested that unlike non-stuttering speakers, people who stutter may process verbal as well as nonverbal material in the same hemisphere—the right hemisphere—which might be the "wrong" hemisphere for language (Moore, 1984).

By making moving X-ray films (cineradiography) of stuttering speakers' faces and oral structures, other experts have determined that the movements involved in speech are slower in people who stutter than in normal speakers, even when speech is fluent. The movements of the jaw, the lips, and the tongue are not coordinated in people who stutter. All these observations suggest that the brains of people who stutter may not be initiating and regulating speech activity in a smooth, efficient, and coordinated manner. Possibly, the nervous system is unstable in these individuals (Zimmermann, 1980).

The bulk of the available evidence does not suggest a gross neurophysiological defect in persons who stutter. Any defect is likely to be subtle and found only in some speakers with the stuttering problem. Most of the neurophysiological research has not identified causes of stuttering. For example, the slow

An old assumption that most stuttering people are born left-handed and were forced to use their right hand is not supported by research.

Handedness is no sure sign of hemispheric dominance for language.

and discoordinated speech movements do not cause stuttering; such movements are stutterings themselves. Therefore, much of the neurophysiological research describes the behavior of nerves and muscles of speech as they produce fluent and stuttered speech. The research does not point out why they behave the way they do.

Defective Auditory Mechanism

Another organic theory of stuttering is that people who stutter might have a defective auditory mechanism. People who stutter can be significantly more fluent when their hearing is **masked** by noise fed to their ears through headphones. Fluency also increases when people who stutter hear their own speech after a slight delay. This **delayed auditory feedback** is arranged mechanically and has been used in treating stuttering. These two findings, among a few others, have prompted speculation that perhaps the portions of the brain that interprets one's own speech production and thus helps regulate it may be defective. It should be noted that most people who stutter have normal hearing, and the auditory problem hypothesized is not in the ear but in the part of the brain that is concerned with hearing.

Proponents of the auditory defect theory assume that people who stutter have a built-in delay in processing one's own speech. That is why delayed feedback of speech induces more fluency because this delay now matches the built-in delay. However, the critics have pointed out that under delayed auditory feedback, the rate of speech is significantly slowed down. We know that when a person who stutters speaks slowly (with or without delayed auditory feedback), fluency improves. Therefore, it is possible that the effects of the delayed auditory feedback may be due to slower speech.

Stuttering and Environmental Factors

So far, we have seen that genes, the brain, nerves, and the speech mechanisms suggest potential problems and possible partial explanations of stuttering. There also have been theories that have tried to explain stuttering on the basis of environmental variables. Human behavior and its disorders have always been grounds for the *nature–nurture* controversy. Is behavior determined by genetic and neurophysiological factors, or is it shaped by environmental factors? These questions have been debated in the context of stuttering as well.

Many kinds of observations suggest that stuttering varies depending on environmental stimuli or events. For example, the greater the size of an audience, the higher the frequency of stuttering. A stimulus associated with increased or decreased stuttering tends to have the same effect on future occasions. For example, in some studies, a colored border placed on a printed page was associated with a high frequency of stuttering. Later, the participants of the experiment stuttered more in the presence of the colored border. In oral reading, when words that were stuttered on the first oral reading of a printed passage were all blotted out, the reader was likely to stutter on the words next to the blotted mark during the next reading (Bloodstein, 1995).

It already has been noted that stuttering varies depending on the listener. An individual who is talking fluently to a child turns to an adult and immediately stutters on the very first word. Another person, who was talking with relative fluency, walks into a fast food place and cannot place an order. Because of these and other kinds of evidence, the influence of environmental events on the frequency of stuttering is unquestionable (Bloodstein, 1995).

There are many environmental theories of stuttering. Only a few of them are presented here.

The Diagnosogenic Theory

A well-known theory of stuttering that explained it on the basis of environmental events is known as the **diagnosogenic theory.** It was proposed by Wendell Johnson, a pioneer-era speech–language pathologist and an early American researcher on stuttering, who said that the origin of stuttering is its parental diagnosis and that stuttering is not in the mouth of the child, but in the ear of the listener (Johnson & Associates, 1959). Johnson's research had convinced him that all speakers are dysfluent, and stuttering speakers are not necessarily more so. Parents, who have very high standards of fluency, or those who do not understand that all children exhibit dysfluencies, diagnose stuttering in their normally speaking child who happens to repeat, interject, revise, and prolong segments of speech like most other children.

If excessive dysfluencies or dysfluencies of certain kinds are not stutterings, what are they? If parents diagnose a nonexistent problem, so what? Johnson was a stutterer himself, so he had suffered too much to think that stuttering was much ado about nothing. For him, the problem of stuttering started *after* the mistaken diagnosis. Due to the diagnosis, the child believes that there is something wrong with his or her speech. Therefore, the child tries to avoid what the parents think is the problem: the dysfluencies, or Johnson's preferred term, **normal nonfluencies.** What the child does to avoid normal nonfluencies is stuttering. In essence, stuttering is not to be confused with dysfluencies. Stuttering is all those actions a child takes in order not to stutter: the facial grimaces, arm swings, foot tappings, tensed movements, and avoidance of words and speaking situations. According to Johnson, what have been earlier described as associated motor behaviors and avoidance responses are stutterings.

Johnson also hypothesized that Native Americans do not stutter because they do not have a word for it. Data show that they stutter and that they have many words for it.

Johnson's theory rested on one crucial assumption: that stuttering children do not exhibit more dysfluencies than nonstuttering children. Unfortunately, his own data and data collected by others have contradicted Johnson's assumption (Bloodstein, 1995). Most of the stuttering children and adults have significantly more dysfluencies than nonstuttering children and adults. Parents diagnose stuttering when there is an increase in the amount and duration of dysfluencies, most likely accompanied by muscular tension and effort.

A variation of Johnson's (Johnson & Associates, 1959) theory assumes that stuttering is due to the child's belief that speech is a difficult task. Proposed by Bloodstein (1984, 1995), the **anticipatory struggle theory** states that stuttering itself is a reaction of tension and speech fragmentation. The child may acquire the belief that speech is a difficult task for many reasons. For example, some children who have problems in language acquisition or speech production (articulation) later develop stuttering. The problems in learning the language or the sound system of the language, combined with the usual pressure to communicate, are likely to instill the belief that speech is a difficult task. Because of this belief, the child comes to anticipate trouble every time certain words must be spoken and begins to struggle while saying them. The child is most likely to fragment the word for the sake of simplicity. Even the child who can produce the whole word is likely to break it apart because of the belief that it is too difficult to produce the whole unit. Such fragmentations are stutterings.

Bloodstein's theory of anticipatory struggle and fragmentation of speech into dysfluent forms is consistent with many observations about stuttering (Bloodstein, 1995). However, we need more research to fully understand how the child comes to believe that speech is a difficult task. Many children who stutter do not show other kinds of communicative problems that may instill such a belief before their onset of stuttering.

Theories Based on Conditioning and Learning

The observation that a person who stutters speaks fluently on some words, in some speaking situations, and at some times but speaks dysfluently on other words, in other speaking situations, and at other times suggests that perhaps the person has been conditioned to behave that way. Therefore, several theories explain stuttering on the basis of conditioning and learning.

A few theorists have suggested that stuttering is a **learned avoidance behavior.** For example, Wischner (1950) suggested that children whose parents negatively evaluate their dysfluencies (or nonfluencies as Johnson would have said) begin to experience anxiety about their speech. This anxiety, which is eventually conditioned to certain sounds, words, the act of speech, and speaking situations, leads to avoidance behaviors called stuttering. This theory, in essence, is similar to Johnson's (Johnson & Associates, 1959). Parents' negative reaction to their children's speech is the beginning of the problem. The main problem with Wischner's theory (and Johnson's theory) is that it is difficult to show that parents react negatively to normal dysfluencies, creating the chain of events leading to anxiety and avoidance (stuttering).

Another learning-based view of stuttering is based on B. F. Skinner's (1953) operant conditioning. A behavior that can be increased or decreased by arranging certain consequences for it is called an operant. **Operants** are purposive and voluntary behaviors shaped, maintained, or increased by consequences called reinforcers or decreased by consequences called punishers or aversive events. A **reinforcer** is any event that, when made to follow a response, increases the frequency of that response. A **punisher** (or an aversive stimulus) is any event that, when made to follow a response, decreases the frequency of that response. Stimuli, including persons, objects, and physical settings, that are associated with a reinforced response are called **discriminative stimuli** (S^D). The response is more likely in the presence of its discriminative stimuli. Stimuli, including people, objects, and physical settings, that are associated with a punished and thus decreasing response are called an **S-delta** (S^Δ).

The operant theory of stuttering is based on some experiments that have shown that stutterings can be *experimentally* increased by reinforcement and decreased by punishment (Bloodstein, 1995; Hegde, 1995). In some experiments, verbal punishers such as "No" and "Wrong" have been used to reduce the frequency of stuttering. In other studies, electric shock has been used. Under shock, however, stuttering has increased in some cases, decreased in others, and shown no changes in a few cases. In still other studies, a blast of noise has been used to reduce stuttering. In essence, like operant behaviors, stuttering can be increased or decreased by presenting various stimuli.

Although the frequency of stuttering can be changed by experimental methods, we need more evidence to support the claim that stuttering is an operant behavior. How stuttering behaviors are shaped and reinforced is still not clear. How this apparently aversive behavior is maintained also is not clear.

Another conditioning theory called the **two factor theory** states that different dysfluencies may have different causes (Brutten & Shoemaker, 1967). According to this view, only part-word repetitions and sound prolongations are stutterings. All other forms of dysfluencies, including word repetitions and interjections, are not stutterings. The theory further states that stutterings, as defined, are due to anxiety, which is classically conditioned, and other forms of dysfluencies are operant behaviors. The two factors of the theory are the two types of conditioning that lead to stuttering and nonstuttering types of dysfluencies.

Classical conditioning, as researched by the Russian physiologist Pavlov, is achieved when one stimulus, say punishment, which naturally evokes a response such as anxiety, is paired with another stimulus, say a speaking situation, which does not normally evoke anxiety. If the punishment and the speaking situation are paired often enough, the speaking situation itself will provoke anxiety. The two-factor theory suggests that stutterers have been conditioned to experience anxiety in speaking situations. This anxiety leads to a disintegration of fluency, which takes the form of part-word repetitions and sound prolongations.

There is some evidence that part-word repetitions and sound prolongations increase or show no change when shock, which presumably induces anxiety, follows them. As noted before, there also is evidence that all kinds of dysfluencies are decreased under punishment, especially the type of punishment known as time-out and response cost, both described in a later section. The studies that reported increases in stuttering have mostly used electric shock and were conducted in the 1960s and 1970s. Since then, investigators have been understandably reluctant to use shock in experiments. Nonetheless, more research is needed to settle this controversy.

Freudian Psychoanalysis

Freudian theory of human behavior is psychological without being learning or conditioning based. The Freudian view of stuttering is that it is a form of neurosis, which is a milder form of mental or psychological disorder (Van Riper, 1982). Phobia or abnormal fear of something is a form of **neurosis.** Freud's theory of neurosis assumes that all neurotic responses are symptoms of unconscious conflicts that have their origins in abnormal psychosexual development in infancy and early childhood. A child who does not normally progress through such stages as the oral, anal, and Oedipus is **fixated** at one of those stages. For instance, an early weaning from breastfeeding or traumatic toilet training may fixate the child at the oral or the anal stage.

When in later life psychological conflicts and frustrations are experienced, the person tends to **regress** to the earlier stage of fixation. Because the behaviors of such infantile stages are not acceptable, the individual **suppresses** them. But the socially unacceptable and hence suppressed impulses get transformed into acceptable neurotic symptoms such as stuttering, phobia, or hysterical reactions.

Some psychoanalysts believe that stuttering individuals' struggles to say a word reflect oral fixations. Stuttering, like smoking or thumb-sucking, is a way of oral indulgence. Other psychoanalysts believe that the explosive release from blocks that stuttering people exhibit suggests anal fixations. Aggressive behaviors are assumed to be a part of the anal stage. Therefore, stuttering also may be an expression of anal-sadistic aggression. That some individuals who stutter spray saliva on their listeners may be interpreted as evidence of latent aggression.

The Freudian theory of neurosis has come under heavy criticism because the treatment based on that theory has not worked. There is very little scientific evidence to show that the psychoanalysis of phobia or stuttering has been effective. In addition, the basic assumptions of the theory cannot be verified by research. Therefore, during the past several decades, the psychoanalytic treatment of stuttering has declined.

Research conducted to determine whether people with stuttering or their parents show neurotic tendencies has also been negative. Stutterers are like other people who do not stutter. The parents of children who stutter are like parents of children who do not.

Summary of Theories on Stuttering

Stuttering has been explained in many contrasting ways. Two broad categories of theories are organic and environmental. These theories are summarized in Figure 6.2.

(continues)

Organic
- Genetic theory: Stuttering or a predisposition to stutter is inherited.
- Cerebral dominance theory: Stutterers lack cerebral dominance for language; interhemispheric conflict.
- Hemispheric processing problems: Stutterers process language in the right, hence the "wrong," hemisphere.
- Defective neural control of speech: Unstable nervous system does not properly control the speech mechanism.
- Defective auditory mechanism: There is a built-in delay or other problems.

Environmental
- Diagnosogenic theory (Johnson): Parental diagnosis causes stuttering, which is avoidance.
- Conditioned avoidance (Wischner): Stutterers are conditioned to avoid negative listener reactions.
- Anticipatory struggle (Bloodstein): Stuttering is a response of tension and fragmentation.
- Operant view: Stuttering is an operantly learned behavior, affected by its consequences.
- Two factor theory (Brutten & Shoemaker): Stuttering is due to classically conditioned anxiety.
- Psychoanalysis (Freud): Stuttering is due to regression to earlier stages of libidinal development.

Figure 6.2. Summary of theories of stuttering.

It is clear that there is no single, satisfactory theory of stuttering. Most of the theories illuminate a certain aspect of stuttering. Researchers know that a theory that takes both the neurophysiologic and environmental factors into account is probably more valid. However, a fully integrated theory that explains all aspects of stuttering on the basis of all known factors that influence it is yet to be developed. Much experimental research must be conducted before such a theory can be proposed. Nonetheless, there is plenty of research information on the potential causes of stuttering.

Stuttering probably has multiple causes. Both organic and environmental factors play a role in its origin and maintenance. It is probably safe to assume that genetic predisposition makes certain individuals vulnerable to stuttering. Some instability of the nervous system, a potential problem in the way the brain executes movements of speech, may be part of this genetic vulnerability. Given the right (but unfavorable) circumstances in which certain environmental factors such as pressure, conditioning, and conflict are operative, stuttering may be likely to develop.

Assessment of Stuttering

The different criteria by which stuttering may be diagnosed have been discussed earlier. To be able to apply those criteria, the speech–language pathologist collects information about the client and measures stuttering and related behaviors. This process of collecting information and measurement is known as assessment. Table 6.2 highlights the procedures that are unique to stuttering assessment.

The Case History and Interview

By taking a case history and interviewing the client, the parents, or both, the clinician seeks to understand the client and his or her stuttering. Information is

Table 6.2

Assessment of Communicative Disorders: Stuttering

1. History of the client, family, and the disorder
2. Interview of the client, family members, or both
3. Orofacial examination
4. Hearing screening
5. Speech and language sampling
6. **Assessment of stuttering and related behaviors**
   a. **Measurement of dysfluencies in conversational speech**
   b. **Measurement of dysfluencies in oral reading**
   c. **Measurement of dysfluencies in home and other situations**
   d. **Assessment of associated motor behaviors and emotions**
   e. **Assessment of avoidance of words and speaking situations**
   f. **Measurement of speech rate**
7. Recommendations
8. Report writing

Note. Procedures unique to stuttering assessment are in bold print.

obtained about the onset, development, and variability of stuttering across time and situations. How the client's educational, occupational, and personal life is affected by stuttering also is explored. The conversation between the clinician and the parents of Brian, at the beginning of this chapter, gives a glimpse of the clinical interview. In the case of adults, the information is most likely provided by the clients themselves.

Measurement of Stuttering

A major task of assessment is to observe the types and frequency of dysfluencies. The clinician also takes note of the client's associated motor behaviors and avoidance and emotional reactions (Hegde, 2001a).

The types and frequency of dysfluencies are measured in both conversational speech and oral reading, if the client is old enough to read. If practical, the clinician also might observe the client's telephone conversation and conversations with other adults. These and other reading and conversational speech samples may be audio- or video-recorded for later analysis. A tape-recorded home sample of conversational speech also may be obtained from the client.

The total number of dysfluencies and their types help establish a **percent dysfluency rate.** The clinician counts either the number of words or the number of syllables in a recorded speech sample. The total number of dysfluencies is divided by the total number of words (or syllables) spoken, and the resulting quotient is multiplied by 100. This gives a percent dysfluency rate for the client. Brian, for example, spoke 925 words and his total dysfluency count was 173, which yielded an 18.7% dysfluency rate ($173 \div 925 \times 100 = 18.7$). A summary of all types of dysfluencies and their individual and total frequencies is then prepared.

Table 6.3 illustrates the type of summary a clinician might prepare about a client's dysfluency types and frequencies. This type of summary statement becomes a part of the **assessment report,** which also includes the case history and other relevant information. The dysfluency rates shown in the table are for Brian, the child described at the beginning of this chapter. Note the summary statements about the associated motor behaviors and avoidance reactions. In addition to such summary statements, some clinicians also might rate the observed stuttering as either mild, moderate, severe, or very severe.

Treatment of Stuttering

The long history of stuttering has produced a lengthy list of therapies, a few of them dangerous, most of them ineffective, but each of them hailed as the cure at one time or another. It appears that almost everything has been tried in the past, including cutting portions of the tongue of people who stutter and putting leaches on them to drain the "bad blood" that presumably caused stuttering.

The current professional treatment of stuttering includes several procedures (Culatta & Goldberg, 1995; Hegde, 2001b; Onslow, 1993). To give an overview of the diverse and often controversial subject of stuttering treatment, five approaches (outlined in Figure 6.3) are described: the approach based on psychological methods, the approach designed to teach fluent stuttering, the approach designed to teach fluent speech, and two approaches of directly reducing stuttering (pause-and-talk and response cost).

Table 6.3

Summary of the Assessment of Brian's Stuttering

Types of Dysfluency	Frequency
Part-word repetitions	26
Whole-word repetitions	16
Phrase repetitions	18
Silent prolongations	24
Sound prolongations	31
Sound/syllable interjections	19
Word interjections	8
Phrase interjections	11
Broken words	7
Silent pauses	13
Total of all types	173
Number of words spoken	925
Percent dysfluency rate	18.7

Associated motor behaviors included eye blinks, knitting of the eyebrows, rubbing the floor with his right foot, lack of eye contact, and general facial tension. Brian avoids talking to strangers and older kids. Has difficulty on words starting with /s/, /m/ /d/, /b/, /k/.

Psychological Methods of Treatment

Psychological methods of treating stutterers include **psychoanalysis, psychotherapy,** and **counseling.** These are methods of treating psychological and emotional problems. Psychoanalysis is a special form of psychotherapy based on the Freudian theory of neurosis. Therefore, not all psychotherapists are psychoanalysts. Many psychotherapists use methods other than psychoanalysis to treat emotional and psychological disorders. Counseling and non-Freudian psychotherapy are similar methods, although psychotherapy generally is more intensive and prolonged. Compared to counseling, psychotherapy is used to treat more serious problems.

Treatment of stuttering with **psychoanalysis** or **psychotherapy** involves talking with the therapist about personal, emotional, and interpersonal problems. In psychoanalysis, the emphasis is on the unconscious, sexual urges supposedly suppressed by the individual. In psychotherapy, the emphasis is on emotional conflicts that may or may not be unconscious or sexual in nature. In either case, it is believed that psychological conflicts are at the root of the problem behaviors and that the patient must resolve these conflicts with the help of the therapist to change his or her behavior.

The effectiveness of psychoanalysis and psychotherapy in reducing stuttering is not documented. These therapies focus almost exclusively on emotions, feelings, and psychological conflicts. They do not directly teach the skills of fluent speech to replace stuttering. After psychotherapy, people who stutter may still not know how to speak fluently. They typically continue to stutter.

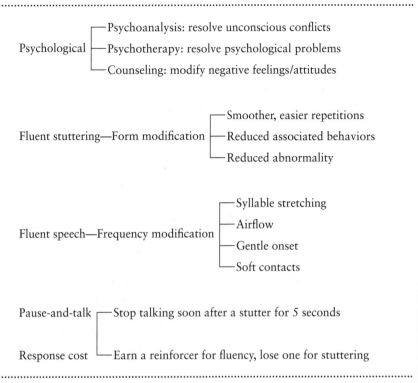

Figure 6.3. Major stuttering treatment procedures.

Counseling, in a general sense, is a part of treating all speech–language disorders (Shipley, 1992; Van Riper, 1973). **Counseling** may consist of the clinician's discussion of the communicative problem, what can be done about it, what kinds of treatment options are available, what the chances are of recovery, and so forth. In a more technical sense, counseling is the use of certain psychological methods to reduce or eliminate a problem. Therefore, in the present context, *counseling* means the use of psychological methods to treat stuttering, not just to offer information of various sorts.

The counselor is a sympathetic listener who understands the client's problems and is willing to offer interpretations and potential solutions. The therapist helps the client see the problem from different points of view and thus encourages a more objective analysis. For example, a stuttering person who believes that most listeners are rude and impatient may be encouraged to see the problem more objectively. The person who stutters may then conclude that his or her feelings and thoughts about the listener reactions were grossly exaggerated.

Because there is no evidence that mere counseling helps reduce stuttering, very few clinicians use it exclusively (Bloodstein, 1995; Hegde, 1985). Clinicians who believe in counseling combine it with other methods that directly teach skills of fluent speech.

Counseling, when used with other methods, may appear effective. However, in such cases, it is difficult to evaluate the true value of counseling. Any improvement seen in stuttering may be entirely due to the other methods because we know that when counseling is used exclusively, no reduction in stuttering is noted.

Teaching Fluent Stuttering

Van Riper (1973, 1982), a pioneer in the treatment of stuttering in the United States, established a method that seeks to teach "fluent stuttering," not necessarily fluent speech. Van Riper's procedure involves a large collection of varied tactics. The basic idea behind his multiple procedures is that normal fluency may not be the appropriate goal for most people who stutter. A majority of clients can be helped only to a certain degree, but not to the degree that they become fluent speakers like nonstutterers.

Van Riper (1973, 1982) believed that lives of stuttering people are difficult mostly because of their compulsive repetitions, endless prolongations, uncontrolled blockages, forceful struggles, helpless avoidances, and contorted facial grimaces. More than the dysfluencies themselves, it is these behaviors that make the speech of people who stutter so strikingly abnormal. Many nonstuttering people also speak dysfluently, but they do not exhibit all those abnormal behaviors. Therefore, if people who stutter can speak with less abnormality, then their speech may be socially more acceptable and their personal lives more tolerable. They might still be more dysfluent than normal speakers, but their speech would not be the focal point of painful social attention.

The major goal of Van Riper's treatment, therefore, was to change the form of stutterings such that they are less abnormal. He called this goal "fluent stuttering." Van Riper taught his clients to reduce muscular tension and speak without bizarre facial expressions, hand and feet movements, and similar abnormal behaviors. When prolongations and repetitions could not be eliminated, Van Riper taught people who stutter to repeat and prolong in an easy, effortless manner. He taught his clients to approach a feared word differently, perhaps by assuming a more relaxed and less abnormal posture. By teaching these and other methods of changing the form of stuttering, Van Riper encouraged his clients to stutter more fluently and in a more socially acceptable manner.

Van Riper's therapy also uses many indirect procedures to help stutterers understand, cope with, and adjust to their problem. Counseling and psychotherapy are a part of his treatment process. He believed in modifying a stuttering person's faulty attitudes and negative emotions along with the form of stuttering.

Van Riper's treatment has helped a great many people. Nonetheless, critics point out that Van Riper's goal of fluent stuttering falls short of normal or near-normal fluent speech. If normal speech is not targeted for treatment, we may never achieve it even if it is technically feasible. Therefore, other clinicians have developed methods to teach normally fluent speech (Hegde, 2001b). These methods are described in the next section.

Teaching Fluent Speech

Currently, many clinicians consider fluency a skill that consists of several components, each of which can be taught to induce stutter-free speech. The components may be taught separately and then put together and practiced in conversational speech. Therefore, unlike Van Riper's (1973, 1982) approach, the technique of teaching fluent speech seeks to reduce the frequency of dysfluencies to near-normal levels. Instead of fluent stuttering, normal sounding fluent speech is the goal of treatment. This type of treatment is also known as **fluency shaping.**

In inducing fluent speech, the clinician teaches several specific skills necessary to maintain fluency. When these skills are learned and practiced, they generally result in much greater fluency. In many cases, the clinician is able to achieve normal sounding fluent speech by teaching some or all of the following skills: modified airflow, gentle onset of sound, slower rate of speech, and soft contact of the articulators.

Modified airflow includes inhalation of sufficient air and a slight exhalation before saying something and having enough air that is exhaled in a controlled manner throughout the utterance. These skills are taught to counter many breathing abnormalities associated with stuttering. As noted earlier, some people who stutter forget to breathe in just before saying something. They run out of air even before they have said two words. Others waste their air by stuttering, even before they have begun to say anything. Some individuals who stutter try to speak while breathing in. Still others breathe in and immediately close their vocal cords so the air is not flowing out; they impound the air in the lungs while trying to talk. Therefore, to counteract all these problems, the clinician teaches the client to inhale and immediately exhale a small amount of air before starting to speak. When speech is begun soon after the exhalation is begun, and an even airflow is maintained throughout an utterance, speech sounds much more flowing and fluent.

Gentle initiation of sound further helps reduce the chance of stuttering. Some forms of stuttering are due to abrupt initiation of sound at the laryngeal level. The vocal cords go into abrupt action usually accompanied by increased tension of the vocal cords and related muscular structures. The result is hard and tensed beginning of speech. To reduce this problem, clinicians teach people who stutter to start the sound gently, softly, and in a relaxed manner.

In teaching **slower rate of speech,** the clinician teaches the client to stretch the syllables to prolong them. When the syllables are prolonged, the rapid and jerky stuttering behaviors are typically eliminated. Though the speech will not sound normal at this stage of treatment, the prolonged speech gives a chance to eliminate the long-standing stutterings. The prolonged speech is excessively slow and monotonous. Later, the clinician allows a gradual return to near-normal rate of speech that is both fluent and normal sounding.

Most clinicians teach a slower rate of speech by instruction, modeling, and positive reinforcement. However, clinicians may use electronic instruments, such as the one illustrated in Figure 6.4, to induce a slower rate of speech. Instruments that help induce a slower rate are known as **delayed auditory feedback devices.** These devices feed back the client's speech to his or her ears with a brief delay. It produces a more familiar echo effect. This effect slows down the speech rate and reduces stuttering. In gradual steps, the amount of delay is reduced. As fluency stabilizes, the delayed auditory feedback is withdrawn.

Finally, teaching **soft contacts of articulators** will make the speech more relaxed and will help further eliminate tensed, dysfluent speech. Many people who stutter jam their tongue against the hard or soft palate and close their lips too tightly. If the contacts between the tongue, the palates, and the lips (articulators) are soft, the speech is more relaxed, smooth, fluent, and normal sounding.

The treatment is usually started at the level of one- or two-word phrases. As the client becomes more proficient in producing the target fluency skills, the length of the utterances is gradually increased until the client talks in sentences. Eventually, the target behaviors are produced in conversational speech.

When the client's conversational speech is stutter-free for a while, the clinician begins to reshape the normal rate, rhythm, and intonation of speech. In gradual steps, the client is allowed to increase the rate of speech (the number of words spoken per minute). Eventually, the client speaks in the near-normal

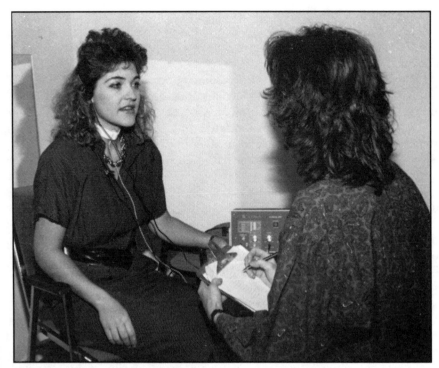

Figure 6.4. An adult stutterer receives treatment with the help of a vocal feedback device that helps slow down the speech.

rate while maintaining fluency. Typically, when the client's rate of speech is normal, the intonations and rhythms also are normal.

The same basic treatment procedure is used with adults and children. However, each person who stutters tends to have a unique pattern of abnormal speech behaviors. Therefore, the clinician carefully selects the particular targets for each client. Some clients may need extra emphasis on proper airflow; others may benefit just from a slower rate. Therefore, the treatment targets and procedures are modified to suit the individual client.

A major difficulty with fluency shaping procedures is that they result in somewhat unnatural sounding speech because many adults who stutter need to maintain a somewhat slower rate to sustain fluency. This slower rate often is not acceptable to clients because it sounds monotonous and socially distracting. Unfortunately, when they increase their rate of speech, their stuttering returns. Therefore, there still is a major problem of maintenance of fluency, especially when adults are treated.

Pause-and-Talk and Response Cost

Treatment research has supported the use of two other behavioral procedures that directly reduce the frequency of stuttering (Hegde, 2001b). Although less commonly employed than the fluency shaping techniques, pause-and-talk and response cost offer certain advantages. The main advantage is that these two techniques reduce stuttering without reducing the rate of speech. Speech sounds natural from the beginning.

Pause-and-talk is a procedure in which a brief duration of silence is strictly enforced immediately following a stutter. In behavioral science, this procedure is described as *time-out*. As soon as a stutter is observed, the clinician says, "Stop," or gives a visual signal (e.g., a red light) and avoids eye contact for 5 seconds. The client immediately stops talking. At the end of the pause (time-out) duration, the clinician reestablishes eye contact and lets the client resume speech. This method can reduce stuttering without affecting speech rate (Ahlander & Hegde, 2000).

Response cost is a procedure in which the client earns a token for fluent productions and loses one for each stuttering. For the client, each stuttering costs a reinforcer, hence the name. At the end of the session, the client exchanges the remaining tokens for a small gift. The methods works very well with young children who may be reinforced with small gifts at the end of each session. This method, too, reduces stuttering without negatively affecting the speech rate (Ahlander & Hegde, 2000).

In reducing stuttering, pause-and-talk and response cost are the two most powerful methods available today. Because of their potential to reduce stuttering without affecting speech naturalness, they deserve careful consideration.

Computer-Assisted Treatment

There have been several efforts to develop computerized treatment programs for people who stutter. Different computer programs to teach such fluency skills as gentle onset of speech and slower rate have been made available from time to time. Other kinds of electronic devices that monitor various aspects of speech production and give feedback to people who stutter also have been available. Unfortunately, no single technological device has stood the test of time. Several instruments that were developed and hailed as the answer to the stuttering treatment problem are currently not available. This may be due to lack of continued research and refinement of the products, which were not sustained in the marketplace.

Although we can expect significant advances in speech science that might make it possible to treat stuttering with electronic instruments in the future, currently clinicians are cautious in recommending expensive instruments that might be quickly dated and go off the market. Clinicians are looking for small, portable, simple, yet advanced instruments that sustain themselves in the marketplace and thus continue to be technologically refined.

Generalization and Maintenance

A significant problem with the current treatment procedures is that it is relatively easy to generate fluent speech in the clinic, but it is hard to achieve maintenance of fluency outside the clinic and over time. This is the problem of **generalization** and **maintenance**. Generalization is evident when a client's clinically established fluent speech is produced at home, the office, or school. The client who is fluent in the clinic but not in other situations shows no generalization. A client who sustains fluency across time without the clinician's presence shows maintenance.

Clinicians take several steps to make sure that their clients generalize and maintain fluency. For example, during the latter stages of treatment, the clinician may take the client out of the formal therapy room and into more informal situations. The clinician and the client may talk while taking a walk. Together, they may visit a restaurant where the client orders food. The client may practice the newly learned skills of fluency while talking on the telephone. Gradually, the client is made to face most speaking situations that were previously avoided.

To promote maintenance of fluency in children, the parents are trained to use some of the treatment procedures at home with their children. For example, in the fluency shaping (fluent speech) techniques, parents might be trained to reinforce the use of somewhat slower rate and proper airflow at home. In the case of pause-and-talk and response cost, parents may be asked to hold informal treatment sessions at home. In the case of adult clients, the spouse, children, and other members of the family also are trained to reinforce fluency and fluency skills at home. Clients might be taught to self-monitor their stuttering and fluency. For example, an adult might be taught to pause soon after a stutter and cease talking for a few seconds. A child might be taught to stop soon after a stutter and slow down the speech to sustain better fluency.

Research on treating stuttering shows that clients who complete most treatment programs benefit to a significant extent. Many people who stutter have an excellent chance of speaking with normal or near-normal fluency. It is especially important to start the treatment early. A child of any age who stutters can be treated. Early intervention is especially important because it can be very successful, and it can prevent the prolonged suffering that is sure to follow if untreated (Onslow, 1993). In sum, the treatment of stuttering is much more effective now than it ever has been in the past.

A person informed about disorders of communication can take steps to help a loved one who stutters. Table 6.4 describes what one should do to get help.

Table 6.4
Stuttering and What To Do About It

1. A child who just begins to stutter typically shows an increase in the number of dysfluencies. The child may or may not show tension and struggle. Most likely, the child will show part-word repetitions, sound prolongations, and an increased amount of other types of dysfluencies.

2. If an adult sounds like a person who stutters, he or she probably is a stutterer.

3. As soon as stuttering is suspected, consult a speech–language pathologist; preferably, find one who specializes in the treatment of stuttering.

4. Do not assume that stuttering will go away even if it had disappeared for a while in the past. Do not take the often-given advice by many people, including certain professionals, that stuttering in young children will disappear if left ignored.

5. Even if an adult had unsuccessful treatment in the past, it is now possible to benefit from treatment.

6. Treatment for stuttering is available in the public schools, many hospitals, college clinics, and private speech and hearing clinics.

7. To get more information about communicative disorders and available services, see the Appendix.

Summary

- Many procedures have been tried in the treatment of stuttering. Many have failed.

- Psychological methods of treatment include Freudian psychoanalysis, psychotherapy, and counseling. These methods have not been successful in eliminating stuttering.

- Teaching fluent stuttering is an approach that assumes that normal fluency is not an attainable goal and that reduced abnormality of stuttering is a realistic goal for people who stutter.

- Teaching the skills of fluent speech, or fluency shaping, is an approach in which stuttering people are taught proper airflow, gentle onset of sound, and reduced rate of speech through stretched (prolonged) syllables. Normal sounding fluency with near-normal rate is then shaped in gradual steps.

- In any teaching method, family members and others should be trained to support fluency outside the clinic.

- Early intervention for stuttering is especially effective.

Cluttering

Another disorder of fluency is called cluttering. Historically, this disorder has not received much attention in the United States, although this is now changing. Much of the early writing on cluttering is in German. It is reported that in Germany, 1.8% of 7- to 8-year-old children clutter. We do not know the prevalence of cluttering in the United States (Simkins, 1973).

Cluttering is a complex disorder of communication with impaired fluency, rapid but disordered articulation, possibly combined with disorganized thought and language production (Daly, 1986; Diedrich, 1984; Simkins, 1973; Wall, 1988). Often, but not always, cluttering coexists with stuttering. The rhythm of the cluttered speech is jerky or stumbling. The tone is often monotonous because the person who clutters speaks without much variation in pitch and stress. The speech is indistinct mainly because of many errors of articulation. However, most people who clutter are able to articulate the speech sounds correctly if they speak at a slower rate. But they just cannot speak at slower rates. Just when a listener thinks that a person who clutters is about to say something, the person will have finished a whole sentence, often swallowing many syllables. The words and syllables are **telescoped** (compressed or deleted). For example, the word *parliamentarian* may be pronounced as "pamerian" and *Japanese* is pronounced as "Japese." On television commercials one can hear speech that is very rapid, yet intelligible, because all the sounds and syllables are articulated. In contrast, the cluttering person's rapid speech is unintelligible mainly because of syllable deletions and other errors of articulation. Also, there are cluttering people whose speech rate is normal or slower than normal, yet unintelligible because of articulation disorders (Diedrich, 1984).

People who clutter also show **spoonerisms,** which is the unintentional interchange of sounds in a sentence. For example, a speaker who clutters might say, "many thinkle peep so" instead of "many people think so" (Simkins, 1973).

Some who clutter may not show disorganized thought and language.

Although cluttering involves poor articulation, it is *not* a disorder of articulation.

The central language imbalance hypothesis is controversial.

Some people who clutter also stutter. But even if they are not diagnosed as stutterers, the speech of people who clutter is full of dysfluencies. They tend to repeat words and phrases. Their speech is full of such interjections as *and, um, uh,* and so forth. Some experts believe that disassociation between thought and language causes the stumbling talk of people who clutter. This problem is often described as a **central language imbalance.** Cluttering individuals repeat much on their own initiative and also at the request of their perplexed listeners. They speak in a hurry, but they take more time saying something because they have to repeat several times before they are understood.

It is often stated that people who clutter, unlike those who stutter, are not concerned about their speech problem. They often are surprised that people do not understand them. Eventually many speakers with cluttering become aware at least of listeners' negative reactions. However, they have great difficulty in self-monitoring their speech. Even when it is demonstrated to them that a slower, better controlled speech is more fluent and intelligible, they find it hard to do on their own. This often gives the impression that they are not aware of their problem.

The causes of cluttering are unknown. Some have speculated that cluttering is a genetically transmitted disorder of speech and language (Weiss, 1964). Others have speculated that cluttering is due to subtle brain damage that affects all aspects of movement (motor behaviors) including speech. No theory has been fully substantiated (Simkins, 1973).

Research on the treatment of cluttering is lacking. Like people who stutter, those who clutter also vary in the number and combination of problems exhibited. Most clinicians have modified various stuttering treatment techniques to treat individuals who clutter. Reducing the rate of speech usually improves the clarity of speech as well as its fluency. A major problem with the treatment of cluttering is that the treatment effects are not generalized or maintained. Techniques known to produce generalized fluency in people who stutter might not be as effective with those who clutter. More research is needed to identify effective treatment, generalization, and maintenance techniques for people who clutter (Simkins, 1973).

Dialogue

Ms. Noledge-Hungry, as usual, visits Professor Speech-Wisely in his office to discuss fluency disorders.

N-H: Dr. Speech-Wisely, it appears that stuttering has many definitions and descriptions. It can be confusing.

S-W: Yes, it can be. That is why it is important to organize the information in some manner. When you understand different ways of diagnosing stuttering, you will have done that. What are the different **criteria for diagnosing stuttering?**

N-H: There are three of them. First, you may diagnose stuttering on the basis of the frequency of all forms of dysfluencies. If dysfluencies exceed a criterion such as 5% of words spoken, then the speaker is a person who stutters. Second, stuttering may be diagnosed when a speaker exhibits part-word repetitions and prolongations on the assumption that these are not found in the speech of normal speakers. Third, you may diagnose stuttering when a speaker's dysfluencies are abnormally long.

s-w: Very good. You should be able to describe the major forms of dysfluencies including part-word, whole-word, and phrase repetitions; sound, syllable, and silent prolongations; interjections of various sorts; pauses; and broken words.

N-H: Besides dysfluencies, clinicians also look for signs of muscular tension and struggle when they measure dysfluencies. Associated motor and avoidance behaviors and negative emotions are not essential to a diagnosis of stuttering. Most stutterers tend to exhibit them anyway. In each case, the clinicians describe them, right?

s-w: That is right. You should also know that stuttering is very likely on the initial sound of a word, initial word of a sentence, consonants, and content words in adults and function words in very young children.

N-H: I found it fascinating that stutterers think that their stuttering is uncontrollable. Is it an involuntary behavior, then?

s-w: Some experts think so, but the evidence is controversial. For the person who stutters, it may seem like their stutterings are uncontrollable. But they can and often do control them. In the treatment sessions, they are taught to control them.

N-H: The prevalence of stuttering has suggested many theories, mostly genetic theories, right?

s-w: Right. Stuttering tends to run in families and is more common in males than in females; several identical twin pairs are **concordant** for stuttering. A stuttering female poses the greatest risk of stuttering to her sons. All of these may suggest that genes are involved in the etiology of stuttering.

N-H: I was surprised at the amount of neurophysiological research on stuttering.

s-w: There is much more than what we have discussed. Researchers have found that laryngeal muscles are too tense and excessively, and often inappropriately, active during stuttering. Many but not all people who stutter are slower than nonstuttering people in phonatory reaction time. Can you summarize the research on brain and stuttering?

N-H: I will try. First, there is the theory that says that people who stutter do not have a dominant cerebral hemisphere to control language. There is conflict between the two hemispheres. Second, there are the hemispheric processing theories, which say that people who stutter process language in their right hemisphere. Most normal speakers process language in their left hemisphere. There is one more, and I am not sure of it!

s-w: The third is a general theory of an unstable nervous system that does not control the speech mechanisms well. Can you summarize the environmental theories of stuttering?

N-H: There also are a variety of environmental theories. Johnson proposed that parents mistakenly diagnose stuttering in their normally speaking child and thus create the problem of avoidance behaviors, which are the stutterings. Bloodstein proposed that stuttering is an anticipatory struggle response. Wischner believed that stuttering is a conditioned avoidance behavior. The operant view of stuttering is that it is a behavior that can be modified by consequences. The two-factor theory states that part-word repetitions and prolongations, which are considered stutterings, are due to classically conditioned anxiety, and other forms of dysfluencies are operantly conditioned. Finally, psychoanalysis suggests that stuttering is a psychological disorder.

S-W: Excellent!

N-H: Thank you! Now about **assessment.** I guess many procedures like case history, hearing screening, checking the oral structures, and the interview are common to assessment of communicative disorders in general, right?

S-W: Right! The case history and the interview focus on the onset and development of stuttering. The main task of assessment is to measure the types and frequency of dysfluencies in conversational speech and oral reading, along with associated motor behaviors. You then count the number of words or syllables spoken and the number and type of dysfluencies exhibited; from this you can calculate the percent dysfluency rate. The diagnosis of stuttering is then made on the basis of one of the criteria discussed earlier.

N-H: I found out that therapies of stuttering are as varied as the theories. And, there were also plenty of therapies that didn't do any good to people who stutter.

S-W: Unfortunately, that is true. How did we classify stuttering treatments?

N-H: We discussed **psychological methods,** which included psychoanalysis, psychotherapy, and counseling. These focus on psychological problems, emotions, attitudes, and similar variables. Generally, these methods are not effective in teaching fluent speech to people who stutter.

S-W: Van Riper's **fluent stuttering method** is the second approach. In this method, the severity and abnormality of stuttering is reduced by teaching people who stutter to speak with less tension and struggle. What is the third major approach?

N-H: The third major approach teaches **fluent speech** by reducing the frequency of stuttering. The client is taught the proper use of airflow, gentle initiation of sound, syllable stretching, and soft contact of the articulators.

S-W: That is right! The final approach involves both **pause-and-talk** and **response cost** that directly reduce stuttering without affecting speech rate.

N-H: To promote **generalization** and **maintenance** of fluency, clinicians move therapy to less formal situations. Parents, spouses, siblings, friends, and others are trained to reinforce fluency in many situations.

S-W: That is correct. Now what about cluttering?

N-H: **Cluttering** is another form of fluency disorder characterized by problems of fluency, excessive rate of speech that causes articulatory breakdowns, and perhaps disorganized thought and language. People have trouble understanding cluttered speech. Some believe that it is inherited, and others believe that it is due to brain damage.

The Outlook

N-H: Dr. Speech-Wisely, do clinicians specialize in stuttering?

S-W: Yes, they do. And of course that is true of any other disorder of communication. Much of the research on stuttering is done by those who have devoted their lives to understanding this fascinating disorder.

N-H: What does it take to specialize in stuttering?

S-W: You specialize at the graduate level, especially at the doctoral degree level.

N-H: I do not know if I should specialize in one of the disorders of communication. But stuttering interests me tremendously. What kinds of courses do you take to specialize in it?

S-W: You take a full undergraduate course on stuttering and its treatment. Then at the graduate level, you take one or more seminars, which will be mostly research oriented. As a doctoral student, you take more advanced seminars and do original research.

N-H: Treating people who stutter must be both interesting and challenging.

S-W: Yes, it is. It also is very gratifying. A child who could not say his or her last name, a man who could not order at a restaurant, a woman who broke into a cold sweat at the thought of saying "hello" are the kinds of people you help to say what they want to say. Once I asked a very bright 9-year-old child to read aloud a paragraph for me. He just stared at the first word for more than a minute, then looked at me with an expression of despair on his face. Then I asked him to try again. He did, but he couldn't. He burst into tears. At the end of the session, he could read by stretching the syllables. The smile he gave me at the end of the session is one of my treasured gifts.

N-H: I imagine you can change their lives entirely by making them more fluent.

S-W: Yes, and that is the biggest reward you get from working successfully with people who stutter. Their social, personal, and emotional lives change so much that they feel like new people. You become a special person in their lives.

N-H: I might think seriously about specializing in stuttering. But first I must decide on majoring in communicative disorders.

S-W: That is right!

N-H: I think I am almost certain that I will. Well, thank you Dr. Speech-Wisely. I will see you in class.

S-W: Bye!

Study Questions

1. Describe the different forms of dysfluencies. Give examples.

2. A 10-year-old child's overall dysfluency rate is 22% of the words spoken. Does this child stutter? Why or why not?

3. An adult person exhibits noticeable part-word repetitions and sound and silent prolongations. Is this person a stutterer? Why or why not?

4. An adult female person exhibits only a few sound prolongations in conversational speech. Her prolongations typically exceed 20 seconds. Is she a stutterer? Why or why not?

5. Is the offspring of a stuttering father or a stuttering mother more likely to stutter? Who experiences the greatest risk, sons or daughters?

6. What is concordance rate? How does it relate to stuttering?

7. Describe a few associated motor behaviors. Are they essential to diagnose stuttering?

8. Within an utterance or a sentence, where are the stutterings more likely to occur?

9. Describe a few avoidance responses of people who stutter. Are they essential to diagnose stuttering?

10. What is anticipation or expectancy?

11. How do people who stutter describe their stuttering?

12. According to people who stutter, what are some of the annoying listener reactions?

13. What is the prevalence of stuttering in school-age children and in the general population?

14. What kinds of laryngeal dysfunctions in people who stutter have been described?

15. What kinds of breathing abnormalities are associated with stuttering?

16. What hemisphere is normally dominant for language?

17. What is the gender ratio among people who stutter?

18. According to some studies, in what hemisphere do people who stutter process language?

19. What is a fiberoptic scope? How is it used in studying people who stutter?

20. What is electromyography? How is it used in studying people who stutter?

21. Describe Johnson's diagnosogenic theory of stuttering.

22. Did Johnson consider dysfluencies to be stutterings? Why or why not?

23. Describe the anticipatory struggle theory of stuttering.

24. When is a behavior an operant?

25. Define reinforcement and punishment.

26. What does it mean to say that stuttering is an operant?

27. What is a discriminative stimulus?

28. How is stuttering defined and explained in the two-factor theory?

29. Who first researched classical conditioning?

30. What is the main task in assessing stuttering?

31. Distinguish between psychotherapy and counseling. How are they used in treating people who stutter? Have they been effective?

32. Describe Van Riper's stuttering treatment approach.

33. Describe the four components of the treatment program designed to reduce the frequency of stuttering.

34. How is the pause-and-talk technique administered? What are its advantages compared to teaching fluent speech (fluency shaping)?

35. What is response cost? How is it administered?

36. What are some of the things clinicians do to help promote generalization and maintenance of fluency?

37. What steps would you take to help if stuttering appears in a member of your family?

38. What is cluttering? How is it explained?

References

Adams, M. R., Freeman, F. J., & Conture, E. G. (1984). Laryngeal dynamics of stutterers. In R. F. Curlee & W. H. Perkins (Eds.), *The nature and treatment of stuttering* (pp. 89–129). San Diego, CA: College-Hill Press.

Ahlander, E., & Hegde, M. N. (2000, April). *An experimental analysis of time-out and response cost in treating stuttering.* Paper presented at the National Treatment Efficacy Research Conference, Vanderbilt University, Nashville, TN.

Bloodstein, O. (1984). Stuttering as an anticipatory struggle disorder. In R. F. Curlee & W. H. Perkins (Eds.), *The nature and treatment of stuttering* (pp. 171–186). San Diego, CA: College-Hill Press.

Bloodstein, O. (1995). *A handbook on stuttering* (5th ed.). San Diego, CA: Singular.

Brutten, E. G., & Shoemaker, D. J. (1967). *Modification of stuttering.* Englewood Cliffs, NJ: Prentice Hall.

Culatta, R., & Goldberg, S. A. (1995). *Stuttering therapy: An integrated approach to theory and practice.* Needham Heights, MA: Allyn & Bacon.

Curlee, R., & Siegel, G. (1997). *Nature and treatment of stuttering* (2nd ed.). Needham Heights, MA: Allyn & Bacon.

Daly, D. A. (1986). The clutterer. In K. O. St. Louis (Ed.), *The atypical stutterer: Principles and practices of rehabilitation* (pp. 155–192). New York: Academic Press.

Diedrich, W. M. (1984). Cluttering: Its diagnosis. In H. Winitz (Ed.), *Treating articulation disorders: For clinicians by clinicians* (pp. 307–324). Baltimore: University Park Press.

Hegde, M. N. (1985). Treatment of fluency disorders: State of the art. In J. M. Costello (Ed.), *Speech disorders in adults: Recent advances* (pp. 155–188). San Diego, CA: College-Hill Press.

Hegde, M. N. (1995). Measurement and explanation of stuttering: A retrospective appreciation of Gene Brutlen's contribution. *Journal of Fluency Disorders, 20,* 205–230.

Hegde, M. N. (2001a). *Hegde's pocketguide to assessment in speech–language pathology* (2nd ed.). San Diego, CA: Singular.

Hegde, M. N. (2001b). *Hegde's pocketguide to treatment in speech–language pathology* (2nd ed.). San Diego, CA: Singular.

Hegde, M. N., & Hartman, D. E. (1979a). Factors affecting judgments of fluency: I. Interjections. *Journal of Fluency Disorders, 4,* 1–11.

Hegde, M. N., & Hartman, D. E. (1979b). Factors affecting judgments of fluency: II. Word repetitions. *Journal of Fluency Disorders, 4,* 13–22.

Johnson, W., & Associates. (1959). *The onset of stuttering.* Minneapolis: University of Minnesota Press.

Jonas, G. (1977). *Stuttering: A disorder of many theories.* New York: Farrar, Straus & Giroux.

Kidd, K. K. (1984). Stuttering as a genetic disorder. In R. F. Curlee & W. H. Perkins (Eds.), *The nature and treatment of stuttering* (pp. 149–169). San Diego, CA: College-Hill Press.

Moore, W. H., Jr. (1984). The central nervous system characteristics of stutterers. In R. F. Curlee & W. H. Perkins (Eds.), *The nature and treatment of stuttering* (pp. 49–71). San Diego, CA: College-Hill Press.

Onslow, M. (1993). *Behavioral management of stuttering.* San Diego, CA: Singular.

Shipley, K. G. (1992). *Interviewing and counseling in communicative disorders*. New York: Macmillan.

Simkins, L. (1973). Cluttering. In B. B. Lahey (Ed.), *The modification of language behavior* (pp. 178–217). Springfield, IL: Thomas.

Skinner, B. F. (1953). *Science and human behavior*. New York: Free Press.

Travis, L. (1931). *Speech pathology*. New York: Appleton.

Updike, J. (1987). Getting the words out. *Asha, 29*, 19–20.

Van Riper, C. (1973). *The treatment of stuttering*. Englewood Cliffs, NJ: Prentice Hall.

Van Riper, C. (1982). *The nature of stuttering* (2nd ed.). Englewood Cliffs, NJ: Prentice Hall.

Wall, M. J. (1988). Dysfluency in the child. In N. J. Lass, L. V. McReynolds, J. L. Northern, & D. E. Yoder (Eds.), *Handbook of speech–language pathology and audiology* (pp. 622–639). Philadelphia: Decker.

Weiss, D. A. (1964). *Cluttering*. Englewood Cliffs, NJ: Prentice Hall.

Wingate, M. E. (1964). A standard definition of stuttering. *Journal of Speech and Hearing Disorders, 29*, 484–489.

Wischner, G. J. (1950). Stuttering behavior and learning: A preliminary theoretical formulation. *Journal of Speech and Hearing Disorders, 15*, 324–335.

Zimmermann, G. N. (1980). Stuttering: A disorder of movement. *Journal of Speech and Hearing Research, 23*, 122–136.

Voice and Its Disorders

Normal acquisition of speech sounds, language structures, and speech fluency may still leave room for a disorder of communication that comprises voice problems. Although speech sounds are more basic than language, voice is even more basic than the speech sounds because voice is necessary to articulate speech sounds. Without voice, there would be no vocal communication. However, certain aspects of voice may be abnormal or unpleasant even when other aspects of verbal communication, including speech, language, and fluency, are within the range of normal variation. In other words, a verbally competent person may have a voice disorder. These disorders, along with normal aspects of voice and how it is produced, are the topics of this chapter.

Louis, the Swan with a Trumpet

In a parable called *The Trumpet of the Swan*, E. B. White, the author of such modern classics as *Charlotte's Web* and *Stuart Little*, captures both the essence of communication and the agony of an inability to communicate.

Louis was one of five Trumpeter cygnets (baby swans). In most respects, Louis was like his brothers and sisters. But he was *different* in one respect: He "came into the world lacking a voice" (White, 1970, p. 35). The parents, already distressed about having a "defective" baby, wonder how he would ever say "ko-hoh" to attract a female swan or cry out in pain or joy. One day, the father takes Louis to an isolated place to see if Louis can say anything at all. No matter how hard he tries, Louis cannot utter a single sound. When the frustrated father says, "I guess you are dumb" (White, 1970, p. 40), Louis feels like crying. The rest of this fascinating story is about how Louis overcomes his speech defect by learning to play a trumpet. Eventually, he is able to play "Beautiful Dreamer, Wake Unto Me" and win his lover's heart.

Nathan, the Talkative Child

While the Trumpeter Louis's story is a parable, the story of Nathan, the human child, is typical of many children and adults who have certain kinds of voice problems. While Louis could not talk, Nathan could not keep quiet.

His young mother, Lydia, a registered nurse, brought Nathan to a speech and hearing center because an ear, nose, and throat specialist had recommended voice therapy for her 4-year-old son Nathan. As they were taken to one of the clinical rooms, Nathan looked a little tense and apprehensive but was trying his best to look brave and cheerful. Nathan was small and thin for his age. He was smiling nervously when asked, "How are you, Nathan?" but he said, "Fine" promptly, somewhat loudly, and with a rough voice.

While the clinician was talking with the mother about Nathan's voice problem, Nathan was restless in his chair. He constantly wiggled, changed his position, and looked briefly at a preschool book that was kept on the table next to him. He carefully examined the sparsely furnished, small therapy room. And then, suddenly, interrupting his mother's conversation with the clinician, Nathan declared, "Mom, I don't see any needles here!" Nathan's voice also indicated a sense of relief.

The mother said that neither she nor her husband ever thought that there might be something wrong with Nathan's voice. On the recommendation of the family physician, she took Nathan to the ear, nose, and throat specialist. The specialist listened to Nathan's voice, examined his larynx, and told the mother that Nathan's hoarse voice was due to small nodules on his vocal folds. The specialist recommended a voice evaluation and therapy for Nathan.

The mother also said that Nathan had excellent verbal skills. He began to talk early and never stopped. The clinician noticed that he talked more like a 10-year-old than a 4-year-old. He talked in long, complex sentences. But the problem at home was that Nathan also talked constantly. He talked while playing alone or with other children. Every night, he talked himself to sleep by recounting the events of the day. He did not need listeners to talk to. He had the greatest, the most attentive, and the ever-present listener: himself. He lectured to himself in the bathroom, shouted to other kids on the playground, bossed his older sister with his extraordinary language skills, and talked to his mother all the time. He even talked incessantly to his newborn baby brother. By early afternoon, the mother would beg Nathan to keep quiet; by late afternoon, she would repeatedly ask him to stop talking; and by evening, she would just leave him alone so that Nathan could bathe himself in his own endless verbal flow.

Talking too much was not the only problem behavior. Nathan loved to play with toy wrestling characters. During this play, he refereed in a loud, harsh, and tensed voice. With bulging chest and strained neck muscles, he announced the winners and the losers, chided those who engaged in foul play, praised the winners, put the losers to shame, and excited the nonexistent audience. In a loud and boisterous voice, he talked to the trees, the flowers, the bees,

The medical specialists of ear, nose, and throat are professionally known as **otorhinolaryngologists**.

the butterflies, the two family dogs, and the four kittens. Simply by talking all the time, he wore out his many cousins, the two grandmothers, and the one grandfather, who firmly believed that speech is silver, but silence is gold. Everyone attributed the grandfather's uncharacteristic and recently acquired belief to Nathan's extraordinary verbal skills.

This excessive talk, combined with an excessively tense manner of speaking, had caused two nodules on his vocal folds. His voice was very hoarse. The hoarseness was so constant that his parents had never heard his normal voice. They thought that his hoarse voice *was* his normal voice.

The Trumpeter swan and Nathan illustrate two kinds of voice problems: lack of voice and overuse of voice (and speech). Unlike the Trumpeter swans, humans tend to lose voice because of some disease such as cancer, which necessitates the surgical removal of the larynx. These and other kinds of voice problems are described in later sections of this chapter.

Voice, the Sound of Speech

Of all aspects of speech, voice is probably the most aesthetic. Voice makes beautiful music. Voice is most closely related to the emotional tone of communication. Voice can reveal whether someone is angry or happy. The speaker does not have to say it in words. For the same reason, listeners also are tuned to the emotional messages hinted by the voice. The voice can hide messages, or give messages that are different from the ones conveyed by the words. For example, a person may be invited to a party, but the tone of that invitation may tell that the person really is not welcome. Therefore, voice helps communicate more than what the words say.

Voice also is unique. Like fingerprints, voice marks a speaker's individuality. An early response a newborn baby learns is to recognize the mother's voice, perhaps because of this vocal individuality. Adults, too, can recognize a person by just listening to voice.

More than any other aspect of a speaker's speech, his or her voice is most closely related to how pleasant or unpleasant that speaker *sounds* when he or she talks. The tone and the quality of the person's voice may not be right; they may be pleasant, unpleasant, interested, or indifferent. The voice may sound too rough, "noisy," too high pitched or low pitched, too loud or too soft. All of these problems cause a subjective feeling of unpleasant voice.

With a few exceptions, voice disorders do not necessarily create communication barriers of the kind experienced by a person who has a language, fluency, or articulation disorder. Nonetheless, a voice problem is no less handicapping to the person who has it. Many voice disorders may be just unpleasant to the listeners. But the person who has a voice problem usually has to contend with many kinds of personal, social, and often medical complications.

Several voice disorders have associated physical (medical) problems. These physical problems can get worse if the voice problem is not treated. Physical problems such as vocal nodules and the resulting voice problems create a vicious circle. When one gets worse, the other becomes a more serious problem.

In many occupational situations, employees with unpleasant voice may not last too long. A sales clerk with a hoarse voice may not sell much. Of course, a career in vocal music would be out of the question. Besides, several occupations require a *sustained* voice because they require sustained speech. Anyone who needs to speak or sing for relatively long periods of time needs to sustain his or her voice. Teachers, preachers, radio announcers, television reporters, cheerleaders, sports coaches, singers, auctioneers, entertainers, talk show hosts, and campaigning politicians, among others, can sustain their job only by a sustained voice that is capable of long and hard performance. Some of these and other occupations also require a pleasant voice.

Unfortunately, the occupations that depend on pleasant and capable voice also are the ones that pose the greatest threat to a healthy voice. People in such occupations are most likely to have one of the voice disorders.

Voice is a complex phenomenon made possible by a highly sophisticated and extremely sensitive structure called the phonatory mechanism. The basics of this mechanism are described in Chapter 3. The following is a summary of that information.

Phonation: Structure

Trachea is popularly known as the windpipe.

The single most important part of the phonatory mechanism is the **larynx,** which is a biological valve located at the top of the trachea. The larynx helps close the entry into the trachea so that food, liquids, and other particles do not enter the lungs. It also helps build air pressure below so that biological functions such as giving birth to a child and getting rid of the body wastes as well as coughing are possible. The larynx probably evolved because of these biological reasons and not for the sake of the Metropolitan Opera.

The larynx is a tubelike structure in the neck that includes various muscles, cartilages, and membranes. It is suspended by the **hyoid bone** and supported by a system of cartilages called the **cricoid, thyroid,** and **arytenoid.** These cartilages keep the larynx in place. They also help the larynx move and make fine adjustments. Being the top ring of the trachea, the cricoid is wide at the back and narrow on the sides and the front. The laryngeal structures, as seen from the front and back, are shown in Figure 7.1.

The thyroid is the largest of the laryngeal cartilages whose frontal prominence is known as the Adam's apple. The thyroid and the cricoid cartilages are attached to each other via the **cricothyroid joint.** As a result, both the cartilages can move back and forth.

The two small arytenoid cartilages are crucial for laryngeal functions because the vocal folds are attached to these pyramid-shaped cartilages. The arytenoids, in turn, are attached to the cricoid cartilage through the **cricoarytenoid joint.** This joint permits circular and sliding movements, which are extremely important for voice and speech production. In essence, the vocal fold movements are made possible by the cricoarytenoid joint.

The larynx is partly a muscular structure. In fact, the vocal folds that vibrate during the voice production are a pair of thin muscles attached to the thyroid and arytenoid cartilages and known as the **thyroarytenoid** or **vocal muscles.** The vocal folds are illustrated in Figure 7.2.

Not only do the vocal folds vibrate, but their posterior ends also move closer to each other (adduct) and move apart (abduct). Two pairs of muscles, the **lateral cricoarytenoid** and the **interarytenoid muscles,** bring the folds together. The major abductor which pulls the vocal folds apart is called the **posterior**

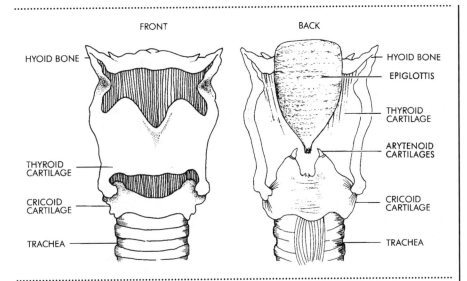

Figure 7.1. The laryngeal structures as seen from front and back.

cricoarytenoid muscle. The adductors and the abductor work in opposition to each other. When the adductors are active, the abductor is not.

The vocal folds also can be lengthened or shortened. This action is performed by the cricothyroid, which is attached to the cricoid and the thyroid cartilages. These actions are important in voice production.

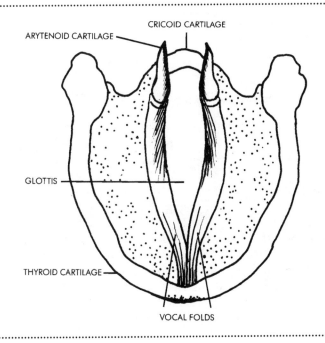

Figure 7.2. The vocal folds.

Phonation: Voice Production

Voice production needs a source of power. The lungs are the source. During exhalation, a column of air moves from the lungs and passes through the opening between the folds, called the **glottis.** In silent breathing, the folds are abducted and inhalation and exhalation smoothly alternate with each other. However, things change when a speaker is about to produce voice or speech.

Vibration of the vocal folds is the key to voice production. Different patterns of vibrations create differences in the voice as perceived by listeners. How the vocal folds are set into vibratory motion has been a fascinating question for many scientists. A generally accepted answer is given by the **myoelastic-aerodynamic theory,** which states that the folds vibrate because of the forces and pressures of air and the elasticity of the muscles (vocal folds). The air flowing out of the lungs is temporarily stopped by the closed (or nearly closed) vocal folds. This builds up pressure beneath the folds (subglottal air pressure). The pressure eventually blows the folds apart. During this process, the folds are set into vibration as well. The air then moves with increased velocity through the glottal opening. The air moves swiftly through the open, but still somewhat constricted, folds. Consequently, the pressure between the edges of the folds decreases. This decreased pressure sucks the folds together. Once again, the subglottal air pressure builds up, which sets the folds into motion. Thus, there is a cycle of opening and closing of the vocal folds. This cycle is repeated more than 100 times each second.

The opening and closing of the folds are aptly described as a cycle because they are repetitive patterns of movements. These cyclic patterns determine many characteristics of voice. The rate at which the folds open and close may be slow or fast. Even at the slowest rate, however, the folds may open and close 70 times a second. The cycle may be as fast as 1,000 times a second. Normally, the vibrations are regular and evenly spaced. Such vibrations help create impressions of a pleasant voice. Irregular vocal fold vibrations cause voice disorders.

The Pitch and Loudness of Voice

The pitch and loudness of voice are names for judgments people make about certain aspects of voice. Therefore, they often are described as **perceptual:** how voice and its characteristics are perceived. Someone's voice could be described as soft or loud, or of low or high pitch. Such subjective judgments, however, have their physical and physiological bases, though most people who make such judgments are not aware of them.

The judgment of **pitch** is largely based on the frequency with which the vocal folds vibrate. At any given time, there is an average rate at which the folds vibrate. This rate often is described as the **fundamental frequency.** In a rough sense, the fundamental frequency also may be considered the habitual or typical frequency for a given individual. The higher the frequency of vibratory cycles, the higher the perceived pitch of the resulting voice.

Three factors affect the vocal fold vibrations: the **mass, tension,** and **elasticity** of the folds. The more massive the folds are, the lower the rate of vibration is and, therefore, the lower the fundamental frequency. The lower the fundamental frequency, the lower the perceived pitch. This is why the male voice is of lower pitch than the female voice. Men's vocal folds are more massive than women's.

Tense vocal folds vibrate faster than relaxed ones. The faster vibrations result in higher frequency, which in turn gives the impression of higher pitch. Thinner vocal folds also vibrate at higher frequency. Women's vocal folds are less massive (thinner) than men's. Therefore, women's pitch is higher.

Mass, length, and elasticity (the tension factor) of vocal folds are closely related. Massive folds are usually longer, too. Longer and massive folds vibrate at a lower rate and thus produce lower pitch. However, when the folds are stretched, they become tensed and thinner, causing higher pitch (Borden, Harris, & Raphael, 1994; Kent, 1997).

Loudness is another characteristic of voice or any kind of sound. Like pitch, loudness also is a perceived (judged) characteristic of voice. While pitch is determined by the frequency of vocal fold vibrations, loudness is determined by the intensity of the sound signal. The more intense a sound signal, the greater its perceived loudness. Sound is actually a disturbance in air particles; it is in the form of waves that move forward and backward in air (or another medium such as water). The extent of such movements is measured as **amplitude.** The greater the amplitude, the louder the voice. These movements of sound waves act upon the eardrums of a listener. The drums themselves are moved back and forth. The higher the amplitude of the sound waves striking the eardrum, the greater the extent of its movement. The greater the extent of movement of the drum, the greater the perceived loudness of the sound.

The sounds of different amplitude are created at the laryngeal level. To produce louder sounds, the speaker closes the vocal folds tightly and creates greater air pressure below them. The tight closure results in greater resistance to the air pressure. Eventually, when the folds are blown apart, the air escapes with increased velocity. Consequently, the air particles (molecules) are displaced to a relatively large extent. It means that the amplitude of the sound wave is large. A relatively large amplitude results in greater displacement of the eardrum and a perception of louder sound.

Voice Quality

While pitch and intensity are related to the physical measures of frequency and intensity, the **quality** of voice is related to the complexity of the sound wave and many other factors, some of which are not easily measured. Nevertheless, we all are aware of the various qualities of voice other than its pitch and loudness. These qualities are of immense clinical significance because they often are deviant in vocal pathologies and voice disorders (Boone & McFarlane, 2000).

Generally speaking, normal laryngeal structures, acceptable vocal habits, appropriate use of the airflow, normal oral–nasal cavities, and good health are all needed to produce normal voice. Poor general health, diseases of the larynx, faulty habits of using the vocal mechanisms, inappropriate use of the airflow, and deviant oral–nasal cavities can contribute to problems of voice quality (Boone & McFarlane, 2000; Wilson, 1987). Three major voice quality problems are harshness, breathiness, and hoarseness.

A **harsh voice** is variously described as unpleasant, rough, and "gravelly" sounding. It is associated with excessive muscular tension and effort. The vocal folds are pressed together too tightly, and the air is then released too abruptly.

The resulting voice sounds harsh and unpleasant. Harshness may be present in loud or soft voice, although it often is associated with weak voice of low pitch (Boone & McFarlane, 2000; Wilson, 1987).

Breathiness results when the vocal folds are slightly open during phonation (see Figure 7.3). Of course, the vocal folds must move toward each other to phonate, but when they do not fully approximate, the voice sounds breathy. The air that escapes through the glottis adds noise to the sound produced by the vocal folds. The air leak and the resulting noise are perceived as breathiness. In extreme cases, only the air leakage may be heard in the absence of phonation (sound).

Voice that is both harsh and breathy is called **hoarse.** Hoarseness can signal serious laryngeal pathology, although it often accompanies the common cold. The predominant component of hoarseness may be breathiness in some cases and harshness in other cases. Hoarseness results from irregular vocal fold vibrations. In such cases, the fundamental frequency of the speaker varies randomly. The pitch of a hoarse voice is typically low and difficult to determine.

Another vocal quality described by some specialists is called vocal fry (Boone & McFarlane, 2000; Wilson, 1987). Vocal fry is heard when the sound is produced in slow but discrete bursts and is of extremely low pitch. By itself, vocal fry is not an abnormal voice quality. But heard to an excessive degree, vocal fry can be abnormal and disturbing.

Resonance

The laryngeal tone does not sound like the voice that eventually comes out of the mouth. The tone is modified by the cavities of the throat, mouth, and nose that lie above the vocal folds. This modification is known as **resonance.** A res-

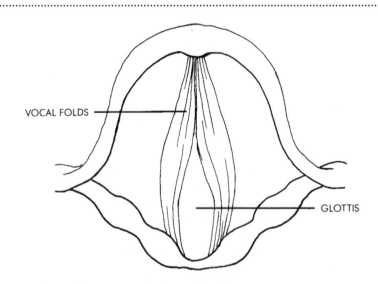

Figure 7.3. Breathy voice is produced when the folds are partly open and partly approximated. Air escapes through the open glottis and adds noise to the sound.

onator does not generate sound; it simply vibrates when sound is passing through it. A resonator reacts to the sound produced by some other structure.

Resonance has two major effects on the laryngeal tone: It reinforces some of the frequencies and dampens others. Consequently, the sound that eventually comes out of the mouth is changed. This change is facilitated by the movements of the tongue, the soft palate, cheeks, and so forth. When these structures move, the size and the shape of the oral cavity are changed continuously. The quality and extent of resonance are determined largely by the shape and the size of the resonating cavities. Therefore, the articulators, by constantly moving around within the oral cavity, contribute to changing resonance characteristics of voice.

Two types of resonance are of particular interest to an understanding of some of the voice disorders. **Oral resonance** is heard when the nasal passage is blocked at the **velopharyngeal port,** which includes the soft palate and the surrounding muscles. When the soft palate moves back and upward, it helps to close the nasal port. Consequently, the nasal passage resonates very little, if at all. **Nasal resonance** is heard when the velopharyngeal port is open. Only three English speech sounds, /m/, /n/, and /ŋ/ (ng) need nasal resonance. All other speech sounds have only oral resonance.

Read more about the velopharyngeal port in **Chapter 8.**

Several structural anomalies, such as **clefts of the palate,** can make it difficult to close the nasal passage. The muscles of the soft palate may be too weak to move swiftly to close the nasal port. Or, the muscles may not have enough mass to achieve an adequate closure. As a result, the voice may sound hypernasal. **Hypernasality** is excessive nasal resonance. Oral speech sounds (such as a /p/ or a /d/) then sound more like nasal sounds.

Read more about clefts and their effects on communication in **Chapter 8.**

In contrast to hypernasality, **hyponasality** is too little nasal resonance on the nasal sounds of a language. When you have a bad cold, your *m, n,* and *ng* do not sound right because there is not enough nasal resonance. Cold infection results in swollen mucus of the throat and nose. Consequently, the nasal passages, which are partially blocked, do not resonate enough. There are other conditions that create hyponasality. They are considered in a later section.

Summary

- The airstream flowing out of the lungs sets the vocal folds into vibration.

- This vibration creates sound waves that travel through the cavities above the larynx.

- These cavities and the structures within them modify the sound.

- When the sound is pleasant and smooth, does not include noise due to air escape, contains the right kind of oral or nasal resonance—not too soft, not too loud—and has appropriate pitch, the voice may be considered normal.

Disorders of Voice

How many adults and children exhibit voice disorders? There have been a few studies made on the prevalence of voice disorders in children, but the results have not always been consistent (Boone & McFarlane, 2000; Wilson, 1987). The estimates of the number of children who exhibit voice problems varies from 3% to 10%. There are no reliable studies on the prevalence of voice disorders in adults. It is thought that about 4% of the population as a whole, including children and adults, may have voice disorders (Boone & McFarlane, 2000). Some people with mild or temporary voice problems may not need voice therapy, but many do.

Voice disorders are classified in different ways. Organic versus psychogenic voice disorders represent one classification. This classification is based on demonstrated or presumed causes of disorders. Such classifications are called etiologic. **Organic voice disorders** are associated with some form of structural deviation or change in the phonatory mechanism. Such disorders may be caused by a physical disease. Paralysis of the vocal folds or vocal nodules, to be described later, illustrate structural deviations or changes. **Psychogenic voice disorders** have their causes in the "mind" of the speaker. There usually is no evidence of a structural pathology. For instance, a person who suddenly loses his or her voice with no physiological or neurological basis is said to exhibit **psychogenic aphonia.**

Organic versus functional voice disorders represent another classification. This also is an etiologic classification. **Organic voice disorders,** as noted, are due to physical diseases such as a tumor or cancer that affects the way the vocal folds work. **Functional voice disorders** are those that are due to misuse or abuse of voice. People who constantly talk or yell develop certain kinds of voice disorders. These disorders are then classified as functional. It is important to note, however, that in functional voice disorders, laryngeal tissue may have been physically damaged. For example, the vocal nodules of a person who yells constantly is an organic condition, although its cause was not organic but behavioral. For this reason, a functional voice disorder is not the same as a psychogenic voice disorder. Vocally abusive behaviors can cause damage to the folds that can be observed, resulting in a functional voice disorder. However, there is no such observable damage in the case of a psychogenic voice disorder.

Disorders of phonation, loudness and pitch, and resonance represent yet another classification. This is a *descriptive classification,* which is based on the dominant characteristic of vocal activity that is disordered. The voice disorders of **phonation, loudness and pitch,** and **resonance** are typically subclassified into functional and organic, as defined earlier. This approach, though not entirely satisfactory, is widely used and adopted here.

Voice Disorders of Phonation

In a majority of voice disorders of phonation, the behavior of the vocal folds is altered. The result is a voice disorder with varying amounts of breathiness, harshness, hoarseness, pitch deviations, and loudness problems. The altered behavior often is associated with some form of structural change in the vocal folds. In some exceptional cases, a voice disorder may be present in the absence of laryngeal structural changes. The suspected or demonstrated reason for a structural change, when present, may be physical (organic) or behavioral (abuse of the vocal mechanism).

It is useful to distinguish the meaning of two terms frequently used in describing voice disorders: aphonia and dysphonia. **Aphonia** means no voice, and it is the name for a particular voice disorder. **Dysphonia,** on the other hand, is a more general term which refers to disordered voice. In essence, any voice disorder, with the exception of aphonia, can be called a dysphonia.

Aphonia

Aphonia is loss of voice. It may have a psychological or a physical basis. Aphonia with a psychological basis is also described as hysterical aphonia because the loss of voice is sudden and the larynx appears structurally normal, especially during the early days of aphonia. There usually is no evidence of neurological damage. Aphonia with a physical basis is usually caused by vocal fold paralysis.

The aphonic patient typically speaks in whispers. The vocal folds are abducted (open) during speech. As a result, there is no phonation, no sound. When there is no vocal fold paralysis, the loss of voice may not be constant, however. At times, the person may be able to speak with voice, although the voice may be breathy or hoarse. In such cases, the person's problem may be an alternating aphonia and dysphonia.

In some cases, aphonia may have its origin in a temporary laryngeal disease, which prevented phonation. A physical injury to the larynx, or an extreme form of throat infection may keep the person from phonating normally for a certain period of time. However, aphonia may persist even after the disease is cured. In a majority of cases of aphonia with no organic pathology, it is thought to be related to stress, anxiety, psychological trauma, and other such factors. The aphonia then becomes a response to a difficult and emotionally taxing situation. Therefore, this type of aphonia is classified as a psychogenic voice disorder.

Aphonia in the absence of paralysis or any other organic cause has been treated with either counseling and psychotherapy or behavior therapy. The clinicians who believe that functional aphonia is psychogenic, because it is due to an unconscious psychological conflict, prefer to treat their clients with counseling or psychotherapy. These clinicians tend to think of aphonia in terms of a neurosis in the psychological or psychoanalytic (Freudian) sense.

Counseling and psychotherapies often are practiced by psychologists and psychiatrists. During the therapy sessions, clients are encouraged to speak freely about themselves and their problems. With the support of a sympathetic listener, the clients are expected to resolve their psychological conflicts. Once the underlying psychological problems are resolved, the voice problem is expected to disappear. With appropriate training, speech–language pathologists also can treat an aphonic client in this manner.

The behavior therapists, on the other hand, do not believe that unconscious forces cause behavior disorders of any kind, including functional aphonia. They believe that most behavior disorders are due to faulty learning and conditioning. Therefore, the behavior therapists tend to treat such disorders as aphonia by modifying their faulty behaviors. This form of treatment requires an analysis of the conditions under which the aphonic behavior is typically present. Most functionally aphonic people can produce voice at times. Whenever the client produces the vocal sound, the clinician may systematically reinforce this behavior and thus increase its duration and frequency. Eventually, the aphonic behavior may be extinguished. Speech–language pathologists who are trained in behavioral analysis and treatment are likely to treat a functionally aphonic client in this manner.

Aphonia due to vocal fold paralysis is described in the next section. Paralyzed vocal folds may not adduct to produce sound. Consequently, the patient is aphonic.

Physically Based Disorders of Phonation

Many disorders of phonation are associated with physical factors. These factors may be infectious or viral diseases, physical trauma or injury, hearing loss, endocrine changes, and factors that affect the central nervous system. Some of the major physical factors associated with voice disorders of phonation are described in the following section.

Paralysis and Ankylosis

The vocal folds, being muscles, can be paralyzed when their nerve supply is cut off. Muscles that are not stimulated by the nerves do not move. This is paralysis.

Read more about cranial nerves in **Chapters 3** and **9.**

Vagus means *wandering* in Latin.

Paralysis of vocal folds may be caused by an accidental injury to the recurrent laryngeal nerve during certain surgical procedures. The paired **recurrent laryngeal nerve** is a branch of the cranial nerve X (vagus); it has wide distribution within the neck and the chest cavity. In fact, the recurrent nerve, as though it did not know its final destination, moves down to the chest cavity and then reverses its course back to the laryngeal area. It supplies many muscles of the larynx. Because of its wide distribution, it is highly susceptible to damage during neck and chest surgery. For example, the nerve may be accidentally cut or injured when the cancerous thyroid gland is removed surgically (**thyroidectomy**). Some diseases also may affect the nerve supply of the vocal folds.

In **unilateral paralysis,** only one of the two vocal folds is paralyzed and assumes a static position. In some cases, the normal fold may move toward the paralyzed fold to make a contact. The voice in such cases may be normal or nearly so. In other cases, the paralyzed fold may be too far away from the middle position. Then the healthy fold cannot move that far to make a closure. This causes aphonia.

Glottis is an opening between the folds.

Paralysis of both the folds, **bilateral paralysis,** may lead to a wide open glottis, causing aphonia. A stroke can cause a bilateral vocal fold paralysis. However, the two paralyzed folds may be positioned close to each other. It is important to note that paralyzed folds can vibrate but not approximate. Because paralyzed folds that are close to each other are already approximated, they can help produce phonation resulting in a near-normal voice.

Even the unilateral paralysis that permits some phonation results in breathy and weak voice. The patient cannot cough vigorously because of the difficulty in achieving the necessary amount of subglottal pressure when the folds cannot close firmly.

In **ankylosis,** the movement of the arytenoids is restricted because of such bone-joint diseases as arthritis. Cancer also may affect the movements of the arytenoids at the cricoarytenoid joints. Recall that the vocal folds are attached to the arytenoids, which are in turn attached to the cricoid cartilage. When this joint is stiffened or fixated, the vocal cords may not come together.

The speech–language pathologist can help patients with unilateral paralysis. The healthy fold can be trained to move farther to meet the paralyzed fold, resulting in improved voice. Sometimes, the paralyzed fold may be injected with Teflon to create a bulge in the fold that helps the folds come together. After such surgical treatment, the speech–language pathologist can train the client to achieve closure and produce voice.

Carcinoma

A 62-year-old man who had cancer of the larynx wrote

> When my doctor told me that I had cancer of the larynx, I did not immediately think of my voice or speech. I did not know how my speech would be affected. All I could think of was "Why me?" and "Why did I ever smoke?" The doctor then told me that I must have an operation soon, in fact one was already scheduled in 3 days. But when he described what this operation would do to my voice—I was going to lose it all—I felt like crying for the first time since the accidental death of my wife several years ago. The sensitive doctor left me alone for a few a minutes. I then pondered my fate and felt alternately relieved that my wife wasn't there to see me like this and sad that she wasn't there to hold my hand. I did not know what to do. Should I have the operation so I can live silently? Or should I refuse it and die like a human who could speak? Sure, the doctor had told me that there are ways to learn speech, but I did not take it seriously. The thought of losing my voice was even more painful than the thought of imminent death.

The larynx is one of the common sites of cancer. Laryngeal cancer is found more frequently in men than in women. In the United States, every year, an estimated 4,000 or more people undergo surgical treatment for cancer of the larynx. Laryngeal cancer accounts for about 3% to 5% of human cancer (Boone & McFarlane, 2000). Smoking is a dominant factor related to cancer of the larynx. A combination of smoking and heavy drinking increases the chances of laryngeal cancer.

Malignant tumors can grow on one or both vocal folds. An early warning sign is hoarseness of voice. The patient may find it difficult to swallow and report pain in the throat. The change in the vocal quality, if heeded promptly, gives an excellent chance for an early diagnosis and treatment of cancer.

Like most forms of cancers, laryngeal cancer may be treated by surgery, chemotherapy, and irradiation. These medical treatments create a need for the services of a speech–language pathologist. For example, the diseased larynx may be partially or totally removed. This operation, known as **laryngectomy**, leaves the patient without the normal mechanism of sound generation. When the laryngeal valve and the surrounding structures are removed, the trachea (the tube through which the air reaches the lungs) becomes disconnected with the neck and mouth. Therefore, the surgeon creates an opening (called a **stoma**) in the lower part of the neck and connects it with the trachea. For the rest of his or her life, the patient must breathe through this opening. The laryngeal and related structures, before and after the surgery (laryngectomy), are illustrated in Figure 7.4.

Laryngectomy is the name of the operation. **Laryngectomee** is a person who has undergone that operation.

Speech for the Laryngectomy Patient. "It is nice to live a little longer, but it is the regained speech that makes me think that I made the right decision to have the surgery," said the 62-year-old cancer patient who was quoted earlier. His surgery was followed by speech treatment. He learned to speak with the help of his esophagus.

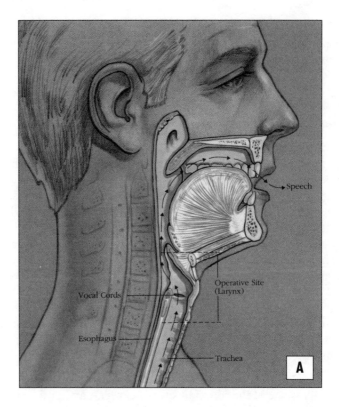

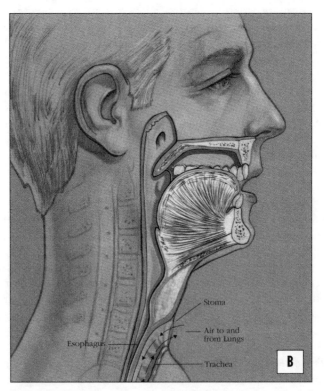

Figure 7.4. The laryngeal and related structures before (A) and after (B) laryngectomy. (Photo courtesy of International Healthcare Technologies.)

The patient who has undergone a laryngectomy usually is referred to a speech–language pathologist for retraining in voice and speech production without the aid of the vocal folds. In medical centers that provide comprehensive services to laryngeal cancer patients, the speech–language clinician is involved from the very beginning of treatment. Before surgery, the clinician will counsel the patient and the family members about the effects of the surgical procedure on voice and speech production. Also, the clinician may reassure everyone concerned about the potential for alternative forms of voice and speech production after surgery.

The patient who has undergone total laryngectomy can still relearn to speak. The patient needs a new source of sound. There are three new sources of sound that a patient can consider: an artificial larynx, which is a handheld electronic instrument; the esophagus, which can be trained to vibrate; and surgical modifications and implanted devices, which are either surgically altered structures in the throat or implanted devices that help produce sound.

An **artificial larynx** is a mechanical device that generates sound. There are a few kinds of such devices. One of them is a **pneumatic device,** which is a curved tube with a vibrator in it. The patient places one end of the tube on the stoma, the surgical opening in the lower part of the neck through which the patient breathes. The other end is placed in the mouth. The exhaled air passes through the vibrator, which generates the sound that is transferred to the mouth. The sound is then modified into speech in the usual manner.

The more popular mechanical device is electronic, the prototype of which is illustrated in Figure 7.5. An electronic larynx (also called electrolarynx) is more convenient than a pneumatic larynx. There are many models on the

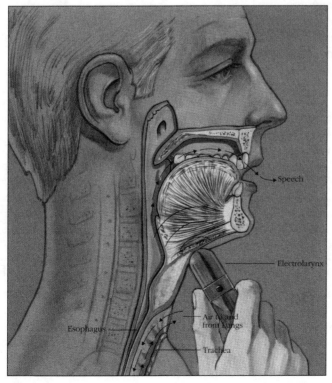

Figure 7.5. An electronic artificial larynx (electrolarynx). (Photo courtesy of International Healthcare Technologies.)

market, but most are handheld units. Some resemble a small flashlight. All generate sound electronically. The vibrating part of the device is pressed against the neck, and the unit is turned on by the thumb. The sound generated by the vibrator is transferred to the mouth. The person then articulates the speech sounds in the usual manner.

The speech produced with the help of an electronic larynx may be monotonous. On some devices, the speaker can change the pitch, and this can help in achieving a more normal-sounding voice. A speaker who is well trained by a speech–language pathologist can produce intelligible speech with the help of an electronic larynx.

The **esophagus,** which is the flexible tube through which food reaches the stomach, also is a source of sound. This muscular tube may be made to produce sound by first inhaling air into it and then releasing it in the form of a belch. The belching sound is then articulated into speech sounds. The speech produced by this means is known as **esophageal speech.**

It is known that some patients with laryngectomy find it hard to learn esophageal speech. However, those who can learn are able to speak surprisingly well. People can easily understand their speech. The patient must first learn to get air into the pharyngeal area. This is accomplished by one of two methods. In the first, the **injection method,** the air is impounded in the mouth as in saying /t/ or /p/. The impounded air is then pushed back into the esophagus. The air is then expelled, which produces vibrations of the soft tissues of the esophagus. Unarticulated, this sound is that of a belch. The sound is then articulated into speech, which does not sound like a belch.

In the second, the **inhalation method,** the patient is taught to inhale rapidly while keeping the esophagus open or relaxed. The inhaled air passes through the esophagus and sets its tissues into vibratory motion. The resulting sound is articulated into speech.

Surgical modifications and **implanted devices** also can be sources of sound. All implanted devices require some form of surgery, but there are surgical procedures that do not include implanted devices. These surgical procedures modify the existing structures in the throat to create mechanisms that help produce sound. In one procedure, the trachea and the pharynx were connected with a tube made from the patient's skin. The tube vibrated when air passed through it. So far, efforts of this kind have not been very successful.

In recent years, methods that combine surgery with a prosthetic device have been used more frequently and with greater success. In one such procedure, known as the **Singer-Blom tracheoesophageal puncture,** a shunt or a tunnel is opened to connect the trachea to the esophagus. The wall separating the two structures is punctured, hence the name of the procedure. To keep this tunnel open, the **Blom-Singer tracheoesophageal voice prosthesis,** illustrated in Figure 7.6, is inserted into it. The device, which is a small plastic tube, has openings on both ends. The prosthetic device is designed to prevent the passage of fluid and food into the trachea. When the stoma is closed, the exhaled air can pass from the trachea to the esophagus. This then sets the esophagus into vibration, resulting in sound production. The patient modifies the sound into speech.

Many laryngectomy patients learn esophageal speech with or without the help of surgical procedures and prosthetic devices. Those who are proficient at it can talk clearly for extended durations. However, most alaryngeal speakers (persons who do not have a larynx) must use relatively short phrases and sentences. Hoarseness is typical of their voice quality. The voice also may lack

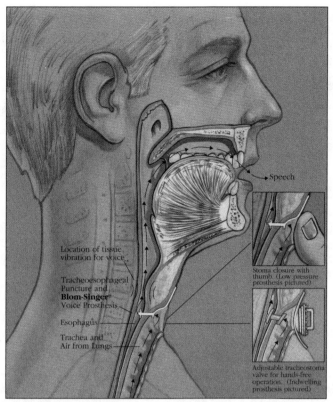

Figure 7.6. The Blom-Singer tracheoesophageal voice prosthesis in place. (Photo courtesy of International Healthcare Technologies. Blom-Singer is a registered trademark of Hansa Medical Products, Inc.)

pitch variations, and the vocal intensity (loudness) also may be limited. With most surgical and prosthetic procedures, the patient must use one hand to close the stoma while speaking. The patient should periodically remove and clean most prosthetic devices. Some patients may find this a difficult chore. Nonetheless, with proper training and family support, most alaryngeal speakers manage their day-to-day communicative needs.

Papilloma

A kind of growth on the laryngeal structures including the vocal folds is called **papilloma.** Some papillomas or papillomata (plural of the singular *papilloma*) are hard and look like warts. The vocal folds can be covered with such wartlike growth. Other papillomas are soft and do not resemble warts. The wartlike papillomas that cover most of the vocal folds are illustrated in Figure 7.7.

Papillomas are found more frequently in children than in adults (Aronson, 1985). Children born to mothers who have genital warts (condyloma acuminatum) may show papilloma of the larynx at the time of birth. Papillomas are not the same as carcinoma, but often a biopsy is needed to distinguish them. Papillomas are thought to be caused by a virus, but this is not known for sure.

Papillomas can create serious breathing problems because they tend to grow quickly and occupy much of the glottal area. Therefore, papillomas can

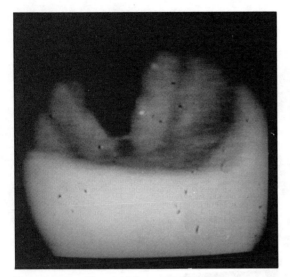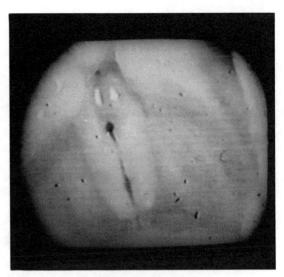

Figure 7.7. Papilloma of the vocal folds. (Photo courtesy of Dr. Stephen McFarlane.)

be life-threatening. The patient's voice will sound breathy and hoarse. Speech clinicians are in a position to notice these early signs of papillomas and refer the patients to medical specialists.

Papillomas are typically treated surgically. The traditional surgical method is to excise the wartlike growths. More recently, ultrasonic and laser surgeries have been used. Unfortunately, the papillomas tend to recur, creating a need for repeated surgery. Some children are reported to have 15 or more operations within a few months (Boone & McFarlane, 2000; Wilson, 1987). Repeated operations weaken the vocal folds and create scar tissues that affect the patient's voice. However, a vaccine developed from a sample of the papilloma may prevent the recurrence of the disease.

After the surgical treatment, voice therapy can help many patients. Voice therapy does not prevent future occurrences of the papillomas, but it can help the patient make the best use of his or her weakened and scarred vocal mechanism.

Laryngeal Trauma

Seen more frequently in children than in adults, **laryngeal trauma** refers to many kinds of injury to the larynx. The most frequent causes of laryngeal trauma include automobile, snowmobile, and motorcycle accidents. Attempted strangulations and bullet wounds also damage the larynx. Young children may suffer trauma by swallowing small toys, pins, glass pieces, eggshells, and other sharp objects. A variety of sports-related accidents can fracture the laryngeal cartilages, crush the larynx, and damage the nerve supply.

Patients who suffer laryngeal trauma undergo immediate surgery in which the laryngeal mechanism is reconstructed. Some patients may recover their voice following successful surgery. In other cases, voice therapy may be needed after the patient recovers from surgery. The kind of voice therapy offered depends on the individual patient, the nature of the trauma, and the type of voice problem. The extent of success depends on the proficiency of the remaining or surgically reconstructed laryngeal mechanism.

Laryngeal Web

The vocal folds are normally covered with a thin membrane. Sometimes, these membranes can grow across and close some or most of the opening between the folds. Such a membranous growth across the folds is called a **laryngeal web.** An incomplete laryngeal web is illustrated in Figure 7.8.

A laryngeal web may be observed soon after birth, in which case it is described as congenital. The web also can develop when the edges of folds are traumatized either by accidental injury or surgery. The treatment is the surgical removal of the web. After the surgery, most people need voice therapy.

Other Conditions

Many other physically based conditions affect voice production. Injury to certain parts of the brain also can cause voice and other speech and language problems. Hearing loss is a major physical cause of voice problems. More detailed descriptions of many physically based disorders of voice can be found in several books on voice and voice therapy (Aronson, 1985; Boone & McFarlane, 2000; Case, 1996; Wilson, 1987).

Abuse-Based Disorders of Phonation

Many disorders of voice are due to vocally abusive behaviors. The sophisticated vocal mechanism works well when used properly. But it is extremely sensitive to abusive practices. Such practices often cause a variety of voice problems.

See **Chapter 10** for hearing and its disorders.

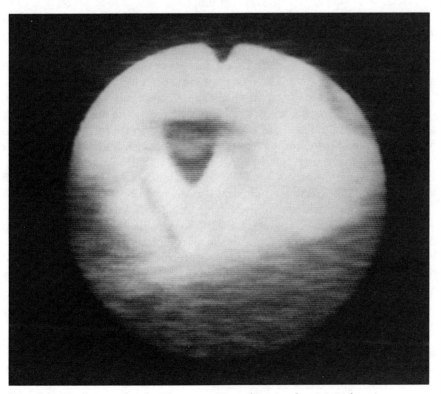

Figure 7.8. The laryngeal web. (Photo courtesy of Dr. Stephen McFarlane.)

People abuse their voice in several ways. The talkative child, like Nathan in the earlier story, learns to abuse the vocal mechanism early in childhood. Such children continue to engage in abusive practices into adolescence and perhaps adulthood. Abusive behaviors include excessive shouting, screaming, cheering, talking, coughing, and throat clearing. Strained and explosive vocalizations and abrupt initiation of sounds (glottal attacks) also are abusive. Finally, talking with inappropriate loudness or pitch is abusive as well.

Many vocally abusive behaviors cause physical damage to the vocal folds and create physical pathologies. The voice problems that result from vocally abusive behaviors are due to such physical damage and pathological states of the larynx.

The majority of the vocally abusive behaviors are associated with excessive muscular effort, tension, and irritation of the folds. Shouting, screaming, and cheering, for example, require excessive laryngeal effort and tension. Many high school cheerleaders may have chronic hoarseness of voice because of vocal fold tension and irritation. Continued tension and irritation of the folds begin to change the structure of the folds. Vocal nodules and injury to vocal muscles and the joints can result. Apparently, a cheerleader's programmed, rehearsed, and excessively overt expression of enthusiasm is perilous to vocal folds.

To talk is to communicate (it is hoped), but excessive talk may be both noncommunicative and dangerous to the health of the vocal folds, as Nathan's story made clear. Prolonged and excessive talking often causes vocal nodules. The risk of inducing pathologic conditions is even greater when continuous and excessive speech also is loud and is of inappropriate pitch. Like excessive talking, excessive singing, especially at unusually high pitch levels, also can induce vocal pathological states and voice disorders.

Noise in speaking environments prompts unusually loud voice. We automatically increase our vocal intensity when we speak in noisy environments. If a person works in a noisy place, the chances are that habitually loud speech is established. As described earlier, louder voice (increased vocal intensity) requires increased subglottal pressure and muscular effort. Increased muscular effort needed to blow the vocal folds apart may cause nodules.

Noise is a part of many environments in which people work. For example, most bars and ballrooms are noisy. People who work in such environments tend to talk louder and at higher pitch. Those who operate noisy machines tend to speak with higher loudness and pitch. Professional gardeners who use power blowers and lawn mowers and people working in various factories and construction sites, among others, are vulnerable to increased loudness and pitch of voice resulting in vocal stress and pathological conditions.

Chronic coughing and throat-clearing, along with explosive vocalizations and abrupt voice initiations, traumatize the vocal folds. Excessive laughing and crying also may induce changes in the vocal folds. All these behaviors require vigorous and abrupt changes in the larynx from a resting position. Laryngeal tumors and vocal nodules may develop in people who initiate voice abruptly and cough incessantly.

The specific type of voice disorder that results from vocal abuse depends on the kinds of structural pathologies induced by those behaviors. Generally speaking, hoarseness of voice is more frequently associated with abusive vocal behaviors. What follows is a description of some of the pathological changes that result from abusive behaviors and the kinds of voice problems that are associated with those changes.

Vocal Nodules

Vocal nodules are small nodes that develop on vocal folds and protrude from the surrounding cells. In the beginning, the nodules are reddish or pinkish. Later on, they appear white or grayish because they become fibrous. Vocal nodules can be unilateral (only one fold has it). Typically, though, they are bilateral; the two nodules sit opposite each other on the two folds. The nodules typically appear at the junction of anterior (frontal) and middle-third portion of the folds. They are well defined in the beginning stages but become more diffuse later because of the inflammation of the surrounding tissue. Figure 7.9 illustrates bilateral vocal nodules.

Vocal nodules are seen most frequently in children who scream and yell on playgrounds and in adults who yell out their enthusiasm for their favorite sports teams and boo the opponents. Singers especially are susceptible to vocal nodules. In fact, the vocal nodules also are known as singer's nodes (as well as screamer's nodes). The nodules develop because of the frequent friction between the two folds. Such friction is necessary to produce the screams of joy and shouts of contempt.

The vocal nodules increase the mass of the folds. Consequently, the folds vibrate at a slower rate. The slower vibration results in lower pitch. The nodules also make it difficult to close the folds. This causes air leakage during phonation, which is perceived as breathy voice. Hoarseness also is a common feature of vocal nodules.

Vocal rest usually clears the nodules. But prolonged abuse of the folds will result in larger and more persistent nodules. Unless the person changes his or her abusive behaviors, these nodules may not disappear. It is the responsibility of the speech–language pathologist to change the vocally abusive behaviors that have caused the nodules and the resulting voice problem. The techniques of voice therapy for the vocally abusive client are described in a later section.

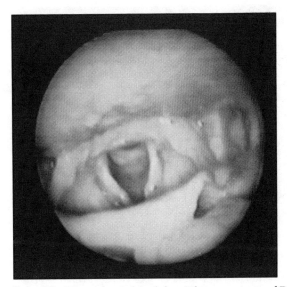 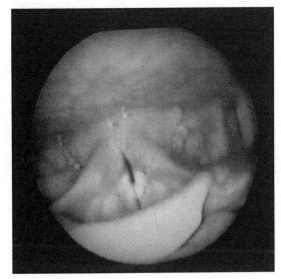

Figure 7.9. Bilateral vocal nodules. (Photo courtesy of Dr. Stephen McFarlane.)

Polyps

Polyps, like nodules, are masses that grow and bulge out from the surrounding tissue. The two types of growths tend to occur at the same site on the vocal folds: the junction of the anterior (front) and middle-third portion of the folds. However, polyps are softer than nodules and may be filled with fluid or have vascular tissue. Polyps tend to be unilateral as opposed to the typically bilateral nodules. Polyps may either have a broad base on the fold or be attached to the fold by a stalk. The broad-based polyp is called **sessile,** whereas the stalk-attached polyp is called **pedunculated.** The two types of polyps are illustrated in Figure 7.10.

It is believed that the traumatic use of the vocal folds results in submucosal hemorrhage (bleeding within the folds), which leads to the formation of tumor-like polyps. Unless the vocally abusive behavior is checked, the polyps usually get bigger. Polyps can be found in other parts of the body, including the nose, the respiratory tract, and the digestive tract.

Polyps are more frequently seen in adults than in children, who are more susceptible to developing nodules. A polyp may develop even after a single episode of screaming and yelling, whereas the development of nodules requires prolonged vocally abusive behaviors (Boone & McFarlane, 2000). Adults who scream at sports events, coaches who yell at the players, and those who supervise noisy children are especially vulnerable to developing polyps.

The effects of polyps on phonation are similar to those of nodules. Breathiness and hoarseness are heard more frequently. Besides, the voice also might sound diplophonic (double voice) because the fold with the polyp may not vibrate at the same rate as the healthy fold.

Polyps are usually removed by surgery. However, voice therapy also is necessary in most cases. The clinician must first identify the vocally abusive behaviors that are responsible for the polyps (and the voice problem). Next, the clinician must help the client change those abusive behavior patterns. The procedures are described in a later section in this chapter.

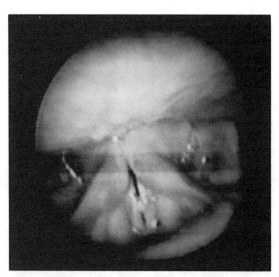 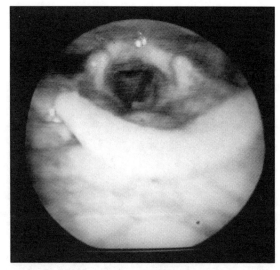

Figure 7.10. Two kinds of polyps: the sessile (left) and the pedunculated (right). (Photo courtesy of Dr. Stephen McFarlane.)

Contact Ulcers

Contact ulcers are sores that develop on one or both sides of the posterior (back) end of the vocal folds. The membranes covering the arytenoids are especially vulnerable because they come in contact with each other. Contact ulcers are seen less frequently than other forms of lesions, but they are seen mostly in adult males. Figure 7.11 illustrates contact ulcers.

A person with contact ulcers is known to talk excessively. The pitch is generally low. The voice is not necessarily loud, but it can be breathy and hoarse. The affected person also is known to initiate voice abruptly and forcefully (hard glottal attacks). The resulting laryngeal trauma is thought to be the cause of contact ulcers.

Contact ulcers need medical attention. The speech–language pathologist, however, must help the client change the faulty methods of initiating and using the voice. The clients must learn to initiate the voice gently and softly. They need to learn to speak at an appropriate pitch. The procedures of modifying vocally abusive behaviors, described in a later section, are used in the treatment of the voice disorder due to contact ulcers.

Vocal Fold Thickening

The vocal folds can be thickened because of vocally abusive behaviors. The site of thickening often is the same as that of nodules and polyps. Speaking with excessive effort, coughing, throat-clearing, and other such actions can thicken the folds. Because the vocal folds thicken slowly and gradually, it is thought that prolonged vocal abuse may be the cause. Eventually, nodules or polyps may appear on the thickened vocal folds.

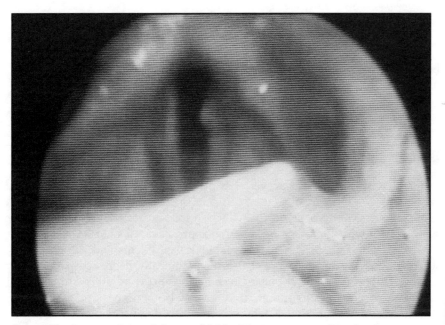

Figure 7.11. Contact ulcers of the vocal folds. (Photo courtesy of Dr. Stephen McFarlane.)

The vocal fold thickening results in breathy voice with lowered pitch. As nodules or polyps appear, the voice becomes increasingly hoarse. The vocal fold thickening can be reduced by eliminating the vocally abusive behaviors.

Traumatic Laryngitis

Some people are prone to have laryngitis when they have an infection that results from a cold or allergy. **Laryngitis** is the inflammation of the membranes of the larynx. The infection also causes a swelling (edema) of the membranes. This is organic laryngitis, which normally does not require voice therapy, although vocal rest is helpful. **Traumatic laryngitis,** on the other hand, is due to vocally abusive behaviors. It is thought that continuous yelling, crying, and loud laughing may be among the causes of traumatic laryngitis. These behaviors irritate the laryngeal structures, which then get swollen. Consequently, the voice is hoarse. In these cases, voice therapy consists of immediate vocal rest and attempts at changing the vocally abusive behaviors.

Voice disorders related to vocally abusive behaviors illustrate the complex and sensitive relation between a person's behaviors and vocal pathological changes. These disorders also illustrate a chain of causes and effects:

- Vocally abusive behaviors, which cause
- Laryngeal tissue changes, which in turn cause
- Voice disorders, which then may cause
- Personal, social, emotional, and occupational problems, which cause additional stress and more vocal strain.

The treatment of these disorders requires both medical and behavioral procedures. The task of a speech–language pathologist is to change the vocally abusive behaviors.

Disorders of Loudness and Pitch

Frequently, the problems of loudness and pitch are a part of other voice disorders. For example, the breathy and hoarse voice is typically of low pitch. Laryngeal pathologies may prevent a loud enough voice. However, a few disorders of loudness and pitch are independent of other problems.

Disorders of Loudness

People's vocal loudness varies. Very few people seek professional help for loud speech unless it is a part of a larger problem, such as excessively loud talk that results in vocal nodules or polyps, which in turn create a voice problem. The typical client who seeks help for a loudness problem talks too softly.

Many clinicians believe that psychological problems underlie faint voice when it exists as an independent disorder. Clinically depressed patients, for example, talk too softly to be heard even under quiet conditions. Frightened or otherwise psychologically traumatized people also may speak in a faint voice. But there also are individuals who speak too softly as a matter of habit and often are surprised that people have difficulty hearing them.

Most cases of inadequate loudness can be treated rather easily. By teaching people to maintain enough air pressure while speaking, and by systematically reinforcing progressively louder speech, the problem can be eliminated or minimized.

Disorders of Pitch

The typical pitch disorder consists of either too high or too low a pitch considering the speaker's age and gender. As stated earlier, the pitch of an average male is lower than that of the average female. The pitch of children is generally higher than that of adults. An unusually high pitch of a man or an unusually low pitch of a woman may be considered abnormal or undesirable.

The **high-pitched male** is probably seen more frequently in speech and hearing clinics than the low-pitched female. This may be so because the typical pitch of the male is the result of a more drastic change than the typical pitch of the female.

Until about age 7, boys and girls do not differ much in their fundamental frequency. At age 1 or 2, both boys and girls have a speaking fundamental frequency (SFF) of about 400 Hz, with a range from 340 to 470 Hz. They continue to have similar SFF until after age 7. At age 7, all children have a fundamental frequency of about 260 Hz, with a range from 220 to 310 Hz. However, the pitches of boys and girls begin to diverge at around age 8, when the SFF of boys is 5 Hz lower (250) than that of girls (255). From then on, the SFF of boys drops more dramatically than that of girls (Wilson, 1987). The biggest single drop takes place around the age of puberty. At age 12, the male (230 Hz) and the female (240 Hz) SFFs are only 10 Hz apart, but at age 13 or 14 they are 50 Hz apart (male, 175; female, 225). From the age of 1 to the age of 18 years, the female SFF is reduced by nearly 50% (from 400 to 205 Hz), whereas the male SFF is reduced by nearly 70% (from 400 to 125 Hz).

As discussed earlier, the pitch is lower when the laryngeal structures are more massive and larger, and it is higher when the structures are thinner and smaller. As children of either gender grow older, the pitch drops because of the increase in the mass and size of their larynx. The increase in the size and mass of the male larynx is proportionately greater than that of the female larynx. Hence, the pitch of the male changes to a greater extent than the pitch of the female. The change takes place over a period of years. The rate of change varies from child to child. The change may be abrupt in some and gradual in others. The process of achieving a lower pitch is associated with pitch breaks, which may be embarrassing or annoying to some boys.

A pitch that is too high for an adult man does not have a physiological basis. Typically, it is not due to a failure of the laryngeal mechanism to grow bigger. The high pitch persists though the larynx has grown normally. Therefore, the persistent high pitch (falsetto) often is described as *functional*.

The most frequently cited reasons for the persistent falsetto are that (a) some boys resist the change; (b) they continue to use the pitch they are used to; (c) they find the new pitch incompatible with their *self-image* or *personality*; (d) they do not feel secure about the adult role they are soon expected to play; and (e) the habit of speaking in a high pitch persists. These are suggestions based on common sense. Their scientific validity has not been established.

The treatment of high-pitched voice in a male is generally successful. The clinician first encourages the client to vary his pitch by saying isolated sounds or words with progressively decreasing pitch. The clinician demonstrates the desirable pitch and asks the client to imitate it. The client receives reinforcement for producing a pitch that is lower than his baseline pitch. In gradual and carefully planned steps, the clinician teaches the client to speak with decreasing pitch levels. Eventually, the client reaches the pitch level judged appropriate for him. The client then systematically practices speech at that level to strengthen it. Using similarly graded steps, the clinician increases the length of utterances from the simpler levels of sounds and words to more complex levels of phrases, sentences, and conversational speech. In most cases, the clinician designs special procedures to make sure that the client uses voice of the lower pitch in situations outside the clinic. The clinician trains parents, siblings, friends, colleagues, and significant others to remind the client to use the new pitch and to reinforce him for doing it.

Persistence of **high pitch in the female** can occur, but it is rare. Because, as noted, the pitch of an adolescent female does not change as dramatically as the pitch of an adolescent male, a higher than normal pitch in a female person is not as noticeable as it is in a male person. However, an extremely high-pitched female voice is noticeable for that reason, and voice therapy may be needed. The treatment procedure remains the same as that described for the high-pitched male speaker.

Pitch disorders due to hormonal changes are more frequent in females than in males. Menstruation, menopause, and virilization (increased masculinity) of the female voice have all been associated with pitch changes. In most cases, pitch changes before and during menstruation are not a major problem. However, such changes are troublesome to professional singers. It is known that a lowered level of estrogen and progesterone before the menses can cause a thickening of the vocal folds. This can lower the pitch and induce some hoarseness as well.

The fundamental frequency of some female speakers changes to a lower level around the time of menopause. Menopause is associated with an increased secretion of androgen (a male sex hormone), which causes a thickening of the vocal folds, hence the lowering of the pitch. Drugs that contain male hormones are sometimes used in the treatment of cancer. For example, uterine cancer in women often is treated with testosterone. Such drugs have a virilizing effect on the female. The drugs also thicken the vocal folds and decrease the vocal pitch. Vocal changes due to medication may be irreversible.

Voice Disorders of Resonance

Resonance is the modification of sound by structures through which that sound passes. In the present context, the resonating structures that lie below and above the larynx modify the laryngeal tone. Many factors affect resonance, but here the concern is on the oral and nasal structures and their corresponding resonance qualities.

Voice disorders of resonance constitute an absence of a desired resonance, inadequate resonance, or inappropriate resonance. These problems can be heard in the case of both oral and nasal resonance.

Disorders of Oral Resonance

Oral resonance disorders are not as well defined as the nasal resonance disorders. Problems of oral resonance are often and primarily related to the position of the tongue during phonation and the extent of the jaw movement (mouth opening). In combination with other subtle oral resonance factors, the tongue positions and jaw movements have the most noticeable effect on oral resonance and its distortions.

The tongue is the biggest structure in the oral cavity. Therefore, its movements continuously change the shape and size of the oral cavity. The shape and size of a cavity are the most important factors in determining its resonance qualities. Therefore, the changes caused by the tongue movements have the most immediate effects on oral resonance.

When the tongue is carried in the front portion of the mouth throughout an utterance, the resulting resonance is described as *thin,* and the person gives a subjective impression of being immature (Boone & McFarlane, 2000). This kind of oral resonance is associated with baby talk, most easily noticed when adults use this kind of speech. The thin resonance is reduced oral resonance because of the forward carriage of the tongue. Limited movements of the lips and the jaw contribute to that thin resonance.

Because it reduces the dimensions of the oral cavity, a retracted tongue that bulges at the back of the mouth during speech also can create oral resonance problems. Known as **cul de sac** (bottom of the sack) **resonance**, it is due to an oral cavity that is partially closed at the back and open in the front. The tongue blocks some of the sound waves generated by the larynx from reaching the oral cavity. The result is a distorted voice and resonance. Individuals with neurological problems and hearing impairment often have difficulty making proper tongue adjustments. Individuals with no organic deviations also might acquire the habit of carrying the tongue too far back in the mouth while speaking, resulting in cul de sac resonance.

Another oral resonance problem results when a person speaks with very little mouth opening. The clenched-teeth speaker greatly reduces the area of the vocal cavity that resonates the laryngeal tone. The result is reduced oral resonance.

The speech–language pathologist can treat most oral resonance problems. In the case of excessive backward carriage of the tongue, the clinician teaches a more normal carriage and movement of the tongue. In the case of cul de sac oral resonance, more forward tongue carriage and movements are taught.

Disorders of Nasal Resonance

Nasal resonance and the problems associated with it are, for the most part, a matter of the workings of the velopharyngeal mechanism, which connects and disconnects the oral and nasal cavities. Several kinds of movements may be involved in the working of this mechanism. For example, the soft palate (velum) moves up and backward to make a contact with the posterior pharyngeal (throat) wall. The posterior pharyngeal wall also may move forward to meet the velum. The sides of the pharyngeal wall also can constrict like a sphincter. All of these movements close the velopharyngeal port and reduce or eliminate nasal resonance on non-nasal speech sounds.

See **Chapters 3** and **8** for more information on the velopharyngeal mechanism.

It must be noted, however, that many vowel sounds, which are considered non-nasal, do contain some nasal resonance, which the listeners may or may not notice but instruments can measure. Thus, when we say that non-nasal sounds lack nasal resonance, we mean only that the *predominant* resonance is oral and that the nasal resonance is not noticeable.

Hypernasality

A person who exhibits excessive nasality (hypernasality) sounds like he or she is speaking through the nose. **Hypernasality** results when the velopharyngeal mechanism does not close the opening to the nasal passage during the production of non-nasal sounds. There are many causes for this lack of adequate closure, but most of them are organic. As a result, the air and sound continue to escape through the nose, adding unnecessary nasal resonance to non-nasal speech sounds.

Cleft palate and associated communication disorders are described in **Chapter 8.**

Cleft palate is a major cause of hypernasality. When the bones of the palate do not fuse, the oral and the nasal cavities are always connected. Individuals with unrepaired palatal clefts tend to exhibit severe hypernasality. Consequently, it often is difficult to distinguish the nasal from the non-nasal sounds in their speech.

Velopharyngeal inadequacy is another cause of hypernasality. Due to many reasons, including the cleft of the soft palate, the muscle mass of the soft palate is reduced. Therefore, the velopharyngeal mechanism is inadequate to achieve a closure.

Adenoidectomy or **tonsillectomy** also can cause hypernasality, especially when the child's velopharyngeal mechanism initially did not have sufficient muscle mass. The adenoids and tonsils are masses that can help compensate for the otherwise inadequate velopharyngeal mechanism. When these masses are surgically removed, the basic velopharyngeal inadequacy may become apparent.

Paralysis of the velum, another organic cause of hypernasality, can be either complete or partial. Obviously, a paralyzed velum will not aid in the closure. Velar paralysis is associated with cerebral palsy, stroke, and such other conditions of neuropathology.

Hearing and its disorders are described in **Chapter 10.**

Deafness also is associated with hypernasality. Most individuals who are deaf have adequate velopharyngeal mechanism. However, during speech, they cannot effectively use that mechanism. Because people who are deaf have difficulty hearing their own voice, they are not able to monitor the degree of nasality in their speech. The result is not only hypernasality, but also hyponasality. Their nasal sounds may sound non-nasal and the oral sounds may sound nasal.

Hypernasality, though often associated with some form of organic defect, can exist with no such defect. This often is described as **functional hypernasality.** If the hypernasality is not excessive, it simply becomes a hallmark of the individual's voice. If it is excessive, the person needs voice therapy. Before treatment begins, the associated organic condition (such as cleft palate) must be surgically or medically treated. Such treatment, however, might not eliminate hypernasality, suggesting a need for voice treatment.

Several techniques help reduce hypernasality. For example, the client can be reinforced for greater mouth opening or a more backward (posterior) tongue position within the mouth. A slightly louder voice or lower pitch also can be targeted. These and other procedures can reduce hypernasality in many cases.

Biofeedback also can be effective in the treatment of hypernasality. In this procedure, electronic instruments that instantaneously display the amount of oral and nasal resonance as the patient talks are used. Such visual displays give immediate feedback to the patient, making it easier to achieve a reduction in nasal resonance.

Hyponasality

A lack of nasal resonance or insufficient nasal resonance on nasal sounds is called **hyponasality (denasality)**. Temporary denasality, often associated with such conditions as cold and allergy, do not need voice therapy.

More serious forms of denasality are due to structural obstructions or deafness. For example, the nasal passage may be fully or partially blocked by nasal polyps, tumors, and other kinds of growth in the nasal cavity.

People who are deaf exhibit hyponasality for the same reason they exhibit hypernasality. Because people who are deaf cannot monitor their own speech and voice production, their nasal resonance is typically missing or misplaced.

In most cases, treatment requires a combination of medical, surgical, and voice therapy techniques. Organic growths and obstructions that create denasality require medical and surgical treatment. Denasality of individuals who are deaf can be treated within a total program of speech and voice therapy. In most cases, immediate mechanical feedback from instruments or verbal feedback from the clinician regarding the presence or absence of nasality will help achieve the desired resonance.

Spastic Dysphonia

A voice disorder whose origin is a subject of much speculation is called **spastic dysphonia.** While some experts consider it a functional disorder, others consider it a neurologically based disorder (Aronson, 1985; Boone & McFarlane, 2000; Wilson, 1987). Because of the controversy, it is described separately.

Spastic dysphonia is more frequently seen in adults than in children. The most severe forms of spastic dysphonia often are seen in people who are 40 years or older. However, it may be found in some teenagers (Wilson, 1987).

The term spastic dysphonia suggests that this voice disorder is associated with unusual muscular tension (spasticity). However, there is usually no evidence of spasticity or paralysis. What is evident is a very tight closure (adduction) of the vocal folds, which prevents the flow of air through the vocal folds. Abduction eventually releases the air, but not in a typically smooth, flowing manner. The airflow and the voice are jerky and strained. The voice gives the impression that the person is almost choked. The voice also is described as strangled, squeezed, choppy, harsh, and breathy. Tremors of the voice also may be heard (Aronson, 1985; Boone & McFarlane, 2000; Wilson, 1987).

Though overadduction is a major problem seen in many spastic dysphonic patients, some may show an opposite trend. In these cases, attempts at speech may be associated with abduction. That is, the folds may remain open, in which case there is no phonation. Some individuals may exhibit both overadduction and abduction. The voice in such people will be perceived as choppy, strained, breathy, harsh, and periodically aphonic.

A significant aspect of spastic dysphonia is its variability. The voice (and speech) may be worse at times and much better at other times. Occasionally, the speech may be near normal. Self-talking and singing may be undisturbed, but talking in social situations may be profoundly affected. The person who is able to talk normally to a pet animal may suddenly find it extremely difficult to talk to a group of people. Most other voice disorders do not show such marked situational variability.

It is not clear what causes spastic dysphonia. Both psychological and neurological causes have been suggested (Aronson, 1985; Boone & McFarlane, 2000; Wilson, 1987). Some case histories have suggested that psychological trauma, such as the death of a loved one, a terrible accident, or marital crisis, is associated with the onset of spastic dysphonia. Other case histories have suggested neurological problems. It is thought that spastic dysphonia is a part of other neurological diseases whose symptoms include fine tremors and **dystonia,** which refers to slow and uncontrollable muscle contractions due to neural damage (Aronson, 1985).

Generally, the traditional methods of voice therapy have not been successful with spastic dysphonia. A relatively drastic method, in which a branch of the recurrent laryngeal nerve is severed, has been tried. This operation produces paralysis of one of the folds (unilateral paralysis), which stays frozen in the middle position. The immobility of one of the folds prevents tight closure of the folds. The resulting voice, however, will be somewhat breathy because of a lack of full closure of the folds. Unfortunately, even this surgical procedure may not be entirely successful. In some cases, the severed recurrent laryngeal nerve may be regenerated with the reemergence of spastic dysphonia. In other cases, spastic dysphonia may return even if the vocal fold remains paralyzed.

A program of modifying the patient's vocal behaviors is probably needed in all cases, including those who have undergone the laryngeal nerve operation. It has been found that spastic dysphonia in its early stage is more successfully treated by such techniques as relaxation training, reducing or eliminating vocally abusive behaviors, breathing exercises, decreasing the vocal loudness, and changing the pitch (Wilson, 1987).

Summary

A summary of voice disorders discussed in this chapter is presented in Figure 7.12. The voice disorders are classified into those of phonation, loudness and pitch, and resonance. Voice disorders may have organic or functional causes. Organic causes of disorders of phonation include various physical diseases of the larynx and the portions of the nervous system that control the phonatory mechanism. Abuse of the vocal behaviors include such activities as screaming and excessive talking. However, abusive behaviors produce voice problems only because those behaviors induce tissue changes in the larynx. These tissue changes are the immediate cause of the voice problem. A majority of the voice disorders of resonance are due to organic causes, including hearing impairment.

Evaluation of Voice Disorders

Adults with voice disorders may seek voice therapy directly from a speech and hearing center. Children with voice disorders often are identified through routine screening procedures that speech–language pathologists conduct in public schools. In many cases, voice therapy may be recommended by a medical specialist, most frequently, the ear, nose, and throat (ENT) specialist. Because voice disorders often are associated with physical pathological conditions,

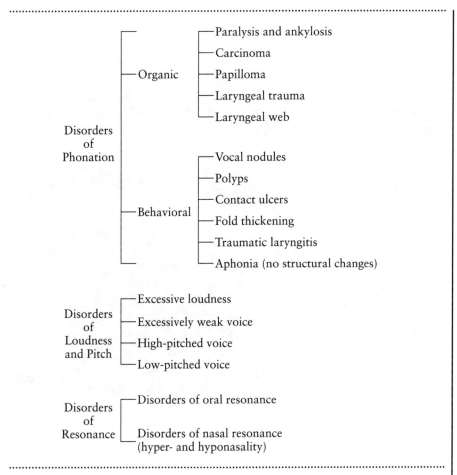

Figure 7.12. A summary of voice disorders.

voice therapy is started only after an ENT specialist completes a medical examination (Hegde, 2001a).

Medical Evaluation

An ENT specialist's medical evaluation will determine whether laryngeal diseases are the causes of the voice problem. The medical specialist uses several methods and instruments to determine the health and the working of the larynx. For example, in **mirror laryngoscopy,** or **indirect laryngoscopy,** the specialist views the laryngeal structures with the help of a small mirror placed in the throat. Various **radiological** (X-ray) procedures are used to detect such conditions as cancer of the laryngeal area and paralysis of the vocal folds.

As illustrated in Figure 7.13, specialists also use fiberoptic nasal or oral **endoscopes** to view the larynx. Endoscopes illuminate internal organs by conducting light to and from an organ via thin fiberoptic tubes. The scope can be inserted either through the mouth (**oral endoscopy**) or through the nose (**nasal endoscopy**). The endoscope can be connected to a video recording machine to make a permanent recording of the vocal mechanism and to see the behaviors of the vocal cords on a television monitor. Speech–language pathologists

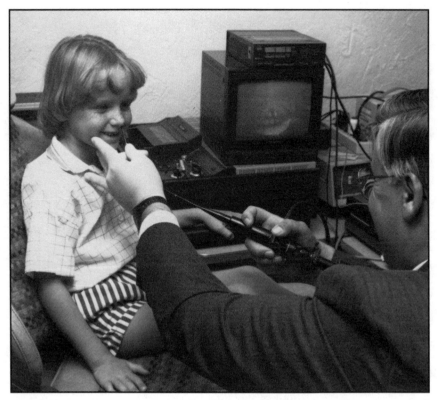

Figure 7.13. An endoscopic examination of the vocal mechanism. (Photo courtesy of Dr. Stephen McFarlane.)

also use endoscopes in the evaluation of voice disorders (Boone & McFarlane, 2000).

Voice Evaluation

The speech–language pathologist makes an evaluation of the voice and its qualities, how the client is using his or her voice, the life conditions affecting the client's voice and its production, and the kinds of behavior patterns related to disordered voice (Case, 1996). This information is essential for treatment planning.

The voice disorder assessment module is illustrated in Table 7.1. As in the assessment of any disorder, the clinician first takes a case history to learn about many important variables. For example, the clinician finds out how the voice problem started, whether any special circumstances were associated with its onset, the client's family and interpersonal relations, whether the disorder has been stable or variable across situations, and so on. The history will also document previous medical or voice treatments, their outcome, the reasons for the current referral, and the general health of the client.

After taking the case history, the clinician may complete the orofacial examination to make sure there are no gross organic defects in the oral region. A hearing screening is then completed. Subsequently, the clinician needs to assess the vocal behaviors of the client. The details of this assessment depend on the particular disorder, although there are some general procedures. Essen-

Experienced clinicians can make valid subjective evaluations of voice, but instrumental measures provide verifiable data.

Table 7.1

Assessment of Communicative Disorders: Voice Disorders

1. History of the client, the family, and the disorder

2. Interview of the client, family members, or both

3. Oral-peripheral examination

4. Hearing screening

5. Speech and language sampling

6. **Measurement/assessment of vocal behaviors:**
   a. **Breath supply**
   b. **Voice quality**
   c. **Pitch and loudness**
   d. **Resonance**
   e. **Muscular tension**
   f. **Variability of the disorder**
   g. **The types and the frequency of vocally abusive behaviors**

7. Recommendations

8. Report writing

Note. Procedures unique to voice assessment are in bold print.

tially, the voice evaluation includes making measurements as well as clinical judgments regarding the client's breath supply, laryngeal tension, voice quality, vocal pitch and loudness, resonance, situational variability, and types and frequency of vocally abusive behaviors (Hegde, 2001a).

With the help of various instruments and clinical judgment, the speech–language pathologist evaluates how the client uses his or her **breath supply** to produce voice. For instance, a client's shallow breathing may require frequent inhalations that interrupt voice and speech. Breathing may be tensed. The flow of air may be inefficient or wasteful. Vocal nodules, for example, make it difficult to sustain the airflow; therefore, the flow rate is higher. In spastic dysphonia, the flow is low because of the tensed and constricted vocal folds.

An assessment of **vocal tension** is made with the help of instruments and by listening to voice. Tension in the neck and facial muscles might be observed as the client speaks. A relatively simple instrument that measures muscle tension is an **electromyographic biofeedback** unit. With the help of surface electrodes fastened onto the skin, the electrical activity of the muscles can be recorded. The relative electrical activity of the muscles is an indication of relative tension. Such biofeedback instruments can be used in teaching the client to relax the speech muscles.

An assessment of **voice quality** is needed in most cases of voice disorders. A change in the quality of voice often is the earliest sign of an organic vocal pathological state. Making clinical judgments by listening to the voice is the most frequent method of assessing the quality. Does the voice sound hoarse, harsh, or breathy? Voice quality assessment requires training in listening and recognizing normal and deviant voice characteristics.

The judgment of breathiness is made when the clinician hears the noise of the leakage of air as the person speaks. The judgment of harsh voice is made when the voice sounds unpleasant, strident, or metallic. A harsh voice is initiated suddenly and with a hard glottal attack. The judgment of hoarseness is made when a combination of breathiness and harshness are heard.

Breathiness, harshness, and hoarseness can be objectively measured by a **spectrograph,** which converts audible signals into printed, visible traces. Normal, breathy, harsh, and hoarse vocal productions can be distinguished by different spectrographic traces.

Pitch and **loudness** are subjective sensations, but they are related, respectively, to the frequency and amplitude of vocal fold vibrations. Because frequency and amplitude are physical events, they can be measured objectively. In addition, the clinician makes judgments about the appropriateness of the pitch and loudness a given client exhibits.

The subjective evaluation of pitch is made in relation to the age and gender of a client. As noted earlier in this chapter, children have higher pitch than adults, and women have higher pitch than men. By listening to the speech of a client and considering the client's gender and age, the clinician determines whether the pitch is too low, too high, or appropriate.

Each person has a typical pitch called the **habitual pitch.** However, the pitch varies within a range, which contains the lowest and the highest notes. Within this range lies an **optimal pitch,** which is judged to be the most comfortable, appropriate, and compatible pitch for the person. People with pitch disorders often tend to speak at a pitch that is too far removed from their optimal pitch.

Sophisticated instruments, such as the **Visi-Pitch** shown in Figure 7.14, may be used to make an objective assessment of the frequency of vocal fold vibrations. The Visi-Pitch displays the frequencies on a computer monitor. It

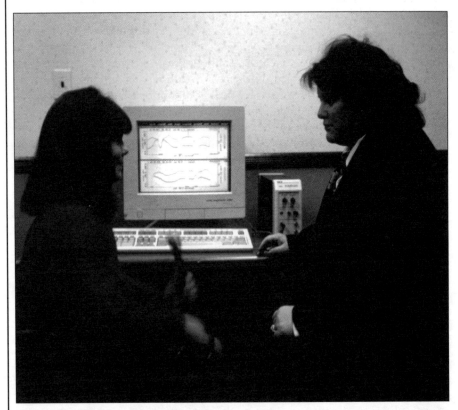

Figure 7.14. The Visi-Pitch instrument used in the assessment of vocal behaviors. (Photo courtesy of Kay Elemetrics Corporation.)

also can show the frequency range, optimal pitch, and habitual pitch. It can give a printout of these factors.

Loudness is a difficult quality of speech to measure and judge. Clients who speak too loudly in many situations may speak more softly in the clinic. There is no particular standard of loudness of speech. It varies depending on the situation. We speak a little louder in noisy situations and whisper in classrooms, churches, and when someone is asleep. People speak softly in some parties but loudly in others.

The clients who cannot speak loudly enough present a different problem. Unusually soft or faint voice is more likely to show in most situations, including the clinic. Weak voice may be due to organic conditions, in which case it is more constant. For example, people with vocal fold paralysis or Parkinson's disease speak in a faint voice.

Oral and nasal **resonance** also is assessed both clinically and with the help of instruments. Most clinicians make this judgment subjectively. Clinicians listen to tape-recorded samples of speech to judge whether the client's speech production includes nasal resonance on non-nasal sounds (hypernasality) or whether nasal resonance is absent on nasal sounds (hyponasality).

Several mechanical instruments may be used to measure oral and nasal resonance. One of them, called the Nasometer, is illustrated in Figure 7.15. With two microphones and a nasal–oral separator, the Nasometer gives a ratio of oral and nasal resonance.

Situational variability of voice disorders is an important factor to assess. Vocally abusive behaviors are situation bound. It is necessary to find out the situations in which such behaviors are more likely to occur. The client or the parents might be asked to observe the variability and report to the clinician. For example, a spastic dysphonic client may keep a pocket notebook in which the

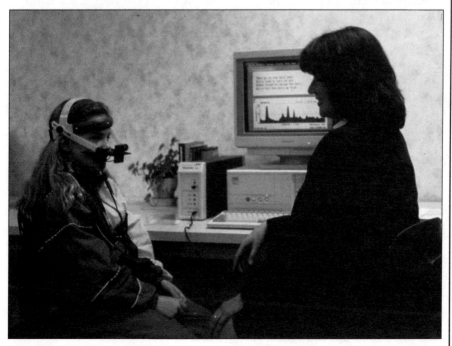

Figure 7.15. The Nasometer used to measure the ratio between oral and nasal resonance. (Photo courtesy of Kay Elemetrics Corporation.)

instances of relatively easy and difficult voice are recorded. The parents of a child with a hoarse voice might note that he or she shouts and yells while swimming with his siblings but is relatively quiet when swimming with the parents.

In the case of vocal abuse, the **types** and the **frequency of vocally abusive behaviors** must be measured before starting treatment. Most adult clients or parents of children are able to help the clinician assess how often shouting, screaming, and loud and excessive talking take place at home. A record of the occurrences of each of these behaviors over a few days gives the clinician the baserate of vocally abusive behaviors. For example, the mother of Nathan, the talkative child described at the beginning of this chapter, was able to document that he spoke for 20 to 35 minutes before falling asleep.

Integration of Assessment Data

The information obtained from various sources, the clinical judgments, and the measurements of various aspects of vocal behavior are integrated and summarized before a treatment plan is developed. An **evaluation report,** which describes all the information collected, is prepared. Many clinicians use rating scales in initially measuring and later summarizing the client's voice and its characteristics. A summary of voice assessment that uses a rating scale is illustrated in Table 7.2.

Treatment of Vocal Abuse

Techniques of treating several varieties of voice disorders were described earlier. In this final section, the treatment of vocally abusive behaviors is described. A majority of voice disorders are due to vocal abuse, which causes many organic laryngeal pathological conditions, including vocal nodules, polyps, traumatic laryngitis, vocal fold thickening, and contact ulcers. Voice disorders in these cases cannot be controlled unless the vocally abusive behaviors are changed. Therefore, clinicians have developed many procedures to change such behaviors and teach more appropriate vocal behaviors (Andrews, 1999; Boone & McFarlane, 2000; Hegde, 2001b; Johnson, 1985; Wilson, 1987). The techniques that help change vocally abusive behaviors often are effective in modifying other kinds of voice disorders that have different origins. Therefore, an understanding of how vocal abuse is treated gives a good idea of the essence of voice therapy.

The otorhinolaryngologist's summary and recommendations, along with the assessment results of the speech–language pathologist, set the stage for modifying the identified vocally abusive behaviors. In the case of Nathan, for example, the otorhinolaryngologist had written that Nathan has "small, bilateral vocal nodules. His voice is chronically hoarse. A history of vocal abuse is evident. A voice evaluation and therapy is recommended." The clinician's observations and the mother's data had shown that Nathan's voice was hoarse almost 100% of the time. He spoke with excessive muscular tension and often initiated voice abruptly. He spoke excessively and loudly, spoke to himself, and frequently screamed and yelled while playing with other children.

Clinicians modify a variety of vocally abusive behaviors in both children and adults. An important goal of voice therapy is to help establish appropriate

Table 7.2

Summary of Voice Assessment Data Using a Rating Scale

....

University Speech and Hearing Center

Client _____ Age _____ Sex _____

Clinician _____ Date/time _____

Rating of Severity

1. Voice quality	Normal	Mild	Moderate	Severe	Profound
Breathy/Harsh/Hoarse	1	2	3	④	5

The client's voice was judged hoarse on 90% of the utterances produced in conversational speech.

2. Pitch

Too high/Too low	1	2	3	④	5

The client's pitch was judged too high on 80% of the utterances produced in conversational speech.

3. Loudness

Too loud/Too soft	1	2	③	4	5

The client's voice was judged too loud during most of the assessment time.

4. Nasal resonance

Hypernasal/Hyponasal	1	2	③	4	5

The client's voice was judged hypernasal on 45% of the utterances produced in conversational speech.

5. Oral resonance

Reduced oral resonance	1	②	3	4	5

The client spoke with limited mouth opening; on most of the utterances, the oral resonance was reduced.

6. Muscle tension

Hypertense/Hypotense	1	2	③	4	5

The client's muscles of the face, neck, and chest were judged hypertense during conversational speech.

7. Abusive vocal behaviors	1	2	3	④	5

Client has a history of vocally abusive behaviors including loud and excessive talking, loud cheering at games, and screaming and yelling while playing with friends.

Comments and Recommendations: The client speaks with excessive muscular tension and effort; voice is excessively hoarse most of the time; there is a history of frequent and severe abusive vocal behaviors. Voice therapy is recommended to reduce the frequency and severity of such behaviors.

....

Note. The comments are for illustration only; a given client may not exhibit all the problems described.

vocal behaviors, some of which are listed in Table 7.3; everyone should learn and maintain those behaviors. In the case of Nathan, the clinician had to reduce his screaming and yelling, his loud self-talk during play and at bedtime, and his overall amount of speech. The clinician had to teach him to play silently, talk less and generally more softly, and to fall asleep without talking too much or for too long.

Both children and adults initially receive explanations of what their laryngeal pathology is and how it may have come about. For example, with the help of pictures and drawings, the clinician illustrates the vocal folds and nodules and explains their relation to vocal abuse in simple terms. Then, the clinician describes the goals of voice therapy for the particular client. In most cases, they include reducing the frequency of vocally abusive behaviors and learning behaviors that help maintain vocal health and desirable vocal qualities. Many clients must talk less, talk softly, reduce or eliminate screaming and yelling, avoid noisy and smoke-filled rooms, and practice more relaxed speech. In addition, clients may have to reduce or eliminate smoking, drink more water to keep the vocal cords moist, reduce or eliminate the intake of alcoholic beverages, and take other steps to maintain vocal health.

Children must be taught to avoid noisy toys, play quietly, and reduce screaming on the playground. In the case of Nathan, for example, the clinician taught him to play with his wrestling characters without loud self-talk. Initially, he was praised for every minute he played with the characters quietly; in gradual steps, he was reinforced for longer durations of quiet play. His mother was trained to reinforce quiet play at home. To eliminate his bedtime self-talk, his mother was asked to give Nathan a token when he was tucked in. He was told he could exchange the token for a small gift the next morning if he did not talk before falling asleep. The very first night the procedure was implemented, Nathan fell asleep without talking to himself. Nathan was also reinforced for quiet sitting for progressively longer durations, something he rarely did. With these and other procedures, his hoarseness was reduced and an examination by

Table 7.3

Take Care of Your Voice! Some Lessons for Everyday Living

1. Get closer! Do not shout. Your voice is not a public address system.

2. Do not try to drown the other voices! Take your turn in conversation.

3. Not too loud! Not too soft! Maintain adequate breath supply.

4. Away from the noisy places! Talk less or not at all under noisy conditions.

5. Do not be a chatterbox! Silence can speak. Let others use the phone.

6. Relax! Don't talk with tension in your neck and chest muscles.

7. Wet your throat! Drink plenty of water.

8. Listen to the Surgeon-General! Do not smoke. Do not drink too much. Avoid smoke-filled, noisy, or dusty places.

9. Cheer your favorite sports team in sign language!

10. Do not shake the building! Cough or sneeze gently and softly. Reduce the frequency of throat clearing.

11. You are not a motorcycle! Teach your child to play quietly.

12. Consult a throat specialist and a speech–language pathologist about voice problems.

the ear, nose, and throat specialist 9 months later indicated an absence of vocal nodules. His voice was judged normal.

Reduction of vocally abusive behaviors takes hard work on the part of the client and his or her family members. In the case of children or adults, family members must watch for the vocally abusive behaviors and discourage the client from exhibiting them. The family members should also be quick in giving positive feedback whenever the client shows vocally appropriate behaviors. To accomplish these goals, the speech–language pathologist works closely with all members of the client's family.

Dialogue

Ms. Noledge-Hungry was eager to talk with Professor Speech-Wisely about voice disorders and her major. She found the subject complex yet very interesting.

N-H: What are the major structures of the larynx that I should remember?

S-W: Remember that the **larynx** is suspended by the hyoid bone and supported by cricoid, thyroid, and arytenoid cartilages. Vocal folds are muscular structures within the larynx, and they form a biological valve with biological functions. What is an important "joint" within the laryngeal structure?

N-H: The **cricoarytenoid joint,** which permits varied movements of the vocal folds because the folds are attached to the arytenoid cartilages. Would you summarize the theory of vocal fold vibrations?

S-W: The most widely accepted theory is the **myoelastic-aerodynamic theory,** which proposes that forces and pressures of air and the elasticity of the folds set the folds into vibration. You must remember the details of this theory.

N-H: Why is it that the pitch and loudness of voice are judgments listeners make?

S-W: Because they really are sensory experiences based on physical events. You hear pitch differences when the frequency of vocal fold vibrations changes. You hear loudness differences when the intensity of vibrations changes. Can you describe voice qualities?

N-H: Yes. Voice quality depends on several factors including the complexity of the sound wave, the amount of noise and air leakage, tension of the vocal folds, and the structure of the laryngeal, oral, and nasal mechanisms. The major voice quality deviations include **harshness, breathiness,** and **hoarseness.** A harsh voice is unpleasant, rough, and "gravelly," caused by too much muscular effort and tension. The breathy voice is phonation with air leakage because of inadequate fold closure; the sound is mixed with the noise of the escaping air. Hoarse voice is a combination of harshness and breathiness. But I am not sure of resonance and its disorders.

S-W: **Resonance** is the modification of sound generated by one structure by other structures, called resonators. The cavities of the throat, mouth, and nose are the major resonators, whereas the vocal folds are the sound generators. Major resonance disorders are **hypernasality,** which is excessive and inappropriate nasal resonance, and **hyponasality,** which is lack of nasal resonance on nasal sounds.

N-H: What is the difference between aphonia and dysphonia?

S-W: **Aphonia** means no voice, and it is a type of voice disorder. **Dysphonia** is any type of voice disorder.

N-H: I found aphonia almost incredible.

S-W: Yes. A speaker with normal voice loses voice and begins to whisper. The loss may be sudden in the case of psychogenic aphonia. Organic aphonia is often caused by paralyzed fold or folds.

N-H: What are some of the physical factors that cause voice disorders?

S-W: The major ones include **paralysis** and **ankylosis, carcinoma of the larynx, papilloma, laryngeal trauma,** and **laryngeal web.** You should be able to describe all of these. Can you name the three sound sources a laryngectomee can use to speak again?

N-H: An electronic larynx, esophagus, and surgically modified sources including prosthetic devices.

S-W: Fine. How is **papilloma** treated?

N-H: By surgery. The surgeon excises the wartlike growths. Unfortunately, many patients need repeated surgery. I was surprised to learn that screaming and yelling can cause physical damage to the vocal folds.

S-W: Yes, they often do. Screaming, yelling, excessive talking, and hard initiation of sound can cause **vocal nodules, polyps, contact ulcers, vocal fold thickening,** and **traumatic laryngitis.** You should be able to describe them.

N-H: I found the treatment for voice disorders based on vocal abuse a very interesting process. You must identify the abusive behaviors and change them. I liked the story of Nathan and how his problem was treated.

S-W: Yes. You should be able to describe the treatment procedure. What are disorders of pitch? How are they treated?

N-H: The pitch that is too high or too low for the person's age and gender is a disorder of pitch. Pitch disorders often are associated with other voice disorders, but an independent pitch disorder is exhibited by the male who has a very high pitch. The higher pitch is changed to lower pitch by instruction, experimentation, and reinforcement for success.

S-W: What about resonance disorders?

N-H: The most frequently observed resonance disorders are **hypernasality** and **hyponasality.** Reduced oral resonance is observed less frequently. Could you summarize spastic dysphonia?

S-W: Hypertensed, strained, and jerky phonation is the main characteristic of **spastic dysphonia.** Some patients overadduct their folds, while others overabduct with periodic aphonia. Still others show a combination of these problems. The causes are not known; both psychological and neurological causes have been suggested. Is there an operation for spastic dysphonia?

N-H: Yes. The surgeon cuts one branch of the recurrent laryngeal nerve, producing paralysis of one fold. This prevents the tight closure and improves voice. But the nerve may regrow in some cases.

S-W: Now, tell me about voice evaluation.

N-H: A medical evaluation is done first. The typical voice evaluation includes a case history; an assessment of the integrity of oral structures; breath supply, muscular tension; voice quality measurements and judgments; analysis of pitch, loudness, and resonance; and measurement of the frequency of vocally abusive behaviors.

S-W: What is the most important element of therapy for voice disorders that are due to vocal abuse?

N-H: Changing vocally abusive behaviors. This aspect illustrates the essence of voice therapy. The clinician systematically reduces the frequency and intensity of abusive behaviors.

S-W: You should be able to describe the procedures. What is an important factor in changing a client's vocally abusive behaviors?

N-H: The cooperation of the client and his or her family. The clinician must train the family members to help modify the vocally abusive behaviors at home. The client must learn to self-monitor voice productions.

The Outlook

Ms. Noledge-Hungry is not sure she wants to major in speech–language pathology. Therefore, she has more questions to ask.

N-H: What are the benefits of studying voice and its disorders for a student who may not major in communicative disorders?

S-W: How you use your voice is a matter of health and disease, which are in turn a matter of your behavior. A good understanding of how your behavior affects the health of your vocal structures can help you immensely. You can take better care of your vocal mechanism by learning and maintaining good vocal behaviors.

You can help prevent voice disorders and many kinds of vocal pathological conditions in your family and friends. If you have children, you can be more sensitive to good and bad vocal behaviors: both seem to get established early in life. From the beginning, you can teach them good vocal behaviors; you can detect signs of problems early and take professional advice before the problems get magnified.

If you enter one of the vocally high-risk professions such as teaching, singing, sports-coaching, broadcasting, preaching, law, politics, and public campaigning, this knowledge will help you sustain your much needed vocal health. Furthermore, in professions such as teaching, this knowledge will help alert young children to possible need for voice evaluation and therapy. A teacher may hear the voice of a child more often than a parent.

N-H: What about a career in health professions? I am leaning in that direction. How can I best use this information?

S-W: If you enter into medical, health, and many human service professions, you can detect early signs of voice problems in your patients and clients and make timely referrals to specialists. For example, Nathan's mother, a professional nurse, could have greatly benefited from a knowledge of voice disorders. At home, she could have detected the signs of Nathan's voice problems sooner and sought help earlier. At work, she could have alerted many of her patients to possible need for voice therapy.

Social workers, clinical psychologists, counselors, and doctors of many branches of medicine can use this knowledge in providing a more effective and broad-based service to their clients and patients. You may not learn much about voice disorders and voice therapy even in medical schools. Therefore, this information is valuable to you.

N-H: What is ahead of me if I do decide on majoring in communicative disorders? What more will I learn? ("Did I see a twinkle in his eyes?" wondered N-H.)

S-W: ("A sign of movement in the right direction, perhaps," thought S-W.) If you decide on majoring in communicative disorders, you will learn more about the voice mechanism. You will gain a better understanding of the anatomy, physiology, and neurology of voice production. You will also take specialized courses on voice disorders. You will start watching the excellent voice therapy that goes on in our clinic, right in our department. Eventually, you will work with individuals who have one of the voice disorders described in this chapter. You will find out that with help and supervision, you can actually treat those individuals. Later on, you may even specialize in voice disorders.

N-H: How do I specialize in voice?

S-W: You will go on for your graduate education in communicative disorders. You will learn more about special kinds of voice problems we did not discuss, and you will learn how to do research on voice and its disorders. You will perhaps go on for your doctoral degree and write a dissertation on a special topic. You will learn advanced techniques of measuring voice and diagnosing voice disorders. You will help refine voice treatment techniques.

N-H: Sounds great!

S-W: (Believing that voice is a mirror held to the deep, dark soul, thinks the student's exclamation, though lacking in conviction, is an encouraging sign.)

N-H: If I wish to spend more of my professional time treating people with voice disorders, where would I work?

S-W: People with voice disorders are treated in public schools, university clinics, hospitals, rehabilitation facilities, and private speech and hearing clinics. If you specialize in treating certain kinds of voice disorders, such as those of the laryngectomee, you may be working in a hospital speech and hearing department.

N-H: Well, thank you, Dr. Speech-Wisely. I think you gave me plenty of useful information. I hope it will help make up my mind about the major.

S-W: I hope so, too.

Study Questions

1. What are the biological functions of the laryngeal valve?

2. What kinds of movements are permitted by the cricoarytenoid joint?

3. Define the terms abduction and adduction.

4. Define glottis.

5. Give a brief description of the myoelastic-aerodynamic theory of phonation.

6. What is pitch? What determines it?

7. Why is the female vocal pitch higher than the male pitch?

8. Is the vocal pitch higher or lower when the vocal folds are stretched and tensed?

9. What is loudness? What determines it?

10. How does a speaker increase his or her vocal loudness?

11. Describe and distinguish harsh, breathy, and hoarse voice.

12. Define resonance and resonator.

13. Distinguish between oral and nasal resonance.

14. Distinguish between hypernasality and hyponasality.

15. What are organic voice disorders? How are they different from functional voice disorders?

16. What is aphonia? What are its suggested causes?

17. What nerve that supplies the larynx may be accidentally cut during thyroidectomy?

18. What is meant by a unilateral paralysis of the vocal folds?

19. Describe ankylosis.

20. Define and distinguish the terms *laryngectomy* and *laryngectomee*.

21. What is a stoma? What is its use?

22. Give a brief description of an artificial larynx.

23. How is esophageal speech produced?

24. What is papilloma? How does it affect speech?

25. What are the causes of laryngeal trauma?

26. What is a laryngeal web?

27. List some of the vocally abusive behaviors.

28. Define and distinguish vocal nodules and polyps. What kinds of effects do they have on voice?

29. What are contact ulcers? What causes them?

30. Distinguish between laryngitis and traumatic laryngitis. Specify their causes.

31. What are some of the causes of faint voice?

32. Give a general description of pitch disorders in the male and the female.

33. What are some of the causes of oral resonance problems?

34. What is cul de sac resonance?

35. Describe how cleft palate can cause hypernasality.

36. Give a brief description of spastic dysphonia. How is this disorder explained?

37. Define dystonia.

38. Give a brief description of the medical evaluation of the voice patient.

39. How does a speech–language pathologist assess voice disorders? List the major procedures.

40. Give a brief description of treatment for vocal abuse.

References

Andrews, M. (1999). *Manual of voice treatment: Pediatrics to geriatrics.* San Diego, CA: Singular.

Aronson, A. E. (1985). *Clinical voice disorders* (2nd ed.). New York: Thieme.

Boone, D. R., & McFarlane, S. C. (2000). *The voice & voice therapy* (6th ed.). Needham Heights, MA: Allyn & Bacon.

Borden, G. J., Harris, K. S., & Raphael, L. J. (1994). *Speech science primer: Physiology, acoustics, and perception of speech* (3rd ed.). Baltimore: Williams & Wilkins.

Case, J. L. (1996). *Clinical management of voice disorders* (3rd ed.). Austin, TX: PRO-ED.

Gargan, W. (1969). *Why me?* New York: Doubleday.

Hegde, M. N. (2001a). *Hegde's pocketguide to assessment in speech–language pathology* (2nd ed.). San Diego, CA: Singular.

Hegde, M. N. (2001b). *Hegde's pocketguide to treatment in speech–language pathology* (2nd ed.). San Diego, CA: Singular.

Johnson, T. S. (1985). *Vocal abuse reduction program.* San Diego, CA: College-Hill Press.

Kent, R. (1997). *The speech sciences.* San Diego, CA: Singular.

White, E. B. (1970). *The trumpet of the swan.* New York: Harper & Row.

Wilson, D. K. (1987). *Voice problems of children* (3rd ed.). Baltimore: Williams & Wilkins.

Speech Disorders and Cleft Palate

- What Is Cleft Palate?
- The Oral Structures: Anatomy and Embryology
- What Causes the Clefts?
- Types of Cleft
- Diseases of the Facial Structures
- Problems Associated with Cleft Palate
- Communicative Disorders Associated with Clefts
- The Cleft Palate Team
- Medical Rehabilitation
- Assessment of Communicative Disorders
- Treatment of Communicative Disorders
- Dialogue
- Study Questions
- References

Typical speech and language problems described in previous chapters need not have their origin in, or be associated with, gross structural problems of the face and mouth. Although many individuals with voice disorders have structural (laryngeal) pathologies, most children who fail to acquire the speech sounds and language structures have normal speech mechanisms. However, many children are born with certain facial and oral structural problems. Such problems create disorders of communication. These structural problems and the resulting disorders of communication are the subjects of this chapter.

Many birth defects produce gross physical deformities that shock the mother the first time she holds her baby. A physician friend of mine, who had delivered a few of those babies in his long career, told the following story of a couple who had a child with cleft lip and palate.

One of my most difficult tasks is to tell a mother that her newborn baby has some kind of birth defect. I have found that it is important to prepare the mother before the nurse shows her the baby with a cleft. Unfortunately, I have also found that no amount of effort to prepare the mother can eliminate the shock she experiences the instant she looks at her deformed baby.

This couple, I shall call Don and Donna, both in their mid-30s, had been wanting a baby for a long time. When Donna got pregnant, they were so pleased with the prospect of having a child that they did not wish to have any of the tests to determine the gender or health of the unborn baby. "We will be

(continues)

happy with any child. We don't care if it is a boy or a girl," they told me. Throughout her pregnancy, Donna was healthy, and of course, very happy. She was having her first baby at age 36, but nothing seemed out of the ordinary.

Donna came to the hospital to deliver a full-term baby. However, complications arose. The labor was prolonged. The baby was not positioned right. I could not reposition the baby, who by now was quite distressed. I decided to deliver the baby by Cesarean section.

When I picked up that little boy and began to clean his mouth, I noticed the bilateral cleft. Attached to the nose, the premaxillary bone and part of the upper lip were sticking out. My cursory examination confirmed my fears: the child had a complete cleft of the hard and the soft palates.

Donna, of course, was sleeping under the influence of anesthesia while I finished my job. The baby was cleaned up and bundled as usual. I told the nurse in charge to get me as soon as Donna woke up and asked to see the baby.

My first task was to break the news to Don. I told him that he had a son, congratulated him, and assured him that Donna was doing fine. Then I asked him if I could see him for a few minutes in my office. As we walked back to my office, he asked, "Is everything OK?" I just told him that there was something to be discussed.

"Don, your son is going to be fine, but you may think otherwise when you see him because he is born with cleft palate."

"That is a birth defect isn't it?" he said and then exclaimed "Oh no!" He went pale and I could see the pain on his face. Soon he asked, "How are we going to tell Donna about this?" I told him that I would talk to Donna before she saw the baby.

Later I showed the baby to Don. Most parents do not take their eyes off of their baby. But Don took one look at the baby and immediately turned his face. I squeezed his hands gently and told him again that surgery could correct the problem. He looked at the baby's face a second time, looked at it longer, but soon he turned away and shut his eyes.

Donna, though only half-awake from her anesthesia, could not wait to see her baby. So I went in. When I asked, "How are you doing?" she said, "Fine, but where is my baby?" "You have a son, and he is in the other room. You can see him shortly, but I must tell you something." She sensed that there was something wrong with the baby. She suddenly became more alert and asked me, "He is OK, isn't he?" I said, "He will be just fine, but he does have a problem. You see, when some babies are born, some parts of the body may not have grown to the extent they normally do. Your son's bones behind the upper lip and in the roof of the mouth did not grow enough. There is an opening in the bones. We call it cleft lip and palate."

"Cleft palate. I know what that is. Oh my God, why, why my son!" she said and began to cry.

I tried to reassure her that surgery could help a great deal and that he would be able to lead a normal life. But I was not sure that she was listening. Fighting her tears back, she just kept staring at me. Eventually, the nurse brought the baby; the father followed the nurse.

Donna looked at her husband whose face told its own story. He went straight to her and gave her a kiss. He stood near the bed and put his arms

(continues)

around her shoulders. The nurse handed the baby to Donna; she looked at the baby's face and tears began to flow. She was staring at the baby's face. She was shaking, biting her lips very hard and not saying anything. After a few minutes, she handed the baby to the nurse. As we looked on helplessly, Donna turned her head to the other side and began to cry softly.

Clefts of the lip, hard palate, and soft palate are a part of a larger syndrome that includes abnormalities of the face, mouth, and head. These abnormalities are called *craniofacial anomalies*. Such anomalies may result in disordered communication. Most of the abnormalities are congenital (noted at the time an affected child is born). They are classified under birth defects. This chapter is about a more common birth defect and the speech problems it causes: cleft of the lip and palate.

What Is Cleft Palate?

A **cleft** is an opening that passes through one or more structures that are normally closed. **Cleft palate** refers to the soft palate and to the bony roof of the mouth with an opening running through them. The upper lip also may have a cleft. There are many kinds of clefts of the lips, the hard palate, and the soft palate.

The clefts appear when the structures of the mouth do not grow enough to move in the right directions and fuse with each other. The growth is typically disrupted during the embryonic stage. Clefts of the soft and hard palate affect speech because the roof of the mouth opens into the nasal cavity. Consequently, the person with a cleft cannot build air pressure in the mouth. Through the cleft, the air escapes into the nose. The sound produced by the larynx also finds its way into the nose. The person sounds like he or she is talking through the nose, and the person literally *is* talking through the nose. To understand this problem, we look at the anatomy and embryology of three structures: the hard palate, the soft palate and pharyngeal wall, and the nasal cavities (nose).

The Oral Structures: Anatomy and Embryology

The oral structures were described in Chapter 3; a review of that chapter follows. More detailed information can be found in books on anatomy and physiology of speech and hearing (Seikel, King, & Drumright, 2000; Zemlin, 1998) or in specialized books on cleft palate (Bzoch, 1997a; Peterson-Falzone, Hardin-Jones, & Kernell, 2001; Shprintzen & Bardach, 1995).

The Hard Palate

The hard palate is covered by a mucous membrane and serves as the bony roof of the mouth and the floor of the nasal cavities. The hard palate is a solid division between the mouth and the nose. Figure 8.1 illustrates the hard palate.

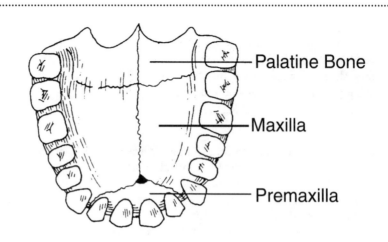

Figure 8.1. The hard palate.

Several bones of the face form the mouth and the nose. The mandible, for example, is the jaw bone that houses the lower set of teeth. A pair of large facial bones called the **maxillae** (the plural form of **maxilla**) forms the major portion of the hard palate. The maxillary bones form the upper jaw as well. The outer edges of the maxillary bones are called the **alveolar process,** which house the molar, bicuspid, and cuspid (canine) teeth. In their embryonic stages, the upper lip and the alveolar process are called the **primary palate.** The central, platelike portions of the maxillary bones are called the **palatine process,** which is embryonically identified as the **secondary palate.** Remember that the secondary palate is the major portion of the roof of the mouth, the hard palate. The upper lip is attached to the maxillary bones.

A small piece of bone, located right under the nose, is called the **premaxilla.** It is a single, triangle-shaped piece of bone holding the front four teeth (the incisors). As shown in Figure 8.1, the premaxilla is attached to the two maxillae. When dissected, the sutures of the premaxilla are seen only in very young children and lower animals. In adults, the premaxilla looks completely fused with the maxillae and no suture lines are seen (Zemlin, 1998). Nonetheless, the maxillae and the premaxilla are embryonically different bones.

Along with the premaxilla in the front and the maxillae in the middle, the **palatine bones** at the back complete the hard palate. The palatine bones meet each other at the midline. The front end of the palatine bones meet the back end of the maxillary bones. The back end of the palatine bones is free. This is the beginning of the soft palate.

The Soft Palate and the Pharyngeal Wall

The soft palate is soft because it is formed by a group of muscles covered with mucosal tissue. It also is known as the velum because it looks like a veil hanging down in the back of the oral cavity at the juncture of the **oropharynx** and **nasopharynx.** A small, cone-shaped uvula is the tip of the velum, which one can see in a mirror. The pharynx and its different sections are illustrated in Figure 8.2.

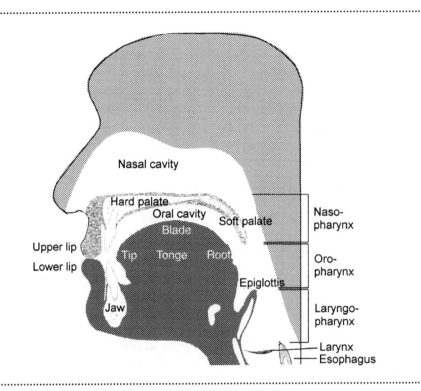

Figure 8.2. The pharynx.

The **pharynx** is an irregular, tubelike structure (cavity). The oral cavity houses the structures of the mouth, and the nasopharynx lies just behind the nasal cavities. The **laryngopharynx** is located above the larynx and below the oropharynx. The oropharynx and the nasopharynx are connected at the back of the mouth where the soft palate is located. The space between the soft palate and the posterior pharyngeal wall (back of the throat) is called the **velopharyngeal port,** an important structure to remember in understanding the speech problems associated with cleft palate.

The soft palate has specialized muscles that stretch it, raise it, and lower it. A pair of muscles called **tensor palatini** stretches it. Another pair called **levator palatini** elevates it. Two muscles, **palatopharyngeus** and **palatoglossus,** lower it.

The **pharyngeal wall,** the muscular ring we know as the throat, consists of several muscles that constrict or relax. The movement of these muscles is important for speech. To close off the nasal passage in producing oral speech sounds, the pharyngeal wall moves forward, and the soft palate muscles move back in a slightly upward direction to make contact with the pharyngeal wall. Such a typical closure of the velopharyngeal port is illustrated in Figure 8.3. In essence, the soft palate and the muscles of the throat help disconnect the nasal cavity from the laryngeal and oral cavities.

The Nasal Cavities

The pair of nasal cavities is divided by septum, which is more flexible (cartilage) at its free, lower end and harder (bone) toward the upper end. Two small

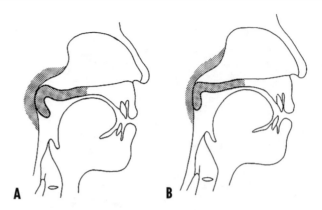

Figure 8.3. Typical velopharyngeal closure in adult males (A) and adult females (B). *Note.* From *Communicative Disorders Related to Cleft Lip and Palate* (p. 17), by K. R. Bzoch (Ed.), 1997, Austin, TX: PRO-ED. Copyright 1997 by PRO-ED, Inc. Reprinted with permission.

nasal bones form the bridge of the nose. For now, it is sufficient to note that the floor of the nasal cavities is the hard palate, especially the maxillary bones.

When the hard palate has an opening in it, then the mouth is directly connected with the nose. Sound traveling from the larynx cannot be shut off from the nasal cavities. When problems such as a cleft of the soft palate and lack of sufficient muscular bulk prevent an adequate closure of the velopharyngeal port, the same effect will result.

The nasal cavity, when coupled with the other cavities, adds nasal resonance to the voice. When it is shut off, you hear mostly oral resonance. Most English speech sounds need only oral resonance. The nasal cavity must be connected to the other cavities only in the production of the three nasal English sounds, /m/, /n/, and /ŋ/ (ng).

Embryonic Growth of the Facial Structures

Clefts of the lip and the palates result because of disrupted **embryonic** and **fetal growth** of the facial structures. Most of the disruptions tend to take place during the embryonic period, which is roughly the first 7 to 10 weeks of gestation. The end of the embryonic period is the beginning of the fetal period.

An embryo grows from within and forms different body parts. By the end of the embryonic period, most of the organs can be identified. These organs grow larger and are more refined during the fetal period, but very few new organs emerge. The most sensitive period of embryonic growth is from the 4th to the 6th week of pregnancy. During this time, the embryo is especially vulnerable to factors that damage its growth or genesis of new organs.

During the first few weeks, embryonic cells multiply, eventually giving rise to three layers of cells from which different organs emerge. By the end of the third week, the top portion of the embryo develops a marked bend, creating a bulge that becomes the primitive forebrain. The bend also creates a groove known as **stomodeum,** which is the primitive mouth and nose.

By the third week, various bulges, also called **prominences** or **processes,** appear in the embryo and give rise to facial structures. Three processes—the frontonasal process, nasomedial process, and nasolateral process—develop into the top, middle, and side portions of the nose; the central part of the upper lip; and the primary palate. Two **maxillary processes** form most of the face, mouth, cheeks, and sides of the upper lip. These processes also evolve into most of the hard palate, the alveolar ridge, and the soft palate. By the end of the 7th week, the upper lip and the primary palate are formed. The embryo is only about 2.5 cm (1 in.) long at this time.

Clefts of the upper lip are possible because the lip does not develop as a single structure. The nose and the midline of the upper lip are formed out of one structure and the two sides of the lip, the cheeks, and the mouth are formed out of another structure. Therefore, the cleft of the lip typically appears at either the right or the left side of the nose.

Two **mandibular processes** result in the lower jaw (mandible), lower lip, and chin. By the end of the 4th or 5th week, these structures are formed and fused. Figure 8.4 shows the frontonasal, nasomedial, nasolateral, maxillary, and mandibular processes in a 6-week-old human embryo.

The growth of the hard and soft palates need more time. The two shelves of the maxillary bone that form the hard palate can be identified at the 5th week of gestation. However, for quite some time, the shelves remain in a vertical position on either side of the embryonic tongue, which lies much higher, actually in the future nose. As the jaw is formed and moved to a lower position, the tongue drops down to its eventual home, the mouth. Then, the palatal shelves begin to move upward to form the roof of the mouth. As they move, the shelves begin to assume a more lateral or horizontal position. They also move toward each other. The major stages of the embryonic fusion of the shelves are illustrated in Figure 8.5.

The shelves of the hard palate fuse at the midline sometime between the 8th and the 9th week. The maxillary shelves also meet the triangular premaxillary bone (the primary palate), which is formed earlier and has been moving backward from the front of the mouth. The three-way fusion between the two maxillary shelves and the premaxillary shelf separates the mouth from the nose. The midline fusion does not take place all at once. Instead, the process of fusion moves from the front to the back portion of the mouth. This is important to remember because the clefts of the palate reflect this embryonic process of front-to-back fusion of the palatal shelves.

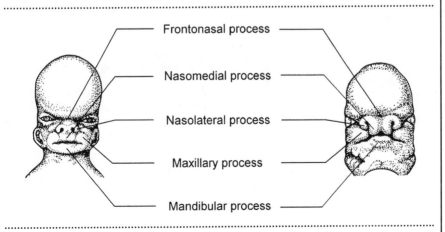

Frontonasal process

Nasomedial process

Nasolateral process

Maxillary process

Mandibular process

Figure 8.4. The embryonic growth of the nose, the maxilla, and the mandible.

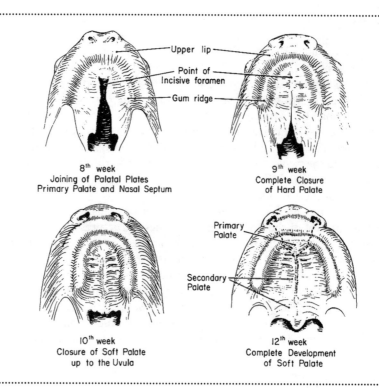

Figure 8.5. A graphic representation of the major stages of palatal fusion during the embryonic period. *Note.* From *Communicative Disorders Related to Cleft Lip and Palate* (p. 27), by K. R. Bzoch (Ed.), 1997, Austin, TX: PRO-ED. Copyright 1997 by PRO-ED, Inc. Reprinted with permission.

The muscular tissue of the soft palate also initially grows as two separated halves. The movement of the palatal bones toward the midline also brings the two halves of the soft palate together. By the 12th week, the muscle mass from the two sides fuse to form the soft palate.

Summary

- A cleft is an opening in certain bony structures that are normally fused.

- A major structure that may fail to fuse during the embryonic stage is the hard palate, which is the roof of the mouth and is formed by a pair of large facial bones called the maxillae.

- The premaxilla, a smaller bone located right under the nose, is in front of the maxillae.

- At the back end, the maxillae are attached to the palatine bones.

- The free, back end of the palatine is the beginning of the soft palate, which is formed by a group of muscles. The soft palate may be lowered or raised.

(continues)

- Along with the movements of the pharyngeal wall, the movement of the soft palate helps to disconnect or connect the pharyngeal cavity with the nasal cavity.

What Causes the Clefts?

Disruptions in the embryonic development cause clefts. The parts that normally fuse together fail to do so. Animal and human research has suggested many possible causes for this failure, but the specific cause in a given case may be unclear. Experts assume that both genetic and environmental factors are potential causes of clefts of the palate and lip.

Genetic Factors

Several observations suggest the importance of genetic factors in the etiology of clefts. First, clefts are associated with many syndromes with known genetic abnormalities. Second, the incidence of clefts varies with ethnic and racial variations.

As genetic research of human abnormalities has advanced, clefting has been found to be associated with more than 400 multiple anomaly syndromes that have a genetic basis. A **multiple anomaly syndrome** is one in which a variety of physical and mental abnormalities are congregated with a single known or suspected cause, often a genetic defect (Shprintzen & Goldberg, 1995). Genetic abnormalities that affect the growth of the face, neck, and head are often associated with clefts. Whereas genetic defects are typically inherited, chromosomal defects need not be; nonetheless, chromosomal defects, too, can cause birth defects along with clefts. Common chromosome disorders consist of an absent (deleted) chromosome or a piece of chromosome, a duplicated chromosome, or an extra chromosome.

Possible influence of genetic factors in causing clefts also is suggested by the differential incidence of clefts and related anomalies in different racial and ethnic groups (Vanderas, 1987). Among the whites in the United States, the incidence reports vary between 1 in 465 births to 1 in 1,235 births, although an incidence of 1 in 750 births is often cited (McWilliams, Morris, & Shelton, 1990). In the United States, the incidence of clefts is the highest in the Chinese (about 4 in 1,000) and it is the second highest in the American Indians (about 3 in 1,000). The incidence is about 2.4 in 1,000 among the Japanese. The incidence of clefts is the lowest in the African Americans (less than 2 in 1,000). The reported highest rate in the United States was for the American Indians in South Dakota at 1 in 220 births, whereas the lowest rate was for the African Americans of upper socioeconomic status in Washington, D.C., at 1 in 8,695 births. The incidence in people of African origin living in Jamaica is among the lowest ever reported: 1 in 8,887 births. The incidence is relatively high among the population of the Hawaiian islands. Various Asian populations, consistent with what is reported for the Chinese, have somewhat higher incidence than that of the white populations.

Read more about ethnocultural variables as they related to communicative disorders in **Chapter 11.**

Clefts only of the upper lip occur less frequently than clefts of the prepalate and the palate (the lip and the palates). However, cleft on the left side of the upper lip is more common than cleft on the right side. Gender also is an important factor. Clefts are found more frequently in males than in females. However, cleft of the palate occurs more frequently in females than in males. Clefts of the lip and the palates are more common in males than in females.

A **familial tendency** for clefting also has been reported. This means that if one member of a family has a cleft, there is a higher than normal probability that others among the blood relatives have clefts. A few scientists have found that among identical (monozygotic) twins, the **concordance rate** for clefts is higher than for ordinary siblings. This means that if one of the monozygotic twin pair has a cleft, the chances are that the other will also have the same defect (concordance). These and other factors suggest that defective genes may cause clefts.

Environmental Factors

Although important in specific cases, genetic causes cannot be established in as many as 75% of people with clefts. Even in monozygotic twins, one of the pair may have a cleft, but the other may be normal. The genetic hypothesis cannot explain this. Therefore, scientists have looked for possible environmental causes as well.

Among environmental factors, both legal and illegal **drugs** seem to be important causes of clefts in infants, although data are scant and it is difficult to draw firm conclusions (Peterson-Falzone, Hardin-Jones, & Kernell, 2001). Alcohol abuse during pregnancy is a known cause of clefts in children (Shprintzen & Goldberg, 1995). Some prescription drugs a pregnant woman might take are known to cause a variety of birth defects, including clefts in children. The drug cortisone has been singled out by many researchers. Maternal cortisone treatment has produced clefts in mice. A few reports have linked clefts in children to the mother's treatment with cortisone, diazepam (or valium, prescribed to treat anxiety), and phenytoins (or dilantin, prescribed to treat epilepsy). Among the illegal drugs, maternal cocaine use has been singled out as the most potent cause of clefts and other congenital abnormalities in children (Shprintzen & Goldberg, 1995).

Radiation also is a demonstrated cause of clefts in animals, but whether it can cause clefts in the human embryo is not clear. Radiation during the early days of pregnancy has been a suspected cause of many forms of birth defects, including clefts.

Maternal **infections** also are suspected environmental causes of clefts. Virus and bacteria in the mother's blood can pass into the fetal blood through the placenta. Strong diseases may abort the pregnancy, but others may cause embryonic and fetal damage or growth deficiencies. Based on limited evidence, mumps, influenza, and other diseases have been suggested as causes of clefts.

Not a single factor has been clearly demonstrated to be the cause of clefts in humans. Most scientists think that clefts have many causes, some genetic and some environmental. A genetic predisposition and certain environmental causes may come together to produce the final effect. This viewpoint, acceptable to many scientists, is known as the **multifactor theory** or **interactionist theory**.

Types of Cleft

Oral and facial clefts vary in location and extent. It can happen that only the lip is affected, or both the lip and the hard palate are affected. Of course, the lip, the alveolar ridge, the hard palate, and the soft palate all can be affected. The opening may be negligible, narrow, or wide. Just a notch on the lip may indicate what could have been a serious cleft. A cleft of the lip may be found on the right or the left side of the nose, or on both sides. A cleft on one side is **unilateral,** and one on both sides is **bilateral.**

Cleft of the hard palate may be found at the midpoint or to the right or the left of the midpoint. In **complete cleft** of the hard palate, the two palatal shelves are totally separated. In **incomplete cleft,** the shelves are partially fused. These different possibilities mix to produce many variations and combinations, making it possible to classify the clefts in different ways. Figure 8.6 shows various clefts of the lip and hard palate.

A classification that was popular for many years was proposed by Veau (1931). He described four types of clefts as follows:

Type I: Cleft of the soft palate only.
Type II: Cleft of the soft and hard palate up to the premaxilla; normal lip and premaxilla.
Type III: Complete unilateral cleft of the soft palate, the hard palate, the lip, and the alveolar ridge; only one side is affected.
Type IV: Complete bilateral cleft of the soft palate, the hard palate, the lip, and the alveolar ridge; both sides are affected.

Clefts are hard to classify because of their wide variations.

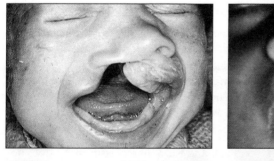 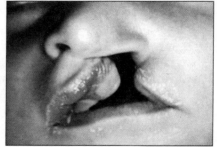
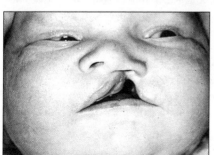 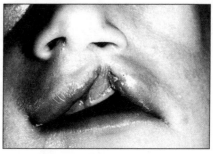

Figure 8.6A. Various clefts of the lip. *Note.* From *Communicative Disorders Related to Cleft Lip and Palate* (p. 22), by K. R. Bzoch (Ed.), 1997, Austin, TX: PRO-ED. Copyright 1997 by PRO-ED, Inc. Reprinted with permission.

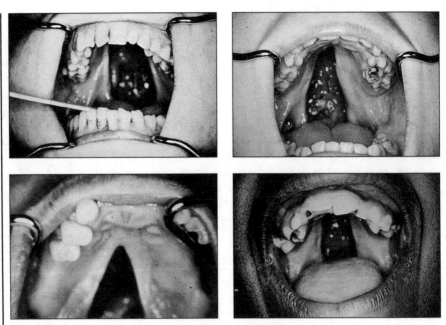

Figure 8.6B. Various clefts of the hard palate. *Note.* From *Communicative Disorders Related to Cleft Lip and Palate* (p. 33), by K. R. Bzoch (Ed.), 1997, Austin, TX: PRO-ED. Copyright 1997 by PRO-ED, Inc. Reprinted with permission.

One problem with this classification is that clefts of the lip or alveolar ridge alone are not included.

In 1959, Stark and Kernahan proposed a new system of classification that many clinicians have used. The system is illustrated in Figure 8.7 and described as follows.

> **Clefts of the Primary Palate.** The hard and soft palates are normal. The lip may be near normal with just a notch, or it may be affected to a significant extent. It may be unilateral or bilateral.
>
> **Clefts of the Secondary Palate.** Normal maxilla and lip. The two palatal shelves have not fused. The cleft may be unilateral, bilateral, or median.
>
> **Clefts of the Primary and Secondary Palate.** The lip, maxilla, hard palate, and soft palate are all affected. These clefts may be unilateral or bilateral.

As with the Veau classification, the Stark and Kernahan classification does not include clefts of the lip or alveolar ridge alone.

Regardless of the limitations of the particular system of classification used, the clinician must describe in detail the cleft of each client and the site and the extent of the deformity. Even within the types, the severity of the deformity varies so much that no system of classification can substitute for a thorough description of symptoms individual patients present. Such a description is even more important when clefts are a part of other craniofacial deformities and specific genetic syndromes.

Rare Orofacial Clefts

There are several syndromes of birth defects with rare orofacial clefts. For example, the midline of the lower jaw may have a cleft. Other rare clefts include

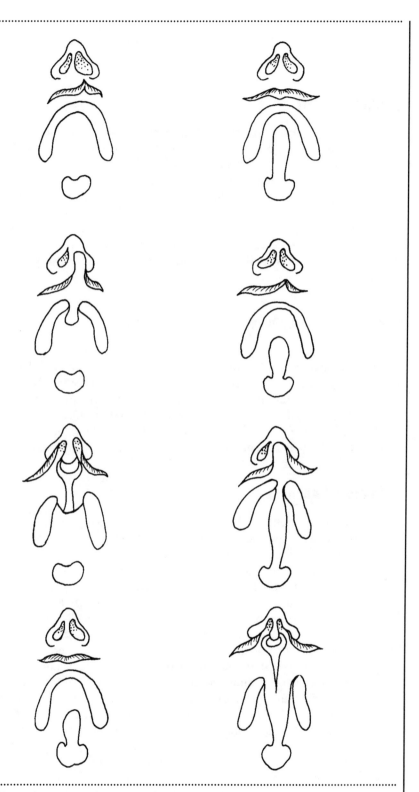

Figure 8.7. Stark and Kernahan's classification of clefts.

lateral or horizontal cleft, which moves from one corner of the mouth to the ear; naso-ocular cleft, which moves from the nose to the eye; and midline cleft of the upper lip or the alveolar ridge.

Submucous Cleft

A type of cleft that may not affect speech in most cases is known as the submucous cleft. The palate appears normal. The tissue covering the palate, however, may hide a cleft of the hard palate, the soft palate, or both. Sometimes, a split uvula, called a **bifid uvula,** may suggest that a cleft is underneath.

The speech can be normal in many cases of submucous cleft of the hard palate. However, in some, the soft palate may not have enough tissue mass, or it may have a cleft that is covered by oral mucosal membrane. The result is that it cannot close the velopharyngeal port adequately. The speech in such patients may be hypernasal. Unless the speech problems are noticeable, submucosal cleft may go undetected.

Congenital Palatopharyngeal Incompetence

Some people are born with a velopharyngeal mechanism that is not adequate to achieve velopharyngeal closure. There is no cleft of any kind, and the muscular mass seems adequate. Nevertheless, the speech of these people is hypernasal.

On closer examination, clinicians have found such problems as a nasopharynx that is too deep or a hard palate that is too short. Occasionally, muscles that are adequate in bulk still do not function to close the velopharyngeal port. This is because the nerves are not properly inserted to the muscles.

Craniofacial Anomalies

In addition to the clefts of the lip and the palates, there are many congenital defects of the skull and face known as **craniofacial anomalies.** Some of these anomalies are associated with clefts, while others are not. Craniofacial anomalies also may be associated with mental retardation, physical deformities, growth deficiencies, sensory defects, and behavior disorders. Disorders of communication often are found in children with craniofacial anomalies. A few examples will illustrate their varied and complex nature.

One of the craniofacial anomalies is known as the **Apert syndrome.** This syndrome is thought to be due to a premature fusing of different bones of the skull in the embryonic stage. A child with this syndrome usually has a longer but flattened face with its midportion underdeveloped. The forehead is usually bulbous. The nose may be saddlelike or beaklike. The eyes may be too far apart, a condition called **hypertelorism.** The hands of the child with Apert syndrome may show fusing of fingers. Consequently, the hands look like mittens.

The palate of children with Apert syndrome is typically high and narrow; in fact, the hard palate is so narrow that it gives the impression of a cleft. Whereas cleft of the hard palate is uncommon, cleft of the soft palate is seen in 30% of the children with Apert syndrome.

Whereas some congenital syndromes of children have a genetic basis, others are due to toxic substances consumed by the pregnant mother. **Fetal alcohol syndrome,** described in Chapter 5, is a primary example. Maternal consumption of alcohol can be detrimental to the fetal growth. Cleft of the lip with or without cleft palate often is noticed in children with fetal alcohol syndrome. The skull may be too small (**microcephaly**). Other physical characteristics include abnormally small jaw (**micrognathia**), underdeveloped midface, short nose, and thin upper lip. Most children with fetal alcohol syndrome show some degree of mental retardation, hyperactivity, and problems of eye–hand coordination and fine motor control. Speech and language disorders often are noticed in such children.

Diseases of the Facial Structures

In addition to congenital syndromes affecting the face, mouth, and skull, various diseases of these structures also affect communication. Such diseases need drastic surgical treatment that alters the structure used for speech.

The upper and the lower jaws, the lips, and the tongue are frequently reported sites of cancer. In many cases, the affected part is removed partially or totally. Thus, a patient may have **maxillectomy** (surgical removal of the upper jaw) or **mandibulectomy** (removal of the lower jaw). In **glossectomy,** the tongue and floor of the mouth also may be removed. In most cases, prosthetic parts are fashioned to replace the natural structure. Prosthetic mandibles and maxillae have been successful to varying degrees in restoring both appearance and function (Peterson-Falzone, 1988a, 1988b). Prosthetic tongues, made out of such materials as silicone rubber with a mobile tip, have also been developed for those who have undergone glossectomy.

Patients who undergo such surgical treatment experience varying degrees of difficulty in producing speech sounds. Even without prosthetic devices, some are able to produce sounds in unusual ways. For example, a patient without an upper lip may produce such bilabial sounds as /p/ and /m/ by labiodental contacts (the upper teeth press gently on the lower lip). Even a small flap of tongue tissue saved by the surgeon may aid in the articulation of speech sounds when unusual methods of producing sounds, called **compensatory movements,** are learned. New methods of producing speech compensate for the structural defect.

Ventriloquists show how speech can be produced in unusual ways.

Problems Associated with Cleft Palate

In addition to problems of communication, which will be described in a later section, clefts in a child tend to create a variety of other problems for both the parents and the child. Because clefts are genetic or congenital, problems begin soon after the birth of the baby. The immediate effects are on the parents, especially the mother. Other problems related to child rearing and child growth follow.

The Child and the Parents

Up to 70% of children born with clefts are not different from those who are born with a normal palate. These children are normal except for the cleft. The remaining 30% of children with cleft may have additional physical or mental problems. Even among them, there are wide individual differences. Whereas one child with a cleft may have just one additional physical abnormality or developmental disability, another child may have a combination of physical deformities including webbed toes, deformed ears, various kinds of facial abnormalities, asymmetry of the skull and other cranial anomalies, unusually small mouth (microstomia), clubfoot, spina bifida, hearing loss, and dental abnormalities. These physical abnormalities may be combined with a variety of developmental disabilities including Down syndrome.

The social and emotional behaviors of children with cleft also vary, as they do in children without cleft. One child might behave normally in most social situations and show appropriate emotional responses. A different child could exhibit temper tantrums, emotionally unstable behaviors, and withdrawal from social situations. Generally, a child with cleft palate but no other physical or mental disabilities tends to exhibit acceptable social and emotional behaviors. There has been no evidence of unusual behaviors or personality traits that are typical of cleft palate children (Peterson-Falzone, Hardin-Jones, & Kernell, 2001). Social and emotional behaviors are more likely to be affected negatively when the child, in addition to cleft palate, exhibits gross facial abnormalities, mental retardation, and other problems.

The academic performance of the child with a cleft is generally comparable to that of other children, unless the child has problems that impede learning. By the time they enter school, most children nowadays will have had some surgical repair of the cleft, though additional functional or cosmetic surgery might be planned for the future. Therefore, the child can be expected to perform adequately and get along with others normally. However, a child with significant facial abnormalities could be underestimated by the classroom teachers. Such negative evaluations could adversely affect the child's academic performance (Peterson-Falzone et al., 2001). Furthermore, the child who continues to exhibit speech and language problems may experience additional difficulties.

As the poignant story of Don and Donna told at the beginning of this chapter indicates, the parents' first reaction to their child with cleft palate is one of shock and disbelief. The magnitude of this response depends upon the extent of the child's structural abnormality. Severe facial deformities and other physical handicaps will overwhelm the parents. Additional physical and mental abnormalities compound the parental response (Peterson-Falzone et al., 2001).

Parental responses depend on how the news is broken to the parents. Most parents would like to be promptly informed of their newborn baby's problems. However, up to 30% of parents of cleft palate babies may not be immediately informed of their baby's problem (Peterson-Falzone et al., 2001). A physician who abruptly and casually announces a newborn's birth defect will shock the mother who is fully conscious during the delivery. One mother reported that as he delivered the baby, the physician said, in a matter-of-fact manner, "Oh, it has a cleft lip . . . and palate, too. Don't worry, it can be repaired" (Gibbs, 1973, p. 16). One researcher found that "Parents, particularly the mothers, are more of an emergency than the affected child and emphasis should be placed on treating the parents—the patient at the moment is the mother" (Slutsky, 1969, p. 426).

Parents generally need more information than they are typically given. At the earliest possible time, the speech–language pathologist should counsel the parents and give them information on rehabilitation. Other parents of children with cleft palate must be involved in a discussion of the child's rehabilitation as soon as possible. In the absence of such information, the parents can be confused, anxious, and even angry. Those professionals who have worked with many parents also have emphasized that soon the reactions of shock and disbelief subside. With early counseling and discussion with other parents of children with cleft, the parents begin to think of facing and handling the problems.

Although there are common patterns of parental reaction, parents differ widely in their immediate and long-term responses to disabilities in their children. Some parents treat their child with disabilities like they treat any other child. Others may react to their child unfavorably. Some parents harbor guilt about having a child who is not normal. Others may take a more objective outlook and offer the special assistance the child needs but not treat the child as someone different. In some extreme cases, parents may reject a child with significant physical and facial abnormalities.

The child with severe cleft needs multiple surgery, prolonged dental and orthodontic treatment, speech–language services, and perhaps otological and audiological consultations as well. Managing and coordinating all these services can put both financial and emotional strain on the child's parents and siblings.

Feeding Problems

An inadequate velopharyngeal mechanism and the opening in the hard palate make it difficult for the child to build up negative air pressure to suck and swallow (and positive air pressure to produce speech). In addition, a severely deformed upper lip with a rotated premaxilla, which may be attached to the nose, can make it extremely difficult to suck. Mothers find it equally difficult to breastfeed such babies.

The cleft in the palate creates other problems as well. Food and fluids tend to find their way into the nasal cavity. The feeding is slow, interrupted, and often frustrating to both the infant and the mother. Because of this, the child may not receive enough food at each feeding and may fail to gain weight at the normal rate. The hungry child tends to cry more often and is generally restless.

When properly instructed, most mothers are able to handle the feeding problems by careful and patient feeding. Feeding the infant while holding him or her in a sitting position is recommended. Bottles that have cross-cut nipples have been helpful in trouble-free feeding. A few specialists recommend special bottles with a plastic prosthetic plate fitted to the nipple. Adequately trained mothers can feed their babies without special appliances.

Middle Ear Disease and Hearing Impairment

Children with palatal clefts tend to suffer from a middle ear disease known as **otitis media,** caused by an infection of the mucous membranes of the middle ear. It is a disease of early childhood; most cases of otitis media are reported before the age of 6. Although only about 5% of all children are susceptible to otitis media, most children with palatal clefts suffer from it.

Problems of hearing are described in **Chapter 10.**

The increased incidence of otitis media in children with cleft palate is not clearly understood. However, as in all cases of otitis media, a malfunctioning eustachian tube is commonly observed in children with cleft palates (Peterson-Falzone, 1988a; Peterson-Falzone et al., 2001). The eustachian tube connects the middle ear with the nasopharynx. The middle ear end of the tube is open, but its other end at the nasopharynx remains closed. This end may be opened by swallowing or yawning. The tube equalizes air pressure within and outside the middle ear, drains fluids that might collect in the middle ear, and ventilates the middle ear. A malfunctioning eustachian tube prevents ventilation and drainage and promotes middle ear diseases. The middle ear chamber may be filled with pus. The tympanic membrane (eardrum) may be sucked in. The result is a type of hearing loss known as **conductive hearing loss.** The degree of loss is typically mild or moderate, and the loss tends to fluctuate.

Approximately 50% of children with cleft palate may suffer from some degree of hearing loss. Children with cleft of the hard and soft palates are more susceptible to experience hearing loss than are those with cleft of the prepalate (premaxilla) and the lip.

The child who does not hear speech sounds well might be delayed in learning to say them. The child might misarticulate some of the speech sounds. Language acquisition also may be delayed.

Dental Problems

Children with clefts of the alveolar ridge are more likely to have dental problems than those with cleft of the hard and soft palates only, who in turn have more problems than children with normal palates. Unrepaired cleft of the prepalate, of course, is likely to produce the most severe dental problems. Even surgically repaired clefts may show more than the usual amount of dental deviations.

The most commonly observed dental abnormalities include insufficient growth of the teeth and the gum tissue (**hypoplasia**), cross bite, protruding premaxilla in the case of bilateral cleft, and growth of extra teeth. In **cross bite,** one arch may be larger than the other arch. For example, the upper arch may be small enough to fit inside the larger, lower arch. But in some children, malocclusion is the most important dental problem.

The term **malocclusion** means that the upper and the lower dental arches are not aligned properly. Normally, the two arches and their corresponding individual teeth are aligned. The alignment is rarely perfect, but significant deviations are classified into *types of malocclusions*. When the two arches are aligned but a few individual teeth of the arches are not, the malocclusion is classified as **Class I,** also known as **neutrocclusion.** The children with cleft, however, are more likely to show **Class II** malocclusion (**distocclusion**) in which the upper set of teeth protrude and the lower set of teeth are pushed back. **Class III** malocclusion (**mesiocclusion**) is the opposite of Class II; the lower arch protrudes in front of the upper arch. Some children with cleft palate are likely to show Class III malocclusion.

Summary

- Clefts, being serious birth defects, may be associated with a variety of problems.

- The parents of cleft babies are initially shocked, but sensitive handling by the physician and counseling by other professionals can reduce this emotional response.

(continues)

- Although many children with cleft grow normally, others may experience many problems of health and growth.

- Problems that are frequently associated with clefts include feeding difficulties, middle ear diseases and the attending hearing impairment, and dental problems.

Communicative Disorders Associated with Clefts

Children with cleft palate are likely to show a range of communicative problems. Here again, individual differences are noteworthy. Some children acquire speech and language with very little deviation, whereas others show considerable delay in learning to speak. Those who do learn may exhibit unintelligible speech. Still others show various degrees of delayed language and distorted speech. There are many reasons for this range of variation.

The children who have clefts that are not severe and who do not have other mental, behavioral, physical, and sensory disabilities have better speech and language skills. Also, those who have received early and comprehensive rehabilitative services exhibit superior speech and language skills than those who have not.

There are two major effects of cleft palate. One is faulty speech production, and the other is faulty voice. A peculiar combination of these two effects creates the distinct cleft palate speech. It is readily distinguished from speech and voice problems of children and adults with normal palates. Language disorders are an additional and more variable problem seen in children with clefts.

Communication skills vary in proportion to the severity of the cleft and associated problems.

Language Disorders

Many children with clefts have normal or near-normal language. Nonetheless, the prevalence of language disorders among these children as a group is higher than that found in children with normal palates. As many as 50% of children with cleft may have some delay or disorder of language. It is possible that some children show language problems because of their hearing loss and not cleft palate.

Compared to those with normal palates, children with clefts are likely to be slower in learning language. They tend to have a smaller and less varied vocabulary and speak in shorter and simpler sentences. Children with clefts might not ask many questions, be hesitant in making requests, be slow in answering questions, and not describe objects, events, or their own emotional experiences (Shames & Rubin, 1979). Clefts also seem to discourage spontaneous speech to some extent in most children (Morris, 1962). These and other language deviations seem to be more pronounced during the early years. As the children grow older, their language begins to resemble that of normal children (Shames & Rubin, 1979). Still, the children with cleft tend to make more grammatical errors than children with no clefts.

In many cases, the language deviations of children with clefts are subtle. Therefore, researchers have paid more attention to what distinguishes the

Chapter 5 describes language disorders in detail.

communicative problems of children with cleft palate the most: the speech and voice disorders.

Speech Disorders

Recall from Chapter 4 that speech disorders refer to errors of articulation and the resulting problem of intelligibility. **Intelligibility** is the clarity of speech as judged by listeners. When a listener says, "I don't understand that speech," we have a judgment of unintelligibility.

Cleft palate tends to create speech disorders, which in turn make it difficult for the listeners to understand the speaker. Many speech sounds are not produced well, others simply are omitted, and some are substituted.

Many children have problems of articulation, and not all of them have clefts. Children with cleft and those without misarticulate many of the same sounds. However, the speech of those with clefts produces a unique effect on the listener. Experts can easily distinguish speech disorders that are associated with clefts from those that are not associated with clefts.

The number and the severity of misarticulations of children with clefts vary. Some children misarticulate fewer sounds and the errors are not severe. Others misarticulate many sounds and the misarticulations are so severe that people cannot understand their speech at all. The severity of the clefts, the age at which the clefts were surgically repaired, the adequacy of the repair, the mobility of the reconstructed oral structures, the quality of the speech services offered to the child, and the presence or absence of other physical and mental handicaps seem to create this variability.

In spite of the variability, some common patterns of misarticulation can be found in children with clefts. These children are likely to misarticulate the following sounds:

/s/, as in *s*oup
/z/, as in *z*ebra
/θ/ (voiceless /th/), as in *th*ink
/ð/ (voiced /th/), as in *th*ose
/ʃ/ (/sh/), as in *sh*oe
/ʒ/, as in bei*ge*
/tʃ/ (/ch/), as in *ch*alk
/dʒ/, as in *j*ob
/f/, as in *f*an
/v/, as in *v*an
/k/, as in *k*ite
/g/, as in *g*irl
/l/, as in *l*amp
/r/, as in *r*un

Many structural problems contribute to defective articulation. In the case of cleft of the primary palate, the alveolar ridge, which houses the upper teeth, may be deformed. Consequently, the frontal teeth, especially the incisors, might not be of normal shape, size, or alignment. Severe forms of malocclusions described earlier can be present. As a result, the child can have difficulty producing certain speech sounds that require precise contact between the lower lip and the upper teeth. For example, sounds like /f/ and /v/, called labiodentals, require such contacts. The deformed alveolar ridge also may cause difficulty in making

Chapter 4 describes articulation disorders in detail.

*Review the information in **Chapter 4** on different methods of producing speech sounds.*

other groups of sounds: the alveolar sounds such as the /s/ and the /z/, and the interdental sounds (/θ/, the voiceless *th*, and /ð/, the voiced *th*).

Cleft of the lip alone may not cause serious errors of articulation. Cleft of the alveolar ridge can cause some errors, while cleft of the hard or soft palates creates the most serious errors. This is because clefts in the palates make it difficult, if not impossible, to build up air pressure in the mouth (intraoral air pressure). Production of many speech sounds requires some amount of intraoral air pressure that may be released slowly or in bursts.

The airflow is stopped at different places for the production of different sounds. For example, the airflow is stopped at the back of the mouth for the production of /k/ (as in *kite*) or /g/ (as in *give*), and then the air is suddenly released. However, in producing /p/ (as in *pot*) and /b/ (as in *boat*), the air is impounded in the mouth by firmly closing the lips. The air pressure within the mouth is increased for a brief duration and then released. But what is not so readily seen is that the velopharyngeal mechanism seals off the nasal passage as well.

Because of either a direct and nonmanipulable connection between the oral and nasal cavity, or an inadequate velopharyngeal mechanism, or both, the air coming out of the lungs will escape through the nose in the case of clefts of the hard or soft palate. As a result, non-nasal sounds will have unwanted nasal resonance. For example, the child's /p/ or /b/ may sound more like /m/. One might think that the child is substituting the /m/ for /p/ and /b/. The word *papa* will sound like "mama," and *Bob* will sound like "mom."

The sound /t/ will sound more like /n/ because both the sounds are made with similar tongue positions. Therefore, *time* may turn into "nime," and *tight* may turn into "nine." The /d/ will be similarly affected. The child says *daddy,* but it sounds like "nanny." The child says *Debbie,* but it sounds like "nemmie." Consequently, the speech is not intelligible to the listener.

Generally, a sound that more or less sounds like /n/ or /m/ may be heard in place of /s/, /z/, /v/, /f/, and many other sounds. Therefore, the word *soup* may resemble "noom"; *zero* may resemble "neno"; *vote* may resemble "mone"; and *fan* may resemble "man."

Compensatory Articulation

A child with cleft palate and velopharyngeal insufficiency tries to produce sounds the way he or she hears them. Because of the organic deficiency, the child will have to produce many sounds in unusual ways, however. A child's (or an adult's) attempt to produce speech sounds in unusual ways because of organic deficiencies is called **compensatory articulation.** This is not to say that the attempts are entirely successful; the speech sounds may still be distorted or otherwise faulty. But that is the best the child can do given the speech structures he or she has.

A commonly observed compensatory articulation is to shift the production of most sounds to the back portion of the oral cavity (Peterson-Falzone, 1988b). The child tries to produce the speech sounds before the air escapes through the nose; to accomplish this, the child tries to produce the sounds, even those that are produced in the front part of the mouth, at the back part of the mouth. Often, attempts are made to produce sounds at the level of the larynx or in the pharynx (throat). For example, the /k/ and /g/ may be produced by pushing the back of the tongue against the back wall of the throat. Some children may substitute a glottal stop for /k/ and /g/. The **glottal stop** is produced by a sudden release of air impounded briefly below the tightly closed vocal folds. It has a coughlike character. Some children produce even such tongue-tip sounds as /s/ and /t/ at the back of the mouth.

The speech–language pathologist working with a child with repaired cleft must correct compensatory articulatory problems. Even when the surgery for the cleft and the velopharyngeal insufficiency is mostly successful, the child might continue to use the old compensatory articulation. The treatment in this case consists of retraining the child to produce the sounds more naturally.

Nasal Emission

Another problem related to faulty articulation of the cleft palate child is called **nasal emission,** which is discharge of air through the nose during speech production. When the child produces sentences without nasal sounds, nasal emission of air may be observed by holding a mirror under the nares (nostrils). The mirror will be fogged by the warm air escaping through the nose. Known as **silent nasal emission,** it is the inaudible leakage of air through the nose during the production of non-nasal speech sounds.

In some speakers, the air escaping through the nasal passage may add noise to speech. This is **audible nasal emission,** which is the noise of the gushing air when it escapes through the nose. Audible nasal emission should not be confused with nasality (or hypernasality). While nasality is nasal resonance of sounds generated by the larynx, nasal emission is friction noise created by the stream of air rushing out of the nasal passage.

Some speakers with cleft palate constrict the nares (nostrils) to control the amount of air escaping through the nose. This attempt is unsuccessful and actually adds a distracting noise that sounds more like a hiss or /h/-like sound. Thus, a cleft palate child's production of *pants* will sound more like "hmans," which starts off with a forcefully expelled puff of air at the beginning.

Resonance and Voice Disorders

The hypernasality heard on the non-nasal sounds produced by a child with cleft palate may not be strictly a problem of articulation. A child without cleft who says "wadio" for *radio* is substituting /w/ for /r/. But the child with a cleft who says "nanny" for *daddy* is not substituting /n/ for /d/; the child's attempts at producing /d/ are not successful because of the air leakage from the nose, turning the /d/ into /n/. Therefore, it is believed that this is a problem of resonance, not articulation, although an ordinary listener may hear substitution of a nasal speech sound for non-nasal sounds.

A pervasive nasal resonance (hypernasality) is characteristic of the speech of a person with unrepaired palatal cleft. Because of the velopharyngeal inadequacy, even the vowel sounds, which are otherwise produced correctly, tend to be hypernasal. Thus, in people with cleft, many faulty articulations are closely related to deviant resonance.

A high proportion of children with clefts have voice disorders, especially hoarseness (Peterson-Falzone et al., 2001). **Hoarse voice** sounds harsh and breathy; the vocal folds do not approximate well enough; and there also may be excessive tension in the folds. Some experts think that when a child tries to compensate for the inadequate velopharyngeal mechanism, the vocal folds may experience excessive strain, resulting in vocal pathology and hoarseness.

Some children with cleft palate speak too softly. This may be because the child has difficulty building air pressure needed to speak with a louder voice.

> Nasal resonance is desirable when not misplaced, but nasal emission is typically undesirable.

Other children might adopt the strategy of speaking softly to control the excessive air leakage through the nose. Too soft voice tends to be monotonous, and this also has been observed in some children with cleft palate.

Summary

- A comprehensive rehabilitation program started very early will prevent or reduce communicative handicaps; still, a certain number of children with clefts experience speech–language difficulties.

- Children with cleft palate may be delayed in language acquisition.

- Disorders of articulation that make the children's speech less intelligible are common. Sounds that require a buildup of air pressure in the mouth are especially hard for children with palatal clefts.

- Speech may be hypernasal because of an inadequate velopharyngeal mechanism. Both silent and audible nasal emission may be present. Some children may develop unusual methods of producing speech sounds (compensatory articulation).

The Cleft Palate Team

The family that has a child with cleft typically faces an array of specialists, because no single specialist can attend to the many needs of the child. The parents often are bewildered by the different specialists and their unique jargon. But each specialist is concerned with a particular aspect of the child's problem.

Besides the services of the plastic surgeon, speech–language pathologist, dentist, and orthodontist, the child needs the help of many other specialists. The otologist (medically trained ear specialist) and the audiologist manage the child's ear diseases and hearing problems. The clinical psychologist provides counseling for the family and makes the psychological assessment of the child. Nurses, pediatricians, social workers, and educational specialists also are involved in the overall rehabilitation planning. The group of specialists who design a rehabilitation program for children with clefts is known as the **cleft palate team.**

The cleft palate team is coordinated by one of the specialists. In some settings, the coordinator is a speech–language pathologist who keeps in touch with the other specialists as well as the parents and the child. This helps the parents because they can contact one person to find out about the total rehabilitation plan drawn for the child. Most cleft palate teams work in a hospital where comprehensive services are offered.

Medical Rehabilitation

Beyond the initial counseling of the parents and managing feeding problems, the first step in the rehabilitation of the child with cleft is to surgically repair the cleft. Surgical repair, though sometimes initiated before the baby leaves the hospital, is completed over a period of several years. During these years, other medical and dental problems are attended to.

Surgery

Although it is the plastic surgeon who performs the surgery, the entire team is involved in this important rehabilitative step. This is because surgery tries to achieve medical as well as nonmedical goals, including better communication and appearance. In fact, the development of speech and language skills is one of the primary goals of plastic surgery of the cleft. Therefore, the speech–language pathologist is especially interested in the type of surgery planned for the child. Some types of surgical repair of the cleft promote better speech than other types.

Lip Surgery

The cleft of the lip is surgically repaired at the earliest possible time. In some rare cases the cleft lip may be operated on before the baby leaves the hospital. Because the baby must withstand the shock of surgery and anesthesia, most surgeons wait until the baby weighs about 4.5 kg (10 lbs) and is about 10 weeks of age. In most cases, the cleft of the lip will have been repaired by the time the child is 6 months old.

Unilateral clefts of the lip are somewhat simpler to correct than bilateral clefts. Wide bilateral clefts with the premaxillary bone attached to the nose present the most difficult challenge to the plastic surgeon. In cases of severe cleft, repeated surgeries may be needed. The initial, or the **primary surgery,** is performed to close the cleft. Subsequent **secondary surgeries** are performed to improve function and appearance.

In cases of unilateral cleft of the lip, which extends to the alveolar ridge, surgeons sometimes graft a piece of bone to close the gap so that the upper dental arch is stabilized. A piece of bone may be obtained from a rib, the hip, or the leg. The piece is then used to fill the gap in the alveolar ridge.

Palatal Surgery

A surgeon's preference and the extent and type of the cleft will determine the procedure selected for a child.

Successful palatal surgery offers many advantages to the child. It improves swallowing and reduces infections of the middle ear. The middle part of the face grows more symmetrically. The dental structures improve and look better. The upper respiratory infections decrease. Most important of all, the palatal surgery improves the chances of learning normal speech and language.

When the child is between 12 and 18 months of age, the primary surgery is done to repair the palatal clefts. Of the several palatal surgical methods, some are named after the surgeons who first performed them. Thus, there is the von Langenbeck procedure or the Schweckendiek procedure. Modifications of procedures by other surgeons or combinations of different procedures create numerous variations. Therefore, there are such procedures as the Veau–Wardill–Kilner procedure or the Dieffenbach–Warren–von Langenbeck procedure. Other techniques have descriptive names: primary veloplasty, the pharyngeal flap procedure, and so on. What follows is a description of a few commonly used procedures.

The **Veau–Wardill–Kilner procedure,** also known as the **V-Y retroposition,** is illustrated in Figure 8.8. The distinguishing feature of this procedure is the lengthening of the palate as the cleft is closed. In many cases, surgical repair of the cleft leaves a short palate that does not aid in the velopharyngeal closure. The speech remains hypernasal. Therefore, the palate-lengthening aspect of the Veau–Wardill–Kilner procedure can aid better speech.

The clefts of the palate are closed by flaps of tissue freed from the palate itself. The thick layer of tissue that covers the hard palate is called the **mucoperiosteum.** In most cases, the cleft remains under the newly moved mucoperiosteum. However, the tough tissue can effectively close the cleft for swallowing and speaking.

In the Veau–Wardill–Kilner procedure, the surgeon first makes an incision on either side of the cleft but along the alveolar ridge, as shown in Figure 8.8A. The surgeon then frees the two flaps of mucoperiosteum that cover the bone underneath. The flaps are attached at the back of the palate to keep the blood supply intact; they are completely free from the bone in the front and to the sides (Figure 8.8B). Next, the edges of the cleft are pared (Figure 8.8C). The two elevated flaps of tissue are then moved toward each other and pushed toward the back of the mouth to lengthen the palate. Thus positioned, the two flaps are sutured (Figure 8.8D). The operation leaves portions of the bony palate exposed (denuded), because the covering has been moved to the site of the cleft and back of the mouth (shaded, triangular space in Figure 8.8D). Eventually, new mucoperiosteum grows over the bone.

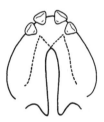

A. Incision on either side of the cleft

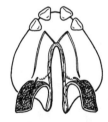

B. Two flaps of tissue freed from the bone

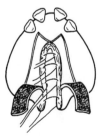

C. Margins of the cleft pared

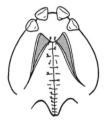

D. Flaps brought together, pushed back, and sutured

Figure 8.8. The Veau–Wardill–Kilner operation.

The V-Y procedure has certain limitations. The lengthening of the palate may not be enough to achieve velopharyngeal closure. The tissue could shrink after the operation, leaving a short palate as usual. There may be growth problems for the midface because of the denuded bone in the front of the mouth.

The **von Langenbeck procedure**, illustrated in Figure 8.9, is one of the oldest of the modern surgical procedures. The surgeon makes an incision along the alveolar ridge on either side of the cleft to release the two flaps from the bone to which the mucoperiosteum is attached. Unlike in the V-Y procedure, the surgeon attaches the two flaps at the front and back; they are freed from the bone only in the middle portion. He or she then brings together the two elevated flaps on either side of the cleft and sutures them. If the cleft is complete, the surgeon may also raise the soft palate tissue from the bone and suture the split velum.

The von Langenbeck procedure is used frequently. Many surgeons have modified this procedure to overcome its shortcomings. One shortcoming is that the palate might be too short and tight. It might not move enough to aid in the velopharyngeal closure. Therefore, the speech disorder could continue to be a problem. In such cases, speech therapy might not be productive.

The soft and the hard palate clefts are typically closed at the same time, although both may need secondary surgeries. In some cases, the cleft of the hard palate is closed first, and the cleft of the soft palate is repaired later. In a variation of this practice, the cleft of the soft palate is first repaired, and then sometime later the cleft of the hard palate is repaired. This is known as the **Schweckendiek procedure**.

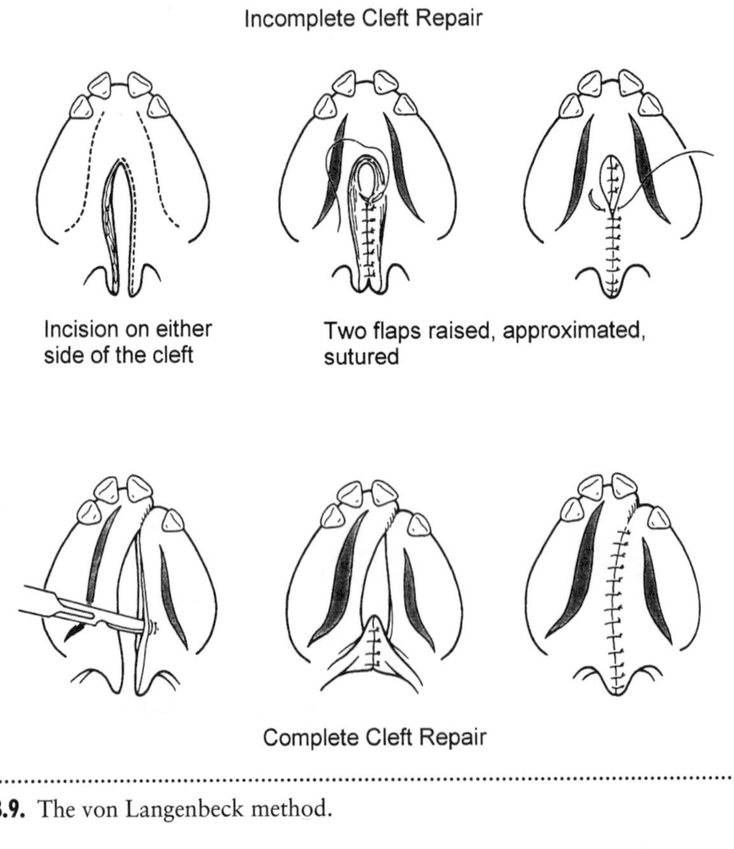

Incomplete Cleft Repair

Incision on either side of the cleft

Two flaps raised, approximated, sutured

Complete Cleft Repair

Figure 8.9. The von Langenbeck method.

Pharyngeal Flap

Some children with wide and complete cleft may be left with an inadequate velum, even after the best possible repair of the hard and the soft palates. The speech is still hypernasal because the short velum (soft palate) does not close the nasal port when non-nasal speech sounds are produced. These children are candidates for a *secondary operation* known as the pharyngeal flap procedure.

In the pharyngeal flap operation, illustrated in Figure 8.10, a muscular flap is raised from the back wall of the throat (technically, the *posterior pharyngeal wall*). The flap of tissue and mucosa is cut, raised, and attached to the velum. The flap is open on either side so that nasal breathing, nasal drainage, and production of nasal sounds are possible. One end of the flap is attached to the throat wall, and the other end is attached to the velum. The flap may be cut and positioned so that either it moves down to attach to the velum (Figure 8.10, right) or it moves up to the attaching point (Figure 8.10, left). The flap that moves down to the velum is known as the **inferiorly based pharyngeal flap** (Figure 8.10, right) and the one that moves up to the velum is known as the **superiorly based pharyngeal flap** (Figure 8.10, left). The pharyngeal flap may or may not move along with the soft palate; in either case, the extra mass of the flap, along with the lateral pharyngeal wall movements, helps close the velopharyngeal port.

A few surgeons use the pharyngeal flap as one of the primary operations. Most often the flap is constructed in a secondary procedure when the child is between the ages of 6 and 12 years (Peterson-Falzone et al., 2001). By this time, the child will have had one or more palatal surgeries. The speech, however, is still hypernasal. The cleft palate team's assessment of the child shows that the velopharyngeal mechanism is inadequate and that extra muscle mass should help. Following such an assessment, the pharyngeal flap operation is carried out.

A majority of children who undergo the pharyngeal flap operation benefit from it. Their speech improves markedly. Speech training will further improve the intelligibility of speech.

The limitations of the procedure are mostly technical. If the flap is too narrow, the velopharyngeal port will continue to be open when it must be closed.

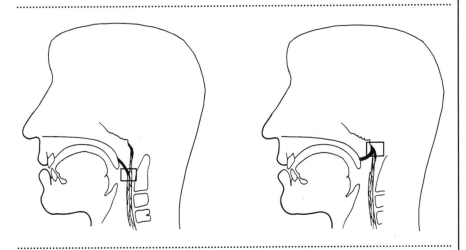

Figure 8.10. The pharyngeal flap operation.

If the flap is too wide, then the person cannot breathe through the nose; he or she will be a chronic mouth breather. The person also may sound hyponasal.

Besides the pharyngeal flap, surgeons have tried other pharyngeal surgical procedures collectively known as **pharyngoplasty** to improve the functioning of the velopharyngeal mechanism. Most of the procedures are experimental, and some are not commonly used in the United States. For example, surgeons have injected Teflon into the pharyngeal wall to make it bulge so it can meet the soft palate better to close the velopharyngeal port. Silicone was implanted in some cases. Muscles and cartilages taken from the patient's body also have been implanted into the pharyngeal wall. In most cases, the improvement in velopharyngeal functioning has not been as marked as it is following the pharyngeal flap procedure (Peterson-Falzone, 1988b).

Orthodontics and Prosthodontics

The dentist takes care of the routine dental problems of children with clefts. However, the special needs of these children require the services of the orthodontist and the prosthodontist.

The **orthodontist** specializes in moving the oral structures with the help of specially constructed devices. To the extent possible, the specialist corrects malocclusions of the upper and lower dental arches, straightens crooked individual teeth, expands the dental arch and the palatal area, and improves the overall appearance and function of the upper and lower jaw. To accomplish these goals, the orthodontist uses many tools including wires, plastic or stainless steel plates, and expanders, retainers, and externally worn appliances. The basic technique of orthodontics is to put pressure on dental structures, dental arches, and the palate to move them in certain directions, expand them to facilitate growth, and make it possible to use other surgical or nonsurgical procedures.

The **prosthodontist** is a specialist who can design and fit many kinds of devices that help improve the function of the oral structures. The prosthodontist's work is **prosthetics**, which is defined as the development and fitting of devices that compensate for missing or deformed structures. A frequently fabricated device is known as an **obturator,** which is an artificial device that helps close an opening.

Cleft of the alveolar ridge may be closed with a plastic prosthetic device that bridges the divided sections of the upper dental arch. Another type of obturator, illustrated in Figure 8.11, helps close the cleft in the palate and aids in the velopharyngeal closure. It has a plate that hugs the hard palate and a bulb that helps close the velopharyngeal port (Figure 8.11A). In the front the plate can hold artificial teeth to replace missing teeth in the cleft of the alveolar ridge. When worn (Figure 8.11B), the body of the plate closes the cleft of the palate. The bulb in the back of the mouth is positioned in the soft palate region, so it helps close the velopharyngeal opening. When the soft palate moves in the backward and upward direction, the pharyngeal walls constrict and the bulb comes in contact with them.

The bulb must be the right size for the individual patient. The prosthodontist makes a trial-size bulb and fits it. The speech–language pathologist helps evaluate the usefulness of the obturator by assessing the speech and resonance qualities of the child before, during, and after fitting the obturator. Based on the results, the speech–language pathologist suggests modifications in the size of the bulb to achieve the best possible results.

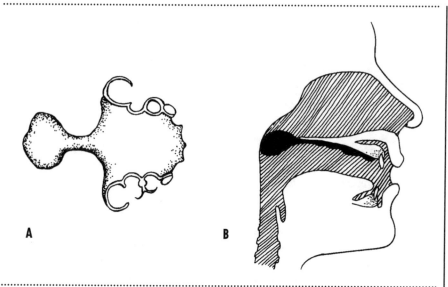

Figure 8.11. An obturator.

The patient must first learn to tolerate the obturator in the mouth. Then the patient must get training in using the appliance for better speech production. Many patients gag when they are fitted with the obturator, mainly because of the bulb at the back of the mouth. With the help of the speech–language pathologist, the child learns to use the obturator for achieving better speech production.

Summary

- Children with cleft undergo multiple surgeries.

- The initial (primary) surgery is done as early as feasible to close the cleft.

- Secondary surgeries are performed to improve the appearance of the child and the functioning of the speech structures.

- The lip surgery is done when the baby is about 10 weeks old and the primary palatal surgery is performed later.

- The clefts are closed by flaps of tissue that are freed from the hard palate and moved and sutured together to close the gap.

- In the Veau–Wardill–Kilner procedure, the freed flaps of tissue are moved back to lengthen the palate.

- In the von Langenbeck procedure, the cleft is closed without lengthening the palate.

- In the pharyngeal flap operation, a muscular flap is raised from the posterior pharyngeal wall and attached to the velum. This flap helps achieve better velopharyngeal closure.

(continues)

- In addition to surgery, orthodontic treatment is needed to correct dental abnormalities.

- To achieve a better velopharyngeal closure, prosthetic devices may be needed.

Assessment of Communicative Disorders

Before starting treatment for disorders of communication, the speech–language pathologist makes a careful assessment of the child's communicative behaviors and speech structures. The clinician takes a case history, interviews the parents, talks to the child, and then takes steps to assess the communicative behaviors of the child. The general procedures of assessment are presented in Table 8.1.

The initial assessment helps establish a treatment program for the child. However, some aspects of assessment are repeated at various stages of rehabilitation. Any time a new prosthetic, surgical, or other procedure is considered for the child, the speech–language pathologist must judge whether it will help the child speak better. The clinician evaluates the effectiveness of surgical, orthodontic, and prosthodontic procedures by comparing speech-related data obtained before and after the implementation of those procedures.

Assessment of Speech and Language

Assessment of speech and language of children with cleft palate generally follows the procedures described in Chapters 4 and 5. The case history, standardized tests of language and articulation, and tape-recorded samples of conversational speech are the major sources of information on the child's speech and language skills. Based on these data, the clinician can determine whether the child

Table 8.1

Assessment of Communicative Disorders: Cleft Palate Speech

1. The history of the client, the family, the disorder

2. Interview of the client, the family members, or both

3. **Orofacial examination**

4. Hearing screening

5. Speech and language sampling

6. Assessment of:
   a. language problems
   b. **articulation disorders and intelligibility**
   c. **voice and resonance problems**
   d. **velopharyngeal functioning**

7. Recommendations

8. Report writing

Note. Procedures unique to the disorders of communication in children with clefts are in bold print.

can produce speech sounds correctly and use words, phrases, and grammatically correct sentences considered appropriate for his or her age.

There also are a few special tests of articulation designed for assessing the speech of people with cleft palate. These include the Iowa Pressure Articulation Test, which is a subtest of the *Templin–Darley Test of Articulation* (Templin & Darley, 1969); the Bzoch Articulation Test (1997b); and the *Miami Imitative Ability Test* (Jacobs, Philips, & Harrison, 1970). These tests help evaluate the production of speech sounds that are especially difficult for the child with cleft palate. As you know, the sounds that require increased intraoral breath pressure (/p/, /b/, /s/, and other sounds) are especially difficult for the person with a cleft palate.

Conversational speech samples and portions of articulatory test responses are used to judge the intelligibility of speech a speaker with cleft palate produces. Most clinicians judge intelligibility based on a percentage of words, phrases, or sentences that can be understood. For example, the clinician might say that "only 50% of the child's utterances are intelligible."

Assessment of Voice and Resonance

Assessment of voice and resonance disorders, described in Chapter 7, requires the use of many procedures, including some electronic instruments. In the absence of costly instruments, the speech–language pathologist makes subjective judgments about the presence and extent of hoarseness, harshness, or breathiness of voice; the appropriateness of the vocal pitch of the client; and the loudness of speech.

A unique aspect of this assessment is the determination of the velopharyngeal adequacy. The presence and the extent of hypernasality is the main basis to make this determination. Typically, speech–language pathologists make clinical judgments of hypernasality. Some clinicians use **rating scales,** which permit such categorical descriptions of hypernasality as *mild, moderate, severe,* and *very severe.* Such instruments as the Nasometer, illustrated in Chapter 7, also can be used to objectively measure nasal resonance.

Many instruments can be used in the assessment of velopharyngeal movement, including some that medical specialists use. Most of the techniques help assess not only the adequacy of the velopharyngeal mechanism but also many other oral and facial structures and their interrelations.

Several radiological procedures help assess the functioning of the velopharyngeal mechanism. **Cineradiography,** for example, yields motion pictures of the speech mechanisms filmed through X ray. The film shows the movements of the tongue, the jaw, and the velopharyngeal mechanism. A related technique is **videofluoroscopy** in which the images are videotaped. **Tomography** is a more recent development in the X-ray technology. Using computers, a tomograph takes three dimensional X-ray pictures of the body. Tomography shows the internal structures of the body better than the traditional X ray. The usefulness of tomography in the assessment of the velopharyngeal mechanism has been demonstrated (Iglesias, Kuehn, & Morris, 1980; Weiss & Blackley, 1981).

Ultrasound also can help evaluate the velopharyngeal mechanism. A beam of ultrasound is sent to the pharyngeal wall, which deflects it back to the machine. The sound signal is displayed on a small television-like screen of an oscilloscope, an instrument that transforms sound into visible patterns. The screen of the oscilloscope shows the movement of the pharyngeal wall.

Read more about endoscopy in **Chapter 7.**

Other procedures used in the assessment of the velopharyngeal mechanism include **endoscopy.** By inserting a small tube through the nose or mouth, the velopharyngeal mechanism and its workings can be observed either directly or on the video screen.

Assessment of Hearing

Assessment of hearing and the work of an audiologist are described in **Chapter 10.**

Assessment of hearing is important because of the high frequency of hearing loss in children with cleft palate. An **audiologist,** who is a specialist in the measurement of normal and impaired hearing, evaluates the child's hearing. Through periodic measurement of hearing, the audiologist on the cleft palate team monitors the hearing of the child. The audiologist may prescribe and fit a hearing aid. The audiologist may hold a few treatment sessions in which the use of the aid from the standpoint of speech is demonstrated for the child. This aspect of an audiologist's work is described as **aural rehabilitation.**

Assessment Report

The speech–language pathologist studies all of the assessment data to determine the treatment program for the child. Each child needs a slightly different emphasis in treatment. An integrative summary of assessment written for the child will help establish the initial and long-range treatment targets.

Summary

- Children with cleft or repaired cleft are assessed repeatedly and over a period of time.

- Speech, language, voice, and resonance problems are assessed before and after treatment and many times during treatment.

- An important part of assessment is the evaluation of the velopharyngeal functioning, as this is closely related to many speech disorders associated with clefts.

- Techniques including cineradiography, videofluoroscopy, tomography, ultrasound, and endoscopy may be used in this part of the assessment.

- Periodic assessment of hearing also is important.

Treatment of Communicative Disorders

Surgical, orthodontic, and prosthodontic procedures directly affect the child's acquisition of speech and language. Therefore, the speech–language pathologist should work with other professionals and help them make decisions that facilitate speech and language behaviors. Whenever the cleft palate team considers a surgical, orthodontic, or prosthodontic procedure, the speech–language pathologist points out how the procedure helps or hinders language teaching and learning. At times, the clinician may prompt discussion on the need for a particular procedure. For example, the clinician may request that an obturator be developed for a child.

In the past, surgeries either were crudely performed or were performed late in the life of a child with a cleft. This tended to cause profound speech, voice, and resonance disorders. Current surgical procedures are much more refined and are performed on younger children. Therefore, the negative effects of the cleft on communication are reduced. Nonetheless, most children who have had cleft palate surgery need some form of speech training because some of the speech problems of the presurgical period tend to persist. The child may not be able to make the best use of the restored velopharyngeal mechanism because of the continued faulty speech habits.

Treatment of Language Disorders

Not all children with clefts need formal and intensive intervention for language problems. Some children might learn language at the usual rate, whereas others might have a slight or a significant language problem. Slight delays in language learning might be corrected by home programs designed to stimulate language. The essence of any home program is frequent parent–child interactions that repeatedly draw the child's attention to the use of language.

The clinician trains the parents to promote language learning in their child. The parents are asked to start the language stimulation early. While feeding, dressing, and playing with the infant, the parents are taught to name things and talk to the infant. For example, while dressing, the infant repeatedly hears the words like *shoes, socks, shirt,* or *skirt.* The parents reinforce the baby's babbling and production of words and phrases by smile, touch, and other responses. The parents model the words and reinforce correct productions or even approximations. The parents are asked to stimulate the production of speech sounds that are especially difficult for a child with cleft palate. For example, words starting with /k/, /g/, /s/, and /z/ can be frequently stimulated so that their production is encouraged and reinforced.

To promote appropriate communicative behaviors in a child with cleft, the speech–language pathologist intervenes as early as possible. The clinician is involved with the parents from the very beginning. The speech–language pathologist periodically evaluates the child's progress in learning the language. If the child is not making sufficient progress, the clinician starts more formal language training in the clinic.

The clinician uses the procedures described in Chapter 5 in implementing a formal language training program. For training, the clinician selects language structures the child does not produce, including words, phrases, sentences, and aspects of syntax and morphological elements. With the help of pictures and objects, the clinician trains a few target behaviors at a time. The clinician shows the pictures or objects, asks questions, models the correct responses, and praises the child for approximate productions. In the beginning, the clinician teaches simple words and phrases, targeting more complex structures as the child makes progress. Procedures designed to help the child produce the newly learned responses at home and other places also are implemented.

Read more about formal language training procedures in **Chapter 5.**

Treatment of Articulation Disorders

Treatment of articulation disorders in children with cleft palate is a major responsibility of the speech–language clinician. Research has shown that children with cleft palate are able to speak better when they receive articulation training than when they do not (Peterson-Falzone et al., 2001).

Read more about treating articulation disorders in **Chapter 4.**

The basic procedures of treating the articulation disorders of the child with a cleft are not different from those described in Chapter 4. However, the child with a cleft must be taught a few special target behaviors that are not necessarily taught to a child without a cleft.

Many children with repaired cleft can produce speech sounds without speech training. For those who do need speech training, early intervention is important. This will prevent the acquisition of faulty methods of sound productions that might persist. When the child's velopharyngeal mechanism is adequate or nearly so, the treatment for articulation disorders is most productive (Peterson-Falzone et al., 2001).

In the beginning, the child produces selected phonemes in isolation, in syllables, or in words. The clinician selects such stop consonants as /p/, /b/, /t/, /d/, /k/, and /g/ and such fricatives as /f/, /v/, /s/, and /z/ for training. Generally, the clinician first teaches the sounds that are produced in the front of the mouth and then those that are produced in the back of the mouth. For example, the labial sounds /p/ and /b/ are more visible than the velar stops /k/ and /g/. The child can see how the labial sounds are made and presumably this helps faster learning.

In all phases of treatment, the clinician gives maximum visual and auditory cues to the child. The clinician and the child may face a mirror so that the child sees the movement of the tongue and the placement of the tongue tip while producing various sounds. The clinician repeatedly models the correct production of the target sound. The child is encouraged to watch the clinician's production, listen carefully, and try to produce the sound.

The child who learns to produce the sound in isolation is asked to produce it in syllables. In gradual steps, the child is trained to produce the target sound at the more complex levels of words, phrases, sentences, and conversational speech. The clinician monitors the child's production of clinically taught sounds in situations outside the clinic to promote their maintenance.

A special target of articulation treatment is to teach the child to direct the flow of air out of the mouth instead of the nose. The child is shown how the air flows out of the mouth while producing a /p/ or a /b/. The movement of a piece of tissue placed in front of the mouth as the clinician produces the target sound might help the child appreciate the direction of air flow. The child might be taught to produce speech with less force. Gentle contact of articulators and a wider mouth opening also can help reduce nasal resonance.

Treatment of Voice and Resonance Problems

Read more about treatment of voice disorders in **Chapter 7.**

Unrelated to their cleft, some children might have voice problems including hoarseness and harshness. The treatment of such disorders does not differ significantly from the treatment of voice disorders described in Chapter 7. However, some voice problems associated with clefts are due to the child's efforts to compensate for the inadequate velopharyngeal mechanism. The child may adopt the strategy of talking too softly or with excessive muscular effort to close the velopharyngeal port. In such cases the clinician teaches socially appropriate loudness and relaxed speech.

The resonance problems of a child with cleft palate need intensive clinical efforts. Some of the techniques including wider mouth opening and easy articulatory contacts described earlier will help reduce nasality. In most cases, more than this is needed to achieve significant reductions in hypernasality. Therefore, clinicians have developed specific techniques to control hypernasal speech.

Even the non-nasal (oral) sounds are produced with variable amounts of nasal resonance. For example, the vowel /a/ tends to be less nasal than the vowel /i/ (the *ee* sound as in *eat*). Among the consonants, such sounds as /r/ and /t/ may be less nasal than /s/ or /z/. Therefore, in reducing hypernasality, the clinician develops practice trials starting with the least nasal sounds and moves on to the most nasal sounds (Sommers, 1983). The sounds are eventually produced in words and phrases. This approach is better suited for children with an adequate postsurgical velopharyngeal mechanism than for those with velopharyngeal incompetence.

Biofeedback instruments may be used in treating hypernasality. These instruments convert one form of energy into another form and display it in either visual or auditory mode. For example, the Nasometer described earlier (and illustrated) in Chapter 7 gives immediate feedback on the amount of nasal resonance in the form of a display on a computer screen. A target level of nasal or oral resonance may be set and the client trained to meet the target.

Summary

- The most intensive treatment is likely to be directed against the articulation and resonance problems of children with palatal clefts.

- Language problems often are mild and are handled through a home management program. Formal language treatment, offered when needed, does not differ substantially from treatment given to children without clefts.

- Speech training is particularly concerned with the stop sounds that are especially difficult for children with palatal clefts. The child also is taught to direct the flow of air out of the mouth instead of the nose. In treating resonance problems (such as hypernasality), biofeedback instruments may be used.

Dialogue

As usual, Ms. Noledge-Hungry walked into Dr. Speech-Wisely's office to discuss cleft palate with the professor. These discussions give her a chance to summarize the information and identify the areas she must study more carefully. Also, she has found these discussions helpful in deciding her major.

N-H: Dr. Speech-Wisely, I was interested in cleft palate because one of our neighbors' sons had it. It is fascinating to learn about this birth defect.

S-W: Yes, it is a birth defect involving the mouth and face, hence the term **orofacial** abnormalities. If the abnormality affects at least one of the eyes and structures above it, as in some cases, you call it **craniofacial** abnormality. And now, tell me, what is a cleft?

N-H: A **cleft** is an opening. We talked about the cleft of the lip, the hard palate, and the soft palate. But do you mind summarizing the anatomy and embryology for me?

S-W: Well, you must remember that at the back of the mouth is the **soft palate**, which is muscular and helps close the **velopharyngeal port.** The **upper jaw** and the **hard palate** are made of two bones called the **maxillae.** The outer edges of these bones house most of the upper teeth and are called the **alveolar process.** A small piece of bone of triangular shape, which lies under the nose, is the **premaxilla.** It holds the front four teeth of the upper arch, and the middle part of the upper lip is attached to it. During the various stages of embryonic development, the structures grow toward each other and fuse. Do you remember why this fusion may not take place in some unborn babies?

N-H: Yes. Some think it may be due to genes because clefts are more frequent among Native Americans and less frequent among African Americans. More boys than girls have clefts. Animal and human research has suggested that various drugs, viral infections of the mother, radiation, and maternal anoxia could cause cleft palate in babies.

S-W: Very good. The next thing to remember is the classification of clefts. You are doing fine if you are about as confused as the experts, but you should know the classifications of Veau, and Stark and Kernahan.

N-H: Veau described four types; Stark and Kernahan described clefts of the primary palate, clefts of the secondary palate, and clefts of both the palates. As a clinician, I should fully describe the cleft of an individual baby.

S-W: Very good. But also remember, there is the **submucous cleft,** which is hidden by the muscular sheet that covers the palates. Then there is the **congenital palatopharyngeal incompetence,** which simply means that the child is born with an inadequate pharyngeal mechanism.

N-H: But isn't it true that some children with cleft palate also may exhibit other gross physical abnormalities?

S-W: True, in some rare cases. Most may be otherwise normal and healthy.

N-H: I was very interested in the family's reaction to cleft palate in the baby. All the shock, guilt, and disbelief. But it is nice to know that there are ways of helping the parents handle their emotional responses. It is important to counsel the parents.

S-W: Absolutely. The new mother soon finds out that the baby has feeding problems. The baby is prone to have middle ear infections, hearing loss, and dental problems. You should know these.

N-H: But how can I summarize the communicative problems of the cleft palate?

S-W: Children with cleft palate might be slow in learning language. But more serious and more common effects of cleft palate are on speech production and resonance. The children have problems articulating speech sounds, especially certain kinds of sounds. You should know the sounds and why they are especially difficult for the child with cleft. The problem of resonance is hypernasality.

N-H: I will remember the sounds, but they are mostly the **plosives** and **fricatives.** Isn't it true that the child misarticulates because it is difficult to build breath pressure in the mouth?

S-W: Exactly. And the child is **hypernasal** because it is not possible to shut off the nasal port while producing non-nasal speech sounds.

N-H: But there also is that **nasal emission.** It is not nasal resonance but just the noise of air escaping through the nose while speaking. Possibly to compensate for the speech difficulties, some children talk too softly or with too much muscular effort.

S-W: That is right. Now tell me about the **cleft palate team.**

N-H: Well, children with clefts have many problems. Many specialists form a team to help them. The team consists of a pediatrician, the oral surgeon, the otologist, the nurse, the dentist, the orthodontist, the prosthodontist, the audiologist, the psychologist, and the speech–language pathologist.

S-W: Excellent. You should be able to describe what each one does. When does the surgeon close the cleft of the lip?

N-H: **Lip surgery** is done when the baby is about 10 weeks of age and weighs about 10 pounds. But I am not sure when palatal surgeries are done.

S-W: The **primary surgery** to repair the cleft of the palate is done when the baby is between 12 and 18 months old. Either the soft palate or the hard palate may be repaired first. Do you remember the two basic surgical procedures?

N-H: Yes, the **V-Y retroposition** or the **Veau–Wardill–Kilner** procedure and the **von Langenbeck** procedure. I think the major difference between the two is that in the V-Y procedure, the flaps of muscles raised from the palate are moved back and toward each other before they are sutured together, whereas in the von Langenbeck procedure, the flaps are moved only toward each other to close the cleft. Also, in the V-Y procedure, the flaps are freed from the bone at the sides and in the front, but in the von Langenbeck procedure, the flaps are freed from the bone only on the sides.

S-W: Excellent. You should also know about the **pharyngeal flap** operation, in which a flap of tissue is raised from the back wall of the throat and sutured to the soft palate to increase its bulk. This flap helps achieve better velopharyngeal closure.

N-H: And then there is **pharyngoplasty** to increase the thickness of the pharyngeal wall. Muscles from other parts of the body may be grafted to the posterior pharyngeal wall. Foreign substances such as silicone, paraffin, and Teflon may be injected into the pharyngeal wall to make it thicker.

S-W: Fine. Now what about the dental specialists?

N-H: The dentist takes care of the routine dental problems. The **orthodontist** aligns the teeth and the jaws, and the **prosthodontist** builds prosthetic devices that close the cleft or increase the efficiency of the velopharyngeal mechanism.

S-W: What is an obturator?

N-H: An **obturator** is a plastic plate that closes the cleft of the palate, but it also may have a bulb at the back that assists in velopharyngeal closure.

S-W: Very good. Now a little bit about the **assessment** of communicative disorders. The speech–language pathologist evaluates the structure and the use of language, errors of articulation, voice qualities, and deviations in resonance. The clinician administers standardized tests, interviews parents, observes the child in the clinic, and takes language samples. Integrating all the information on hand, the clinician designs speech, language, voice, and resonance treatment programs for the child.

N-H: What about the tests of articulation?

S-W: It is good to remember the names of a test or two. The Iowa Pressure Articulation Test, a subtest of the *Templin–Darley Test of Articulation* (Templin & Darley, 1969), and the Bzoch Articulation Test are good examples. You should also know the techniques of assessing the craniofacial structures and functions. These include **cineradiography, tomography, ultrasound,** and **endoscopy.**

N-H: And the assessment of hearing loss. Audiologists on the team evaluate the hearing of the child and determine if the child needs aural rehabilitation.

S-W: Yes. The audiologist selects and fits a hearing aid if one is needed. He or she counsels the parents and the child and helps them cope with the problems of hearing impairment.

N-H: Not all cleft palate children need language therapy, right?

S-W: Right. Most children are likely to show a slight delay in learning language. These children are best helped with a home program in which the parents stimulate, evoke, and reinforce language in the child. The important task here is to train the parents in the home program and have them implement it.

N-H: When the home program is not effective, the speech–language pathologist treats the child's language. I think I have a pretty good idea of language therapy because we discussed it before in the class. You treat the language disorders in a child with cleft palate in roughly the same way that you treat the language problems in children without cleft.

S-W: That is correct, and you can say that about **articulation treatment** as well. You select the target speech sounds; provide plenty of visual, auditory, and kinesthetic cues on how to produce them; model the correct responses; and encourage the child to imitate your productions. The child is praised for correct productions or approximations. The treatment moves from more "visible" to less "visible" sounds and from a simple level of sounds or syllables to more complex levels of words, phrases, sentences, and conversational speech.

N-H: But what about some special procedures used with children with cleft palates?

S-W: They are special target responses, not really special procedures of treatment. The child with cleft palate is taught to direct the flow of air through the mouth and not through the nose. The child is taught to speak without much oral breath pressure and muscular effort. Gentle articulatory contacts are encouraged. The nares may be closed during the production of non-nasal sounds, but this should not be done too frequently.

N-H: I understand that the treatment of resonance problems, hypernasality for the most part, requires special procedures.

S-W: Yes, the **biofeedback** procedures have been relatively more successful in the treatment of voice and resonance disorders than in the treatment of other disorders of communication. Instruments such as the Nasometer can be useful in giving the client immediate feedback on the amount of oral and nasal resonance. But you should not forget nonmechanical procedures either. Often, the clinician does not have costly mechanical devices.

N-H: Right. It is possible to experiment with the client and reinforce whenever the speech is less nasal. I like the idea of constructing a hierarchy of sounds that are least to most nasal and have the client practice them.

S-W: That is very good.

The Outlook

Ms. Noledge-Hungry wanted to ask a few more questions about majoring in communicative disorders (CD) and specializing in cleft palate. So she went on with it.

N-H: Well, Dr. Speech-Wisely, what more will I learn about cleft palate if I major in communicative disorders?

S-W: You will learn plenty because cleft palate is a complex condition that belongs to a much broader area of birth defects. In advanced courses at the undergraduate and graduate levels, you will study oral anatomy more thoroughly than you have done in this class. You will study embryology in more detail. You will also study variations of surgical procedures and find out how they affect communication. You will, of course, find out more about the speech, language, voice, and resonance disorders and how to treat them.

N-H: I can see there is much to learn. Do we get to see a cleft palate team in action and work with cleft palate children?

S-W: Yes you do. Most university programs in communicative disorders have an arrangement with a hospital so that the student clinicians can watch the activities of a cleft palate team. Advanced student clinicians may be a part of the team. The students may be able to do their clinical internship in a hospital and learn about all aspects of cleft palate rehabilitation.

N-H: I would like that. Can a student clinician watch cleft palate surgery?

S-W: Yes, with the permission of the surgeon. You can watch the work of most other members of the team and discuss their and your problems with them.

N-H: What about speech–language therapy? Where will I work with children who have clefts?

S-W: You may be able to work with a child who has clefts in our own speech and hearing clinic on the campus. If not, you may work with them during your internship at the hospital or at one of the medical centers out of town.

N-H: If I specialize in cleft palate, will I work in a hospital?

S-W: Most likely. Cleft palate teams work in hospitals where comprehensive medical, communicative, social, and psychological services are provided. Occasionally, clinicians in university clinics and in private practice also may work with children with repaired cleft. In such cases, the clinician stays in touch with the cleft palate team that referred the client.

N-H: Sounds good, Dr. Speech-Wisely. What are we going to discuss next?

S-W: We are going to talk about a group of communicative disorders that have their origin in neurological damage. I know you will enjoy that.

N-H: I sure hope so!

Study Questions

1. What are congenital abnormalities?

2. What are orofacial and craniofacial abnormalities?

3. The major portion of the hard palate is formed by a pair of bones called _____.

4. A small piece of bone located right under the nose is called _____.

5. The soft palate also is known as _____.

6. Give a brief description of the structure and function of the velopharyngeal port.

7. The pair of nasal cavities is divided by _____.

8. The primitive (embryonic) mouth and nose are called the _____.

9. Give a brief description of the embryonic growth of the facial structures.

10. What is a cleft?

11. What are some of the causes of clefts in humans?

12. How did Veau describe the varieties of clefts?

13. Give a brief description of Stark and Kernahan's classification of the clefts.

14. What is a submucous cleft?

15. What is congenital palatopharyngeal incompetence?

16. Define the following terms:

    Ablation

    Maxillectomy

    Mandibulectomy

    Glossectomy

17. Describe the problems of and solutions for feeding babies born with clefts of the palates.

18. What kinds of middle ear problems are common in children with clefts?

19. What is malocclusion? Give brief descriptions of the three types of malocclusions.

20. Give a brief description of the speech problems of children with cleft palate.

21. What is compensatory articulation?

22. Define nasal emission.

23. What kinds of resonance and voice problems are found in children with cleft palate?

24. Name the specialists who serve on a cleft palate team.

25. When is the lip surgery performed to repair a cleft lip?

26. What are the goals of palatal surgery in children with clefts?

27. Give a brief description of the Veau–Wardill–Kilner procedure of cleft palate surgery. What is its major strength?

28. Describe the von Langenbeck procedure of cleft palate surgery. What is its major drawback?

29. What is the pharyngeal flap operation? Why is it performed?

30. Define pharyngoplasty.

31. Distinguish between an orthodontist and a prosthodontist.

32. Describe the major assessment procedures used in evaluating a child with cleft palate.

33. What is hypernasality?

34. How are biofeedback instruments used in treating hypernasality of cleft palate children?

35. What kinds of speech sounds may be initially taught to a child with repaired cleft?

References

Bzoch, K. R. (1997a). Clinical assessment, evaluation, and management of 11 categorical aspects of cleft palate speech disorders. In K. R. Bzoch (Ed.), *Communicative disorders related to cleft lip and palate* (4th ed., pp. 261–312). Austin, TX: PRO-ED.

Bzoch, K. R. (Ed.) (1997b). *Communicative disorders related to cleft lip and palate* (4th ed.). Austin, TX: PRO-ED.

Gibbs, J. M. (1973). Cleft palate babies: One mother's experience. *Nursing Care, 1,* 19–23.

Iglesias, A., Kuehn, D. P., & Morris, H. L. (1980). Simultaneous assessment of pharyngeal wall and velar displacement for selected speech sounds. *Journal of Speech and Hearing Research, 23,* 429–446.

Jacobs, R. J., Philips, B. J., & Harrison, R. J. (1970). A stimulability test for cleft palate children. *Journal of Speech and Hearing Disorders, 35,* 354–362.

Khan, A. (2000). *Craniofacial anomalies: A beginner's guide for speech–language pathologists.* San Diego, CA: Singular.

Morris, H. L. (1962). Communication skills of children with cleft lip and palate. *Journal of Speech and Hearing Research, 5,* 79–90.

Peterson-Falzone, S. (1988a). Speech disorders related to craniofacial structural defects: Part 1. In N. J. Lass, L. V. McReynolds, J. L. Northern, & D. E. Yoder (Eds.), *Handbook of speech–language pathology and audiology* (pp. 442–476). Philadelphia: Decker.

Peterson-Falzone, S. (1988b). Speech disorders related to craniofacial structural defects: Part 2. In N. J. Lass, L. V. McReynolds, J. L. Northern, & D. E. Yoder (Eds.), *Handbook of speech–language pathology and audiology* (pp. 477–547). Philadelphia: Decker.

Peterson-Falzone, S., Hardin-Jones, M. A., & Kernell, M. P. (2001). *Cleft palate speech* (3rd ed.). St. Louis, MO: Mosby.

Seikel, J. A., King, D. W., & Drumright, D. G. (2000). *Anatomy and physiology for speech, language, and hearing* (2nd ed.). San Diego, CA: Singular.

Shames, G., & Rubin, H. (1979). Psycholinguistic measures of language and speech. In K. Bzoch (Ed.), *Communicative disorders related to cleft lip and palate* (2nd ed., pp. 202–223). Boston: Little, Brown.

Shprintzen, R. J., & Bardach, J. (1995). *Cleft palate speech management: A multidisciplinary approach.* St. Louis, MO: Mosby.

Shprintzen, R. J., & Goldberg, R. (1995). The genetics of clefting and associated syndromes. In R. J. Shprintzen & J. Bardach (Eds.), *Cleft palate speech management: A multidisciplinary approach* (pp. 16–43). St. Louis, MO: Mosby.

Slutsky, H. (1969). Maternal reaction and adjustment to birth and care of the cleft palate child. *Cleft Palate Journal, 6*, 425–427.

Sommers, R. K. (1983). *Articulation disorders*. Englewood Cliffs, NJ: Prentice Hall.

Stark, R. B., & Kernahan, D. A. (1959). A classification of cleft lip and cleft palate based upon newer concepts of embryology. *Cleft Palate Bulletin, 9*, 45–46.

Templin, M. C., & Darley, F. L. (1969). *The Templin–Darley Test of Articulation* (2nd ed.). Iowa City: Bureau of Educational Research & Service, University of Iowa.

Vanderas, A. P. (1987). Incidence of cleft lip, cleft palate, and cleft lip and palate among races: A review. *Cleft Palate Journal, 25*, 171–183.

Veau, V. (1931). *Division palatine*. Paris: Masson.

Weiss, C., & Blackley, F. (1981). Feasibility of using computerized tomography in diagnosing nasopharyngeal closure. *Journal of Communication Disorders, 14*, 43–50.

Wells, C. G. (1971). *Cleft palate and its associated speech disorders*. New York: McGraw-Hill.

Zemlin, W. R. (1998). *Speech and hearing science* (4th ed.). Needham Heights, MA: Allyn & Bacon.

Neurologically Based
Communicative Disorders

What is the experience of an accident inside the head? An artery of the brain ruptures. Suddenly, the brain, that model of complex and superb organization, is thrown into chaos. A patient who recovered from a severe stroke described it this way:

> In a split-second, everything you have known about yourself and the world around you is thrown into a chaos. It is noise in your head, it is confusion in your mind, it is dull pain in your body, but you may not know where it hurts. You wonder whether you are already dead and this is the life after death. You wonder whether you are floating on the clouds or drowning in a deep sea. The faces, the places, the things, the sounds, and the colors of your life suddenly lose all meaning. This is what scares you the most. (An anonymous patient's report following recovery)

Sorting Out the Neurologically Based Communicative Disorders

For several communicative disorders, we cannot readily find a cause in the person's nerves or muscles. As pointed out earlier, some children's misarticulations or difficulty in learning language are disorders of this kind.

Communicative disorders described in this chapter are different. Some individuals have a neuromuscular system that is not working properly because of disease or injury. Consequently, the individuals have various communicative problems. Because of the involvement of the neuromuscular system, their communicative problems are described as **neurologically based**. Some adults described in this chapter either have a language problem called **aphasia,** which is due to such internal causes as strokes, which typically damage the left hemisphere, or speech problems called **motor speech disorders,** which also are due to internal neurological problems. Some adults have a **right-hemisphere syndrome,** which is due to injury to the right side of the brain, caused by such internal causes as strokes and tumors. Other adults have a variety of conditions that are associated with degenerative brain diseases and are grouped under **dementia** including communicative disorders, attentional deficits, and memory problems. Still others have communicative and cognitive deficits due to externally induced **traumatic brain injury.** The children described in this chapter have a disorder of communication due to brain injury sustained during infancy or the prenatal period. These children are diagnosed to have **cerebral palsy.**

Because it is the neuropathological features that bring aphasia, motor speech disorders, right-hemisphere syndrome, dementia, traumatic brain injury, and cerebral palsy together for this chapter, we must first review a few basic structures of the brain and certain peripheral nerves that are involved in language and speech functions. Although there is a separate chapter on the anatomy and physiology of speech and hearing (Chapter 3), the following section makes this chapter self-sufficient. To gain a better understanding of the neurophysiology of speech and language, the student must read one of the several excellent sources (Bhatnagar & Andy, 1995; Calvin & Ojemann, 1980; Love & Webb, 1996; Seikel, Douglas, & Drumright, 1997; Webster, 1999; Yorkston, Beukelman, Strand, & Bell, 1999; Zemlin, 1998).

The Brain and Language

A convoluted mass of gray cells, the brain has stimulated the normally prosaic neuroscientists to be poetic. It is the human brain, we are reminded, that is responsible for our art, culture, literature, sense of beauty. Our sense of excitement at studying the brain is probably due to the brain itself (Calvin & Ojemann, 1980).

The **central nervous system** has two structures: the **brain** and the **spinal cord.** Another nervous system is called the **peripheral nervous system,** through which the central nervous system keeps in touch with the environment. Sensory impulses flow into the central nervous system via the peripheral nervous system, which also carries impulses from the brain to the muscles and end-organs of the body.

The **cerebrum** is the largest, the most complex, and the topmost portion of the central nervous system. It is covered by membranes called **meninges.** The cerebrum is protected by the bony skull and cushioned by the surrounding **cerebrospinal fluid.**

Gyrus and **sulcus** are the singular forms of gyri and sulci, respectively.

The two halves of the cerebrum are known as the **hemispheres,** which are connected by a thick band of nerve fibers. The right hemisphere controls the left half of the body, and the left hemisphere controls the right half. The topmost layer of the hemispheres is called the **cortex,** which means the bark of a tree in Latin. It is a folded layer of specialized tissues. If the cortex were taken out of the skull and stretched out, it would be almost impossible to repack it. Many ridges and valleys (grooves) on the surface of the cortex help distinguish various landmarks on it. The ridges are called **gyri,** and the grooves are called **sulci.** They are due to the complicated folding of the cortical tissue.

The Lobes of the Cortex

A **lobe** is an area of the cortex, and each cortex (hemisphere) has four of them: the **frontal, parietal, occipital,** and **temporal.** Figure 9.1 shows the four lobes of the cortex.

The Frontal Lobe

The **frontal lobe** lies behind the forehead. It is the largest of the four lobes. Its boundaries are the central sulcus (also known as the Fissure of Rolando) at the back and the lateral cerebral fissure (also known as the Fissure of Sylvius) at the bottom. In front of the central sulcus is the precentral gyrus whose general area also is known as the **primary motor cortex,** or **primary motor area,** shown in Figure 9.2. The back end of the frontal cortex, then, contains the primary motor area.

The primary motor area controls movement; because speech is movement, it is an important area for speech. Specific parts of this area control particular parts of the body. The foot, for example, is controlled by the topmost layer, whereas the tongue is controlled by the bottommost layer. Of all the areas that govern different parts of the body, those that govern the hands and the mouth are the largest. This may be so because of the complex skills the human hands and the mouth perform. Speech is a complex motor skill, hence a relatively large area of the primary motor area controls it.

The frontal lobe also contains an important center for motor speech control named after the French neurosurgeon, Paul Broca, who discovered it in the 1860s. Damage to **Broca's area** (the area surrounding the inferior, or lower, frontal gyrus) is thought to cause one kind of aphasia, described in a later section. Figure 9.2 shows Broca's area.

It is thought that to a large extent, motor speech production is planned, programmed, and executed by the frontal lobe. Therefore, the frontal lobe is important in motor speech production and in understanding motor speech disorders.

The Parietal Lobe

The parietal lobe is found at the downward slope of the head at the back. Its boundaries are the central sulcus in the front, an arbitrary line that divides it

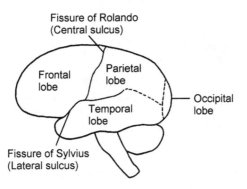

Figure 9.1. The four lobes of the cortex.

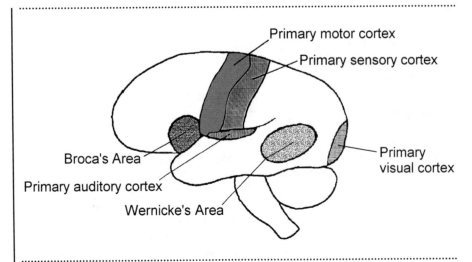

Figure 9.2. The major functionally related areas of the cortex.

from the occipital lobe at the back, and the lateral cerebral fissure below. The main function of this lobe is sensory. The senses of touch, pressure, and positions of the body or particular muscle groups are controlled by the **primary sensory cortex** of the parietal lobe. As shown in Figure 9.2, the primary sensory cortex lies behind the primary motor cortex. The central sulcus separates the motor and sensory areas.

Damage to one side of the parietal lobe causes a person to "ignore" or "forget" the other side. A business executive with a left side damage neatly combed his hair on the left side, but the hair on his right half of the head would have put a punk rock musician to shame.

The Occipital Lobe

The occipital lobe, also known as the visual cortex, is behind the parietal lobe. It contains the **primary visual area** as shown in Figure 9.2. The eyes send their sensory information to this lobe where it is analyzed and integrated. Damage to the parietal lobes can cause many kinds of visual difficulties including an inability to recognize printed words (alexia) and even blindness when the eyes themselves are perfectly healthy.

The Temporal Lobe

The **temporal lobe** is the most important lobe for hearing and language.

The temporal lobe is shaped like the thumb of a fist. It lies below the parietal and frontal lobes and in front of the occipital lobe. The temporal lobe contains two areas important for hearing and language, both shown in Figure 9.2. The first is the auditory cortex or the **primary auditory cortex** (or area) which receives and analyzes auditory stimuli. This is the main area concerned with hearing. The second is **Wernicke's area,** a small portion of which extends to the parietal lobe. Wernicke's area is concerned with language comprehension. In most people, damage to Wernicke's area in the left temporoparietal lobe causes a kind of aphasia that also is named after Wernicke. Patients with Wernicke's aphasia speak fluently without making sense and do not understand spoken or written language.

The Brain Stem

The brain stem is down from the cerebral cortex. It can be thought of either as the head of the spinal cord below or as the tail of the cortex above. Illustrated in Figure 9.3, the brain stem is a part of the central nervous system. The **medulla oblongata (medulla)**, which is the uppermost portion of the spinal cord or the lowermost portion of the brain stem, is noteworthy because it controls breathing, heart rate, and other vital and mostly automatic activities of the body. The medulla is important for speech not only because it controls breathing but also because it contains neural pathways that move up and down to carry messages to and from the brain. Damage to this part of the brain stem may cause many speech difficulties. These neural pathways are described in the next section.

The **pons** lies just above the medulla and connects the brain stem with the cerebellum (not cerebrum) and its two halves. The structure sitting on top of the medulla is called the **midbrain** or **mesencephalon.** It lies in between the cerebrum and the lower parts of the brain. The midbrain's main function is to link the higher and the lower centers of the brain.

The Cerebellum

The cerebellum looks like a little cerebrum and is attached to the back side of the brain stem; it lies below the cerebrum. This structure is important for speech because it regulates and coordinates movement of the body, including fine and complex movements necessary to produce speech. The cerebellum is illustrated in Figure 9.4.

The cerebellum does not generate motor impulses; it only coordinates and regulates motor impulses. It helps control posture, locomotion, and purposeful

Damage to the cerebellum causes problems in balance and a speech disorder called **dysarthria,** described later.

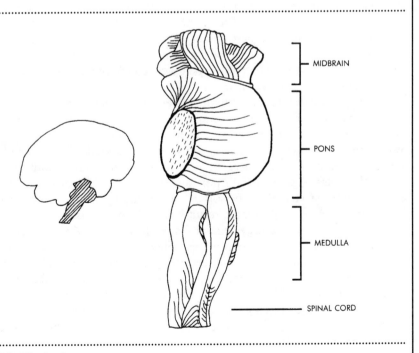

Figure 9.3. The brain stem.

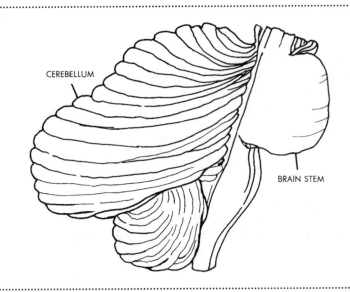

Figure 9.4. The cerebellum.

movement. It is believed that the motor cortex may often generate impulses that are too strong to achieve a balanced target movement. The cerebellum inhibits those excessive impulses to a certain degree so that the movement is well coordinated.

The Pyramidal and Extrapyramidal Pathways

As noted, the frontal lobe of the brain contains the primary motor area that controls movement as well as Broca's area, which controls speech production. Two neural pathways link these and other cortical structures with various muscles including those of speech. The pathways carry impulses originating in the brain to those muscles. The pathways are called the pyramidal and the extrapyramidal pathways or systems.

The **pyramidal system** is a bundle of nerve fibers that primarily originate in the motor cortex and travel without interruption to the brain stem and spinal cord (the reason they also are known as the direct system). It is the primary pathway to carry impulses for voluntary movement of all kinds. The pyramidal system has different tracts of fibers, some of which are more important for speech than others. Damage to certain portions of the pyramidal system can cause paralysis of the larynx, pharynx, soft palate, tongue, lips, and face. Many motor speech disorders, described later, result from such paralysis.

The fibers of the **extrapyramidal system** (also called the indirect system) have a diffuse origin in the cortex. The fibers of the system take an indirect route to their final destination in the sense that the fibers have multiple synaptic connections and relay stations. The indirect pathways descend down to the pons, cerebellum, and basal ganglia. The pons and the cerebellum have been described earlier. The **basal ganglia**, shown in Figure 9.5, are a major structure of the indirect motor pathways. They are located just below the cortical layer and just above the brain stem.

The pyramidal system is also called the **direct system,** and the extrapyramidal system is also called the **indirect system.**

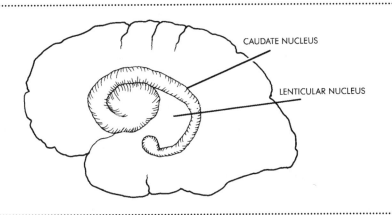

Figure 9.5. The basal ganglia.

The basal ganglia receive impulses from the motor cortex and relay information back to it. Basal ganglia are thought to help program movement patterns and, along with other structures of the indirect motor system, help maintain muscle tone and posture. When this system is damaged, the patient exhibits abnormal muscle tone and posture and involuntary movements (tremors).

The motor fibers of both the pyramidal and the extrapyramidal systems have their origin in the cerebral cortex. The fibers of both the systems that connect with the brain stem and spinal cord nuclei also are called the **upper motoneurons.** They are distinguished from the **lower motoneurons,** which are tracts that originate in the brain stem and the spinal cord and make connections with various muscles. A lesion in either the upper motoneuron or lower motoneuron causes paralysis. However, a lesion in the upper motoneuron causes a kind of paralysis known as **spastic paralysis.** The muscles in this case are too rigid and have too much tone. To the contrary, a lesion in the lower motoneuron causes **flaccid paralysis.** Lacking in tone, the muscles are too soft and flabby.

The Peripheral Nerves That Control Speech Production

The **peripheral nervous system** includes the cranial nerves, the spinal nerves, and portions of the autonomic nerves. These are described in Chapter 3. We will not be concerned with the autonomic nerves here as they mostly regulate the smooth muscles and glands inside the body.

Closely related to the autonomic nervous system, the 31 pairs of the **spinal nerves** are attached to the spinal cord. The nerves exit from the spinal cord and move on to the particular muscles to which they are attached. Several spinal nerves are important for speech because they control muscles of breathing.

The **cranial nerves** play a major role in speech production. The cranial nerves emerge out of holes (foramina) in the base of the skull. The nerves exit at different levels of the brain stem and the uppermost portion of the spinal cord. Therefore, the nerves are numbered according to the vertical order in which they leave the skull.

See **Chapter 3** for a brief description of the autonomic nervous system.

Most cranial nerves carry either sensory impulses from the peripheral sense organs to the brain (**sensory nerves**) or motor impulses from the brain to the muscle (**motor nerves**). Some nerves do both (**mixed nerves**).

There are 12 pairs of cranial nerves. Of these, 6 pairs, the cranial pairs I, II, III, IV, VI, and VIII, are not involved in speech production (see Chapter 3 about their function). As the following summary shows, the remaining six pairs control muscles of speech to varying extents:

- **Trigeminal nerve (V)** is a mixed nerve that is sensory to the upper jaw, the lower jaw, and the tongue. As a motor nerve, it controls the movements of the lower jaw and the tongue.
- **Facial nerve (VII)** is a mixed nerve. As a sensory nerve, it picks up sensations of taste. As a motor nerve, it controls many movements and facial expressions including wrinkling of the forehead, tight closure of the mouth, retraction of the corners of the mouth, and cheek movements.
- **Glossopharyngeal nerve (IX)**, a mixed nerve, is sensory to the tongue but motor to the pharynx. Therefore, movements of the throat muscles are controlled by this nerve.
- **Vagus nerve (X)**, the "wandering" nerve, is mixed, is complex, and serves many organs including the heart, the lungs, and the digestive system. It serves also as a sensory nerve for the muscles of the larynx and throat. One of its branches, known as the (paired) **recurrent laryngeal nerve,** serves most of the intrinsic muscles of the larynx. A damaged recurrent laryngeal nerve paralyzes one or both of the vocal folds.
- **Accessory nerve (XI)** is a motor nerve, but it is mixed in a different sense. It is both a spinal and a cranial nerve. It helps control the muscles of the pharynx (throat), the soft palate, the head, and the shoulders.
- **Hypoglossal nerve (XII)** is a motor nerve controlling the movements of the tongue.

The Study of Brain–Language Relations

The crowning achievement of the brain, as pointed out by many neuroscientists, is language. But how did scientists find out that particular groups of cerebral cells control particular aspects of language?

Autopsy is one method clinical scientists use to find out which areas control what functions. For example, Broca and Wernicke found out about specific areas that control certain language functions through autopsies of their former patients. In this method, clinical scientists keep a careful record of the language and related disturbances of neurologically sick patients. When the patient dies, the scientists dissect the brain to study the pathological changes in the tissue and their locations. The scientists then relate specific language disturbances recorded earlier to specific areas of the brain that show signs of damage or decay.

Another method clinical scientists use is more reliable and yields more direct data because the patient who supplies the information is still alive and hopes to live a long time. These are, for the most part, patients who suffer from severe epileptic seizures, the kind known as the *grand mal*. These seizures handicap some individuals to such an extent that they become candidates for brain surgery. On the operating table, the neurosurgeon cuts the scalp and carefully folds it over. Surgical saws and drills help cut open the necessary portion of the skull. The removed portion of the skull is saved and later replaced. This is done with local anesthesia, as the skull and the brain tissue are not sensitive to pain.

The neurosurgeon specializes in brain surgery.

Therefore, the patient is fully conscious, perhaps annoyed a bit by the noisy drilling and sawing. More important, the patient can talk and move parts of the body during the operation.

The neurosurgeon's task is to remove the damaged cells of the brain that are causing epileptic seizures but without causing speech problems (dysarthria), language problems (aphasia), or paralysis. In essence, the neurosurgeon does not wish to remove brain cells that control speech, language, and movement. Therefore, the neurosurgeon must first map the brain for language before reaching for the surgical knife.

The neurosurgeon uses a pair of thin silver wires connected to an electric stimulator to stimulate areas of the brain. The areas that control movement induce movement when stimulated. The hand or the lips, for example, may move upon stimulation of specific brain tissue. However, when stimulated, the areas that control speech do not produce speech; instead, speech is interrupted or confused. Therefore, the brain is stimulated when the patient is talking. For example, a patient is looking at a video screen that shows an object, and the patient is about to name the object shown. The surgeon then stimulates certain areas in the frontal and temporoparietal lobes. The patient then says, "It is a . . . well, . . . it is a . . . I know what it is. It is uh . . . . Well, I can't get that." The patient may be trying to say a simple word like *book,* but the word is elusive. The area stimulated controls naming. The mapping of the cortical areas goes on like this.

The frontal and the temporoparietal lobes of the left hemisphere are mostly involved with language. Within these areas, specific groups of cells might specialize in particular aspects of language. For example, an area in the frontal cortex controls grammar; another area in the same cortex controls facial movements, including those of speech. Certain sites in the temporoparietal lobe control short-term memory for verbal material (remembering what you read or heard a few minutes ago).

The sites of particular language functions (grammar, short-term memory) are not the same for all individuals, a fact not mentioned in many books. The only relatively stable area across individuals seems to be the back portion of the frontal area that controls speech production. The rest of the language functions may be localized in different parts of the frontal and temporoparietal lobes. In fact, Calvin and Ojemann (1980, p. 29) wrote, "The individual pattern of language localization seems to be quite variable, perhaps as variable as individual appearance." It is good to commit this striking statement to your long-term memory.

The two hemispheres and their four lobes are structurally similar but not identical. In a majority of people, the left hemisphere is slightly larger than the right hemisphere; the enlarged portions are concerned with speech, language, and writing. Such anatomical facts and the pathological changes observed in stroke patients have supported the idea that in a majority of cases, the left hemisphere is dominant for language.

In recent years, the left brain–right brain dichotomy has been a topic of both popular and technical writing. The idea that the left brain controls language and logic and the right brain controls musical performance and spatial ability is becoming widely known. However, it must be remembered that humans do not have two unrelated brains on each side of the head. The brain is an integrated network of cells. The two hemispheres are connected by corpus callosum, association fibers, and other structures through which they communicate. Injury to any one area is likely to have a widespread effect.

Two Canadian surgeons, Penfield and Roberts, did pioneering work on brain and language.

Read Calvin and Ojemann (1980) for a lucidly written description of brain mapping.

Broca's area and Wernicke's area also are connected through a band of fibers.

Summary

- Language, which is more conceptual and abstract than speech, is the function of higher cortical centers.
- The frontal lobe of the cortex is more directly involved in speech–language production.
- The temporal lobe is more directly involved in speech–language comprehension.
- In most persons, the left cerebral hemisphere exerts a greater influence on language.
- The brain stem contains the neural pathways that conduct motor and sensory impulses to and from the brain.
- The pyramidal and the extrapyramidal systems control the movements of various muscles, including those involved in speech.
- The cerebellum is a coordinator of movement.
- Cranial nerves (V, VII, IX, X, XI, and XII) are involved with speech production. Spinal nerves that control breathing also are important for speech.

We now turn our attention to language, speech, memory, attention, intellectual, and related problems that are caused by damage to various parts of the brain, especially those that are involved in the regulation of language and speech.

Aphasia

Strokes, which are the most common causes of aphasia, strike more than half a million people in the United States every year. After heart diseases and cancer, strokes are the third leading cause of death in the country. About 2 million people who have survived a stroke live in the United States, and roughly half of them have aphasia.

A Physician's Story of Aphasia

The anonymous patient quoted at the beginning of this chapter was a 52-year-old pediatrician who had a busy practice until the night he had the stroke. He had a hectic day at the office and came home very tired at 7 P.M. On his way home, he thought that he did not feel good, but he could not pinpoint anything. He dismissed the thought by telling himself that he was just too tired. He remembered that he had started the day very early. At 6 A.M., he had to visit one of his patients in the hospital. At the office, he had no relief until he closed it. He had to skip lunch to visit another sick baby he had hospitalized. He was very hungry. So while driving home, he prescribed himself a hearty dinner for his hunger and a chat with his wife, his comfortable

(continues)

La-Z-Boy, and the bulky evening newspaper for his vague and unsettling feeling, dominated by fatigue.

He and his wife talked about their day and ate their dinner. He helped his wife to load the dishwasher. While doing this, he suddenly broke a glass, and found that instead of placing the glass in the top tray of the dishwasher, he had smashed it against the tiled edge of the countertop. He wondered for a second about it, but he dismissed it as an accident.

Soon he settled himself in his comfortable chair and began to read the newspaper. The thought that he still did not feel well recurred, and he wondered why his prescriptions were not working. He did not say anything to his wife as his feelings were vague. As he read the paper, his vision became a bit blurry; he could not concentrate on the stories. He kept reading, struggling, and wondering a bit. Then he wanted to tell his wife something so he turned around to see where she was; not seeing her, he stood up to find her, still holding a section of the paper in his hand.

He thought he was going to take a step forward, but the newspaper slipped out of his hand, and he slowly crumbled to the floor. The soft thud his fall made brought his wife running to the living room where she found her husband on the floor. Apparently, he was in some pain, but what struck her the most was the dazed expression on his face.

The physician had had a stroke.

He was soon on his way to the hospital in an ambulance. Later he was told that he had a second stroke before reaching the hospital. He found that he could not sign his name on the admission papers; to his amazement, all he could do was to scribble like a 2-year-old. Looking at his writing, the physician thought of a poorly drawn network of nerve fibers. He tried to talk to his wife, the attending physician, and the nurses who surrounded him, but all he could say was to endlessly repeat "shucks." Stronger expletives that he had avoided all his life began to flow freely out of his mouth. Sometimes he did not know he was uttering obscenities, and at other times what came out of his mouth surprised him. At times, he could not remember his or his wife's name. When he did remember, he could not say them right. Jumbled, tangled, and confused, his expressions did not make much sense.

The physician had aphasia.

Aphasia: What It Is and What It Is Not

It is not possible to define aphasia in a sentence or two. It is better described than defined. **Aphasia** is a language disorder associated with brain injury; an impairment in understanding and formulating complex, meaningful, and ordered or sequenced elements of language including words, phrases and sentences; a difficulty in remembering words, saying the correct words, or saying words in correct syntactic order; a difficulty in talking grammatically; difficulty in reading and writing in conjunction with the described oral language problems; and difficulty understanding or expressing through gestures (Benson & Ardila, 1996; Brookshire, 1997; Darley, 1982; Davis, 2000; Hegde, 1998; LaPointe, 1997; Payne, 1997; Rosenbek, LaPointe, & Wertz, 1989).

What aphasia is not also can be described briefly: It is not a speech disorder of neurological origin; it does not necessarily suggest a deterioration in

Read Kopit's play *Wings* for a fascinating literary account of aphasia.

intelligence (dementia) found in some progressive neurological diseases; it is not the confused language or mutism found in some neurologically impaired patients (Damasio, 1981; Darley, 1982); and it is not the bizarre language of the schizophrenic patients.

The description is not comprehensive and applies to most but not all patients. What follows is an elaboration of the problems mentioned and description of additional problems.

Communicative Problems of the Patient with Aphasia

The behaviors of patients with aphasia show both variability and complexity. For the expert who invents a technical name for any kind of difficulty, the language of patients with aphasia has been especially exciting. As will be discussed shortly, most of the difficulties of people with aphasia have been given technical names and are evident in speaking, reading, writing, and understanding language.

Spoken Language

A majority of patients with aphasia are willing to talk. Unlike the person who exhibits mutism due to psychological, behavioral, or neurological reasons, patients with aphasia make great efforts to express themselves. But their efforts are full of mistakes, which add up to a great variety.

Anomia. Difficulty in naming things, objects, and people is called **anomia.** It is a basic problem people with aphasia face. Patients who recover from aphasia often have reported that they knew what they wanted to say but had difficulty finding the right word for it. When they cannot think of the right word, they try hard to somehow get that word activated. Some patients show such struggle in their face that the listener gets the impression that they are trying to literally squeeze the word out of their exhausted brain.

A patient with aphasia who cannot find a word may be able to talk about it in the fashion of beating around the bush. A patient, when asked to name the picture of a pair of shoes, said, "Well, it is made up . . . well, leather. It has lace on them. You wear it on your feet. . . ." He repeatedly pointed to his own shoes, but could not name them.

A wrong response, dredged up after much effort, may persist even when the patient realizes the mistake. A patient who said "hat" when shown a picture of a *house,* went on like this: "Hat. Shucks, no. Hat. No, that is not it. Hat. No, you live in it. Hat." Then he gave up in frustration and dismay.

Paraphasia. A word substitution problem is called **paraphasia.** It is found frequently in people with aphasia who can talk fluently and grammatically. But the words they cannot remember are easily substituted with wrong or unusual words. Some substituted words *sound* like the correct words; hence, the problem is called **phonemic paraphasia.** These are word substitutions based on phonemic similarity. A patient asked for a *hiss* instead of a *kiss* from his wife; another asked for *loose* when she wanted *juice.* Other examples include *gun* for *fun, life* for *wife,* and *fixed* for *mixed.*

Some other substituted words have meanings similar to the correct words. This is known as **verbal paraphasia.** In this case, words that tend to appear together in everyday usage cause confusion; the patient uses a wrong word of the pair. For example, a woman with aphasia constantly referred to her husband as "wife"; another man referred to his daughter as "son"; another person, holding a pen in his hand and wanting a piece of paper, repeatedly asked for "pen." At other times, two words of a paired expression may be reversed. *Sidewalk* may become *walk side* and *walkie-talkie* may be turned around to *talkie-walkie.*

Another kind of paraphasia is called **neologism,** which is the creation of new words, often meaningless in the case of patients with aphasia. Patients simply use a "word," often quite confidently, but the word is their pure creation. It does not exist in the language. A patient with aphasia looked at a computer in a clinic room and called it an "ibmash." A chair was a "ponty," and a pen was a "badle."

Agrammatism. Another major characteristic of patients with aphasia, **agrammatism,** is the omission of certain grammatical elements. The speech sounds like a telegram, in which articles and other grammatical words are omitted. Patients with aphasia also omit many grammatic morphemes that are essential to understand the meaning of utterances. For example, the plural /s/ inflection, past tense inflection *ed*, articles, conjunctions, and prepositions might be omitted.

The agrammatic patient speaks in short phrases and struggles to say them. The patient is not fluent; the speech is full of pauses and other forms of dysfluencies. The patient speaks in broken sentences and thus appears to have lost control on the basic structure of his or her language. The speech lacks the normal patterns of intonation.

Jargon. Relatively fluent but irrelevant or meaningless speech is called **jargon** in aphasia literature. Its patterns of intonation are normal. It is the opposite of the fragmented agrammatic speech. The patient responds almost readily to questions asked; the speech follows the normal syntactic arrangements, the "sentences" are relatively long, and the expressions are smooth and free flowing. But the meaning is either irrelevant to the preceding question or totally obscure.

A patient who was asked, "What did you do this morning?" said, "Fine. Everything is just fine so I plan to go for it right away." This is an example of an irrelevant speech; it could have been meaningful in response to some other question. But the response of another patient illustrates the meaningless variety of jargon. When asked to name her home town, a 63-year-old woman replied, "Try head shoe, OK, it is make back, but really awful. It is so make back head in morning so you can. Try it!"

Some jargon contains neologistic "words" created by the patient and mixed with already incomprehensible utterances. In response to the question, "What is your occupation?" an English literature professor with aphasia replied this way: "You see what I do is quite nice to go exactly to the grocery, but it is perfectly *entequin*. Not in the least, though it is a job I like to do in the education of young *quintoes* as you can imagine the problem I have in the morning. It is the *trandone* that you and I are concerned with."

Verbal Stereotypes. Some patients with aphasia, especially those who are severely affected, seem to get stuck with a few stereotypic expressions. The patients give the same response to any question they face. The response might be "yes," "no," "That is right," or "I see." In some cases, however, a patient's stereotyped expression may be an obscene word. To the dismay of the family members, a gentleman or a lady who has never used such a word before may routinely, promptly, and with a straight face say the word in response to every question.

Jargon is technical (hence often incomprehensible) language in everyday usage.

Some patients may have **neologistic stereotypes** that are not meaningful in any context. In response to most questions asked, a 68-year-old man with aphasia either said "Gutty, gutty, gutty" or "Ledder, ledder, ledder."

Summary

- Some patients with aphasia struggle too much while trying to say something; such patients often exhibit agrammatism, anomia, and paraphasia.

- Other aphasic patients talk fluently but do not make sense; such patients often exhibit jargon and neologism.

- The profoundly affected patients say very little or use verbal stereotypes including the neologistic variety.

Writing and Reading

The writing problems of a person with aphasia are called **agraphia.** Some patients cannot write anything. Most appear as forgetful in writing as in speaking. The letters are poorly formed or nothing more than a meaningless scribble. The writing is full of mistakes even when the preferred hand is not paralyzed. Some patients cannot write what they can say perfectly. Others make the same kind of mistakes in both speaking and writing. They may omit words, use neologisms and jargon, delete grammatic morphemes, and use wrong word arrangements.

Reading problems are called **alexia.** Some patients with aphasia do not recognize even the simplest of printed words. Patients may not read the words they use in speech. Those who can, might make the same kind of mistakes in their reading and speaking. A patient may read the word *son* as "daughter," which may be a confusion based on paired usage. Another may read the word *horse* as "luddy," a case of neologism.

Comprehension of Spoken Speech

Not understanding the speech of other people is a significant problem of the patient with aphasia even when the patient appears to pay close attention to what is told. Some patients may give stereotypic responses ("Yes"; "I think so") that mislead the speaker into thinking that they understand what is spoken to them. This thinly disguised problem is easily exposed when the clinician asks "What is your name?" and the patient replies, "I think so!"

Some patients with aphasia have special sensory deficits that can be independent of their aphasia. Injury to the sensory areas of the brain can cause various types of **agnosias,** which are difficulties in understanding the meaning of sensory information. Thus, aphasia may coexist with agnosia. In **auditory verbal agnosia,** the patient can hear, but cannot recognize the meaning of words unless the object the word names is shown. In **visual agnosia,** the patient cannot tell what it is by looking at something; he or she must hear the sound it makes or touch and feel it to say the word.

Many people think that the patient with aphasia does not understand spoken language because of no response or wrong responses. However, the writings of people who have recovered from aphasia suggest that on many occasions they understood what was spoken to them, they thought they gave the correct response, and then they wondered why the speaker kept asking the same stupid question (Armstrong, 1979; Hodgins, 1964). Only after the recovery does a patient realize that he or she did not respond to questions or said something meaningless.

To Classify or Not To Classify Aphasia

The discoveries of Broca in 1861 and Wernicke in 1874 prompted the idea that there are different types of aphasia. Broca's patient was nonfluent, whereas Wernicke's patient was fluent but had marked difficulty in understanding speech. Ever since, experts have argued whether aphasia is a single disorder or whether there are different types. Over the years, more than two dozen classifications have been proposed (McNeil, 1988). Currently, among those who believe in classifying aphasia according to its symptoms, etiology, or both, the Boston classification, summarized in Table 9.1, is popular. This classification has two broad categories: the fluent and the nonfluent aphasias, and each category includes different aphasias (Goodglass & Kaplan, 1983a).

Other clinicians have argued that there is only one kind of aphasia. In most patients with aphasia, speaking, understanding, reading, writing, and gesturing are all impaired to some extent, although some symptoms may be more subtle than others (Calvin & Ojemann, 1980; Darley, 1982; Schuell & Sefer, 1973). Anatomically, the motor speech area and the auditory speech area are closely connected. In fact, brain cells that specialize in speaking and understanding can

Table 9.1

Types of Aphasia According to the Boston Classification

Types	Characteristics
Nonfluent aphasias	
Broca's aphasia	Agrammatism; effortful speech; short phrases; lacks intonation; nonfluent; presence of apraxia; good comprehension; impaired repetition; mostly expressive (motor) problems.
Transcortical motor aphasia	Spontaneous speech characteristics similar to Broca's except good imitation of speech, even long sentences.
Global aphasia	All language functions affected; severe deficits in comprehension and production; verbal stereotypes; the most severe form of aphasia.
Fluent aphasias	
Wernicke's aphasia	Fluent but meaningless speech; impaired auditory comprehension of speech; jargon, neologism; good articulation and intonation.
Conduction aphasia	Somewhat fluent speech; only minor comprehension problems; marked difficulty in repeating words and phrases.
Anomic aphasia	Marked word-finding problem; near-normal language; good comprehension.

be found in both the frontal and temporoparietal cortex (Calvin & Ojemann, 1980).

Some patients may have problems in addition to their aphasia, thus giving a picture of some unique set of symptoms. For example, a patient with aphasia may have paralysis or weakness of the speech muscles, giving rise to a disorder called **dysarthria,** to be described later. In such a patient, aphasia may seem to include different symptoms, but those are the symptoms of dysarthria, not aphasia (Darley, 1982).

Some researchers have questioned the validity of long-established beliefs regarding Broca's aphasia (Mohr, 1980). It has been pointed out that, curiously, Broca's first and most celebrated patient may not have had Broca's aphasia. Broca was a staff physician in a large nursing home in Paris where the first patient he reported on was a man named LeBorgne, but better known as "Tan-tan" because he could not say anything but "Tan-tan." In essence, a severe case of nonfluent aphasia. When Tan-tan died, Broca did an autopsy on him, removed the entire brain for examination, but did not dissect the brain. The famous brain can be viewed in its intact form in a Paris museum. The often-cited pathological tissue changes in the frontal cortex were not actually observed in this first patient (Calvin & Ojemann, 1980).

It also is known that damage limited to Broca's area does not cause nonfluent Broca's aphasia, but apraxia. The early symptom is mutism, which rapidly improves, but the regained speech is full of articulation errors. The language is relatively intact (Darley, 1982). The traditional Broca's aphasia is caused by extensive brain injury not limited to Broca's area (Mohr, 1980).

Causes of Aphasia

A cause of a disorder or disease often is a sequence or chain of events. The etiology of aphasia provides a superb illustration of causal chains. For example, the immediate cause of aphasia is brain injury, but brain injury has many causes. The source of injury may be external, such as in the case of automobile accidents, or internal, such as in case of a stroke, which is technically known as the **cerebrovascular accident.** As noted before, stroke is the most common cause of aphasia.

Strokes, in turn, are caused by many factors. High blood pressure, high levels of blood cholesterol, and cerebral arteriosclerosis are among the most frequent causes of stroke. **Cerebral arteriosclerosis** is the hardening of the cerebral arteries, which become thickened. Elasticity of the arteries is lost or reduced and their walls are weakened. Therefore, the flow of blood is restricted.

The brain tissue dies within 3 minutes of blood interruption.

The cerebral arteriosclerosis is only an element of the chain of causes. The immediate cause of a stroke is due to other factors. For example, the actual stroke may be due to an **embolus,** which can be a blood clot, fatty materials, or an air bubble that forms a wedge-shaped obstruction of the blood flow (**embolism**). The traveling embolus eventually blocks the flow of blood in one of the smaller arteries. Lack of blood supply cuts off the oxygen to the brain cells, which are then damaged.

Another immediate cause of stroke is **thrombosis,** which is the presence of a blood clot at the point of its origin. The **thrombus,** or the stationary blood clot, blocks the flow of blood and thus causes a stroke.

Yet another immediate cause of stroke is **aneurysm,** which is a sacklike bulging on the wall of a weakened artery. The bulge may eventually rupture, causing **cerebral hemorrhage.** The brain cells in the hemorrhaged area are damaged because of a lack of blood flow and oxygen supply.

Epilepsy, meningitis, encephalitis, brain tumors, and accidents during brain surgery are all potential causes of brain injury.

A stroke often leaves the person paralyzed, although not all patients with aphasia are paralyzed. For example, patients with Wernicke's aphasia might not show obvious signs of neurological damage. These patients usually are not paralyzed. However, paralysis is due to damage to a hemisphere that is on the opposite side: injury to the left hemisphere produces paralysis on the right side of the body. In all of the right-handed people, and in some left-handed people as well, injury to the language-dominant left hemisphere, which paralyzes the right side of the body, produces aphasia. Injury to the right hemisphere produces aphasia in only 3% of the general population (Calvin & Ojemann, 1980). This is a portion of the left-handed people whose right hemisphere is dominant for language.

Assessment of the Patient with Aphasia

Before designing a treatment program for aphasia (or any other disorder of communication), the patient's communicative problems should be assessed. The assessment module, presented in Table 9.2, highlights procedures that are unique to assessing patients with aphasia. These procedures help determine the nature and extent of aphasia.

Case history, results of neurological and other medical examinations, careful observation of the patient's speech and general behavior, and listening to what the patient says and how the patient talks are important in determining the nature and extent of aphasia (Davis, 2000; Helm-Estabrooks & Albert, 1991;

Table 9.2

Assessment of Communicative Disorders: Aphasia

....

1. History of the client, the family, and the disorder

2. Interview of the client, the family members, or both

3. Orofacial examination

4. Hearing screening

5. Speech and language sampling

6. **Measurement/assessment of:**
    a. **general language performance**
    b. **functional communication**
    c. **auditory comprehension**
    d. **oral expressive language**
    e. **reading and writing skills**
    f. **gestures and other nonverbal means of communication**
    g. **conversational skills**
    h. **specific aspects of language (phonological, semantic, syntactic, morphological, and pragmatic)**

7. Recommendations

8. Report writing

....

Note. Procedures unique to assessment of aphasia are in bold print.

Rosenbek et al., 1989). Clinicians might use one of several standardized tests, including the *Minnesota Test for Differential Diagnosis of Aphasia* (Schuell & Sefer, 1973), the *Boston Diagnostic Aphasia Test* (Goodglass & Kaplan, 1983b), the *Porch Index of Communicative Ability* (Porch, 1981), and the *Western Aphasia Battery* (Kertesz, 1982).

On most tests, the clinician asks the patient to name a set of pictures, point to a particular picture, repeat sentences or phrases, recite the days of the week, describe the use of objects, answer specific questions, read a story and summarize it, and write a few lines. Through these and other tasks, the clinician evaluates the patient's understanding of spoken speech, use of grammatical and syntactic features, articulation, and other aspects of communication. Based on some test results, the severity of aphasia might be rated as either mild, moderate, or severe. Potential areas of brain injury and the type of aphasia may be suggested.

Beyond standardized tests and language samples, clinicians use functional assessment tools. **Functional assessment** concentrates on how the patient communicates in everyday situations, including how the client interacts with health care workers. Several functional assessment tools are now available. One such tool, *Functional Assessment of Communication Skills for Adults* (Frattali, Thompson, Holland, Wohl, & Ferketi, 1995), helps assess how a patient communicates in social situations, expresses basic needs, reads and writes, and makes daily planning. Note that such an approach does not emphasize grammatical accuracy. It is concerned with naturalistic communication.

Treatment of Aphasia

The language performance of most patients with aphasia improves to some degree without much help from a speech–language pathologist. This is known as **spontaneous recovery.** The rate of recovery is generally faster during the first few weeks after the stroke, and the rate eventually slows down and becomes negligible after 6 months. Therefore, treatment of aphasia should be started as soon as possible. Early and continued treatment can be expected to increase the rate of recovery and help achieve sustained improvement in language behaviors.

Many procedures are used in the rehabilitation of people with aphasia. Details of treatment targets and procedures may be found in books on aphasia (Brookshire, 1997; Chapey, 1994; Davis, 2000; Hegde, 1998; Helm-Estabrooks & Albert, 1991; LaPointe, 1997; Rosenbek et al., 1989). Only a few essential features of treatment are summarized here. The goals of treatment may vary depending on the individual patient. But in all cases, *functional communication*—effective communication in natural settings—is the goal of all aphasia treatment. If this goal can be achieved by teaching the clients use of language, gestures, writing, signing, printed messages on a board, or an electronic keyboard, so much the better. The clinician's main goal is to help the patient regain as much language as possible and learn new skills that compensate residual problems (Rosenbek et al., 1989). In the beginning, individual therapy is the most effective. After establishing certain communicative behaviors, group therapy can be used to strengthen them and to encourage social interactions.

Based on the results of assessment, the clinician selects certain target behaviors for the particular patient. For example, the clinician may determine that teaching recognition and production of selected words is best for a given client. Recognition may be defined as correctly pointing to a particular picture when a set of pictures is presented. For another client, functional communication involving verbalizing simple requests (e.g., "water, please") and names of family members may be judged appropriate.

Stimuli to the selected verbal responses are then prepared. They can be pictures, drawings, actual objects, or specially created situations. A baseline of the patient's performance is established. **Baselines** are measures of what the client can and cannot do without treatment and help determine whether the patient is improving. If the patient is not showing improvement, the clinician changes the target behaviors, the treatment procedures, or both.

The selected target behaviors are then trained in individual sessions. The patient is asked to listen to the clinician's production of a word to encourage auditory recognition. The patient is encouraged to imitate the clinician's productions. The patient is positively reinforced for attentive listening, imitative responses, and other correct responses.

The task is made progressively more complex. For example, the patient who can recall single words or give single-word responses to questions may be moved to the next level of therapy in which two-word phrases are taught. A patient who can request "water" may be taught to say "water, please" or "some juice, please." In successive stages, more complex responses may be taught. But in teaching complex language, the clinician never loses the sight of functional communication in everyday situations. If a client cannot learn complex and grammatically correct language, he or she still can learn means of communicating basic needs and expressing simple messages.

When the patient begins to give correct responses reliably, the clinician implements procedures designed to promote generalization and maintenance of those responses. The family members are trained to evoke and reinforce newly learned verbal responses at home. Patients with aphasia need support from the family members to maintain relearned communicative behaviors. Procedures similar to these have been described by Holland (1970) and LaPointe (1985). This approach makes use of the concepts and methods of **programmed learning** and **behavioral principles**.

Some clinicians believe that auditory stimulation is the first and the most important element of treatment (Schuell, Jenkins, & Jimenez-Pabon, 1964). It is thought that the person with aphasia knows vocabulary and grammar but has lost the auditory connection to linguistic symbols. Accordingly, the emphasis is not so much on having the patient produce specific verbal responses, but on having the patient listen to language spoken slowly and in simple sentences. While receiving intense auditory stimulation through language, the patient may be encouraged to make any kind of communicative response including pointing, gesturing, saying a word along with the clinician, and imitating.

Counseling the family of patients with aphasia is an important aspect of treatment. Aphasia profoundly alters the interpersonal relationships. The stroke and the resulting aphasia are devastating to the patients and their families alike. The family members need to know that there is hope for the patient and that, with concerted effort by the physician, the speech–language pathologist, the physical therapists, and other specialists, the patient with aphasia can be rehabilitated to a significant extent. The family members also should know that they play a major role in rehabilitating the patient. The patient with aphasia needs emotional support, patience, and positive feedback. The speech–language pathologist helps the family members understand these and other problems and solutions. The clinician counsels them and suggests methods of supporting, encouraging, and reinforcing the patient's attempts at communication.

Summary

- An intact brain is necessary for proper formulation, expression, and comprehension of language.

- Aphasia is a language disorder due to brain injury caused by accidents and many diseases including brain tumor and cerebral vascular pathologies. The disorder includes problems in comprehension, formulation, and expression of language as well as those in reading and writing.

- Some patients with aphasia talk fluently but do not make much sense; others struggle to say a word or to form a sentence.

- Specific problems exhibited by patients with aphasia include anomia, paraphasia, agrammatism, jargon, verbal stereotypes, agraphia, alexia, and agnosia.

- Whereas some experts believe that aphasia is a single, complex disorder that affects all aspects of language use, others believe that it can be classified into several varieties. Accordingly, the two categories of aphasia are the fluent and the nonfluent.

- Many treatment procedures are available to help a patient with aphasia recover some or most of the lost language skills.

Motor Speech Disorders

Neurological damage can cause not only aphasia, a central language disorder, but also speech disorders, which are distinguished from each other and from aphasia. Speech disorders that result from central or peripheral nervous system damage are called **motor speech disorders** or **neurogenic speech disorders**. There are two major categories of motor speech disorders: apraxia of speech and dysarthria.

Verbal Apraxia

Apraxia is a neuromuscular disorder of sequenced movement of body parts in the absence of muscle weakness or paralysis. There are different kinds of apraxia. When the patient cannot move the muscles of the throat, soft palate, tongue, and cheek for nonspeech purposes, the disorder is called **oral apraxia**. A patient with oral apraxia may not be able to stick the tongue out or lick the lips when asked to do so. But while eating ice cream on a cone, the patient has no difficulty in making the same movements, suggesting that there is no paralysis or muscle weakness. The action is possible, the muscles are capable, and the actions are exhibited at other times. However, as a response to a verbal request, the patient's movements are clumsy and confused.

Some patients cannot comply when requested to move their hand to wave good-bye or to show how a hammer is used. On their own, they may be able to execute these movements. This is called **limb apraxia.**

A difficulty in initiating and executing the movement patterns necessary to produce speech when there is no paralysis, weakness, or discoordination of speech muscles is called **verbal apraxia** or **apraxia of speech.** A distinct problem of articulating speech sounds is the predominant result of this movement disorder. A disturbed prosody also may be present (Brookshire, 1997; Darley, Aronson, & Brown, 1975; Duffy, 1995; Ferrand & Bloom, 1997; Freed, 2000; Haynes, 1985; Kearns & Simmons, 1988; Kent & Rosenbek, 1983; Wertz, 1985; Yorkston et al., 1999).

A patient with apraxia of speech has difficulty positioning the articulators (the tongue and the lips) correctly. The patient seems to be unsure of the movements necessary to produce a certain sequence of speech sounds. The patient makes many errors of articulation, recognizes the errors, and makes repeated attempts to correct the errors. But each attempt might result in a different kind of mistake. Such variability of errors across trials is a significant feature of apraxia of speech.

The patient with verbal apraxia makes more errors on consonants than on vowels; the most errors are found on consonant clusters (e.g., /dr/ in *drinking* or /str/ in *streets*). For example, a patient who was asked to say *strategy* produced the following responses: "Statir . . . Tatar . . . Strkeg . . . Stratipy . . . Satirigy . . . I can't do it." Phonemes and words that are used more frequently are produced with greater accuracy than those that are used less frequently. The speech sounds of a word may be produced out of sequence. When asked to say the word *California,* for example, a patient with apraxia produced the following attempts: "Lala . . . Hala . . . uh . . . Calfa . . . Calanor . . . Calforfa . . . Halfnora . . . I can't get that." This illustrates the variable mistakes on repeated attempts and the frequent switching of the phonemic sequence of the target word. Complex or longer words are more difficult than simpler or shorter words.

Patients with verbal apraxia are able to produce the same words at other times, especially when it seems automatic. Their speech at times is well articulated. At the end of the session, the patient who could not say *California* upon request, remarked freely and easily, "I can't believe the amount of trouble I had on *California!*"

The apraxic speech may not sound normal because of the disturbed rhythm and intonation. This may be due to the broken, dysfluent, and repetitive speech attempts because normal rhythm and intonation are associated with speech that flows smoothly.

Verbal apraxia can occur without other kinds of speech or language problems. However, it is most frequently associated with aphasia. These patients, then, have a language disorder and a speech disorder, both due to neurological damage.

In the absence of aphasia, a patient with verbal apraxia can handle the structures of language well. There are no unusual problems with the morphological and syntactic aspects of language. The person who cannot say a word can write it. The articulatory problems are not due to word finding problems that are seen in patients with aphasia.

Verbal apraxia in adult patients is associated with various kinds of neuropathological factors that have been well documented. However, some experts believe that children also exhibit apraxia, including verbal apraxia (Hall,

Jordan, & Robin, 1993). This problem is known as **developmental apraxia.** Currently, the concept of developmental apraxia is controversial because neurological injury or diseases in children thought to have this disorder are not documented. Researchers do not fully agree on the symptoms of developmental apraxia either (Thompson, 1988). Children who are diagnosed with developmental apraxia most often show numerous errors of articulation, including such unusual errors as added sounds (e.g., "clat" for *cat*), prolongation of sounds, and repetition of sounds and syllables (Hall et al., 1993).

In adult patients, verbal apraxia is thought to be the result of a lesion in the central motor programming area, such as Broca's area in the left frontal lobe (Darley et al., 1975). It is hypothesized that a motor speech programmer in the brain plans and executes various movement patterns necessary for speech. When the working of this programmer is impaired by brain injury, the patient has difficulty in positioning the articulators and moving them according to a plan necessary for producing words.

Other experts have hypothesized that verbal apraxia is due to a disordered phonological system (Klich, Ireland, & Weidner, 1979; Marquardt, Rinehardt, & Peterson, 1979; Shewan, 1980). Accordingly, verbal apraxia is caused by the errors in the sound system of language represented in the brain. Phonological impairment, described in Chapter 4, is a disorder of the sound system of a language. Such an impairment induces errors of articulation. Therefore, the articulatory problems of the patient with verbal apraxia may be explained on this basis. Some scientists have cautioned that it is too early to conclude on the nature of verbal apraxia and that more research is needed to resolve the issue (Kent & Rosenbek, 1983).

Treatment of Verbal Apraxia

The main target of treatment for a patient with verbal apraxia is the sequenced production of speech sounds and motor planning needed for this task. Modification of vocal and resonance qualities may be of secondary concern.

Initially, nonspeech movements of the tongue or lips may be practiced, especially if the patient also is orally apraxic. Once the patient begins to consistently produce selected nonspeech movements (such as gently biting the lower lip or opening the mouth) upon request, movements of target speech sounds are practiced. For each patient, procedures that facilitate correct responses are discovered and practiced by the patient again and again. For example, some patients articulate a difficult word when they say it along with the clinician; others can imitate after the clinician has modeled it; still others can say the word or make an isolated sound only when the clinician shapes the lips or pulls the jaw down with his or her hand. Some patients include an omitted syllable when the clinician puts an extra emphasis on them; others respond better when spoken to at a slower rate. Thus, for each patient, what works is first determined and then repeatedly practiced.

During therapy, the patient is provided with multisensory stimulation. The patient hears correctly articulated speech sounds; possibly sees the movements of the articulators; and feels the different positions of the tongue, lips, and soft palate when he or she produces different speech sounds and syllables. After the patient learns simpler sounds and words, more difficult sounds and words are taught. More complex movement patterns of consonant clusters are trained last. Improved articulation on semiautomatic, everyday expressions ("Good morning"; "How are you?"; "I am fine") also are practiced and reinforced.

In gradual steps, the clinician models words, phrases, and sentences. The patient receives reinforcement for correctly imitating them. Eventually, more accurate productions in evoked (spontaneous, not imitated) speech are strengthened.

Patients with severe apraxia who have very little speech and do not respond to the best efforts of the clinician may be candidates for nonverbal modes of communication. For example, patients who do not also have severe limb apraxia may learn a form of sign language or other forms of nonverbal communication described later in the chapter.

Dysarthria

Dysarthria is a group of speech disorders due to paralysis, weakness, or incoordination of the speech muscles. In this respect, it is unlike verbal apraxia and aphasia. The patients with dysarthria alone have no difficulty with the structure of language. They may have a good vocabulary and good control on syntax and morphological features of language. They give appropriate answers to questions. They can write the words that they cannot say well. The patients can read as usual, and the reading comprehension is good. In this respect, dysarthria is like apraxia. However, unlike apraxia, dysarthria is a speech disorder associated with problems in speech muscle control. There is no such problem in apraxia (Brookshire, 1997; Darley et al., 1975; Duffy, 1995; Ferrand & Bloom, 1997; Freed, 2000; Yorkston et al., 1999).

There are different types of dysarthria. Therefore, the plural form, dysarthrias, often is used. The different types are caused by lesions in different parts of the brain, the pyramidal and the extrapyramidal motor pathways, and the peripheral nerves that supply speech muscles. Many kinds of neurological diseases cause these lesions.

The different types of dysarthria share many common speech problems. They tend to show deviations in respiration, phonation, resonance, articulation, and prosody. As the following summary shows, all of the neurophysiological speech processes and functions are affected in dysarthria:

- **Respiratory problems.** The dysarthric patient may not have enough breath supply to speak adequately. Breathing may be forced and audible.
- **Phonatory problems.** The patient's vocal pitch may be too high or too low. There may be pitch breaks. The voice may not be loud enough, or there may be abrupt variations in loudness. Voice may sound breathy or harsh. It also may sound hoarse (both breathy and harsh).
- **Resonance problems.** Modification of the laryngeal tone by the cavities of the throat, nose, and mouth may be abnormal. The typical symptom is hypernasality.
- **Articulatory problems.** Errors of articulation are more consistent than in apraxia, but they may still show some variability. Speech sounds may be omitted, distorted, or imprecisely formed. Both consonants and vowels may be abnormally prolonged.
- **Prosodic problems.** The person with dysarthria may have a rate of speech that is too slow, too fast, or abnormally variable. Syllables may be stressed or unstressed, both inappropriately.

The muscular problems of the patient with dysarthria are due to many neurological diseases and traumatic injury. Different neuropathological factors create different clusters of neurological and speech problems, though most patients with dysarthria share some common symptoms as described. Some patients with dysarthria, for example, have a lesion in the lower motoneurons. This results in **flaccid** (flabby) muscles. A dominant problem of a patient with flaccid paralysis is hypernasality. Other patients with dysarthria may have lesions in the upper motoneurons, resulting in **spastic paralysis** (stiff and rigid muscles). Such patients have slow and imprecise articulation. Still others may have lesions in the extrapyramidal system, causing reduced movements of the body (**hypokinesia**). These patients may have speech that is too soft and lacking in stress and emphasis. Lesions of the extrapyramidal system also can cause increased movement (**hyperkinesia**) and a different set of speech problems including imprecise articulation (Darley et al., 1975; Duffy, 1995; Freed, 2000).

Treatment of Dysarthria

Treatment of dysarthria takes place in the context of a neurological disease or trauma. Some of the diseases are progressive with no medical treatment. Therefore, the type of speech treatment and the extent of improvement under treatment will depend on many factors, including the nature and the severity of the disease or trauma and the level of the patient's motivation for improved communication. In cases of irreversible and severe neurological diseases, the most the speech clinician can accomplish is to help the patient make the best use of the affected speech mechanism and to teach skills that somehow compensate for the neuromuscular deficit. In all cases, the clinician counsels and supports the patient and his or her family.

The **specific speech treatment goals** for patients with dysarthria include modification of the problems of (a) posture, tone, and strength of muscles; (b) respiration; (c) phonation; (d) resonation; (e) articulation; and (f) prosody. When these efforts are not productive or are judged unsuitable for a given patient, the clinician may teach nonverbal modes of communication (Kearns & Simmons, 1988; Rosenbek & LaPointe, 1985; Wertz, 1985; Yorkston et al., 1988).

Posture, tone, and **strength** of muscles are improved by a variety of physical exercises, some of which are implemented by a physical therapist. Excessive muscle tone (hypertonia) may be treated with relaxation training. The speech–language pathologist determines the most useful and medically safe postural adjustments that are related to speech. For example, a patient whose neck muscles are weak may use a neck brace that will help keep the neck straight while talking. This usually has a beneficial effect on speech.

Modification of **respiratory problems** also may be facilitated by postural adjustments and muscle training. The physical therapist guides the patient through exercises that strengthen the abdominal muscles of breathing. The patient may be trained to sustain exhalation for longer periods of time to produce longer as well as louder utterances.

Modification of **phonation** involves several procedures. A patient with paralyzed vocal folds may be treated surgically; the paralyzed fold may be injected with Teflon to make it bulge so that the movement of the normal fold

There is more about Teflon injection of paralyzed folds in **Chapter 7.**

is sufficient to make contact. However, if the problem is one of hyperadduction of folds (too tight closure), relaxation training might be useful.

Modification of **resonance** problems typically consists of reducing hypernasality. Generally, the treatment includes both behavioral training to achieve the velopharyngeal closure and prosthetic approaches. In the case of severe hypernasality, a palatal lift prosthetic device, which is a small plastic plate fitted over the hard palate, may be used. Its back portion extends into the soft palate and lifts it to make a contact with the back throat wall to close the nasal passage. This reduces hypernasality.

Further information on resonance problems is in **Chapter 7.**

Modification of **articulation** may be achieved to some extent by improved breath support, phonation, and resonation achieved through other procedures. Modeling correct articulation is a commonly used method of articulation training. Initially, the patient might imitate as the clinician models the target syllables, and later the patient might imitate after the clinician has completed the modeled production. A collection of methods called phonetic placement might help patients who experience great difficulty in moving the articulators into correct positions. In one such method, the clinician manipulates the lips and the tongue to demonstrate correct movement patterns needed to produce target syllables.

Treatment of articulation problems is discussed in **Chapter 4.**

Modification of **prosody** is achieved by changing the patient's pitch, loudness, rate of speech, and stress. Often, too high or too low a pitch may not be treated at all because the overall intelligibility of speech is not affected by such pitch problems. The patient also might begin to speak louder when he or she learns to speak with better breath support and muscular effort. In some cases, loudness may have to be trained behaviorally by reinforcing progressively increased loudness of speech. In some extreme cases, the patient might have to use a small, portable amplifier that makes the speech louder for listeners.

Finally, some patients simply cannot communicate verbally, in spite of best efforts from the speech–language pathologist. These patients are then taught alternative modes of communication, including various forms of sign language and communication through electronic communication boards.

Summary

- Motor speech disorders are due to neurologic involvement and include apraxia and dysarthria.

- Apraxia is an impairment of movement patterns needed to produce speech. This impairment is due to a motor programming problem and not to muscle weakness or paralysis.

- Dysarthria is a disorder of respiration, phonation, articulation, resonance, and prosody in patients who have suffered central or peripheral nervous system damage. There are six types of dysarthria: the flaccid, the spastic, the ataxic, the hypokinetic, the hyperkinetic, and the mixed.

- Motor speech disorders are contrasted with aphasia, which is a central language disturbance.

- Treatment of motor speech disorders is somewhat new and more research is needed. Most patients show improvement with treatment.

Right Hemisphere Syndrome

While it was known for a long time that the left hemisphere of the brain controls language, the functions the right hemisphere controlled remained a mystery until recent times. However, such diseases as cerebrovascular accidents (strokes), tumors, and various neurological diseases that affect the left side of the brain also can affect the right side of the brain. Studies of people whose right hemisphere was thus damaged have produced information on the functions of this hemisphere (Brookshire, 1997; Myers, 1999; Tompkins, 1995).

It is now known that the right hemisphere controls such visual functions as facial recognition, drawing, and copying; such spatial awareness as right and left side awareness; maintaining attention and readiness to respond to stimuli (arousal); orientation to space and geographic location; recognition of other people's emotional expressions; and certain aspects of communication. What follows is not a comprehensive description of symptoms but a sampling of symptoms that highlight the uniqueness of the right hemisphere syndrome (Brookshire, 1997; Hegde, 1998; Myers, 1999; Tompkins, 1995).

- **Left-neglect.** A striking feature of right hemisphere syndrome is the patients' tendency to neglect the left side of their body or what is in the left visual field. The patients might read only the right side of a printed book, bump into things or people on their left side, copy only the right side of a drawing, deny the existence of their paralyzed left arm or leg, comb only the right side of the head, and use only the right side pockets of pants or jackets.
- **Facial recognition deficits.** These deficits, also known as **prosopagnosia,** include failure to recognize familiar faces (e.g., those of family members) or familiar stimuli (e.g., a carpenter's failure to recognize his hammer or a writer's failure to recognize her pen).
- **Attentional deficits.** Impaired attention may be evident in reduced readiness to respond to stimuli, difficulty in giving sustained attention to a task, and difficulty in giving selective attention (e.g., paying attention only to selected pictures while ignoring others when several are displayed).
- **Disorientation.** This may take the form of spatial disorientation (e.g., the patients might be unable find their way in their own home) and geographic disorientation (e.g., the patients might believe that they are in a different city or hospital than they are actually in).
- **Affective deficits.** These include difficulty in comprehending emotions other people express (especially by their facial expressions and tone of voice) and confusion about emotions expressed in printed pictures.
- **Communicative deficits.** Pure linguistic (language-based) deficits are less common in patients with right hemisphere damage. Their attentional deficits, disorientation, and left-neglect complicate their communication. The more common communicative deficits include a monotone; emotionally flat speech; difficulty in narrating stories; concentrating on irrelevant details while narrating events; failure to grasp abstract, alternative, or implied meaning of messages; problems in maintaining a topic of conversation; excessive talking; and impulsive speech.

Assessment of patients with right hemisphere syndrome includes systematic observations, having the patients perform selected activities (e.g., reading aloud or copying drawings and geometric shapes), administration of standardized tests, and assessment of communication skills. Specialized tests are available to assess visual neglect, attentional deficits, and communication problems (Hegde, 1998).

Treatment of patients with right hemisphere syndrome involves two main approaches. In one approach, specific skills (e.g., turn-taking in conversational speech, copying drawings, and reading without neglecting the right side of the printed page) might be targeted for treatment. In another approach, processes thought to underlie such skills might be the target of treatment. This approach emphasizes cognitive rehabilitation (Brookshire, 1997; Hegde, 1998; Myers, 1999; Tompkins, 1995). For example, attention, which underlies various skills (such as reading and copying), may be the treatment target.

Dementia

Dementia is a serious and expensive health problem that affects older people. Chances of developing dementia increase with advancing age. The prevalence rate of dementia in people under 60 years of age is only 1%, whereas it may be as high as 25% in the population over 65. In the decade of the 1980s, the national *annual* cost of caring for people with dementia was $30 billion.

In a majority of cases, **dementia** is a neurological syndrome associated with persistent or progressive deterioration in intellectual functions. In these cases, the course of dementia is not reversible, and the patient gets progressively worse. In a few cases, dementia may be stable. In some other cases, dementia may be reversible. For example, dementia due to vitamin B_{12} deficiency may be reversed, significantly improved, or stabilized (Bayles & Kaszniak, 1987; Cummings & Benson, 1992; Payne, 1997).

There are many varieties of dementia. However, we will limit ourselves to highlighting a few common types to give a glimpse of this complex problem. Dementias are often classified into the *cortical, subcortical,* and *mixed* types. In recent years, dementia due to infections, especially that due to human immunodeficiency virus (HIV), has received much attention. Cortical dementias include the dementia of the Alzheimer's type (DAT) and dementia associated with Pick's disease. Among the subcortical dementias, that associated with Parkinson's and Huntington's diseases is the most noteworthy. Mixed dementia, in which both cortical and subcortical structures are involved, may be found in people who have suffered repeated strokes with bilateral brain damage (Brookshire, 1997; Cummings & Benson, 1992; Hegde, 1998).

Alzheimer's disease produces the most common form of cortical dementia. **Alzheimer's** is a neurological disease of the elderly characterized by several brain abnormalities. Among these, neurofibrillary tangles, neuritic plaques, and granulovacuolar degeneration are the most important. A nerve cell's body, dendrites, and axons contain filament-like structures called **neurofibrils.** When those fibrils are thickened, twisted, and looped, they are called **neurofibrillary tangles. Neuritic** or **senile plaques** are degenerated minute areas of cortical or subcortical tissue. Nerve cell degeneration due to small fluid-filled cavities are called **granulovacuolar degeneration.**

In **cortical dementias,** the neuropathology is found mostly in the cortical regions of the brain.

Dementia in patients with Alzheimer's disease progresses slowly. Mild symptoms of the initial stage slowly intensify and become progressively more debilitating. Major symptoms include loss of memory for both recent and remote events; generalized intellectual deterioration; restlessness, agitation, and hyperactivity; loss of mathematical and arithmetic skills; disorientation to place, time, and person; difficulty in self-care (e.g., dressing, bathing); wandering; lack of tact, judgment, and social appropriateness of actions resulting in uninhibited behavior; bewildered facial expression; difficulty managing such daily routines as shopping and cooking; eventual profound intellectual deterioration and complete lack of bladder control.

Communicative disorders found in patients with DAT, especially in the more advanced stages, include naming problems; difficulty in understanding speech; difficulty in generating a list of words that begin with a specific letter; repetitious, empty, and meaningless speech; inability to maintain a topic of conversation; incoherent and rapid speech; echolalia (repeating what is heard); impaired reading and writing skills; inattention to social conventions (e.g., greeting, farewell); and even mutism in the terminal stage.

In **subcortical** dementias, the neuropathology is found in structures *below* the cortex.

Of the several varieties of subcortical dementias, the one associated with Parkinson's disease is common. It is more common in males than in females. **Parkinson's disease**, popularly known as shaking palsy, is a slowly progressing neurological disease in which the nuclei in the brain stem are degenerated, the sulci in the frontal portion of the brain are widened because of neuronal loss, and dopamine production in the corpus striatum is reduced. Dopamine is a *neurotransmitter*, so called because it is a brain-produced chemical that helps transmit messages across neurons. Dementia is not a certain outcome of Parkinson's disease; it is found in only 35% to 55% of patients who have the disease. L-Dopa (levodopa) treatment can improve intellectual functions but cannot arrest the eventual and inevitable deterioration.

Symptoms of Parkinson's disease include slow voluntary movements or even immobility, tremor in resting muscles that gets worse with stress, rigidity in the muscles of the limb and trunk, masklike face, disturbed posture, muscle weakness, and festinating gait (taking short, accelerating steps). Symptoms of dementia associated with Parkinson's disease include deterioration in general intellectual functions; memory problems; impaired reasoning, word-list generation, and problem-solving skills; and flat affect and depression.

Communication problems associated with Parkinson's dementia include monotonous voice quality; faint voice; long pauses in speech, especially at the beginning of sentences; dysarthric speech; severe naming and language comprehension problems, especially in the late stage of the disease; and naming problems characterized by extremely small handwriting.

Dementia associated with **Huntington's disease** (also known as Huntington's chorea) is another subcortical variety that might have a genetic basis. Half the offspring of an affected person may have this disease. The major neuropathology is loss of neurons in the frontal and parietal regions of the brain. The dominant neurological symptoms include *chorea*, which refers to involuntary, irregular, spasmodic movement of the limbs, neck, head, and facial muscles. Other neurological symptoms include a gait that resembles dancelike walking; uncontrollable and ever-increasing facial grimaces and head-nodding; lurching, halting, and faltering movements; slow movements; and eventual loss of most voluntary movement. Behavioral or psychiatric symptoms include complaining, nagging, eccentricity, irritability, emotional outbursts, a false sense of superiority, mood swings (depression and euphoria), suspiciousness (paranoia), and suicidal tendencies. Deterioration in all intellectual activities characterize their dementia. Beginning with impaired word-list generation, the communication deficits advance into naming problems, dysarthria, and eventual muteness (total lack of speech).

There are several varieties of **infectious dementias** that are due to infections that attack the central nervous system. Of these, **AIDS dementia complex,** which is due to human immunodeficiency virus that causes *acquired immuno-deficiency syndrome* (AIDS), has been the most devastating in its prevalence rate and seriousness of symptoms. The terminal stage of AIDS has been a form of subcortical dementia and death, although in recent years, progress has been made in the treatment of the disease. Ironically, as the AIDS patients have been living longer because of improved treatment, the longer life span also has raised the incidence of AIDS dementia complex (Larsen, 1998).

The neurological symptoms of AIDS dementia complex include gait disturbances, tremor, headache, seizures, lack of muscle coordination, rigidity and general weakness of muscles, facial nerve paralysis, and lack of bowel and bladder control (incontinence). Dementia symptoms include memory and attentional problems, slow thinking, apathy, loss of interest in work, social withdrawal, confusion, hallucination, and delusion in some cases. Communication problems are less serious, although mutism may be evident in the final stages (Larsen, 1998).

Assessment of all forms of dementia is a multidisciplinary task. Among others, medical, behavioral (psychological), and speech–language pathology specialists are involved in a comprehensive assessment of patients with dementia. A firm and final diagnosis of dementia is possible only after an autopsy because noninfectious dementias are not reliably diagnosed with such laboratory tests as blood or urine analysis. Communicative disorders are assessed by speech and language sample, an analysis of discourse, and a careful analysis of patients' language use. Combined with an assessment of intellectual functions and general behavior, one can determine the extent of dementia.

Rehabilitation or treatment of patients with dementia consists mostly of a program of *clinical management* because the course of the underlying diseases cannot be reversed or checked. Various specialists support the patient and his or her family members through repeated counseling sessions in which they are educated about the course of the underlying diseases, medical treatment options, and management of daily, and typically deteriorating, symptoms. Patients are encouraged to develop strategies that compensate for their deficits. For example, patients might be taught to have a simple daily routine that is more easily managed; use various reminders (such as alarms and written reminders) to combat the memory problems; keep a checklist of things to do; carry a card with name, address, and telephone number so if they wander they can be relocated; and so forth. The family members might be taught a variety of skills to manage the deteriorating patient as well as they can. These skills might include speaking clearly, distinctly, and in simple sentences; talking about the things here-and-now; asking simple *yes* or *no* questions; approaching the patients slowly as they tend to get easily alarmed; and so forth.

Another form of infectious dementia is associated with **Jakob-Creutzfeldt** disease, popularly known as the mad cow disease.

Traumatic Brain Injury

Traumatic brain injury (TBI) is a major, expensive, sometimes fatal, and often lifelong health and rehabilitation problem, costing the nation up to $25 billion a year. Each year 2 million people in the United States suffer head injuries, 500,000 of them are hospitalized, and 90,000 or more may have permanent disability. The prevalence of TBI is the highest in the age group of 15 to 19 years and is more common among males than females (Bigler, 1990; Bigler, Clark, & Farmer, 1997; Hartley, 1995; Hegde, 1998) .

Unlike such internal causes as strokes, tumors, and degenerative diseases that affect brain function, traumatic brain injury is due to external factors. **Traumatic brain injury** is injury to the brain sustained by physical trauma or external force. Automobile accidents cause up to 50% of all cases of TBI. Other causes include various kinds of accidents (e.g., falls, which are more common among the elderly and industrial accidents), violence (including gunshot wounds to the head), and drug abuse.

Trauma to the head may cause different kinds of injuries. Some are called **penetrating brain injuries,** in which the skull is fractured or perforated, the meninges are torn, and the brain tissue is damaged. Foreign substance (e.g., glass fragments) may enter the brain to cause such additional problems as infection. Penetrating brain injuries also are known as open head injuries as there usually is an open wound in the head. Bullets, knife stabbing, blows to the head, and automobile accidents cause penetrating brain injuries.

Nonpenetrating brain injuries, also known as closed head injuries, involve indirect damage to the brain with intact meninges. The skull may or may not be fractured, and there is no brain penetration of foreign objects. Frequent causes of nonpenetrating injuries include blunt blows to the head and back-and-forth movement of the brain within the skull. The brain moves within the skull when the head rapidly moves forward and then moves back, such as in an automobile accident. When the brain moves within the skull, the tissue at its base gets torn because of the bony projections on the base of the skull. Hitting the skull in the front and back, the brain gets further damaged. Injuries that result from a brain moving within the skull are known as **acceleration/deceleration injuries.** A stationary head also may receive a trauma. For example, an automobile may crash down on the head of an automechanic lying on the floor. Such injuries sustained by stationary heads are known as **nonacceleration injuries.**

A majority of patients who need long-term rehabilitation are those who receive nonpenetrating brain injuries. Penetrating brain injuries create acute medical conditions but not necessarily a need for long-term rehabilitation. Therefore, much effort in the rehabilitation of patients with TBI is directed toward nonpenetrating injuries.

Traumatic brain injury causes a sequence of neuropathological events. Blood may accumulate in the brain or within the different meningeal layers, causing death of brain tissue. The pressure within the brain may increase, partly due to swelling of the brain tissue. Breathing difficulties may limit oxygen to the brain, also causing the death of brain tissue. Some patients may develop seizures.

The **effects of TBI** are varied. Some patients initially lose consciousness, which they slowly regain. Nearly all patients are inconsistent, disorganized, disoriented to time and place, distracted, restless, and irritated. Impaired *memory* and *reasoning* skills are typical of patients with TBI. **Communication deficits** are not purely linguistic; language problems are not as severe as other kinds of communication problems. Grammar of patients with TBI, for example, may be intact. Initial and persistent communication deficits include the following:

- **Dysarthria,** more likely the spastic variety when the damage is bilateral (both sides of the brain)

The meninges are the protective layers of membrane that cover the brain.

- **Confused language,** which may include irrelevant and incoherent talk

- **Difficulty in language comprehension,** especially when the spoken language is complex or abstract

- **Pragmatic language problems,** including difficulty in conversational turn-taking, initiation of conversation, and maintaining a topic of conversation

- **Rambling speech** (difficulty in being concise)

- **Difficulty in understanding facial expressions and gestures,** possibly due to lack of attention

- **Reading and writing difficulties,** which may partly be due to lack of attention and distraction

Assessment of patients with TBI includes a detailed case history to find out the pretraumatic levels of cognitive and communicative skills, evaluation of medical records including medical prognosis for recovery, evaluation of the patients' current medical condition, systematic observation of the patients, and administration of assessment tools. Assessment is a continuous process because the patients with TBI continuously change as their medical condition improves. An initial assessment is done at the bedside to assess the degree of responsiveness to environmental stimuli and events. This assessment might include such activities as eye opening, reflexive motor responses such as pulling the examiner's hand away from painful stimulation, and verbal responses to simple questions. Several standardized tests are available for initial and subsequent assessment.

Assessment of communicative deficits focuses on the previously listed symptoms. The clinician samples the presence of dysarthria, confused language, spoken language comprehension problems, naming difficulties, and pragmatic language problems.

Treatment or rehabilitation of patients with TBI includes both cognitive and communication approaches. In cognitive rehabilitation, clinicians target such skills as improved attention and memory. In communication treatment, clinicians target such skills as increased orientation to space, time, and person; paying attention to communication partners and the patient's surroundings; improved memory for daily routines and names of family members; better narrative skills; and turn-taking, topic maintenance, and topic initiation in conversation. By initially simplifying treatment tasks, the clinician positively reinforces even small improvements and systematically increases task complexity. In the case of children, activities related to schoolwork may be incorporated into therapy. For example, comprehension of material read from the child's grade-level books may be a part of treatment. Writing assignments appropriate to the child's grade also may be incorporated.

In the case of severe TBI, patients may have residual effects that no amount of rehabilitation can eliminate. In such cases, the clinician teaches a variety of skills that will help compensate for the deficits with which the clients have to live. For example, to compensate for residual memory problems, the clinician may teach a client to write down directions needed to complete such activities as preparing a meal. Another patient who has difficulty understanding spoken speech might be taught to ask questions seeking repetition or clarification. The clinician might teach some patients to use various electronic devices (e.g., digital watches with alarms) that remind them of activities and appointments. Working with families, teachers, and employers to educate them about the persistent special needs of the patient is an important aspect of TBI rehabilitation.

Dysphagia

Dysphagia is the term for disorders of swallowing food and liquids. These disorders also are known as *deglutition* disorders. They are not disorders of communication. However, in medical settings, speech–language pathologists assess and help manage patients who have several kinds of swallowing disorders (Groher, 1997; Hegde, 2001a, 2001b; Logemann, 1998).

Swallowing food is a complex activity that involves several stages, including chewing of the food, preparing it for swallow, initiating the swallow, propelling the food through the pharynx, and passing the food through the esophagus. A patient may have difficulty with any or all of these activities necessary for swallowing food. Except for esophageal swallowing disorders, which are handled medically, speech–language pathologists are involved in the assessment and management of swallowing disorders (Hegde, 2001a, 2001b).

Swallowing disorders have many causes including

- Strokes that affect the motor control of structures involved in swallowing

- Tumors of the mouth and throat (pharynx) and neurological diseases such as Parkinson's

- Surgical or radiation treatment of oral, pharyngeal, and laryngeal cancer

- Any form of brain, head, neck, and gastrointestinal surgery

- Traumatic brain injury, polio, and cerebral palsy

Swallowing disorders often are classified according to the different stages of swallow. For example, some swallowing disorders involve difficulty in chewing food (mastication) because of a weak tongue that cannot move food in the mouth and impaired movement of the jaw. This is the *disorder of mastication*. Normally, chewed food is prepared for swallow by turning the food into a bolus, and some patients cannot accomplish this. They cannot hold the bolus in the mouth before swallowing it. The food may enter the airway ("the wrong track"), resulting in *aspiration*.

In the disorder of the next phase, known as the *oral phase*, the food may be moved more toward the front of the mouth in preparation for swallow. This is opposite the normal movement of food toward the back of the mouth. Normally, the oral phase is followed by the *pharyngeal phase* in which the food is reflexively propelled down through the pharynx. Thus in the disorder of the pharyngeal phase, the patient may have difficulty propelling the food through the pharynx because of impaired reflexive action of the muscles of swallow in the pharynx. Food may enter the nose and airway. Food may coat the pharynx. Paralysis of the pharyngeal muscles is the most frequent cause of this condition.

Finally, there is the *esophageal phase* of swallow, in which the food is propelled through the esophagus and down into the stomach. This stage is not under voluntary control and the associated disorders are managed medically. The main problem of this stage is that the food is propelled back from the esophagus and into the pharynx.

Assessment of swallowing disorders involves medical specialists and speech–language pathologists. Besides screening for communication disorders, the speech–language pathologist evaluates swallowing disorders by administering *test swallows,* involving liquid and solid food of various consistencies. These test swallows help evaluate the kinds of problems the patient has. Among other techniques, the clinician also may conduct a *videofluorographic assessment* of swallow. In this technique, low dosage radiation (X ray) is used in videotaping movements involved in swallowing.

Treatment of swallowing disorders may be both indirect and direct. Food is not used in *indirect treatment,* in which efforts are made to strengthen the muscles involved in swallowing by various *oral-motor exercises.* For example, tongue exercises may be prescribed to strengthen its range and force of movement. Lip exercises may be prescribed to strengthen lip closure necessary to hold the food in the mouth while chewing it.

In *direct treatment,* food and liquid are used to promote better swallowing. Disorders of different stages of swallow require different strategies. For example, in treating disorders of mastication, the clinician may teach the patient to keep the food in the side of the mouth, where the muscle strength is greater. In treating disorders of the oral preparatory phase, the clinician may teach a patient to tilt the head forward to keep the food in the front of the mouth until ready to swallow and then to tilt the head back to promote the swallow. In treating disorders of the oral phase of the swallow, the clinician may teach a patient to hold the food at the back of the tongue before initiating a swallow. In treating disorders of the pharyngeal stage of the swallow, the clinician may teach the patient to tilt the head forward while swallowing to compensate for a delayed or absent swallowing reflex.

Cerebral Palsy

Two popular books written by Marie Killilea, *Karen, A True Story Told by Her Mother* and *With Love from Karen,* tell the story of a child with cerebral palsy and her family. Incidentally, because Karen was born in the 1940s, the first book also gives a rare account of the recent history of the rehabilitation of children with cerebral palsy written from the standpoint of parents.

When the Killileas noticed that there was something the matter with their daughter, they began to look for help, which was hard to find in the early 1940s. The pediatrician did not tell the parents anything until Karen was a year old and, even then, only after the parents pressed for an answer. He said that Karen might have cerebral palsy and that "a cerebral palsied child would never sit up, use his hands, or walk" (Killilea, 1952, p. 27). He confessed that in the medical school, he was not taught much about it.

Not fully accepting this heartbreaking prediction, the parents began their search for help, going from one specialist to another and traveling across the country and to Canada. The first specialist told them that children with cerebral palsy do not have any "mentality." Another specialist told the parents to leave Karen in an institution with a "good-size insurance policy" to pay for the care.

Karen was already 2½ when the next specialist who "knew the answer" saw her. His answer? Perhaps the parents could consider taking Karen up on top of a mountain and leaving her there.

Nowadays, the parents of children with cerebral palsy get more enlightened advice from the experts.

What Is Cerebral Palsy?

Cerebral palsy is characterized by brain injury, resulting paralysis, and attending problems of physical growth, locomotion, communication, and potential sensory deficits. Therefore, cerebral palsy is a name for a group of neurological problems caused by brain injury. Cerebral palsy is a disorder of childhood, especially of the first 2 years of life. In fact, its origin may be prenatal or congenital. Cerebral palsy is not a progressive disease; it is chronic. In fact, some children with cerebral palsy improve as they grow older. Cerebral palsy is not the name of a disease; it refers to the effects of a chain of events.

Again, in understanding cerebral palsy, it is essential to remember the basic facts of neuromotor control of speech. The motor cortex, the pyramidal and the extrapyramidal motor systems, and the cerebellum are the main structures that are damaged in cerebral palsy.

The incidence of cerebral palsy is variously estimated to be 1 to 6 per 1,000 births. In the United States, there are at least 750,000 people with cerebral palsy. Most of them are under 21 years of age.

Some Causes of Brain Injury

Brain injury in children has many causes. The cause may occur during pregnancy (prenatal), during childbirth (perinatal), and soon after birth (postnatal).

Infections the pregnant woman suffers are a major **prenatal** source of brain injury. Rubella, mumps, and influenza in the mother, especially during the early period of pregnancy, can damage the fetal brain. Other prenatal causes include anoxia and Rh incompatibility. For example, by restricting the fetal blood supply, a mother's anemia may cause fetal anoxia (reduced supply of oxygen) and brain injury. If the mother has Rh negative blood (unusual) and the child has Rh positive blood (usual), the mother's blood may produce some antibodies that will affect the fetal blood and result in fetal brain injury.

A sick pregnant woman who is exposed to too many X rays, too much radiation, or large amounts of anesthesia might have a brain-injured child. Accidents during pregnancy are a major source of fetal brain injury. While the incidence of fetal brain injury due to infections has decreased over the years, the incidence due to car accidents has increased.

Perinatal causes of brain injury include prolonged labor, breach delivery (wrong position of the baby), too fast a delivery, and structural damage to the head by the use of forceps. Fetal brain hemorrhage due to any of these and other causes eventually injures portions of the brain by the formation of blood clots that prevent the free flow of cerebral blood. Premature babies are more likely to suffer brain injury than full-term babies. In fact, the incidence of cerebral palsy is about three times higher among the prematurely born than the full-term born.

Postnatal causes of cerebral palsy also are numerous. Auto accidents, once again, play a major role. Other causes are infections or diseases including mumps, scarlet fever, measles, whooping cough, meningitis, and encephalitis. Meningitis is a diseases of the meninges, a membrane covering the brain. Encephalitis results in inflamed brain cells. Both cause brain injury.

Postnatal anoxia, another frequent cause of brain injury, results when a baby does not breathe soon after birth. Vascular diseases that reduce the cerebral blood supply can damage the brain cells for the same reason. Numerous poisoning agents including lead and mercury also are important causes.

The Major Types of Cerebral Palsy

There are several ways of classifying cerebral palsy. One classification is based on the body parts that are paralyzed. When only either the left or the right half of the body is affected, it is called **hemiplegia;** when only the legs are involved, it is called **paraplegia;** when only one limb is affected, it is called **monoplegia;** when *either* the legs *or* the arms are involved, it is called **diplegia;** when all four limbs are involved, it is called **quadriplegia.**

A common classification of cerebral palsy has three types: spastic, athetoid, and ataxic. Unlike the other classification, which is based on the number of limbs paralyzed, this one is based on other neurological symptoms.

The Spastic Type

Roughly 60% of the children with cerebral palsy are of the spastic type—that is, the major symptom is spasticity of the muscles. **Spasticity** is increased tone or rigidity of muscles. Spastic muscles are stiff, possibly because muscles that oppose each other's actions, known as **antagonistic,** are simultaneously active. The muscle contractions are abrupt, jerky, rigid, slow, and labored. The arms, thighs, and feet might show inward rotation or the arms might be drawn upward, toward the neck. The head also might be drawn back and rotated to one or the other side of the body. The abnormal gait of these children is described as the "scissors gait" because the thighs are drawn inward and the legs tend to show some degree of crossover. Toe-walking also is common.

Spasticity is caused by injury to the **pyramidal motor pathways,** or the cortical centers of motor control. The injured higher centers fail to control the impulses generated by the lower centers, including the brain stem and spinal cord. These lower centers are generally responsible for muscle tone. In the absence of regulation by the higher centers, the lower centers send excessive impulses to the muscles, causing rigidity, stiffness, and jerky movements.

The Athetoid Type

The main symptom of this type is **athetosis,** which is characterized by slow, involuntary, writhing, and wormlike movements. When sitting quietly, the athetoid movements are subsided and the child may look near normal. However, when the child tries to do something, such as reaching for an object or talking, the involuntary movements overwhelm the purposeful, coordinated, serial movements. The movements are disorganized. The feet are rotated inward, and the fingers are overextended. The head is drawn back, the mouth is open, and there may be drooling.

Athetosis is caused by injury to the **extrapyramidal motor pathways,** especially to the basal ganglia. Through a network of diffused pathways, the basal ganglia help plan movement patterns and modify cortical motor impulses. When the basal ganglia are injured, the cortical impulses are not modified. The result is athetosis.

The Ataxic Type

Disturbed balance and movement are the two major kinds of problems of **ataxia,** resulting in abnormal gait. The child stands and walks with wide-spread legs to maintain the easily disturbed balance. While walking, the child's neck may be pushed forward and both the arms drawn backward. This gives the appearance of a birdlike posture.

A child with ataxia has movements that are clumsy, awkward, uncoordinated, and misdirected. The flabby and weak muscles lack proper tone (hypotonia). The hypotonus muscles lack adequate force and rate when they move; they cannot maintain the needed direction.

Injury to the **cerebellum** causes ataxia. The cerebellum serves two main functions. First, it maintains the body's balance with the help of the semicircular canals in the inner ear. An injured cerebellum cannot coordinate the impulses received from the inner ear. Therefore, the balance is disturbed. Second, the cerebellum coordinates movements through the **kinesthetic** or **proprioceptive** sense. The kinesthetic sense makes it possible to constantly monitor the tone of the muscles, body positions, direction of movements of body parts, rate and force of movements, and so on. The position and movements of one's toes inside shoes is known precisely because of the kinesthetic sense, monitored by the cerebellum. When it is injured, the automatic sensing of the spatial arrangement of the body parts is impaired. This impairment causes the kinds of movement problems found in the person with ataxia.

Speech and Language Problems in Cerebral Palsy

The basic speech problem of the individual with cerebral palsy is dysarthria. To distinguish the dysarthria of children with cerebral palsy from that of adult patients, the term **developmental dysarthria** is used. Because cerebral palsy is due to injury to the motor systems, there should be no language problem. However, a coexisting lesion in the language centers of the brain or a more widespread brain injury can cause language problems as well.

Some children with cerebral palsy are slow in acquiring language. Some may never attain the normal level of language behavior. However, this delay or disorder may be due to several other factors, including mental retardation and hearing impairment, that may coexist with cerebral palsy.

The developmental dysarthria of children with cerebral palsy includes problems of articulation, respiration, voice, fluency, and prosody. Typically, the children are not able to articulate speech sounds correctly. The sounds that are made with the help of the tip of the tongue (/s/, /z/, /l/, /r/) are especially troublesome because of the difficulty in moving the tongue tip. The speech can be slow and labored. Lacking in rhythm, it can sound monotonous. In severe cases, the speech might be unintelligible because of the weakness of the muscles of the lips, tongue, soft palate, and jaw.

Many children with cerebral palsy have breathing abnormalities. For example, these children may breathe more rapidly than normal and may have reduced vital capacity (the total amount of air that can be expelled from the lungs after a deep inhalation). These breathing abnormalities may be responsible for some of the voice problems of children with cerebral palsy. Smooth voice initiation may be difficult, and it may not be possible for the child to sustain vocalization. Because the airflow is not consistent, the pitch and loudness of voice may vary unpredictably.

The slow and effortful speech of children with cerebral palsy does not flow naturally and easily; therefore, the speech is not very fluent nor does it have the normal prosodic features. Short phrases and frequent interruptions of speech due to muscle discoordination also add to the quality of generally nonfluent, nonrhythmic speech.

Related Problems

Among the many related problems of children with cerebral palsy, intellectual deficiency, hearing impairment, visual impairment, behavior disorders, and epilepsy are important (Bottenberg & Hanks, 1986).

Intellectual deficiency, a consequence of brain injury, is found in 50% of children with cerebral palsy; the degree of deficiency varies across children, depending on the extent of brain injury. Many children, however, have normal or superior intelligence.

Hearing impairment also is more common in children with cerebral palsy, especially in the athetoid type, than in the general population. The cochlea, the auditory pathways, and the auditory areas of the brain may all be affected, resulting in different kinds of hearing loss. Some of the speech and language problems of children with cerebral palsy may be due to their hearing loss.

Visual impairments also tend to be associated with cerebral palsy. An often noted problem is **strabismus,** in which the eyes cannot focus together. It may be either of the convergent (the eye deviates toward the nose) or divergent (eye deviates outward) variety. Another common visual problem is **hemianopsia** (hemianopia), which is a loss of vision in one half of the visual field in one or both eyes. Children with cerebral palsy have difficulty maintaining visual focus because of their various involuntary movements.

Behavior disorders of various sorts are frequently associated with brain injury. The child may be highly distractible, causing problems in learning. Strong and sometimes inappropriate emotional responses and temper tantrums may be noted. Not enjoying social interactions, the child may withdraw. Some children and adolescents may set unrealistic goals for themselves, while others are difficult to motivate.

Epilepsy is a seizure disorder commonly found in individuals who have brain injury, including those with cerebral palsy. The precipitating (immediate) cause of epilepsy is an excessive electrical discharge of a group of brain cells called the **epileptic focus.** The abnormal impulses set off a series of convulsions in the body.

In the **grand mal** variety of epilepsy, the person loses consciousness, falls to the ground when standing or sitting, and has violent convulsions of the body. In the less severe **petit mal** variety, there is no loss of consciousness and there are no convulsions. Instead, there is a momentary loss of attention and interruption of whatever the person is doing at the time of an attack. Being unaware of these attacks, the person resumes the activity.

Rehabilitation of Children with Cerebral Palsy

Rehabilitation requires the efforts of different specialists. Therefore, it typically takes place in a hospital with a rehabilitation department. The team of specialists evaluates the physical, sensory, psychological, behavioral, and communicative problems and the potential of a child with cerebral palsy and designs a program of rehabilitation. As summarized here, each specialist then implements his or portion of the program:

- **Pediatrician.** Probably the first to identify cerebral palsy, the pediatrician refers the child to a neurologist for examination.
- **Neurologist.** This specialist in nerve diseases evaluates the child and diagnoses cerebral palsy and its type.
- **Orthopedic surgeon.** This specialist in the function and disorders of the skeletal system provides the needed corrective surgery to achieve better balance and more coordinated movement and gait. The surgeon also advises on the use of braces that achieve similar goals.
- **Physical therapist.** This specialist in rehabilitating body functions through a variety of procedures designs and implements a program of muscle training and exercises to increase the tone, strength, and movement potential of paralyzed or weakened muscles.
- **Otorhinolaryngologist.** This specialist diagnoses and treats the child's ear, nose, and throat problems.
- **Audiologist.** This specialist in hearing and its disorders evaluates the hearing loss and designs a program of rehabilitation.
- **Speech–language pathologist.** This specialist evaluates and treats communicative disorders.
- **Clinical psychologist.** This specialist evaluates the child's intellectual level and evaluates and treats behavioral problems.
- **Occupational therapist.** This specialist in vocational and personal skills teaches a variety of behaviors including the use of tools (a pair of scissors, for example), dressing, driving, typing with the help of modified typewriters, and other vocational skills.
- **Ophthalmologist.** This specialist makes an assessment of visual problems and designs and implements medical and corrective procedures.
- **Social worker.** This specialist helps coordinate the various services that different private and government agencies offer. The social worker also finds financial help as the expensive and prolonged rehabilitation of the child with cerebral palsy is beyond the reach of many families.

In the educational setting, the **special education specialist** plays an important role in the rehabilitation of children with cerebral palsy. Many children with mild cerebral palsy are educated in regular classrooms. These children may receive such special services as speech–language therapy and physical therapy. However, children who are more severely affected need the services of reading specialists, teachers who specialize in teaching students with disabilities, and, when needed, the deaf educator. These children may be educated in special classes designed to help students with physical and mental disabilities.

Speech and Language Services

The speech and language problems of children with cerebral palsy vary from a few errors of articulation to near-total lack of speech. Some of these children have normal speech and language, but many need treatment for speech disorders, language disorders, or both. Those who receive treatment for both do so for a prolonged period.

Speech and **language treatment** techniques described in Chapters 4 and 5, respectively, are appropriate for children with cerebral palsy. Speech training involves teaching the correct production of erred speech sounds in words, syllables, and conversational speech. In some cases, teaching the child to speak at a slower rate improves the speech intelligibility. Language stimulation or treatment involves initially teaching simple functional words (e.g., *mommy, daddy, milk, juice, shoes, car, truck, cat, doll*) and systematically expanding the skills by teaching phrases and sentences and conversational speech. What distinguishes treatment of children with cerebral palsy is the need for considering additional targets such as muscle movements, shaping those movement patterns that result in better speech, and controlling various abnormal movements.

The speech–language pathologist works closely with the physical therapist in teaching better control of speech muscles. Some clinicians advocate the development of "reflex inhibiting postures." The best known method of teaching postures that inhibit reflexive and uncontrolled movements of the limbs is the **Bobath** method (Bobath & Bobath, 1967). The child is placed and firmly held in a position that inhibits a particular kind of reflex. For example, the child whose elbows and knees are flexed and drawn toward the body may be made to lie flat on his or her stomach with the arms fully extended over the head, on either side of the ears. The position is exactly opposite to that of flexion because the entire body is extended. A child whose typical reflex is extension may be held in a position of flexion. For example, the child may be made to sit with bent knees. These and other reflex inhibiting postures help the child overcome the typical abnormal postures. Some of the postures improve breathing and induce relaxation, which should facilitate speech and voice training.

Nonspeech Communication

For children with the most severe form of cerebral palsy, it is extremely difficult, if not impossible, to teach speech and language. The mastery of the complex movements of the vocal folds, the soft palate, the tongue, and the lips necessary to produce speech may be an unrealistic target for such children. Even with intensive efforts, some may remain speechless. In recent years, nonspeech forms of communication for the speechless have been researched.

Manual modes of communication, including **American Sign Language,** have been taught to children with mental retardation and autism who have some degree of motor control. However, the speechless children with cerebral palsy whose hands are paralyzed cannot form signs, which require fast and sequenced hand movements. For such children, **communication boards** are more practical. A communication board contains words (traditional orthography) or various forms of symbols. On a board that contains words, the client who can read points to a word such as *mother, hungry,* or *bathroom.* The words may be combined to form phrases or sentences. The words of a phrase or sentence are pointed to in the correct sequence. The "listener" reads the words pointed to and understands the message.

Symbols are more practical than words because most clients who need communication boards are not able to read. Two well known sets of symbols have been researched. One set consists of symbols that are more or less abstract shapes, some more geometric than others. The other set consists of symbols that are pictorial; a word is represented by a picture that suggests an object or person. A picture or a symbol that looks like the object it is supposed to suggest is called **iconic.** An abstract geometric shape that suggests a person or object is **noniconic.** Iconic symbols are direct. Just by looking at them, one knows their meaning. The more abstract (and arbitrary) noniconic symbol must be matched with what it suggests to establish its meaning.

See **Chapter 10** for more on American Sign Language.

In teaching language to chimpanzees, the behavioral psychologist David Premack (1971) developed a set of geometric symbols. The chimps learned to use them and formed novel combinations and did some limited "talking" with Premack. These symbols were later adapted for teaching nonvocal speech to the speechless and are known as the **Carrier symbols** (Carrier & Peak, 1975). The Carrier symbols are the most geometric, abstract, and noniconic of the symbol systems. However, they are movable shapes that can be physically arranged and rearranged like words to form sentences. The child with cerebral palsy who cannot move them can point to the symbols to communicate.

The other symbol system, developed by Charles K. Bliss, was suggested as an international language (Bliss, 1965). Known as **Blissymbolics**, the system has been used in teaching nonspeech communication to children with cerebral palsy. Blissymbolics are a combination of semi-iconic and abstract symbols. The symbols are printed characters posted on a communication board. Under each symbol, the word it suggests is printed. As the client talks by pointing to the symbols, the listener understands by reading the words under them.

The Carrier and the Bliss symbols are nonpictorial compared to the pictorial **rebus system**. A rebus is a picture of an object or a person, hence the name, rebus system. Charlotte Clark and her associates have published a set of 818 rebuses, which has been researched in teaching nonvocal speech to the speechless (Clark, Davies, & Woodcock, 1974). A rebus is iconic. It may be more easily learned than the other noniconic or less iconic systems (Clark, 1981). Figure 9.6 shows examples of the Bliss, the Carrier, and the rebus symbols.

Communication boards pose problems for the individual with severe forms of cerebral palsy who cannot point with the hands. Such individuals may use *pointers* that are fixed to the head or the feet when these are mobile. The combined efforts of biomedical engineers and speech–language pathologists have helped refine the technology of communication boards and the mode of client responses. For example, electronic pointing or activating devices have been researched. Eye movements or a beam of light from a mechanical device fixed on the forehead can send signals to an electronic communication board. Those signals can activate stored messages. In the coming years, we can expect rapid progress in electronic communication boards connected to sophisticated computers, which will display the messages on video screens or print them out.

Summary

- A disorder of early childhood, cerebral palsy refers to a complex set of neuromuscular and communication problems due to brain injury; it is a chronic condition that improves as the child grows older.

- Many prenatal, perinatal, and postnatal factors are associated with cerebral palsy.

- Cerebral palsy is classified into the spastic (characterized by rigid muscles), the athetoid (characterized by slow, writhing involuntary movements), and the ataxic (characterized by disturbed balance) types.

- Delayed language, disorders of articulation, disturbed prosody, and problems of voice may all be associated with cerebral palsy. Hearing impairment, visual problems, behavior disorders, and epilepsy, among others, also may be associated with cerebral palsy.

(continues)

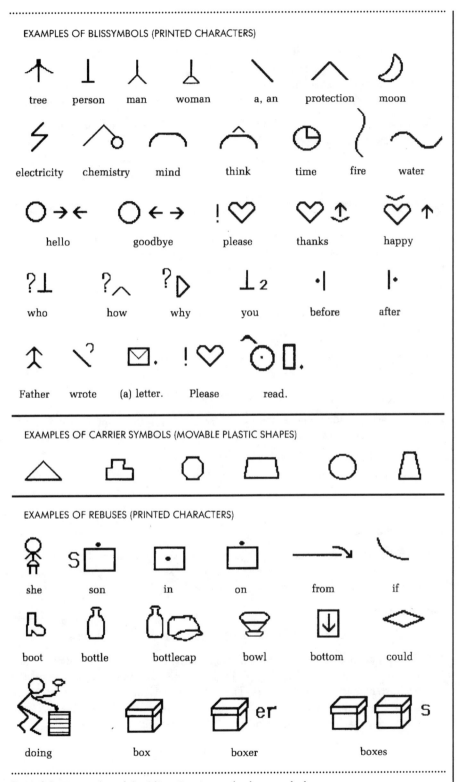

EXAMPLES OF BLISSYMBOLS (PRINTED CHARACTERS)

tree   person   man   woman   a, an   protection   moon

electricity   chemistry   mind   think   time   fire   water

hello   goodbye   please   thanks   happy

who   how   why   you   before   after

Father   wrote   (a) letter.   Please   read.

EXAMPLES OF CARRIER SYMBOLS (MOVABLE PLASTIC SHAPES)

EXAMPLES OF REBUSES (PRINTED CHARACTERS)

she   son   in   on   from   if

boot   bottle   bottlecap   bowl   bottom   could

doing   box   boxer   boxes

Figure 9.6. Examples of the Bliss, Carrier, and rebus symbols.

- Children with cerebral palsy need services from many specialists including neurologists, orthopedic surgeons, physical therapists, otorhinolaryngologists, audiologists, speech–language pathologists, psychologists, and social workers. The speech–language pathologist treats the multiple problems of communication including the often prominent disorders of articulation.

- Some very profoundly involved children need to be taught nonverbal means of communication.

Dialogue

The student, Ms. Noledge-Hungry, who read the chapter carefully, walked into Professor Speech-Wisely's office to discuss the information. The professor loved these dialogues. Any opportunity to give a lecture on neurogenic communicative disorders was exciting to the professor.

N-H: Dr. Speech-Wisely, I think I know the answer, but why "neurogenic" communicative disorders?

S-W: Neurologically based communicative disorders are problems of speech, language, or both that are caused by **neurological damage** of one kind or the other.

N-H: They include both speech and language disorders, then?

S-W: Yes. They include aphasia, apraxia, dysarthria, and the communicative problems of children with cerebral palsy. You know which one of them is exclusively a language disorder?

N-H: Yes. **Aphasia** is a language disorder, and **apraxia** and **dysarthria** are speech disorders. The children with **cerebral palsy** may have both speech and language disorders.

S-W: But what is common to them?

N-H: Some kind of neural damage. However, aphasia, apraxia, and cerebral palsy are caused by central nervous system damage, whereas dysarthria is caused by either central or peripheral nervous system damage.

S-W: That is true.

N-H: Could you summarize the major structures of the central nervous system?

S-W: The **spinal cord** and the **brain**. The spinal cord is a neural network contained within the spinal column. The brain is contained within the skull, and the **brain stem** is its lowermost part. The left and the right halves of the brain are called the **cerebral hemispheres**. The topmost layer of the hemispheres is called the **cortex**. Each hemisphere controls the opposite side of the body.

N-H: What are the lobes of the brain?

S-W: Each hemisphere is divided into **four lobes**: the **frontal, parietal, occipital,** and **temporal**. The frontal lobe contains the **primary motor area** and **Broca's area**. Both are important for speech production. The frontal lobe controls much of our purposeful behaviors. The parietal lobe controls sensations through its **primary somesthetic area**. It also is concerned with speech because some speech areas overlap the parietal and temporal lobes. The occipital lobe, which has the **primary visual area**, is mostly concerned with vision. The temporal lobe contains the **primary auditory area** and **Wernicke's area,** which is important for understanding the meaning of sound and speech. Wernicke's area extends to the parietal lobe. The most important parts to remember are the speech areas of the frontal and temporoparietal lobes.

N-H: What should I remember about the **brain stem?**

S-W: You should know its major parts: the **medulla,** the **pons,** and the midbrain. Through the brain stem, the neural pathways move up and down the brain. The medulla controls automatic body functions (heart rate, breathing). The pons bridges the two sides of the cerebellum and connects the cerebellum with the cerebrum. The midbrain links the higher centers with the lower centers of the brain.

N-H: I know there are three motor control mechanisms, but . . .

S-W: Yes, but they are in addition to the motor control centers of the frontal cortex. They are the **cerebellum,** the **pyramidal motor system,** and the **extrapyramidal motor system.** The cerebellum coordinates and regulates motor impulses generated by other structures. It controls posture, locomotion, balance, and movements. The pyramidal motor system carries motor impulses to the muscles without relay stations. The extrapyramidal system carries motor impulses to the muscles through relay stations (other structures). The system also can give feedback to the brain regarding movements in progress. What is the most important structure of the extrapyramidal system?

N-H: Could it be the **basal ganglia?**

S-W: Precisely. OK, then what is the other nervous system?

N-H: The **peripheral nervous system,** which consists of **spinal** and **cranial nerves.** There are 31 pairs of spinal nerves, some of which are of special interest to us because of their involvement in breathing.

S-W: Good. What about the cranial nerves?

N-H: I knew I had to memorize these, Dr. Speech-Wisely! There are 12 pairs of cranial nerves. Of these, one pair, the acoustic nerve, carries auditory impulses to the brain. Six other pairs are concerned with speech: the **trigeminal** (V), the **facial** (VII), the **glossopharyngeal** (IX), the **vagus** (X), the **accessory** (XI), and the **hypoglossal** (XII).

S-W: Excellent! We now move on to aphasia. You know that it is a language disorder caused by brain injury due to trauma, diseases, and stroke. Now, tell me about the causes of strokes.

N-H: I remember **embolism,** which is due to a traveling embolus which obstructs blood supply to a part of the brain; **thrombosis,** which is a stationary blood clot; **aneurysm,** which is the bulging of a weakened artery that ruptures and causes cerebral hemorrhage. The book described so many speech problems of patients with aphasia. How can you summarize them?

S-W: Well, patients with aphasia forget names (**anomia**); substitute words they can't remember or say (**paraphasia**); create nonexistent words on the spot (**neologism**); omit grammatical words (**agrammatism**); produce grammatical but meaningless speech (**jargon**); and use a phrase or two repeatedly (**verbal**

stereotypes). Problems of writing (**agraphia**), reading (**alexia**), and speech comprehension also are common. You tell me how aphasia is classified.

N-H: I knew you would hit me with that! A classification I know includes **three types of fluent aphasia**—Broca's, transcortical, and global—and **three types of nonfluent aphasia**—Wernicke's, conduction, and anomic. Several clinicians do not believe in classifying aphasia into types.

S-W: That is true. The sooner the budding speech–language pathologist learns to live with controversies, the better it is.

N-H: I am not sure how to summarize the treatment of aphasia.

S-W: I can understand that because it is not very easy. No matter how you summarize it, some clinicians will be unhappy with it because different clinicians probably treat them somewhat differently. The treatment of aphasia consists of many procedures. Speech fluency, naming skills, recognition of objects, and speech comprehension can all be improved by treatment that proceeds from simple to more complex verbal tasks.

N-H: Can I say something about motor speech disorders? The two types of motor speech disorders are apraxia and dysarthria. **Apraxia,** being a central movement disorder, affects speech but not language. The speech movements are clumsy and groping. Errors are inconsistent but common on consonants and consonantal clusters. I know there are two theories of apraxia, but . . .

S-W: One theory says that it is a disorder of motor planning, and the other theory says that it is due to inadequate representation of the sound system of the language. What do you think?

N-H: Don't we need more research to come to conclusions?

S-W: Yes. I wish experts had your restraint. **Dysarthria,** the other speech disorder, is caused by weakness or paralysis of the speech muscles associated with the central or peripheral nervous system damage. Many neurological diseases damage the nervous systems. Dysarthria affects articulation, respiration, phonation, resonance, and prosody.

N-H: I understand that treatment of motor speech disorders is somewhat new and more research is needed.

S-W: That is true. In apraxia, improvement in sequencing the motor responses is the treatment target. The patients with dysarthria can be trained to improve their posture, articulation, voice, prosody, and speech breathing patterns. Now, what is a right hemisphere syndrome?

N-H: It is a collection of disturbances due to right hemisphere damage.

S-W: What are some of the major symptoms of right hemisphere damage?

N-H: An interesting symptom is left-neglect. Other symptoms include facial recognition deficits, attentional deficits, disorientation, difficulty in understanding emotions others express, and certain communication deficits.

S-W: Very good. It is important to remember that right hemisphere damage does not cause the same kinds of language problems seen in people who have sustained left hemisphere damage.

N-H: Yes. Right hemisphere damage results in such speech problems as flat tone and various pragmatic problems.

S-W: Excellent! What about dementia?

N-H: I have been reading a lot about dementia in popular press these days. I understand President Reagan has it. Dementia refers to progressive intellectual and behavioral deterioration due to neurological diseases and some infections such as HIV.

S-W: Correct! What is the neuropathology of dementia of the Alzheimer's type?

N-H: Three types of pathologies were described: neurofibrillary tangles, neuritic plaques, and granulovacuolar degeneration.

S-W: Very good! Make sure you can define them. What are some of the communicative problems of DAT?

N-H: Alzheimer's patients may have difficulty in naming, speech comprehension, topic maintenance, coherent narration of events, and reading and writing, among others.

S-W: You should be able to summarize the other forms of dementia. Now, tell me something about **traumatic brain injury, or TBI.**

N-H: It is a serious and expensive national problem. It is externally induced trauma to the brain. TBI may be penetrating or nonpenetrating. Penetrating TBIs involve fractured skull, torn meninges, and damaged brain tissue. Nonpenetrating TBIs involve indirect damage to the brain with intact meninges.

S-W: Excellent! You also should know about acceleration/deceleration injuries and nonacceleration injuries found in nonpenetrating TBIs.

N-H: Yes. I guess you want me to know all the symptoms of TBIs including dysarthria, confused language, rambling speech, language comprehension deficits, and so forth.

S-W: You are right! Also, you should be able to summarize assessment and treatment information as well.

N-H: I find cerebral palsy to be very complex. Can you summarize it for me?

S-W: Sure. Brain injury, resulting paralysis of the limbs, and the associated problems of physical growth, locomotion, communication, and potential sensory deficits characterize **cerebral palsy.** It is a disorder of early childhood. Any factor that can induce brain injury in the fetus or the newborn can cause cerebral palsy. Do you recall some of the causes?

N-H: Yes, maternal **rubella, anoxia, head injury,** and **meningitis.**

S-W: OK, what about the types of cerebral palsy?

N-H: There are three major types of cerebral palsy: the **spastic,** the **athetoid,** and the **ataxic.**

S-W: Both speech and language problems may be found in people with cerebral palsy. You should be able to describe some of the problems. What are some of the related problems found in children with cerebral palsy?

N-H: Hearing loss, mental retardation, visual impairment, behavior disorders, and epilepsy. Now, let me see if I can remember the names of all those professional people who help the child with cerebral palsy. There are neurologists, orthopedic surgeons, otorhinolaryngologists, audiologists, speech–language pathologists, and . . .

s-w: Physical therapists, occupational therapists, and clinical psychologists. The speech–language pathologist works on language as well as speech production. Treatment is typically prolonged. You should be able to summarize the treatment procedures described in the text. The most severely affected children might be taught nonverbal communication including symbol systems like the Carrier system and the Bliss system.

The Outlook

N-H: Dr. Speech-Wisely, of all the neurologically based communicative disorders, I find aphasia the most interesting. When I was small, my grandmother had a stroke. I do not remember much, but she could not speak much and struggled to say things. She may have had the nonfluent aphasia, I think. Anyway, if I do decide on majoring in communicative disorders, what more will I learn about aphasia and other neurologically based disorders?

s-w: There is a whole lot to learn. You will take separate courses on the anatomy and physiology of speech and hearing. You will learn more about neurology in general and the neurology of the central nervous system in particular. You will understand more about language functions of the brain.

N-H: What about all those diseases of the nervous system we only discussed briefly?

s-w: Yes, you will read more about neuropathology. You will study aphasia in greater detail. In fact, we have a required graduate course on aphasia and a more advanced seminar on aphasia and its treatment. You may take both of those courses.

N-H: What about clinical practice? Do graduate students get to work with patients with aphasia?

s-w: Sure, in our own speech and hearing clinic on the campus, we see quite a few patients with aphasia every year. But we also have an internship program at two of the local hospitals. You will observe many patients with aphasia being treated by different specialists including speech–language pathologists. The hospital has a rehabilitation unit where you can also see the treatment of children with cerebral palsy. There, for a full semester, you work under the supervision of a staff clinician.

N-H: A little bit scary.

s-w: You will be ready, though in the beginning it is a bit scary. It is so for everyone, remember. But you will have had good course work and well-supervised clinical practice before you do your internship elsewhere.

N-H: How does one specialize in aphasia?

s-w: You should probably go on for your doctoral degree in speech–language pathology and make an intensive study of neurology and speech–language pathology, with specialization in aphasia. Many excellent graduate schools offer special programs in aphasia. You can find a program affiliated with a medical school as well.

N-H: I was talking to a friend of mine who is thinking about nursing. She told me that all this information on aphasia will be very useful to her.

S-W: Sure. Nurses, general physicians, psychologists, and many other health and human service professionals will find information on neurologically based communicative disorders useful in their work.

N-H: What are some of the places where speech–language pathologists treat clients who have neurologically based communicative disorders?

S-W: A majority of them are treated in speech and hearing departments or clinics of large hospitals. They also are treated in college clinics and private speech and hearing clinics.

N-H: Well, the more I learn about speech–language pathology, the more I want to major in it. What is coming up next?

S-W: The next topic we are going to discuss in the class is hearing and its disorders. It is about audiology, the twin profession of speech–language pathology.

N-H: Something new, again!

Study Questions

1. Name the two structures of the central nervous system.

2. What are the two nervous systems?

3. The two halves of the cerebrum are known as _____.

4. The _____ on the cortex are called gyri and the _____ are called sulci.

5. Name the four lobes of the cortex.

6. In what lobe do you find the primary motor area?

7. In what lobes do you find Broca's area and Wernicke's area?

8. Name the major structures of the brain stem.

9. What functions are controlled by the medulla?

10. What functions are controlled by the cerebellum?

11. Give a brief description of the pyramidal and extrapyramidal pathways.

12. Basal ganglia is a major structure of the _____ motor pathways.

13. Name the six pairs of cranial nerves that are involved in speech production.

14. What is aphasia? Give a brief description.

15. Define the following terms:
    Anomia

    Paraphasia

    Agrammatism

    Jargon

    Verbal stereotypes

    Agraphia

    Alexia

    Agnosia

16. Distinguish between Broca's and Wernicke's aphasia.

17. What is CVA? How is it related to aphasia?

18. Define the following terms:

    Arteriosclerosis

    Embolus

    Thrombosis

    Aneurysm

    Cerebral hemorrhage

19. Give a brief description of treatment of aphasia.

20. What are motor (neurogenic) speech disorders? How are they distinguished from aphasia?

21. Define and distinguish the following terms: apraxia and dysarthria.

22. How is verbal apraxia explained?

23. What are some of the causes of dysarthria?

24. Give a brief description of the different types of dysarthria.

25. What specific treatment goals are set for dysarthric patients?

26. List the functions of the right hemisphere.

27. Compare the communication problems found in people with left hemisphere damage with those found in people with right hemisphere syndrome.

28. What is prosopagnosia?

29. Define dementia and give a description of its classification.

30. Specify the neuropathology of dementia of the Alzheimer's type.

31. Summarize the symptoms of Huntington's disease.

32. What are the neurological symptoms of AIDS dementia complex?

33. What is the focus of rehabilitation of patients with dementia?

34. Distinguish penetrating from nonpenetrating brain injury.

35. What is meant by the statement that in TBI, communication deficits are not purely linguistic?

36. Define cerebral palsy. What are some of its causes?

37. Give a brief description of the following types of cerebral palsy:

    Spastic cerebral palsy

    Athtoid cerebral palsy

    Ataxic cerebral palsy

38. What is developmental dysarthria found in the child with cerebral palsy?

39. Describe at least two related problems of the child with cerebral palsy.

40. Name at least four specialists on a team of experts who treat children with cerebral palsy.

41. Give a brief description of speech and language services offered to children with cerebral palsy.

42. What are communication boards?

43. What are Carrier symbols?

44. Distinguish between Blissymbolics and the rebus system.

45. What is meant by iconic?

References

Armstrong, A. O. (1979). *Cry Babel*. Garden City, NY: Doubleday.

Bayles, K. A., & Kaszniak, A. W. (1987). *Communication and cognition in normal aging and dementia*. Austin, TX: PRO-ED.

Benson, D. F., & Ardila, A. (1996). *Aphasia: A clinical perspective*. New York: Oxford University Press.

Bhatnagar, S. C., & Andy, O. J. (1995). *Neuroscience for the study of communicative disorders*. Baltimore: Williams & Wilkins.

Bigler, E. D. (Ed.). (1990). *Traumatic brain injury*. Austin, TX: PRO-ED.

Bigler, E. D., Clark, E., & Farmer, J. E. (Eds.). (1997). *Childhood traumatic brain injury: Diagnosis, assessment, and treatment*. Austin, TX: PRO-ED.

Bliss, C. (1965). *Semantography*. Sydney, Australia: Semantography Publications.

Bobath, K., & Bobath, B. (1967). The neuro-developmental treatment of cerebral palsy. *Journal of American Physical Therapy Association, 47,* 1039–1041.

Bottenberg, D. E., & Hanks, J. M. (1986). Language and speech of physically handicapped children. In V. A. Reed (Ed.), *An introduction to children with language disorders* (pp. 201–219). New York: Macmillan.

Brookshire, R. (1997). *An introduction to neurogenic communication disorders* (5th ed.). St. Louis: Mosby Year Book.

Calvin, W. H., & Ojemann, G. A. (1980). *Inside the brain*. New York: New American Library.

Carrier, J. K., Jr., & Peak, T. (1975). *Non-SLIP (Non-Speech Language Initiation Program)*. Lawrence, KS: H & H Enterprises.

Chapey, R. (Ed.). (1994). *Language intervention strategies in adult aphasia* (3rd ed.). Baltimore: Williams & Wilkins.

Clark, C. R. (1981). Learning words using traditional orthography and the symbols of rebus, Bliss, and Carrier. *Journal of Speech and Hearing Disorders, 46,* 191–196.

Clark, C. R., Davies, C. O., & Woodcock, R. W. (1974). *Standard rebus glossary*. Circle Pines, MN: American Guidance Service.

Cummings, J. L., & Benson, F. D. (1992). *Dementia: A clinical approach*. Newton, MA: Butterworth-Heinemann.

Damasio, H. (1981). Cerebral localization of the aphasias. In M. T. Sarno (Ed.), *Acquired aphasia* (pp. 27–50). New York: Academic Press.

Darley, F. L. (1982). *Aphasia*. Philadelphia: Saunders.

Darley, F. L., Aronson, A., & Brown, J. R. (1975). *Motor speech disorders*. Philadelphia: Saunders.

Davis, G. A. (2000). *Aphasiology: Disorders and clinical practice*. Needham Heights, MA: Allyn & Bacon.

Duffy, J. R. (1995). *Motor speech disorders: Substrates, differential diagnosis, and management*. St. Louis, MO: Mosby.

Ferrand, C. T., & Bloom, R. L. (Eds.). (1997). *Introduction to organic and neurogenic disorders of communication*. Boston: Allyn & Bacon.

Frattali, C. M., Thompson, C. K., Holland, A. L., Wohl, C. B., & Ferketi, M. M. (1995). *Functional Assessment of Communication Skills for Adults (ASHA FACS)*. Rockville, MD: American Speech-Language-Hearing Association.

Freed, D. B. (2000). *Motor speech disorders: Diagnosis and treatment*. San Diego, CA: Singular.

Goodglass, H., & Kaplan, E. (1983a). *The assessment of aphasia and related disorders* (2nd ed.). Philadelphia: Lea & Febiger.

Goodglass, H., & Kaplan, E. (1983b). *Boston Diagnostic Aphasia Test*. Philadelphia: Lea & Febiger.

Groher, M. E. (1997). *Dysphagia*. Boston: Butterworth-Heinemann.

Hall, P. K., Jordan, L. S., & Robin, D. A. (1993). *Developmental apraxia of speech: Theory and clinical practice*. Austin, TX: PRO-ED.

Hartley, L. L. (1995). *Cognitive-communicative abilities following brain injury.* San Diego, CA: Singular.

Haynes, S. (1985). Developmental apraxia of speech: Symptoms and treatment. In D. F. Johns (Ed.), *Clinical management of neurogenic communicative disorders* (pp. 259–266). Boston: Little, Brown.

Hegde, M. N. (2001a). *Hegde's pocketguide to assessment in speech–language pathology* (2nd ed.). San Diego, CA: Singular.

Hegde, M. N. (2001b). *Hegde's pocketguide to treatment in speech–language pathology* (2nd ed.). San Diego, CA: Singular.

Hegde, M. N. (1998). *A coursebook on aphasia and other neurogenic language disorders* (2nd ed.). San Diego, CA: Singular.

Helm-Estabrooks, N., & Albert, M. L. (1991). *A manual of aphasia therapy.* Austin, TX: PRO-ED.

Hodgins, E. (1964). *Episode: A report on the accident inside my skull.* New York: Atheneum.

Holland, A. L. (1970). Case studies in aphasia rehabilitation using programmed instruction. *Journal of Speech and Hearing Disorders, 35,* 377–390.

Kearns, K. P., & Simmons, N. N. (1988). Motor speech disorders: The dysarthrias and apraxia of speech. In N. J. Lass, L. V. McReynolds, J. L. Northern, & D. E. Yoder (Eds.), *Handbook of speech–language pathology and audiology* (pp. 592–621). Toronto: Decker.

Kent, R. D., & Rosenbek, J. C. (1983). Acoustic patterns of apraxia of speech. *Journal of Speech and Hearing Disorders, 26,* 231–249.

Kertesz, A. (1982). *Western Aphasia Battery.* New York: Grune & Stratton.

Killilea, M. (1952). *Karen: A true story told by her mother.* New York: Dell.

Killilea, M. (1983). *With love from Karen.* New York: Dell.

Klich, R. J., Ireland, J. V., & Weidner, W. E. (1979). Articulatory and phonological aspects of consonant substitutions in apraxia of speech. *Cortex, 15,* 451–470.

Kopit, A. (1978). *Wings.* New York: Hill & Wang.

LaPointe, L. L. (1985). Aphasia therapy: Some principles and strategies for treatment. In D. F. John (Ed.), *Clinical management of neurogenic communicative disorders* (2nd ed., pp. 179–242). Boston: College-Hill Press/Little, Brown.

LaPointe, L. L. (Ed.). (1997). *Aphasia and related neurogenic language disorders* (2nd ed.). New York: Thieme Medical.

Larsen, C. R. (1998). *HIV-1 and communication disorders: What speech and hearing professionals need to know.* San Diego, CA: Singular.

Logemann, J. A. (1998). *Evaluation and treatment of swallowing disorders.* Austin, TX: PRO-ED.

Love, R. J., & Webb, W. G. (1996). *Neurology for the speech–language pathologist* (3rd ed.). Boston: Butterworth-Heinemann.

Marquardt, T. P., Rinehardt, J. B., & Peterson, H. A. (1979). Markedness analysis of phonemic substitution errors in apraxia of speech. *Journal of Communication Disorders, 12,* 481–494.

McNeil, M. R. (1988). Aphasia in the adult. In N. J. Lass, L. V. McReynolds, J. L. Northern, & D. E. Yoder (Eds.), *Handbook of speech–language pathology and audiology* (pp. 738–786). Toronto: Decker.

Mohr, J. P. (1980). Revision of Broca aphasia and the syndrome of Broca's area infarction and its implications in aphasia therapy. In R. H. Brookshire (Ed.), *Proceedings of the conference on clinical aphasiology* (pp. 1–16). Minneapolis: BRK.

Myers, P. S. (1999). *Right hemisphere damage.* San Diego, CA: Singular.

Payne, J. C. (1997). *Adult neurogenic communication disorders: Assessment and treatment.* San Diego, CA: Singular.

Perkins, W. H., & Kent. R. D. (1986). *Functional anatomy of speech, language and hearing.* Boston: Little, Brown.

Porch, B. E. (1981). *Porch Index of Communicative Ability.* Austin, TX: PRO-ED.

Premack, D. (1971). Language in chimpanzee? *Science, 172,* 808–822.

Rosenbek, J. C., & LaPointe, L. L. (1985). The dysarthrias: Description, diagnosis, and treatment. In D. F. Johns (Ed.), *Clinical management of neurogenic communicative disorders* (2nd ed., pp. 97–152). Boston: College-Hill Press/Little, Brown.

Rosenbek, J. C., LaPointe, L. L., & Wertz, R. (1989). *Aphasia: A clinical approach.* Boston: College-Hill Press/Little, Brown.

Schuell, H., Jenkins, J. J., & Jimenez-Pabon, E. (1964). *Aphasia in adults: Diagnosis, prognosis, and treatment.* New York: Harper & Row.

Schuell, H., & Sefer, J. (1973). *Differential diagnosis of aphasia* (Revised ed.). Minneapolis: University of Minnesota Press.

Seikel, J. A., Douglas, W. K., & Drumright, D. G. (1997). *Anatomy and physiology for speech, language, and hearing* (Expanded ed.). San Diego, CA: Singular.

Shewan, C. M. (1980). Phonological processing in Broca's aphasia. *Brain & Language, 10,* 71–88.

Thompson, C. K. (1988). Articulation disorders in the child with neurogenic pathology. In N. J. Lass, L. V. McReynolds, J. L. Northern, & D. E. Yoder (Eds.), *Handbook of speech–language pathology and audiology* (pp. 548–591). Toronto: Decker.

Tompkins, C. A. (1995). *Right hemisphere communication disorders: Theory and practice.* San Diego, CA: Singular.

Webster, D. W. (1999). *Neuroscience of communication* (2nd ed.). San Diego, CA: Singular.

Wertz, R. T. (1985). Neuropathologies of speech and language: An introduction to patient management. In D. F. Johns (Ed.), *Clinical management of neurogenic communicative disorders* (2nd ed., pp. 1–96). Boston: College-Hill Press/Little, Brown.

Yorkston, K. M., Beukelman, D. R., Strand, E. A., & Bell, K. R. (1999). *Management of motor speech disorders in children and adults* (2nd ed.). Austin, TX: PRO-ED.

Zemlin, W. R. (1998). *Speech and hearing science: Anatomy and physiology* (4th ed.). Englewood Cliffs, NJ: Prentice Hall.

Hearing and Its Disorders

The universe out there may be silent, but our world is full of sounds without which the human existence would not be the same. Sound is an event in the physical world. Looking or finding the source of a sound is a natural tendency of all organisms because the information so gathered may be of survival value (Yost, 1994). Normally, sounds of the physical world that surround us are an integrated part of our existence. Without them, we might be lost, confused, temporarily disoriented in time and space, and may find our ordinary experience strange, annoying, even fearful. Various sounds of time and the seasons make us feel at home, make us feel right. Sounds help us keep in touch with reality. Sometimes we prefer the silence and quiet to sounds that surround us. However, when silence and quiet are biologically imposed, the human experience is profoundly altered.

This chapter is about **biologically imposed silence and quiet.** This form of silence and quiet, imposed by an impaired auditory mechanism, is called **hearing impairment.** The experience of imposed quiet and silence is difficult for people who hear to imagine, and difficult for people with hearing impairment to describe. A person born with deafness has not fully experienced the world of sound, so it is hard to describe what is missed. But there are brilliant exceptions. We have some touching pieces of writing by people who are deaf or hard of hearing. For example, consider the poem called "Silence," written by Robert Smithdas (1966), a poet who is deaf and blind:

There never was a silence
as deep as this one is:
A silence filled with circling thoughts
and spanless distances.

Death never had a stillness
like this one that I know.
Where space and time stand idle
and my brain rocks to and fro!

Acoustics: The Study of Sound

Acoustics, a branch of physics, is the study of sound as a physical event. When sound is studied as a psychological experience of hearing, it is called **psycho-acoustics.**

Abstract physical events called sound cause the human experience of hearing. These events cannot be seen unless they are made visible through scientific instruments. Some of the basic facts of sound are the following:

- The source of sound is mechanical vibrations of some object.
- The vibrations create waves of disturbance in the molecules of a gas, a liquid, or a solid object.
- The waves then travel through a gas, a liquid, or a solid, which are called a medium.
- The medium must be elastic to carry the sound.
- To be called a sound, the disturbance of the molecules must be audible.

The **sound,** then, is "an audible disturbance of a medium produced by a source" (Borden, Harris, & Raphael, 1994, p. 30).

It is from the standpoint of human experience that the sound is defined as an **audible** disturbance of a medium. In this sense, sound is an event that generates auditory sensory experience. However, there are sounds (disturbances of molecules) that humans cannot hear; such sounds do not generate sensory experience in the human ear. Only some animals can hear those sounds. Of course, there are sounds that no biological organisms can hear. Also, there are sounds even if no one is there to hear them. Therefore, objectively speaking, a disturbance of molecules need not be audible, and sounds exist even if they are not heard, but the quoted definition is useful in understanding human hearing and its disorders.

The Source of Sound

Vibrations of an elastic object are the source of sound. There are many sources of sound, strings of a guitar and vocal folds among them (Speaks, 1999). The vibrations of a tuning fork provide a simple illustration of a source of sound. When struck, a tuning fork vibrates at a single frequency. A tone of a single frequency is called a **pure tone.** In this case, **frequency** is the number of times a cycle of vibration repeats itself within a second.

The vibrations happen in **cycles.** As Figure 10.1 shows, the cycles of a vibrating tuning fork consist of back-and-forth movements of its tines (prongs). In one cycle, the two tines first move toward each other, then back to their resting position, and then away from each other, and then back to their resting position. Another cycle then begins. Therefore, at the end of one cycle is the

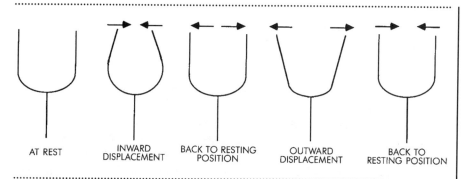

AT REST INWARD DISPLACEMENT BACK TO RESTING POSITION OUTWARD DISPLACEMENT BACK TO RESTING POSITION

Figure 10.1. A single cycle of vibration of a tuning fork.

beginning of another. Thus, the repeated patterns of movements, measured per second, are the cycles. The vibrations of a tuning fork are described as **simple harmonic motion,** resulting in a tone of single frequency which repeats itself.

Unlike the sounds of a tuning fork, the sounds surrounding us are rarely simple. We simultaneously hear many sounds of differing frequencies. Also, the movements of many vibrating objects are complex. When two or more sounds of the same frequency are added, the result is a pure and simple tone. However, when two or more sounds of **differing frequencies** are added, we have a **complex tone.**

The vibrations that make up a complex tone may be periodic or aperiodic. As illustrated in Figure 10.2, **periodic** vibrations have a pattern that repeats itself at regular intervals. **Aperiodic** vibrations have no such pattern. Aperiodic complex signals are mostly noise of various sorts. Many such signals are perceived as unpleasant.

The Sound Waves

When the prongs of a tuning fork move back and forth, the nearby air molecules also move back and forth. As a result, the molecules lying next to the molecules that moved back and forth now begin to move. In this manner, the molecules lying farther and farther away from the vibrating object move. Such to-and-fro movements of molecules of a medium (e.g., air or water) caused by a vibrating object are called **sound waves.**

Note that the molecules that surround the vibrating object do not move from point A to point B. It is the transfer of energy, not matter, that occurs. The

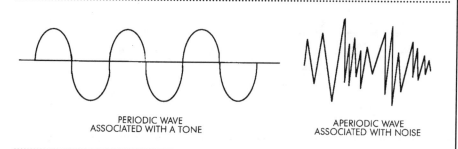

PERIODIC WAVE ASSOCIATED WITH A TONE   APERIODIC WAVE ASSOCIATED WITH NOISE

Figure 10.2. Periodic and aperiodic sound waves.

molecules, while remaining where they are, just swing back and forth. Such swings disturb adjacent molecules, which in turn swing back and forth, thus disturbing the molecules next to them, and so on. The sound moves because of the to-and-fro movements of molecules.

The to-and-fro movements of the molecules change the air pressure because the movements consist of a place where the molecules are compressed together and a place where they are further apart (rarefaction). Thus, regions of air mass compression and rarefaction alternate, creating cyclical variations. As shown in Figure 10.3, a single **cycle** consists of one instance of **compression** and one instance of **rarefaction** within a second. A more recent name for the cycles per second (cps) is **hertz**, abbreviated Hz. (Heinrich Hertz was a German scientist who studied electromagnetic waves.) For example, 100 Hz means that there are 100 cycles of compression and rarefaction in one second. It means the same as 100 cps. A tone of a single Hz is illustrated in Figure 10.3.

Compression means that the molecules are *dense* and **rarefaction** means that they are *thin*.

Frequency and Pitch

The human ear cannot respond to the entire range of the frequency of sound vibrations. The ear of an average, healthy, young adult can respond to frequencies in the range of 20 Hz to 20,000 Hz. Several animals can hear sounds of much higher frequency; for example, dogs can hear special whistles that humans cannot hear.

Variations in the frequency of vibratory cycles create the sensation of different pitch. When the frequency changes, we hear a difference in pitch. Therefore, **pitch** is often described as the *perceptual correlate* of changes in frequency. It means that frequency is physical, but pitch is perceptual. In this context, the term *perceptual* may be understood as a matter of sensation. Sounds of higher frequency create sensations of higher pitch, and those of lower frequency create sensations of lower pitch. However, we are more sensitive to changes in lower frequencies (below 1000 Hz) than in higher frequencies. At higher frequencies, larger frequency changes are needed to perceive changes in pitch.

Read **Chapter 7** for information on pitch as it relates to vocal fold vibrations.

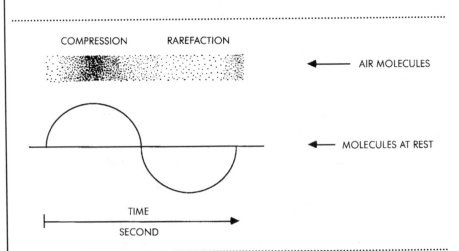

Figure 10.3. A tone of a single Hz (1 cps) has one instance of compression and one instance of rarefaction of air molecules in 1 second.

Intensity and Loudness

Sounds vary not only in frequency, but also in intensity. Intensity is related to **amplitude,** which is the extent of displacement of the molecules in their to-and-fro motion. The greater the range of displacement, the higher the amplitude of sound. And the greater the amplitude of sound, the higher the intensity of sound. The movements of the diaphragm of a loud speaker illustrate the concept of amplitude: When the volume is increased, the diaphragm begins to bulge out more than at a lower volume. Figure 10.4 illustrates tones of different amplitude in the context of different frequency.

The physical characteristic of intensity of a sound determines the psychological sensation of **loudness** of that sound. Therefore, intensity is a physical event, and loudness is a perceptual event. Loudness is a sensation, just like the pitch of a sound. The higher the intensity of a sound, the greater its perceived loudness.

The human ear is sensitive to a wide range of sound intensity. Measured on a **linear scale,** which has a zero and whose numerical increments are equal, the human ear is sensitive to perhaps 10 trillion units of intensity. Measuring intensity with such a large range of numbers is cumbersome. Therefore, scientists use a **logarithmic scale,** in which one number is multiplied by itself a specified number of times. On a logarithmic scale, the ear is sensitive to 130 units called **decibels** (dB). A decibel is 1/10 of a Bell, the basic unit of measurement named after Alexander Graham Bell, the famous American inventor of the telephone and an early educator of students who are deaf.

Read **Chapter 7** for information on loudness as it relates to vocal fold vibrations.

Sound Pressure Level and Hearing Level

The decibel is a relative measure; it helps compare the intensity of one sound against the other, a standard. The decibel also is a measure of sound pressure. The value of **sound pressure** is the square root of the power, which is measured in **watts.** The pressure is measured in terms of **pascals,** or **pa.** Therefore, the intensity of a sound is expressed in terms of decibels at a certain **sound pressure level,** abbreviated **SPL.** For example, the intensity of normal conversational speech varies between 50 and 70 dB SPL. Very intense sounds, such as

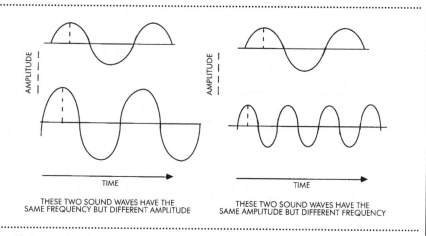

THESE TWO SOUND WAVES HAVE THE SAME FREQUENCY BUT DIFFERENT AMPLITUDE

THESE TWO SOUND WAVES HAVE THE SAME AMPLITUDE BUT DIFFERENT FREQUENCY

Figure 10.4. Amplitude in the context of frequency.

those of a lawn mower, may be as high as 100 dB SPL. The intensity of live rock concerts may reach 115 to 120 dB SPL. A sound of 140 dB SPL induces pain.

The sound pressure level must be distinguished from **hearing level (HL)**, which is the lowest intensity of a sound necessary to stimulate the auditory system (Martin & Clark, 2000; Stach, 1998). However, the auditory system is not equally sensitive to all frequencies at the same intensity. The human ear is most sensitive to sounds of 1000 to 4000 Hz. Therefore, to stimulate the auditory system, tones of 1000 to 4000 Hz need to be less intense than tones of other frequency. This differential sensitivity of the ear to different frequencies creates unnecessary complications in the measurement of hearing and hearing loss. To overcome this problem, scientists first determined the sound pressure levels required to stimulate the auditory system at different frequencies in a large number of healthy people. Then, those sound pressure levels were considered the 0 dB hearing level. For example, to stimulate the healthy normal ear of a young adult, a sound of 250 Hz must have a sound pressure level of 25.5 dB. For the same purpose, a sound of 1000 Hz needs only 7 dB SPL. In measuring hearing with an audiometer (described later), the actual SPL values needed to stimulate normal auditory systems at those two frequencies were set at zero, though in once case (250 Hz) the SPL value is higher than in the other (1000 Hz). Similarly, for all the frequencies that are tested on an audiometer, the amount of energy needed to stimulate the auditory system has been set at zero.

> Remember that zero on an audiometer dial for a given frequency does not mean no sound energy.

Summary

- Acoustics is the study of sound.

- Sound consists of disturbances of a medium due to a vibrating source.

- Vibrations occur in cycles; the number of times a cycle of vibration repeats itself in a second is the frequency of vibration.

- A cycle of vibration also is known as Hertz (Hz).

- Psychoacoustics is the study of sensory (psychological) experiences of sound.

- The pitch of a sound is a sensation determined by the frequency of vibrations.

- Loudness also is a sensation determined by the intensity of the sound signal.

- The sensitivity of the human ear to sound is measured in terms of a unit called decibel (dB).

- The lowest intensity of a sound needed to stimulate the auditory system is called the hearing level (HL).

- The human ear is differentially sensitive to sounds of different frequency; the minimum sound pressure levels needed to stimulate the ear at different frequencies, although unequal, is arbitrarily set at zero.

Anatomy and Physiology of Hearing

As described earlier, sound waves travel through the medium of air, solid objects, or liquid. However, without a functioning biological system, the sound would not be heard and understood. Therefore, a brief description of the biological mechanism of hearing, which includes the ear, the auditory nerve, and certain portions of the brain, follows.

The Ear

The human ear is divided into three sections: the outer ear, the middle ear, and the inner ear. Figure 10.5 illustrates the three sections of the ear and their major parts.

The Outer Ear

The visible **auricle** or **pinna** and the **external auditory canal** are parts of the outer ear. Although its role in hearing is limited, the pinna funnels the sound to the ear canal and helps localize sounds. The external auditory canal (or meatus) leads to the eardrum, at which the outer ear ends. The external auditory canal moves inward with a slight upward angle. In adults, the length of the canal has a range of 2 to 3 cm.

The external auditory canal has special cells that secrete cerumen (wax) that trap small insects that may try to crawl into the middle ear. The cerumen also filters dust. Being an air-filled cavity open at one end, the canal acts as a resonator of the sound it receives. It boosts the high frequency sounds.

The Middle Ear

The middle ear is an air-filled cavity; the outer and the middle ears are separated by the **eardrum** or **tympanic membrane,** which is thin, elastic, and cone shaped. It is tough yet flexible and highly sensitive to sound pressure variations. While the entire tympanic membrane responds to the sounds of low frequencies, only specific portions of it respond to high frequency sounds.

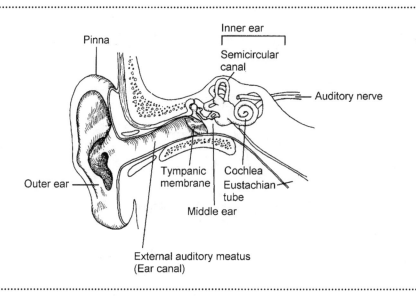

Figure 10.5. The human ear.

The tympanic membrane can be easily damaged. A hairpin or a similar object, inserted in the ear, can rupture it. Explosions and sudden pressure changes also can rupture it. Although a damaged or punctured eardrum may heal spontaneously, repeated ruptures cause scar tissue, which reduces its mobility. The tympanic membrane is illustrated in Figure 10.6A.

Past the tympanic membrane lie the most important structures: the three small bones forming the **ossicular chain** of the middle ear, illustrated in Figure 10.6B. The first and the largest of the bones is called the **malleus** because it resembles a hammer. One end of the malleus is embedded in the tympanic membrane. Because of this attachment, the vibrations of the membrane are transmitted to the malleus.

The malleus is attached to another bone called the **incus**, also known as the anvil. This in turn is attached to the third bone called the **stapes** or stirrup. The other end of the stapes is inserted into the oval window, a small opening that leads to the inner ear.

The ossicular chain transmits sound efficiently and without distortion. The chain also amplifies the sound by about 30 dB before transmitting it into the fluids of the inner ear. Sound loses some of its intensity when it moves from a

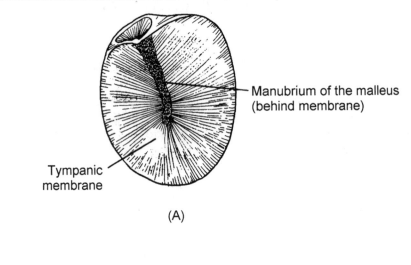

Manubrium of the malleus (behind membrane)

Tympanic membrane

(A)

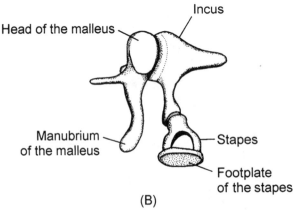

Incus

Head of the malleus

Manubrium of the malleus

Stapes

Footplate of the stapes

(B)

Figure 10.6. The tympanic membrane and the ossicular chain of the middle ear.

medium of air to a medium of fluid. The middle ear, as noted, is filled with air; the inner ear is filled with fluid. Without this amplification by the ossicular chain, the sound reaching the inner ear would be very soft.

Another important structure of the middle ear is the **eustachian tube,** also known as the **auditory tube,** which connects the middle ear with the **nasopharynx.** The nasopharynx is the part of the back throat that opens into the nasal passage. The eustachian tube helps maintain equal air pressure within and outside the middle ear. The nasopharyngeal end of the tube can be opened by yawning or swallowing. This lets fresh air into the middle ear. As we will find out shortly, infection also can gain access to the middle ear through the eustachian tube, causing hearing problems.

The Inner Ear

The inner ear is the most complex of the three divisions of the ear. It begins with the oval window, which is a small opening in the bone that houses the inner ear. Through the stapes, the inner ear receives the mechanical vibrations of the sound.

The inner ear is a system of interconnecting tunnels called **labyrinths** in the temporal bone. The tunnels are filled with a fluid called **perilymph.** Two major structures with two separate functions are found in the inner ear. One structure, known as the **vestibular system,** contains three **semicircular canals** and is concerned with balance, body position, and movement. Therefore, we will not be concerned with this system here. The other structure, important for hearing, is called the **cochlea.** The semicircular canals and the cochlea are illustrated in Figure 10.7.

> Note that the inner ear serves two unrelated functions: hearing and balance.

The cochlea is snail shaped; it is a coiled tunnel filled with another kind of fluid called **endolymph.** The floor of the cochlear duct, known as the **basilar membrane,** contains the **organ of Corti,** which bathes in the endolymph and contains several thousand **hair cells,** which respond to sound. The sound reaches the cochlea as disturbances in the fluid of the inner ear, created by the mechanical force of the stapes bone. Due to this force, the basilar membrane vibrates. The different portions of the basilar membrane respond best to

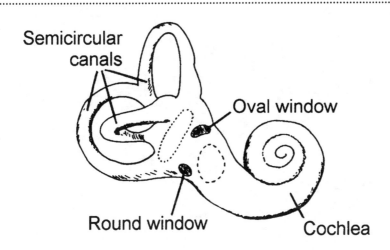

Figure 10.7. The semicircular canals and the cochlea.

sounds of different frequencies. The membrane is thinner, narrower, and stiffer at the base than at the tip. The tip is thicker, wider, and more lax than the base. Sounds of high frequency stimulate the base and those of low frequency stimulate the tip. In either case, the stimulating sound signals set off waves in the fluid, which in turn create movements of the membrane.

Within the organ of Corti, an energy transformation takes place. The mechanical forms of vibrations are transformed into electrical impulses. These electrical impulses are carried to the brain by the acoustic or the auditory nerve.

The Acoustic Nerve and the Brain

The **acoustic nerve** is a bundle of neurons with two branches. The **vestibular branch** is concerned with the body equilibrium. The **auditory** or **acoustic branch,** which supplies the many hair cells of the cochlea, is concerned with sound transmission. It carries the electrical sound impulses from the cochlea to the brain.

A **meatus** is a tunnel.

The acoustic nerve also is called the cranial nerve VIII. Cranial nerves are those that are housed within the skull. From the cochlea, the right and the left branches of the acoustic nerve leave the temporal bone through the **internal auditory meatus** and enter the brain stem. At this level, most of the nerve fibers from one side (ear) cross over to the other side; some continue on the same side. Therefore, the brain can compare the sounds received from each of the two ears. This helps localize the sound.

From the brain stem, the acoustic nerve fibers project sound to the final destination, the temporal lobe of the brain. The temporal lobe contains the primary auditory area, which is responsible for receiving and interpreting sound stimuli. The temporal lobe with its primary auditory area is shown in Figure 10.8. Whether it is speech, noise, or environmental sounds of various sorts, it is the brain that finally interprets the meaning of what is heard.

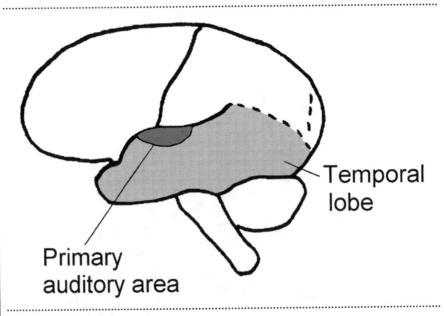

Figure 10.8. The temporal lobe and the primary auditory area.

Summary

- The human ear is divided into an outer, a middle, and an inner section.

- The pinna and external auditory canal make up the outer ear.

- The tympanic membrane and the ossicular chain, being the two most important structures of the middle ear, conduct sound to the inner ear.

- The semicircular canals of the inner ear are concerned with the sense of balance.

- The cochlea, with its organ of Corti that contains the hair cells that respond to sound, is the most important inner ear structure of hearing.

- The acoustic nerve, which carries the sound impulses to the brain, supplies the hair cells.

- The sound is received and interpreted by the brain, particularly the primary auditory center of the temporal lobe.

Normal Hearing

Neurophysiologically, normal hearing is made possible by the ear, the auditory nerve, and the auditory areas of the brain. However, normal hearing is a set of complex skills, most of which develop over a period of time. Also, normal hearing involves two types of sound conduction: air and bone conduction. Therefore, in this section, auditory development will be described along with air and bone conduction of hearing.

Auditory Development in Children

Signs of auditory development can be traced during the fetal period. A 20-week-old fetus responds to sound. The heart rate of the fetus increases when sound is presented through the mother's abdomen. The fetus does not grow in silence. In one study, the mother's pulse as heard by the fetus was measured at 72 dB, a high level of noise the fetus constantly hears for months before birth (Bench, 1968). Also, the mother's abdomen can transmit external sound to the fetus.

The newborn baby can already respond differently to sounds of different pitch and loudness. The infant becomes quieter when presented with low frequency sounds and more active in the presence of high frequency sounds. The infant's heart rate increases in response to louder sounds.

The newborn soon begins to give overt responses to sound and to discriminate between different sounds, including speech sounds. Babies give many responses to sound stimuli. For example, a sound stimulus presented to a baby at rest will evoke such activity as an eye blink or opening of the eyes. A startle response involving an abrupt movement of arms and legs also may be evoked. To the contrary, a baby's ongoing arm and leg movements or crying may stop when a sound is heard.

Read **Chapter 4** for speech sound discrimination in infants.

By the 3rd or 4th month, the baby begins to make a head turn toward the source of sound. This response becomes more precise by the 6th or 7th month. A 3-month-old baby responds to the mother's voice and speech more consistently than to someone else's voice and speech. If a baby can turn on a switch that activates a tape recorder to play sounds, voices, or music, even 8- or 9-month-old babies will quickly learn to turn on the tape recorder (Friedlander, 1970). As babies grow older, their responses to auditory stimuli become more precise. The babies can better localize sounds and discriminate among them.

A healthy baby has exceptionally good hearing. In fact, young babies hear better than adults. Unfortunately, age, the noises of the workplace and of the general environment, and various diseases that affect the functioning of the hearing mechanism take their toll on hearing.

Air and Bone Conduction of Sound

In normal hearing, sound is conducted to the inner ear by two means. One of them is air conduction, and the other is bone conduction. As noted, the sound waves striking the eardrum are transmitted to the ossicular chain, which moves the fluids of the middle ear. These movements cause vibrations in the basilar membrane of the cochlea. The hair cells supplied by the acoustic nerve respond to these vibrations, and the sound is carried by the nerve to the brain. In this process, and for the most part, the sound travels through the medium of air. Therefore, **air conduction** is transmission of sound through the medium of air.

The fluids of the inner ear are housed in the skull. We already know that vibrating bones can conduct sound, as does the ossicular chain of the middle ear. Similarly, the larger bones of the skull also conduct sound because they vibrate in response to airborne sound waves. These vibrations cause movements in the fluids of the inner ear. This is **bone conduction.** Therefore, bone conduction is transmission of sound through the medium of vibrating bone or bones. Normally, the air- and bone-conducted movements are integrated. It is only in certain kinds of hearing loss that the two can be distinguished.

We normally hear our own voice through a combination of air and bone conduction. However, it is possible to feel the difference between the air- and bone-conducted sounds. For example, when a person listens to his or her own speech played by a tape recorder, the voice does not sound the same. This is because the sound coming out of the tape recorder travels through the air and strikes the eardrum. The person is now hearing his or her own voice mainly through air conduction. Therefore, it sounds unusual.

As will be described shortly, the distinction between air and bone conduction is important in diagnosing hearing disorders.

Disorders of Hearing

Hearing impairment is a major health and educational problem. As the population grows older, the number of individuals with hearing loss also grows larger. It is estimated that 7% to 12% of all newborn babies are at risk for hearing impairment (ASHA Committee on Infant Hearing, 1988; Mahoney & Eichwald, 1987). Factors that place a child at risk include family history of childhood hearing impairment, certain maternal diseases such as syphilis during pregnancy, and anatomic malformations of the head or neck. Children without any known risk factors also are susceptible to hearing impairment. It is estimated that 1 in 1,000 to 1 in 3,000 newborn babies who are not at risk are hearing impaired (Coplan, 1987).

Hearing impairment can be very mild, causing no significant problems in communication, or it may be severe to profound, causing major problems in speech comprehension and production. The range of hearing loss in dB HL and the corresponding categories are shown in Table 10.1.

The term **hearing impairment** includes the hard of hearing and the deaf. The child who is **hard of hearing** has a hearing loss within the range of 16 dB and 75 dB. Most children who are hard of hearing acquire speech and oral language with variable proficiency. The adult who is hard of hearing has a hearing loss within the range of 25 dB and 75 dB.

Children and adults who are **deaf** are those who cannot hear or understand conversational speech under normal circumstances. Their hearing loss exceeds 75 dB, and in many cases the loss may be greater than 90 dB. In people who are deaf, the acquisition of oral language is severely impaired. As described in a later section, their speech and language are likely to show many problems.

Hearing Impairment: Types and Causes

Based on their nature or the causes, hearing disorders are classified into conductive, sensorineural, and mixed types. Central auditory disorders are a special type.

Conductive Hearing Loss

In **conductive hearing loss,** the efficiency with which the sound is conducted to the middle or inner ear is diminished. Abnormalities of the external auditory

Table 10.1

The Range and Categories of Hearing Loss with the Corresponding dB HL

Up to 15 dB	Normal hearing in children. In adults, the upper limit of normal hearing may extend to 25 dB.
16 to 40 dB	Mild hearing loss in children: difficulty hearing faint or distant speech; may cause language delay in children. In adults, the range is from 25 to 40 dB.
41 to 55 dB	Moderate hearing loss: delayed speech and language acquisition; difficulty in producing certain speech sounds correctly; difficulty following conversation.
56 to 70 dB	Moderately severe hearing loss: can understand only amplified or shouted speech.
71 to 90 dB	Severe hearing loss: difficulty understanding even loud and amplified speech. Significant difficulty in learning and producing intelligible oral language.
91+ dB	Profound hearing loss: typically described as deaf; hearing does not play a major role in learning, producing, and understanding spoken speech and language.

canal, the eardrum, or the ossicular chain of the middle ear are the frequent causes of conductive hearing loss.

In pure conductive hearing loss, the inner ear, the acoustic nerve, and the auditory centers of the brain are all working normally; the bone conduction also is normal or near normal. Note that the term *normal bone conduction* refers to the bones of the skull and not the bones of the middle ear (the ossicular chain). Even when the bones of the ossicular chain are not conducting sound, the bones of the skull will. Therefore, conductive hearing loss is never profound; there is always some hearing left because of the bone conduction. For this reason, a person with conductive hearing loss can hear his or her own speech well. Consequently, the person tends to talk too softly, especially when there is background noise. The person does not hear this background noise too well, so it seems quieter than it does to his or her listeners.

See **Chapter 8** for cleft palate and associated problems.

The causes of conductive hearing loss are many and include birth defects, diseases, and foreign bodies that block the external ear canal. Some children born with cleft palate and other facial and cranial birth defects may have **aural atresia,** in which the external ear canal is completely closed. Another birth defect is called **stenosis,** in which the external auditory canal is extremely narrow. Consequently, all or most of the sound waves may not strike the eardrum.

A fairly common infection of the skin of the external auditory canal, known as **external otitis,** also is a cause of conductive hearing loss. Found often in swimmers, this infection results in the swelling of the tissue of the external auditory canal. Consequently, sound transmission is reduced.

In some rare cases, **bony growths** may appear in the external ear canal. Such growths block the sound. Tumors grown in the external auditory canal can do the same.

However, the two most common causes of conductive hearing loss are otitis media and otosclerosis. **Otitis media,** also known as **middle ear effusion,** is an infection of the middle ear, often associated with upper respiratory infections. It is common among children; adults rarely suffer from it. It is sometimes noted even in the newborn. There are three varieties of otitis media: serous, acute, and chronic.

Five percent of children under 10 years of age suffer from **otitis media.**

In **serous otitis media,** the middle ear is inflamed and filled with thick or watery fluid. The eustachian tube that connects the middle ear cavity to the nasopharynx is blocked. Normally, the tube remains closed but opens briefly when we swallow or yawn. As it opens, fresh air enters the middle ear and thus keeps it supplied with oxygen. A blocked eustachian tube creates an airtight middle ear; soon the air there is thinned out and the pressure is reduced. The greater air pressure outside the ear begins to push the tympanic membrane inward. This reduces its mobility. The retracted membrane does not vibrate efficiently. The result is conductive hearing loss. Serous otitis media may be treated with medical and surgical means. Insertion of small tubes through the tympanic membrane often ventilates the middle ear and restores normal hearing.

Acute otitis media has a sudden onset due to infection. A quick buildup of fluid and puss results in moderate to severe pain. The child has fever and may have vertigo as well. The buildup of pressure in the middle ear may rupture the tympanic membrane, giving a sudden relief. Puss is discharged from the ruptured membrane. Acute otitis media is treated with medical and surgical procedures. Drugs may control the infection. In the surgical treatment, known as **myringotomy,** a small incision in the tympanic membrane is made to relieve the pressure.

In **chronic otitis media,** the tympanic membrane is permanently ruptured with or without middle ear diseases. Many patients may have a painless but foul-smelling discharge from the ear. Depending on their size and location, perforations of the tympanic membrane cause varying degrees of conductive hearing loss. Chronic otitis media associated with infection may be treated with antibiotics. In addition, there are several surgical procedures, including **myringoplasty,** in which the perforated eardrum is surgically repaired.

Mild and nonrecurrent otitis media may not cause permanent hearing loss. Chronic disease is more likely to induce permanent hearing loss. Even mild and fluctuating conductive hearing loss associated with prolonged middle ear infections in young children can adversely affect their speech and language development (Shaw, 1994).

The other common cause of conductive hearing loss, **otosclerosis,** is a disease of the bones of the middle ear, especially the stapes whose footplate is attached to the oval window. In most cases, the disease is inherited. Otosclerosis is more common in women than in men. The disease, often aggravated during pregnancy, starts as a new, spongy growth on the footplate of the stapes. The stapes then becomes rigid, and the footplate does not move enough into the oval window to create pressure waves in the fluid of the inner ear. The stapes also can become too soft to vibrate due to a disease called **otospongiosis.** An ear surgeon might remove the diseased or fixated stapes in an operation called **stapedectomy.** In place of the removed stapes, the surgeon might place a synthetic prosthesis made of wire or Teflon. In most cases, this operation improves hearing dramatically.

Sensorineural Hearing Loss

The middle ear may conduct the sound to the inner ear, but the hair cells in the cochlea or the acoustic nerve may be damaged, preventing the brain from receiving the neural impulses of sound. This is called **sensorineural hearing loss.**

The damaged hair cells and the acoustic nerve are not repairable. Therefore, the sensorineural hearing loss is permanent. This type of loss varies from very mild to profound deafness. Because of the inner ear damage, bone conduction also is impaired. Therefore, people with sensorineural hearing loss have difficulty not only hearing others but also hearing themselves. Consequently, the person tends to talk louder. These features of sensorineural hearing loss contrast with those of conductive loss.

The degree of sensorineural loss is not the same across all frequencies. Some frequencies are more adversely affected than others. Generally, sensorineural hearing loss tends to be greater for higher frequencies than for lower frequencies.

Sensorineural loss, especially the more profound kind affecting many deaf people, has a severe effect on the acquisition of speech and language. Articulation of speech sounds and language structures can be affected.

The causes of sensorineural loss are many. Some causes are prenatal; they are mostly due to what the mother does during her pregnancy. Certain drugs a mother takes, especially during the 6th and 7th weeks of pregnancy, can cause cochlear damage in the fetus. Certain drugs a child takes also can damage the cochlear hair cells or the acoustic nerve fibers. Drugs that damage the ear are called **ototoxic.** Antibiotic drugs of the "mycin" family (streptomycin, kanamycin, neomycin) are especially ototoxic. Physicians prescribe these powerful antibiotic drugs only when severe infections threaten a patient's life. Unfortunately, the drug that saves a life also may produce an undesirable side effect of profound hearing loss.

Ototoxic literally means poisonous to the ear.

Noise is another health hazard that can induce sensorineural hearing loss. Prolonged exposure to such intense noise as that heard in airfields may permanently damage the cochlear hair cells. Loud music, noisy toys, firecrackers, and explosives have the same effect. Noise-induced sensorineural hearing loss tends to be worst between 3000 and 6000 Hz.

Various **infections** also can cause sensorineural hearing loss. Though not a major cause any more in the United States, maternal rubella is a well-known cause of fetal cochlear damage, resulting in congenital sensorineural hearing loss. Among the early childhood infections, meningitis is especially likely to cause sensorineural hearing loss. **Meningitis** is an inflammation of the meninges due to viral infection. The **meninges** is a thin membrane covering the brain and the spinal cord. Virus and bacteria causing infection of the brain and the spinal cord can easily find their way into the inner ear through the internal auditory meatus. The poet Robert Smithdas, whose poem "Silence" was quoted earlier, was deafened by meningitis at the age of 5.

In some children, **birth defects** might be the cause of sensorineural hearing loss. The cochlea or the auditory nerve might not have developed normally by the time the baby is born. Portions of the inner ear might be missing.

In other children, **syphilis** contracted from the mother at the time of birth can cause inner ear damage. **Anoxia,** or lack of oxygen during delivery, also can damage the inner ear.

In some rare cases, the acoustic nerve develops a **tumor,** which causes sensorineural loss. The tumor, called **acoustic neuroma,** can retard nerve conduction of sound impulses to the brain.

Old age also is associated with sensorineural hearing loss. Hearing impairment in the elderly is called **presbycusis,** which is an effect of aging, not a disease. However, it is not clear whether it is the age, the cumulative effects of environmental noise, or other factors that affect the hearing. There is no particular age at which presbycusis has its onset; it varies among individuals. Some show signs of presbycusis earlier than others. The extent of loss also varies.

Meniere's disease is another condition that causes fluctuating sensorineural hearing loss. In most cases, hearing is impaired only in one ear. It is seen mostly in adults. The symptoms of Meniere's disease include spells of dizziness or vertigo, hearing loss, and **tinnitus,** which is various kinds of annoying noises in the ear. The patient may feel fullness in the ear. The symptoms might disappear on their own and return without warning. No cure for this disease is available.

Some sensorineural hearing loss is amenable to medical and surgical treatment, but much is not. Most of those who have sensorineural loss rely on amplification of sound, early education, and speech and language therapy. A later section describes these and related rehabilitative services.

Mixed Hearing Loss

Mixed hearing loss results when both the middle and the inner ear do not function properly. Any of the several conditions that cause conductive and sensorineural hearing loss can, in some combination, adversely affect both air and bone conduction and thus create a mixed hearing loss. However, the bone conduction is less affected than the air conduction.

Central Auditory Disorders

Hearing loss resulting from problems in the outer, middle, or inner ear (excluding the auditory nerve) is a **peripheral hearing problem.** However, auditory problems also may result from damage to the **central auditory system,** which begins at the brain stem where the auditory nerve terminates and includes the fibers that project sound to the auditory centers of the brain, and those brain centers themselves. **Central auditory disorders** are those that are due to a lesion or lesions in the central auditory system. Tumors, various kinds of brain damage, and degenerative diseases affecting the central auditory structures can cause central auditory disorders.

Patients with central auditory disorders tend to complain about tinnitus and unusual auditory sensations. The patients have trouble localizing sounds and following complex instructions. There may be a dramatic loss of interest in music (Musiek, 1985). An interesting factor of central auditory disorder is that there may be no significant peripheral hearing loss. The routine hearing test may not reveal any problem. Of course, in some cases, both a central and a peripheral hearing loss coexist.

Central auditory disorders affect complex auditory performance. That is why the term *auditory disorders* (instead of hearing loss) is used. Generally, the patient hears but does not understand speech under certain difficult conditions. For example, background noise may make it extremely difficult to understand speech. Difficulty in understanding distorted speech is another major symptom. In some of the central auditory tests, speech may be periodically interrupted, masked with noise, compressed in time, presented at low intensity, or filtered by eliminating certain frequencies of speech. Everyone has some difficulty in understanding speech so distorted, but those with central auditory disorders have a greater amount of difficulty. When there is a lesion in the temporal lobe of the brain, for example, filtered speech test scores may be poorer in the ear opposite the damaged side (contralateral) than in the ear on the side of the damage.

Several other procedures are available to diagnose central auditory disorders. They are valuable because in many cases, an early diagnosis of auditory brain damage can be made only with the help of central auditory tests.

> There is speculation that learning disorders in children may be due to central auditory disorders.

Summary

- Individuals with hearing impairment may be hard-of-hearing or deaf.

- People who are hard-of-hearing have some useful hearing; as children, they are able to acquire oral language and use it for communication.

- People who are deaf have a more serious hearing problem; they cannot hear or understand conversational speech.

- Hearing loss may be conductive, sensorineural, or mixed.

- In conductive hearing loss, the efficiency of the outer ear or the middle ear to transmit sound to the inner ear is diminished. A frequent cause of conductive hearing loss is middle ear infection.

- In sensorineural hearing loss, the hair cells of the cochlea or the acoustic nerve or both are not functioning properly. Consequently, the brain does not receive sound. Many factors, including toxic drugs, infections, and noise, can induce sensorineural hearing loss.

- Mixed hearing loss includes a conductive and a sensorineural component.

Assessment of Hearing Loss

Hearing disorders are a concern of many specialists. The **otologist** is a medical specialist who diagnoses and treats ear diseases. An audiologist has extensive training in the administration of various diagnostic tests of hearing. Therefore, this chapter is not only about hearing and its disorders but also about audiology and audiologists.

Audiology and Audiologists

Audiology and speech–language pathology are twin professions. **Audiology** is the study of hearing, its disorders, and the measurement and management of those disorders.

An **audiologist** is an expert in hearing and its disorders. He or she has special training in the assessment of hearing disorders and rehabilitation of individuals with hearing impairment. Audiologists and speech–language pathologists are typically trained in the same university departments; they share many academic courses before they branch out to specialize. What follows is a description of what audiologists do in the assessment and rehabilitation of individuals with hearing impairment.

Audiometry

Audiologists use instruments called audiometers to measure hearing loss. An **audiometer** is an electronic instrument that generates and amplifies pure tones, noise, and other stimuli for testing hearing. Advanced audiometers are totally computerized. The audiometer generates tones at various frequencies (Hz). The audiologist can select the frequency and vary the intensity of the sound stimulus. An electronic audiometer being used in testing is illustrated in Figure 10.9.

The person to be tested sits in a specially constructed soundproof booth, of the kind illustrated in Figure 10.10. This eliminates or reduces interference from ambient noise in the environment. In testing air conduction, the person wears headphones that deliver the sound stimulus directly to the ear. The person holds a switch in his or her hand and presses it whenever a tone is heard. The response lights up a small lamp on the audiometer. To indicate that he or she heard the tone, the person may also raise a hand.

The pure tone hearing testing is done to determine the threshold of hearing for selected frequencies. A **threshold** is an intensity level at which a tone is faintly heard at least 50% of the time it is presented. Each tone is presented more than once to establish a threshold for it.

The audiologist tests hearing at selected frequencies. Typically, a tone of 1000 Hz is first presented because it is most easily detected. Next, tones of 2000, 4000, and 8000 Hz are tested in that order. Finally, tones of 500 and 250 Hz are tested. The reason for selecting these frequencies is that they are most important for speech. Most human speech sounds are in the frequency range of 100 to 8000 Hz.

The two ears are tested, starting with either ear. The person is asked to listen to faint sounds and press the response switch as soon as the sound is heard. To begin with, the sound is generally presented at 30 dB. If the person

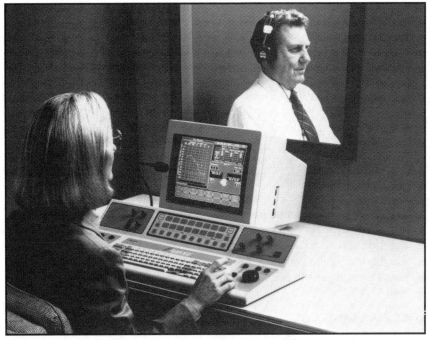

Figure 10.9. An electronic computerized audiometer. (Photo courtesy of Nicolet Instrument Corporation.)

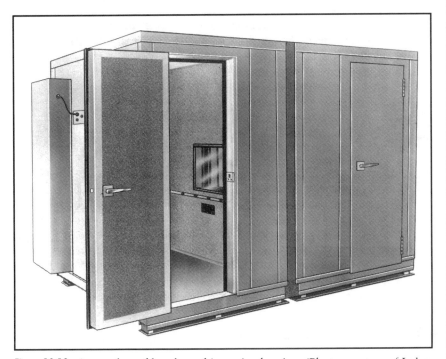

Figure 10.10. A soundproof booth used in testing hearing. (Photo courtesy of Industrial Acoustic Company, Inc.)

does not respond, the intensity is increased in steps until the person responds. If the person responds to the initial presentation, the intensity is reduced in steps until the person no longer responds. The intensity is then increased until the response is once again observed. In this procedure, the threshold is determined by moving down to its level, going below it, and moving up to it. Different audiologists use slightly different procedures to establish pure tone thresholds.

Hearing by bone conduction is tested to assess the sensitivity of the sensorineural portion of the auditory mechanism. In this test, a bone vibrator is placed on the forehead or behind the test ear. The bones of the skull vibrate when the sound strikes them. This vibration stimulates the fluids in both the inner ears. Therefore, it is hard to determine which ear heard the sound and which did not. To overcome this problem, the audiologist introduces noise through a headphone in the ear not being tested. The noise is made strong enough to mask the tone heard in the opposite ear. Even in air conduction testing, masking is used when hearing in one ear is markedly better than the other ear. The better ear is masked when the poorer ear is tested so that the patient does not respond simply because the sound is heard in the better, nontest ear.

Speech Audiometry

A person's pure tone thresholds do not indicate how well he or she understands speech and discriminates between speech sounds. To find this out, the audiologist administers **speech tests.**

In speech audiometry, the audiologist first determines the **speech reception threshold,** which is the lowest level of hearing at which the person can understand 50% of the words presented. Two-syllable words called **spondees** (e.g., *birthday, baseball*) are on this standardized list. Either the audiologist says the words or a tape player built into the audiometer plays them. In either case, the person hears the words through the headphones and either says them or writes them down. The lowest hearing level (measured in decibels) at which the person correctly identifies 50% of the spondee words is the **spondee threshold** (ST) for that person.

In another speech test, how well a person can discriminate between words is assessed. The **word discrimination** (or word recognition) score is established by having the person correctly repeat such monosyllabic words as *day* and *cap.* Because the purpose of this test is to determine not the threshold but comprehension of speech, the words are presented at a level of loudness that is comfortable to the person being tested. The percentage of presented words correctly repeated by the person is the speech discrimination score. This score helps identify those individuals who can hear but cannot understand speech. Those who have sensorineural hearing loss are likely to show this problem.

More complex speech tests are used in the diagnosis of central auditory disorders. Previously described tests that involve distorted speech are examples of such complex central auditory tests.

Measurement of Acoustic Immittance

The hearing tests described so far require the participation and cooperation of the person tested. In some way, the person must indicate that the test tone was heard. There are techniques, however, in which the person need not do anything. In these techniques, a sound stimulus may automatically elicit a response of the peripheral or the central hearing mechanism. A technique of this kind is acoustic immittance.

Acoustic immittance refers to a transfer of acoustic energy (Hall, 1992; Martin & Clark, 2000; Stach, 1998). When a sound stimulus reaches the external ear canal and strikes the eardrum, an energy transformation takes place. The eardrum and the middle ear structures offer some resistance to the flow of sound energy. This resistance is known as **impedance.** A counterpart of impedance is **admittance,** which is a measure of the amount of energy that flows through the system. Both very high and very low impedance suggest auditory pathology. For example, a broken ossicular chain may show low impedance, whereas a fixated stapedial bone may result in unusually high impedance.

Acoustic immittance is most commonly measured with an electroacoustic instrument known as an **impedance meter** or an **impedance bridge.** Such an instrument makes it possible to place a sound stimulus in the external ear canal with an airtight closure and measure changes in the acoustic energy as the sound stimulates the auditory system. The instrument also helps create either positive or negative air pressure within the canal. Acoustic immittance is altered by such air pressure changes. When immittance is measured by this method, it is known as **tympanometry.**

The impedance meter also can be used to measure a simple reflex response of the muscles attached to the stapes bone. Known as the **acoustic reflex,** it is elicited in both the ears by a relatively loud sound presented to either ear. The reflex response involves a stiffening of the ossicular chain, presumably to protect the ear from potential damage. Acoustic reflex testing is a valuable tool in detecting middle ear diseases, including those that are not associated with hearing loss.

Electrophysiological Audiometry

Another objective measure of the working of the auditory mechanism is electrophysiological audiometry. In response to sound, the cochlea, the acoustic nerve, and the auditory centers of the brain generate electrical impulses that can be measured. These impulses are recorded as changes in the background electrical activity of the brain. Such electrical changes produced by sound stimuli are known as **auditory evoked potentials.** Generally, abnormal patterns of electrical activity in response to sound indicates a potential hearing loss.

The measurement of the electrical activity of the cochlea in response to sound is called **electrocochleography.** The electrical activity in the auditory nerve, the brain stem, and the cortical areas of the brain is recorded in a technique known as **auditory brain stem response** (see Figure 10.11). This test is useful in determining the hearing sensitivity as well as neurological functioning, especially in newborn infants with a high risk for hearing loss. The auditory brain stem response also is useful in detecting brain stem diseases.

Testing Infants and Young Children

Testing infants with the traditional audiometry is not possible because they cannot give a voluntary response. However, early intervention can reduce the effect of hearing loss on language acquisition, so it is important to detect it as

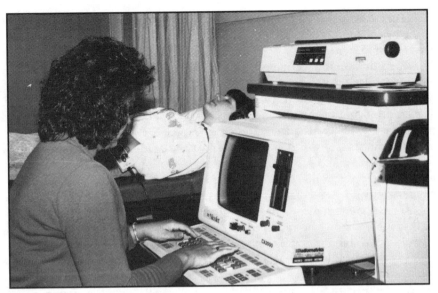

Figure 10.11. A computerized instrument to measure auditory brain stem response.

soon as possible. Therefore, audiologists have researched different methods of testing infants and young children.

Many infant hearing testing procedures depend mostly on reflexive responses that loud sounds tend to elicit in infants. The audiologist may use bells, toys, or electronic instruments to produce sound and elicit reflexive responses. These responses include the auropalpebral reflex, the startle reflex, and arousal. In the **auropalpebral reflex,** the infant quickly closes the eyes as the sound is presented; if the eyes are already closed, the eyelids tighten. In the **startle reflex,** the entire body shows sudden movement that suggests a jumping response. In **arousal,** an active infant becomes suddenly quiet upon hearing a loud sound, or a quiet infant shows sudden activity. Procedures like these are most useful in testing hearing of infants from birth to age 6 months.

With older infants, **localization audiometry** may be used. Older infants turn their head to localize sound. This response is measured by presenting sound from different directions and noting the infant's response.

Operant audiometry is based on operant conditioning.

Through traditional audiometry, it often is difficult to establish hearing thresholds in children who have mental retardation, behavior disorders, or hyperactivity. In such cases the traditional audiometric procedures are modified in some ways. One of the modified procedures is called **operant audiometry,** in which a child's hearing is tested by conditioning voluntary responses to sound stimuli. To begin with, a tone of sufficient loudness is presented. An audiometer, specially designed for this procedure, senses the child's correct response and automatically dispenses a token or lights up a puppet to reinforce the child. The child's response in the absence of sound stimuli are not reinforced. The intensity of the sound stimuli is decreased gradually until the conditioned response disappears. The intensity is then increased until the conditioned response appears again. In this manner, the thresholds for different frequencies are established by identifying the intensity level at which the response is consistent.

Electrophysiological procedures and immittance procedures, as noted before, do not require a voluntary response. Therefore, they, too, can be used with infants and young children.

Hearing Screening

Testing children or adults with a complete battery of hearing tests is time-consuming. Still, it is important to identify children and adults who might have a hearing problem. A somewhat quick and preliminary method of accomplishing this goal is called **hearing screening.**

In hearing screening, the sound is presented at 20 or 25 dB hearing level and only the frequencies of 500, 1000, 2000, and 4000 Hz are tested. Hearing screenings are done in a quiet room. Most children in the public schools are routinely screened this way. Acoustic immittance also may be a part of hearing screening. Those who fail the screening test are scheduled for detailed audiometric testing.

Meaning of Test Results

The audiologist looks at the test results and information gathered from all sources before making recommendations about the rehabilitation of the person with hearing impairment being tested. The result of a single test is not as meaningful as the combined results of several tests; history of the patient; educational, social, and occupational demands made on the patient; report from medical specialists including an otologist; and direct observations of the patient's conversational speech.

The hearing loss can be judged to be mild (15 to 40 dB), moderate (41 to 55 dB), moderately severe (56 to 65 dB), severe (66 to 89), or profound (90 dB plus). The loss may be **unilateral,** meaning that the loss is found in only one ear, or it may be **bilateral,** meaning that both ears are affected. The degree of loss may be the same in the two ears, or there may be a difference between the ears.

The results of air conduction and bone conduction tests are recorded on a graph called an **audiogram** (see Figure 10.12). A typical audiogram shows the hearing level in decibels for both the air-conducted and bone-conducted tones for the tested frequencies. Note that in Figure 10.12 the hearing loss across the tested frequencies does not vary much. The hearing loss ranges from 35 dB HL at 250 Hz in the left ear to 45 dB HL at 1000, 2000, and 4000 Hz; the rest of the tested frequencies show a 35 dB HL loss. Also note that the bone conducted hearing is normal in both the ears. When the sound is delivered directly to the inner ear through bone conduction, there is no hearing loss; but when it is delivered to the outer ear, there is a hearing loss. A person with this kind of an audiogram may experience a slight but not a serious problem in speech comprehension or production.

Figure 10.13 shows an example of a sensorineural hearing loss. Recall that in sensorineural hearing loss, both the air conduction and bone conduction are affected. Also recall that when the hearing is not significantly better in one ear, there is no need to use the masking noise. Therefore, in this audiogram, unmasked bone conduction thresholds are represented by different symbols. The audiogram shows that the hearing is better for some frequencies than for others, a characteristic of sensorineural loss. In this example, the degree of hearing loss in the two ears is comparable. A person with such a hearing loss is likely to experience difficulty in speech perception (understanding what others say). The person hears speech in a distorted manner and his or her speech or word discrimination scores will be lower than normal. This kind of hearing loss also can produce varying degrees of speech production problems.

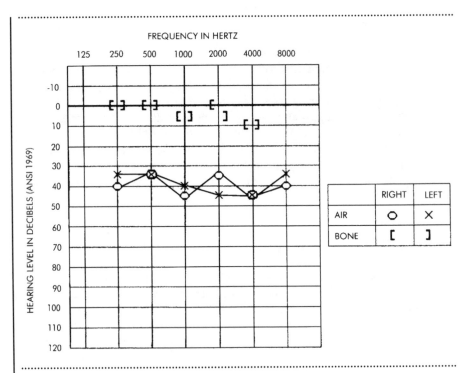

Figure 10.12. An audiogram showing conductive hearing loss.

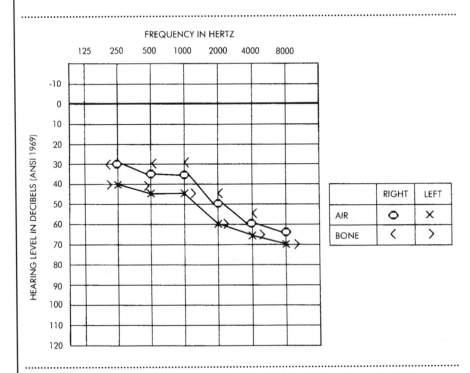

Figure 10.13. An audiogram showing sensorineural hearing loss.

Figure 10.14 is an example of an audiogram showing mixed hearing loss. Because the thresholds are higher than the normal when the sound is delivered directly to the cochlea (bone conduction), a sensorineural component is evident. However, the air conduction thresholds also are elevated (higher than normal); the difference between the air conduction and bone conduction thresholds suggests a conductive hearing loss as well.

Figure 10.15 shows an audiogram of noise-induced hearing loss. This type of loss is sensorineural, indicated by a difference in the air conduction and bone conduction thresholds. In noise-induced hearing impairment, a greater loss is typically evident between 3000 Hz and 6000 Hz. This is an important diagnostic sign of noise-induced hearing loss.

Summary

- Audiologists are the specialists who evaluate hearing impairment and design and implement aural rehabilitative programs.

- Audiologists use many procedures to assess various aspects of hearing and its disorders. With the help of audiometers, hearing thresholds are established by presenting sounds of varying frequency and intensity.

- A threshold is an intensity level at which a test tone is faintly heard in at least 50% of its presentations.

(continues)

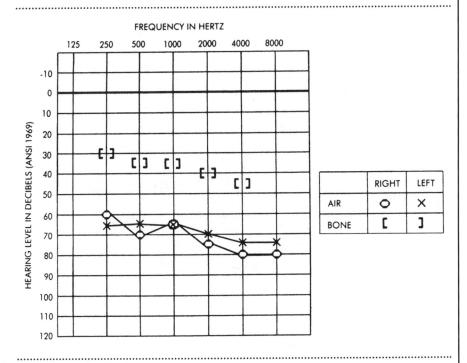

Figure 10.14. An audiogram showing mixed hearing loss.

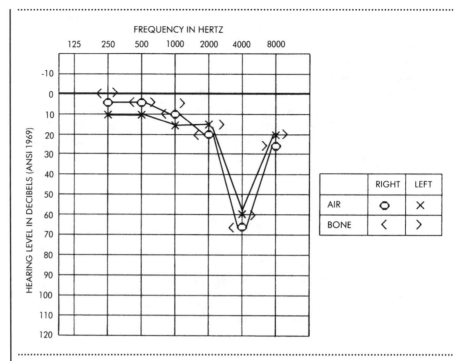

Figure 10.15. An audiogram showing noise-induced hearing loss.

- Both air and bone conduction are tested to determine whether the loss is conductive, sensorineural, or mixed.

- In addition, various speech stimuli are used to establish the speech reception threshold and word discrimination scores.

- Audiologists use many other procedures to assess the functioning of the hearing mechanism. In acoustic immittance, the amount of resistance offered to the flow of sound by the eardrum and the middle ear is measured. In electrophysiological audiometry, the electrical impulses generated by sound in the cochlea, the acoustic nerve, or the auditory centers of the brain are measured.

- In light of the case history and other information, the audiologist interprets the various test results.

Hearing, Speech, and Language

Without normal hearing, the child may readily learn gestures, signs, and other modes of manual communication but not spoken language. The child who somehow manages to learn speech will have difficulty in accurately producing it.

Hearing helps the acquisition and production of speech and language in at least two ways. First, hearing makes the infant aware of the sounds of the environment and those of speech. Also, hearing makes it possible to understand spoken language. Unless we hear and understand speech, we may not be able to produce it without special help.

Second, hearing is necessary to monitor one's own production of speech and language. We hear ourselves speak and, therefore, we can monitor how we are speaking as well as what we are saying. Through self-monitoring, we make sure that we produce the sounds accurately, that we use proper sentence structure, and that our voice is appropriately loud or soft. Not hearing his or her own speech, the person with hearing impairment, especially the person who is deaf, is not able to monitor speech, language, and voice productions.

Communicative Disorders of People with Hearing Impairment

The extent of the various adverse effects of hearing impairment on speech, language, and voice depends on many variables. The age at which the loss is sustained is important. **Congenital** hearing loss has a greater effect than the loss suffered in adult life. Children who have acquired normal speech and language before the onset of hearing loss do better than those who sustain the loss before speech is acquired (prelingual children).

The degree of hearing loss also is important. The greater the loss, the more severe the consequences for speech and language acquisition. Severe loss sustained before the acquisition of speech produces the most devastating effects. In essence, the most severe disorders of communication are found in **prelingually** and **profoundly deaf** children.

How early in life professional help is given and to what extent the parents learn to help their child who is deaf also can make a difference. The child who receives comprehensive services early in life will speak better than the child who does not receive those services until later. Needless to say, the quality of these services is another factor. The children whose parents have learned to help the child speak at home do better than those whose parents do not help the child at home. Finally, the presence of other handicapping conditions (blindness, mental retardation, brain damage) can make it even more difficult for the child who is hearing impaired to acquire speech and language.

The **speech disorders** of people with hearing impairment are numerous. Children have difficulty learning the speech sounds simply because they cannot hear them well. Consequently, children with hearing impairment may omit certain speech sounds, especially the /s/ in all contexts. Because children with hearing impairment depend on visual feedback of speech production, sounds produced at the back of the mouth, which are less visible, are especially difficult for them. These children frequently omit such sounds in word initial positions and less frequently in word medial and final positions. Children with hearing impairment may produce many final consonants with so little force that the listener does not hear them. For instance, the word *most* is heard more like "mos" because of the weak production of the final consonant.

Omission of one of the sounds in blends of two or more sounds also is common in the speech of speakers who are deaf. Thus, the word *strike* may sound

A **congenital disorder** is noticed at birth or soon thereafter.

The problems of speech sound production also are known as **articulation disorders.**

like "sike," with a distorted /s/, or it may even sound like "ike" because both /s/ and /t/ are missing.

Persons who are profoundly deaf distort almost all consonants that they do produce. Even the vowels might be distorted, partly because of the unnecessary nasal resonance on them. In addition to the sounds already mentioned, people who are deaf are likely to misarticulate /ʃ/ (sh), /tʃ/ (ch), /f/, and /θ/ (voiceless *th*).

Substitution of one speech sound for another also is common among hearing impaired speakers. People who are deaf most frequently substitute voiced sounds for the voiceless, and voiceless sounds for the voiced. For example, /p/ and /t/ are voiceless sounds (absence of vocal fold vibration), but /b/ and /d/ are voiced sounds (presence of vibration). The person who is deaf is most likely to substitute /b/ for /p/ and /p/ for /b/, and /d/ for /t/ and /t/ for /d/. Consequently, the word *pat* is heard as "bat" and *bat* is heard as "pat"; the word *time* is heard as "dime" and *dime* is heard as "time."

In another type of substitution, nasal sounds are used instead of oral sounds, and oral sounds are used instead of nasal sounds. The nasal /m/ may take the place of oral /b/, resulting in "moat" for *boat,* and the oral /b/ may take the place of the nasal /m/, resulting in "bother" for *mother.*

The **voice, rhythm,** and **resonance** of people who are deaf are unique. The voice can be breathy and harsh. It may sound as though it is simply reverberating in the throat, often described as "throaty" voice. Generally, the voice is flat and monotonous. It lacks the normal intonation patterns, the ups and downs of voice that give it a pleasant quality. The pitch is generally too high and loudness can vary unpredictably. This is probably due to too high or too low tension in the vocal folds.

The rhythm of speech also is abnormal. The speaker who is deaf tends to produce the words of a sentence in a disconnected manner. The words do not flow as the person is likely to pause between words: "Let/ us/ go/ to/ the/ beach." Consequently, the speech sounds choppy. In many cases, this choppiness is due to an unusual effort to articulate all of the sounds as adequately as possible.

Although some individuals who are deaf learn to use oral language well, many prelingually deaf individuals are likely to exhibit problems of oral language. The **oral language disorders** of individuals who are deaf include difficulty in learning and using elements of grammar and sentence structure. Sentences may be incomplete or grammatically wrong. Grammatic morphemes are typically omitted. For example, the plural inflection *s* may be missing in speech ("two book" instead of "two books"). Articles and other grammatical parts also might be missing. It is thought that such small elements of grammar (e.g., the plural *s*) might not be emphasized in speech; also, people who are deaf are not likely to hear them, even when such elements are produced with emphasis.

It should be noted that *oral language disorders* of people who are deaf do not mean that they are not able to communicate. People who are deaf may be competent communicators. A well-organized system of non-oral communication, such as American Sign Language, might make it possible for them to communicate effectively. In fact, many people who are deaf may not consider their oral language deficiencies a handicap. They just communicate with an alternative system of signs and symbols. With more free availability of interpreters who "translate" sign language to oral language and oral language to sign language, individuals who are deaf and those who are not can communicate effectively.

The writing of deaf persons shows problems similar to those found in their oral language.

Summary

- The degree of communicative handicap depends on the extent of the hearing loss.

- Individuals who are deaf show the most serious oral communicative problems.

- While children who are hard-of-hearing are likely to be delayed in oral language development, those who are profoundly deaf may fail to acquire oral language.

- Disorders of articulation, voice, rhythm, and resonance are all observed in people who are deaf.

- People who are deaf may still communicate effectively with a well-organized system of non-oral communication (e.g., American Sign Language).

Rehabilitation of People with Hearing Impairment

The rehabilitation of people with hearing impairment requires the services of many specialists. While those with mild hearing loss need just a few services, those who are deaf need the most diverse as well as intense services. The otologist monitors the health of the ear. This medical specialist prescribes medication for middle ear diseases and performs such ear surgeries as tympanoplasty and stapedectomy.

The audiologist is responsible for **aural rehabilitation**, which includes an evaluation of the hearing loss, an assessment of the communicative needs of the person, prescription and fitting of a hearing aid, and counseling the person with hearing impairment and his or her family (Kelly, Davis, & Hegde, 1994). The speech–language pathologist teaches speech and modifies the problems of speech, voice, and rhythm. In the school, the educator of the deaf, who is a special education specialist, teaches children with hearing impairment the academic subjects and certain methods of communication, including American Sign Language. A vocational counselor who specializes in the rehabilitation of individuals with disabilities assists people who are deaf in finding suitable employment.

Amplification

An important part of the aural rehabilitation of people with hearing impairment is amplification of sound and speech. Before the age of mechanical amplification of sound, the only thing people could do while talking to individuals with hearing impairment was to speak louder. This has not always been a successful strategy of communication between people with hearing impairment and those with normal hearing. The age of mechanical amplification of sound, especially with miniaturized instruments, has made it much easier and more efficient for people with hearing impairment to hear speech and sound, and thus communicate more effectively with others.

Hearing Aids

The development of modern hearing aids has greatly reduced the educational and social disability of hearing loss. The present-day electronic hearing aids are small, often weighing less than 14.2 g (¹/₂ oz). Most of the traditional hearing aids are instruments that amplify sound and deliver it to the ear canal. A majority of hearing aids in use today are analog devices, contrasted with later developed digital aids.

Types of Hearing Aids. **Analog** hearing aids create patterns of electric voltage that correspond to the sound input. All analog hearing aids have the same basic components: a microphone, an amplifier, a receiver, a power source (batteries), and volume control. An earmold, not strictly a part of the hearing aid, is necessary to use the aid.

The **microphone** picks up the sound, and the **receiver** delivers the sound to the ear. Called **transducers**, both the devices convert one form of energy into another. A microphone converts the sound energy into electrical energy; the receiver, housed in an earmold, converts the electrical energy back to sound waves. The **amplifier,** to which the electrical signals are fed, increases their intensity (makes them louder) and delivers them to the receiver.

The quality of hearing aids has improved dramatically because of advances in all aspects of hearing aid technology. Smaller and more highly sensitive **electret condenser microphones,** amplifiers that amplify sound with little or no distortions, and earmolds that are custom made to comfortably fit a person's ear have all led to greater acceptance of hearing aids.

The **concha** is the small shell-shaped area just before the entrance to the auditory canal.

Several types of hearing aids are now available. The **body-worn** type is the older, currently less popular model. Bigger than the newer types of aids, body-worn aids may be worn by the person on or under a shirt or blouse. Popular in the 1950s, the **eyeglass hearing aids** have the receiver, microphone, and amplifiers built into the frame of the eyeglass. The sales of body-worn and eyeglass varieties have dropped to less than 2% in recent years. More popular are the **behind-the-ear (BTE)** aids that fit behind the pinna. They can be used in a classroom with separate amplification. Therefore, many school children with hearing loss use the BTE aids. The more recently developed **in-the-ear (ITE) models.** are smaller units that fit within the concha of the external ear. Smaller than the ITE models are the **in-the-canal (ITC)** types. This type can be fitted more deeply into the auditory canal. Therefore, compared to the ITE models, ITC models are less visible. However, their small control buttons for adjusting the volume and other functions make them inappropriate for many older adults with reduced manual dexterity. Still smaller and barely visible when worn are the **completely-in-the-canal (CIC)** aids. The CIC aids terminate very close to the tympanic membrane. With less feedback and wind noise, CICs allow normal use of telephones. However, some people with very small ear canals cannot use them. Figure 10.16A illustrates the behind-the-ear, in-the-ear, in-the-canal, and completely-in-the-canal hearing aids, and Figure 10.16B shows how these aids are worn. Figure 10.17 shows how an audiologist fits a behind-the-ear aid.

Recently developed **digital hearing aids,** illustrated in Figure 10.18, contain the microcomputer technology. Whereas the microphone of a traditional analog hearing aid creates a continuously variable voltage pattern that is similar (analogous) to the sound input, a digital aid rapidly samples the input signal and converts each sample into a binary system of zeros and ones. The numbers are then processed by a computer housed in a unit worn on the body. The

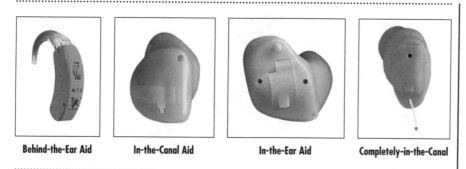

Figure 10.16A. Behind-the-ear, in-the-canal, in-the-ear, and completely-in-the-canal hearing aids. (Photos courtesy of Siemens Hearing Instruments, Inc., Piscataway, NJ.)

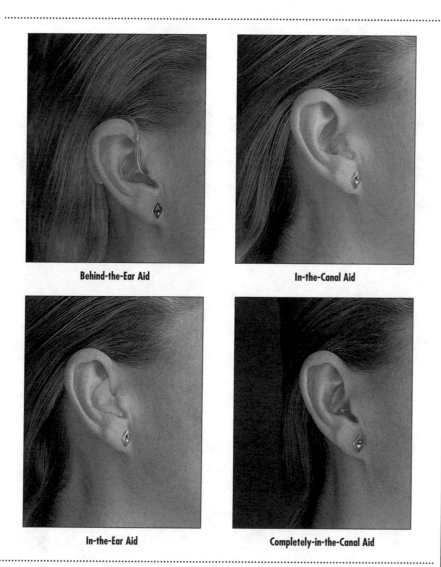

Figure 10.16B. How the hearing aids are worn. (Photos courtesy of Siemens Hearing Instruments, Inc., Piscataway, NJ.)

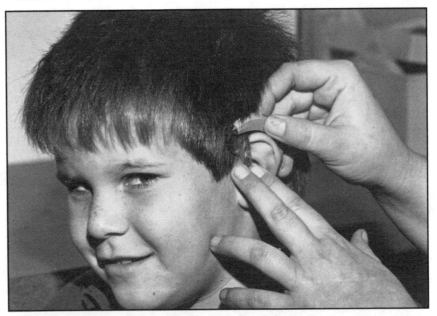

Figure 10.17. An audiologist fits a behind-the-ear hearing aid on a child.

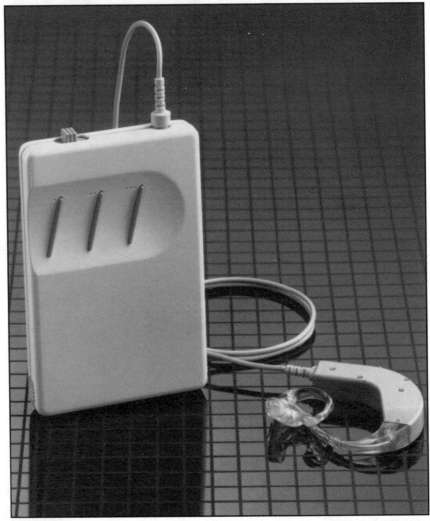

Figure 10.18. A digital hearing aid. (Photo courtesy of Nicolet Audiodiagnostics.)

digital aids are more flexible than the analog aids and are easily modified to suit the individual patient's pattern of hearing loss and communicative needs. Digital processing helps amplify selected frequencies for which the loss is greater. Compared to analog hearing aids, digital aids more effectively reduce annoying loud noises, such as those created by slamming doors or barking dogs. Finally, digital aids more clearly separate speech from background noise (Alpiner & McCarthy, 1993).

Currently, the digital aids are bigger than behind-the-ear or in-the-ear analog aids. They also consume much energy and are expensive. Therefore, the usage of digital aids is still relatively low. However, the problems of digital aids are expected to be solved in the near future. Miniaturized digital aids that are power-efficient can significantly enhance the usefulness of amplification to persons with hearing impairment. Meanwhile, "hybrid aids," known as **digitally controlled analog (DCA) aids,** which combine the analog features with digital sound modification technology, have been introduced. These hearing aids may be coupled to a computer that contains a person's hearing loss data. The computer can program the hearing aid to better suit the loss characteristic to give the most benefit from the aid (Hull, 1997; Martin & Clark, 2000; Stach, 1998).

Selection of a Hearing Aid. One should buy a hearing aid only after medical and audiological consultation. An otologist's ear examination might reveal a physical condition that might contraindicate the use of amplification. The audiologist administers various diagnostic hearing tests that help determine the type and the extent of loss. Subsequently, the audiologist conducts a hearing aid evaluation to select a suitable aid.

The **hearing aid evaluation** is a procedure in which aids of different makes and models are tried to determine the best aid for a given person. A suitable aid improves the threshold of sound and speech reception and the ability to discriminate between words.

A hearing aid can be purchased from one of several sources. Some audiologists dispense hearing aids. Other audiologists, who do not dispense hearing aids themselves, might write a prescription for a particular aid and send the client to a qualified hearing aid dealer who is not a clinical audiologist. The client purchases the aid from the dealer. Ideally, the client should return to the audiologist to make sure that the selected aid was the best choice and that the client understands its proper use. Some people directly contact a hearing aid dealer to purchase an aid. Such people will not have received the professional advice of a clinical audiologist.

Cochlear Implants

Many individuals who are profoundly deaf cannot benefit from even the most powerful hearing aid available today. For such people, a newer technology of implantable hearing aids, better known as *cochlear implants* might be of some value.

Cochlear implants are electronic devices surgically placed in the cochlea and other parts of the ear that deliver the sound directly to the acoustic nerve endings in the cochlea. The name suggests that the entire device is within the cochlea, but this is not the case. There are components outside the cochlea but within the ear. Other components are worn on the body.

The major difference between a more traditional hearing aid and a cochlear implant is that the hearing aid delivers amplified sound to the ear

Cochlear implants are among the few surgical options available in aural rehabilitation.

canal, but a cochlear implant delivers electrical impulses, converted from sound, directly to the auditory nerve. The implant has four major parts: a microphone, a signal processor, an external transmitter, and an implanted receiver.

The microphone picks up the sound and converts it into electrical impulses. It is either worn on the body or mounted on an earmold and worn in the ear canal; it is connected to the processor. The processor is housed in a small box that can be worn on a belt or placed in a pocket. The battery-operated processor suppresses distracting noise and selects sounds that are useful to understanding speech. These sounds are then sent to an external transmitter. The external transmitter is a magnetic coil worn on the skull, somewhat like the behind-the-ear hearing aid. Behind the external transmitter, just under the skin, another (internal) magnetic coil is implanted. The two magnetic coils are attracted to each other. A ground electrode is implanted somewhere outside the cochlea; active electrodes are placed inside of it. Through the skin, the external transmitter sends the signal to the implanted receiver (the internal coil and the electrodes), which stimulates the auditory nerve.

Initially developed cochlear implants had a single channel (only one active electrode). More recently developed implants have multiple channels or electrodes. The device illustrated in Figure 10.19 has an array of 22 electrodes that stimulate the fibers of the auditory nerve.

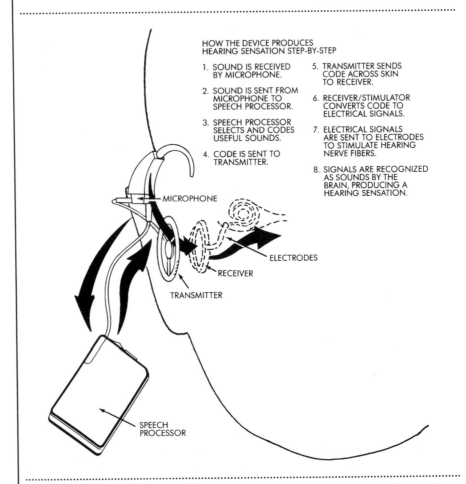

HOW THE DEVICE PRODUCES HEARING SENSATION STEP-BY-STEP

1. SOUND IS RECEIVED BY MICROPHONE.
2. SOUND IS SENT FROM MICROPHONE TO SPEECH PROCESSOR.
3. SPEECH PROCESSOR SELECTS AND CODES USEFUL SOUNDS.
4. CODE IS SENT TO TRANSMITTER.
5. TRANSMITTER SENDS CODE ACROSS SKIN TO RECEIVER.
6. RECEIVER/STIMULATOR CONVERTS CODE TO ELECTRICAL SIGNALS.
7. ELECTRICAL SIGNALS ARE SENT TO ELECTRODES TO STIMULATE HEARING NERVE FIBERS.
8. SIGNALS ARE RECOGNIZED AS SOUNDS BY THE BRAIN, PRODUCING A HEARING SENSATION.

MICROPHONE
ELECTRODES
RECEIVER
TRANSMITTER
SPEECH PROCESSOR

Figure 10.19. A multiple-channel cochlear implant. (Courtesy of Cochlear Corporation.)

Candidates for cochlear implants are selected after extensive tests and examinations conducted by a team of specialists including otologists, audiologists, and speech–language pathologists. As a surgical procedure, putting the implant in place poses some risks including postsurgical infections and possible nerve damage causing facial paralysis. It is currently used only with people who are profoundly deaf with minimal or no hearing and who cannot benefit from hearing aids. The implants can help recognize various environmental sounds. Due to more recent developments, implants may soon be helpful in understanding and producing speech as well. Because of continued research and development, cochlear implants have potential to help many people who are hearing impaired.

Auditory Training

The purchase of a hearing aid (or insertion of an implant) is only the beginning of aural rehabilitation of a person with hearing impairment. Both children and adults need training in the use of the aid, because in the beginning, the amplified sound does not mean much. People who are hearing impaired are used to quiet and silence. The hearing aid (or implant) suddenly changes that. Even the best hearing aids are not high fidelity; they distort sounds to some extent. The sounds and noises the person hears for the first time may be confusing, even irritating. Therefore, without counseling and auditory training, expensive hearing aids, once bought and tried, might never be used.

Auditory training is an aural rehabilitation program designed to train people with hearing impairment to listen to amplified sounds, recognize their meanings, and distinguish one sound from the other. The auditory training of an adult with hearing impairment begins with the **hearing aid orientation.** The person is instructed in the use and care of the hearing aid. How to put it on, how to adjust the volume, and how to change the batteries are some of the basics of this hearing aid orientation. Then the person is trained to listen to various environmental sounds and speech and discriminate between them.

Adults with disorders of articulation may receive speech treatment with the help of a **desktop auditory trainer,** which is often more powerful and effective in amplifying the speech than the hearing aid. Figure 10.20 shows an adult with hearing impairment receiving speech treatment with the help of an auditory trainer.

With very young children, auditory training might be a separate educational or clinical program. The children who are prelingually deaf need the most extensive and perhaps the most prolonged auditory training, the goal of which is to help them make use of their residual hearing. Using a desktop auditory trainer, children are trained in small groups. A teacher of the deaf, an educational audiologist, or a speech–language pathologist might conduct this training. Each child wears a pair of headphones; the teacher's speech is fed to an amplifier through a microphone; and the amplified sound is fed to the earphones and the child's ear. In this arrangement, the movements of the child and the teacher are limited because their earphones are plugged to the trainer.

A different auditory trainer, shown in Figure 10.21, is wireless. Known as the **Frequency Modulated (FM) auditory trainer,** the wireless system can be used in individual or group treatment sessions. As shown in the figure, an FM auditory trainer includes a transmitting unit with a microphone and a receiving unit with a headphone set. The teacher and each of the children wear both

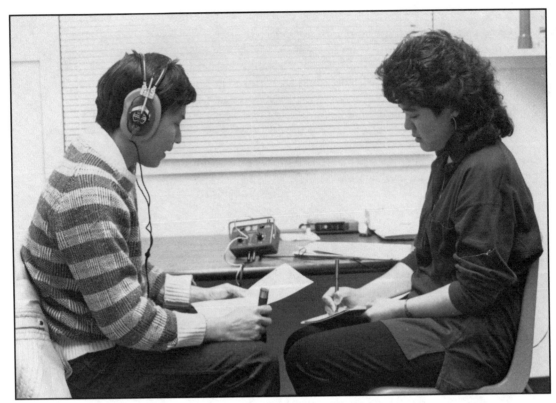

Figure 10.20. An adult receives speech treatment with the help of an auditory trainer.

the receiving and transmitting units so that they can hear and talk to each other. The signal is transmitted wirelessly, along a radio frequency carrier wave. Therefore, the teacher and the students can move around in the classroom.

Whatever the mechanical device, the goals of the auditory training with young children are the same. The children with hearing impairment should learn differences between sounds. The teacher starts with some common and gross sounds of the environment. The children listen to bells, whistles, and horns and to the sounds of animals, vehicles, toys, telephones, and kitchen appliances. The teacher talks about the sounds, describes their origin, and

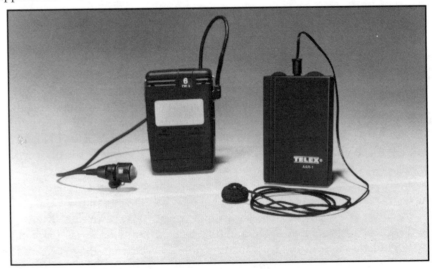

Figure 10.21. A wireless FM auditory trainer. The unit to the left is a transmitter and the one to the right is a receiver. (Photo courtesy of Telex Corporation, Inc.)

shows pictures of the objects. Initially, the teacher contrasts dramatically different sounds; later, he or she contrasts similar sounds. In this process, the children learn to respond differently to different stimuli.

Teaching discrimination between speech sounds is an important aspect of auditory training. Here, too, very different speech sounds are contrasted first, and similar sounds are contrasted next. The children need most practice trials on pairs of sounds and words that are similar to each other. For example, the children might quickly learn the difference between /s/ and /p/ or between /s/ and /a/. The members of these pairs are acoustically different and are made by visibly different movements of the articulators. But the difference between /s/ and /ʃ/ (sh) or that between /t/ and /d/ is more difficult for children with hearing impairment to learn because the visible cues are not grossly different, and the children do not hear the acoustic difference very well. Similarly, such word pairs as *name/tame, time/dime,* and *sock/shock* are difficult to distinguish. Sound and word pairs such as these are selected for auditory training.

The teacher uses all kinds of sensory channels to make the children appreciate the nature of each sound or the word and understand how one differs from the other. The teacher routinely uses mirrors, charts, films, drawings, pictures, and other kinds of visual aids along with modeling of the sounds and words. The children hear the differences; they see the differences in the movements of the tongue, lip, and jaw. The children also feel the difference in speech sounds. By placing their fingers on their throat, the children feel the laryngeal vibrations when they produce voiced /z/ and learn that such vibrations are absent when they produce voiceless /s/.

Eventually, auditory training moves on to phrases and words. The children repeat or write down what the teacher says. The teacher immediately corrects mistakes and reinforces children for their correct responses. Initially using simpler phrases and sentences, the teacher gradually and systematically teaches more complex phrases and sentences.

Speech-Reading

Even those who are able to make the best use of their residual hearing through amplification may not be able to hear all the sounds of conversational speech. This is the most important reason for the social isolation of people with hearing impairment. They might be alone among people because they do not hear some or all of the conversation around them. Soon they stop trying to mix with the hearing people. But if people with hearing impairment can understand speech, they enjoy social situations even when they do not talk much. Therefore, it is necessary to teach the hard of hearing a visual method of understanding speech.

Speech-reading, previously known as lipreading, is understanding speech by looking at the face of the speaker even when all of the sounds of speech are not heard. It is comprehension enhanced by visual cues that supplement the auditory cues.

In speech-reading, the listener with hearing impairment watches the movements and the shape of the lips, the jaw, and the tongue to the extent possible. The listener will also watch facial expressions, gestures, and hand movements of the speaker to understand the total message. While speech-reading, the listener may be getting the benefit of the auditory training as well. When phrases and sentences are the targets during auditory training, the emphasis is on speech-reading.

Some sounds are easier to speech-read than others. Obviously, the sounds that are produced with visible movements of the articulators are easy to speech-read. Therefore, sounds can be described as more or less "visible," although sounds are not visible. In English, no more than 30% of sounds are visible on the face. The most visible sounds include /p/, /b/, /m/, /f/, and /v/, the sounds that are classified as labials. The lip movements are predominant in making these sounds. Unfortunately, some of these sounds look similar on the lips and hence confuse a speech-reader. For example, the lip movements of /p/, /b/, and /m/ are similar.

Movements of other sounds are less visible and similar to each other, causing greater difficulty for the speech-reader. For example, the tongue movements of /t/ and /d/ on the one hand and /s/ and /z/ on the other are less visible and more similar. The movements of /k/ and /g/ and /ŋ/ (ng) also are similar, but in conversational speech they are not visible at all.

People with profound deafness who are experienced in speech-reading can understand 30% to 60% of simple words. Their comprehension of running conversational speech is not as good. It is difficult to comprehend stress, intonation, and rhythm based on speech-reading. Speakers who talk fast and without much mouth opening or those with heavy mustache and beard are difficult to speech-read. Speakers whose faces are not well lighted present similar problems.

Cued Speech

Even under the best of circumstances, speech-reading is not as efficient as hearing the speech. A procedure that supplements and improves speech reading is called **cued speech,** which is speech produced with manual cues that represent the sounds of speech.

Cued speech is not sign language because it is limited to eight hand configurations (signs) for consonants and four for vowels (Cornett, 1967). Note, also, that it is not the people with deafness who use cued speech; it is the person who speaks to those with deafness who makes hand gestures that correspond to the consonant or the vowel classes being used.

Research has shown that a speaker's cued speech improves speech comprehension by people who are deaf. In one study, correct speech-reading of syllables increased from 30% without the cues to 84% with the cues (Nicholls & Ling, 1982).

The problem with cued speech is that speakers must learn the cues and should be able to talk and cue simultaneously. To solve this problem, scientists are researching mechanical devices that give cues automatically as the speaker talks. One such device, known as the Upton Eyeglass, contains miniature lights mounted on a specially designed eyeglass (Upton, 1968). Different lights light up for different kinds of sounds. For example, a set of lights indicate whether the sound is voiced or voiceless. More research is needed to evaluate the usefulness of this and similar devices in understanding conversational speech.

Tactile Speech-Communication Aids

Devices that stimulate the auditory mechanism of people with profound deafness might not be useful because of lack of useable residual hearing. If the person with profound deafness also is blind, the visual means of understanding speech is useless. Tactile speech-communication aids may be useful to such persons.

Tactile speech-communication aids are devices or methods that promote the comprehension of speech by means of touch. Tactile (touch) sense is substituted for hearing. Figure 10.22 shows a tactile aid (also known as a vibrotactile aid) which has a receiver and two wrist-worn vibrators, which provide tactile feedback of speech sounds. The human skin does not respond too well to sounds of different frequencies. Therefore, the vibrator should generate patterns of stimuli that stand for different speech sounds.

Tactile aids are a good supplement to speech-reading. Those who are profoundly deaf and those who are deaf and blind might use them. Simple tactile aids have a single channel that transforms the acoustic signal into a mechanical signal that stimulates the skin. These aids help detect environmental sounds; some are able to give basic information on sound frequency. Research has shown that young children with deafness who are fitted with single-channel tactile aids produce more vocalization and learn words faster (Proctor & Goldstein, 1983).

More complex multichannel tactile aids have multiple stimulators. Different aids stimulate different parts of the body. For example, some stimulate the arm, others stimulate the abdomen. Some stimulate the skin mechanically, others electrically.

The Tadoma Method for People Who Are Deaf and Blind

In addition to using tactile aids, people who are deaf and blind, and who thus cannot benefit from hearing aids and speech-reading, may learn to communicate

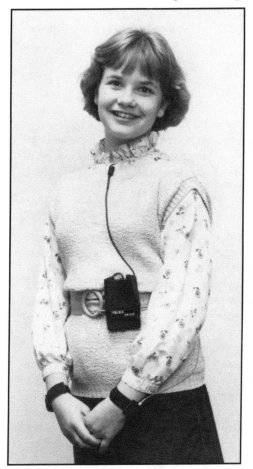

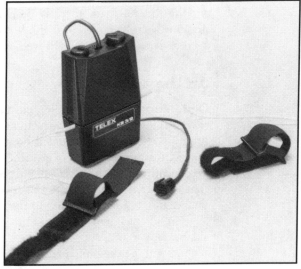

Figure 10.22. A three-channel vibrotactile aid with a belt-pack receiver and two wrist-worn vibrators. (Photos courtesy of Telex Corporation, Inc.)

with a method called Tadoma. **Tadoma** is a method in which the person who is deaf and blind places his or her hand on the speaker's face to feel the vibrations of speech production.

The basic procedure was originally used in Norway by Hofgaard in the 1890s; therefore, it also is called the Hofgaard Method (Norton et al., 1977). Alcorn, an American instructor who in the 1920s taught two children who were deaf and blind, *Tad* Chapman and *Oma* Simpson, named it the Tadoma (Alcorn, 1932). The technique has been used with people who are deaf with normal vision as well.

The listener places his or her right hand on the face of the speaker. The thumb is gently placed on the lips; the index finger is placed on the lower part of the cheek (or the jaw); and the other fingers fan out to touch the throat so that the laryngeal vibrations can be felt. When both the hands are used, the right hand feels the vibrations of the lips and the cheek, and the left hand feels the laryngeal vibrations on the throat.

The Tadoma method can be used to teach speech production to children who are deaf or deaf and blind. The child's hand is placed on the teacher's face, and a simple word is spoken. The teacher then physically demonstrates the action in such a way that a child who is deaf and blind can understand. For example, with the child's hand on the face, the word *sit* may be spoken, and immediately the child would be physically guided to the sitting position. If the spoken word is the name of an object, the teacher places the object in the child's hand to feel it. With repeated trials of this kind, the child understands the meaning of felt vibrations on the face.

The Tadoma method is useful but limited. People who are deaf or deaf and blind must be close to the person talking. The method cannot help people grasp the environmental sounds.

Verbal Communication Training

Hearing aids, speech-reading, cochlear implants, auditory training, tactile aids, and the Tadoma method are all designed to help people who are deaf in understanding speech spoken to them. But to communicate more fully, those people need to express themselves as well, and this requires training.

Oral Language Training

Oral (verbal) language training must begin as soon as possible. The early auditory training is integrated with language stimulation. The language stimulation program is better implemented both at home and in a clinical or educational setting. A team consisting of a speech–language pathologist, an audiologist, and an educator of the deaf typically directs home language stimulation programs that the parents implement. The speech–language clinician demonstrates language stimulation techniques to the parents.

Parents of infants who are deaf might think that it is useless to talk to the infant, play music, sing songs, or buy musical toys. But, in fact, the parents of a child with hearing impairment should do more of these and more often. The child should not be socially isolated. The parents are encouraged to speak to the infant as much as possible. While washing, feeding, and playing with the baby, the caretaker names things, describes the activity, and talks continuously. The parents talk slowly but naturally, using simple words and short sentences.

Visual stimulation is integrated with the auditory stimulation. The parents show the objects and name them at the same time. Actions and movements are demonstrated when they are named or described. Any vocal response the baby makes is reinforced by the parents with a smile, touch, hug, kiss, or gentle tickle. At all times, the parents and others who speak to the baby with hearing impairment make sure that the baby is watching their face and that their face is fully lighted. The articulatory movements are made visible to an extent, but the movements are not exaggerated.

Speech–language pathologists implement more formal language therapy programs. In carefully planned steps, the clinician teaches simple and complex words, grammatical features, sentence structures, and the use of language in social contexts. Supplemented with amplification and auditory training, the procedures of language treatment described in Chapter 5 are used with suitable modifications.

Speech, Voice, and Rhythm Training

The faulty articulation, high-pitched voice, hypernasality, and choppy rhythm of children with hearing impairment need additional training. The speech–language clinician provides this training.

Amplification, auditory training, and language stimulation pave the way for more systematic articulation training. Most of the procedures used to teach auditory discrimination of sounds are used in articulation production training as well. For example, the client is taught to produce differently words in such pairs as *chalk* and *shock, time* and *dime,* and *goat* and *coat.* Production of sounds that are omitted or distorted also is trained. General procedures of articulation training described in Chapter 4 can be used with suitable modifications. A combination of amplification and maximal visual cues is used in all treatment sessions.

Voice and rhythm problems of children who are hard of hearing are treated with or without the aid of mechanical devices. Instruments of biofeedback can be used to monitor vocal qualities. Simple instruments that show the fundamental frequency of vocal fold vibration can be used to lower the pitch of the voice. A smoother flowing speech is demonstrated. The client is encouraged to maintain proper airflow throughout utterances. This improves the flow of speech as well. The client is taught to smoothly join the words of an utterance instead of pausing in between.

Nonverbal Communication Training

Experts agree that verbal communication should be taught to children who are hard of hearing, but they disagree on what should be taught to children who are deaf. Some experts think that verbal communication must be given a good chance before deciding to teach nonverbal communication to those who are deaf. These experts advocate intensive and early efforts to teach language. In deaf education, this is the **oral approach.**

Others believe that verbal communication is an unrealistic goal for most children who are congenitally deaf. The sooner the children learn a nonverbal system of communication, the better it is for them. These experts advocate that early in life, a comprehensive sign language system must be taught to children who are deaf. According to this view, a comprehensive sign language system is the standard means of communication in the community of people who are deaf. Such a system of communication is part of the deaf culture. This is the **manual approach.** Still other experts think that teaching both verbal and nonverbal means of communication is the best alternative. This is the approach of **total communication.**

This historical controversy is not covered in detail here. The cliché, that this controversy has produced more heat than light is true; there is very little controlled clinical or educational research that shows the superiority of one method over the other. Most speech–language pathologists and audiologists tend to argue that verbal communication must be given a serious chance before deciding to teach nonverbal communication. Nonverbal communication isolates people who are deaf from the highly verbal hearing world in which they live. People, including the hearing members of the deaf person's family, typically do not know a sophisticated method of nonverbal (manual) communication.

It must be acknowledged that best efforts to teach verbal communication might fail in case of many people who are deaf. It is recognized that such an acknowledgment is itself offensive to those who advocate the use of sign language because in their judgment, sign language is not reserved for those who fail to acquire verbal communication; rather, it is a preferred method of communication for every child and adult who is deaf (Moores, 1978). In any case, at least some children who are deaf must be taught nonverbal means of communication. Nonverbal communication can be sophisticated and satisfying as well. Although many people who are deaf are not able to communicate with many hearing people, they can with other people who are deaf and who know the nonverbal system.

Typically, it is the deaf educator, not the speech–language pathologist or audiologist, who teaches the different methods of nonverbal communication to children who are deaf. Educators of the deaf have comprehensive training in all aspects of educating deaf children, including nonverbal communication.

Students might be interested in knowing that many universities accept a course in ASL as a substitute for a foreign language requirement.

Among nonverbal means of communication, sign language is perhaps the most developed. There are many sign languages, just as there are many spoken languages. The best known of the nonverbal communication systems is the **American Sign Language (ASL).** It is widely used in the United States and Canada. There are variations in ASL, and there is no single definition of it (Moores, 1978). Its origin is the French sign language, but it has been modified in many ways. ASL is considered a separate language, not a manual version of English. In many colleges and universities, students can take ASL as a separate or foreign language.

ASL uses signs to express ideas and concepts; a sign is a set of more or less complex hand and finger movements. Each sign expresses a complete idea. Different signs are made in quick succession much like different words are spoken in succession. However, the order of signs may not conform to the order in which the corresponding words are spoken in English. Some grammatical categories may be omitted in signing.

The **finger spelling** method is different from ASL. While ASL uses integrated movements to express ideas, finger spelling uses fingers to spell each word, much like writing in the air. It is talking through the manual alphabet. Each letter of the English language has a finger configuration to represent it. Each letter of the word to be used is finger spelled by making the appropriate movements. The word arrangements in finger spelling follow the order of English language.

The **Rochester method** is a combination of finger spelling and oral speech. Signs are not used in this method; the oral aspect of it is traditional English. Several schools for the deaf use this procedure.

The **total communication method** uses speech, signs, and finger spelling simultaneously. People who are deaf are taught speech and language along with a sign system. In the United States the frequently used sign system is ASL. Although ideal in theory, total communication in practice is more manual than oral. Spoken speech of those who use total communication is not very intelligible to listeners who do not know the sign language.

Assistive Listening Devices for Adults with Hearing Impairment

In recent years, significant advances have been made in providing technological assistance to adults with hearing impairment. These devices go beyond the traditional hearing aids described in the previous sections. Such devices do not necessarily replace the hearing aids. Rather, they help overcome some of the limitations of traditional aids and thus help improve the quality of life of individuals with hearing impairment (Hull, 1997; Stach, 1998).

Hearing aids are most effective when the people wearing them and those who communicate with them are in close physical proximity. If the communication partners are physically apart, a hearing aid provides much reduced benefit to the person who wears it because the signal is severely downgraded by the environmental noise. Thus, a person with hearing impairment watching television shows or the one trying to hear a lecture or a sermon in a large room will benefit much less from a traditional hearing aid.

Devices that help people with hearing impairment in various communicative situations are known as **assistive listening devices (ALDs)**. Any device that directly transmits a speech signal from the speaker's mouth to the listener's ears will overcome some of the limitations of a hearing aid. An FM auditory trainer, described in a previous section, is such a device. Therefore, adults with hearing impairment also may use an FM system as an assistive listening device. An FM system directly transmits auditory signals to a receiving unit worn by the listener. Thus, the signal is not affected by the noise in the room. The FM receiver can be coupled to the listener's hearing aid. In this case, the speech signal is directly delivered to the hearing aid through such means as an induction neck loop used with the telecoil (T-coil) of a hearing aid. In this section, we shall take a brief look at some of the other devices adults with hearing impairment might find useful.

Infrared light also can be used to transmit signals, including speech and sound. Most television remote control units transmit signals through infrared light. Similarly, without cables, computers can transmit data to a printer through infrared transmission. **Infrared listening systems** include a transmitter that sends messages on pulses of light and a receiver that receives and decodes those messages. Larger infrared transmitters can be installed in such large listening areas as a concert hall, theater, house of worship, and classroom. Smaller transmitters can be used in homes to view television and to listen to music.

Infrared signal *receivers* come in different forms, but the most common type is an "under-the-chin" unit that a person wears. The unit includes earphones through which the person receives sound. The listener can adjust the volume of sound on the receiver. Infrared receivers also can deliver the sound to a hearing aid. Figure 10.23 shows an infrared receiver. The person using it inserts the earphones into the ears, and the center part rests on the chest, right under the chin. Its base keeps it charged.

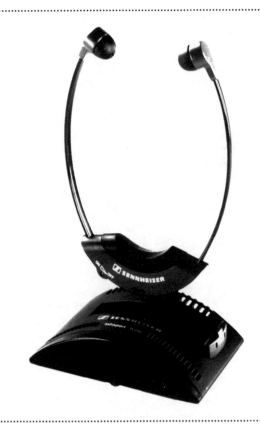

Figure 10.23. An infrared receiver that may be used in conjunction with a transmitter. (Photo courtesy of Siemens Hearing Instruments, Inc., Piscataway, NJ.)

Various kinds of **signaling** or **alerting devices,** also known as **environmental adaptations,** have been developed to help individuals with hearing impairment. Such devices include those that amplify the ringing of a telephone and the phone-transmitted voice. Such visual alerting devices as a flashing light also may signal an incoming telephone call, smoke or fire alarm, baby's cry, ringing of a door bell, or noise of an alarm going off. Some devices alert a person with hearing impairment to various environmental events by physical vibrations. For example, vibrations of a bed may act as an alarm.

Text telephones (TTs) or **telecommunication devices for the deaf** (TDDs) are other examples of helpful assistive devices. In using a TT, the two communication partners type in their messages, and the typed messages are displayed on a small screen built into the telephone. A person with normal hearing without a TT can communicate with a person who is deaf via a relay service. Staff at this service will type in the message spoken by the hearing person and verbally relay back what the person with a hearing impairment types in.

A *hardwire device* physically connects a listener and a talker through a sound carrying wire.

While watching television in the family room, a person with a hearing impairment needs audio signal intensity (volume) that is higher than what the rest of the family needs. This discrepancy may be solved by a **hardwire device,** which includes a small amplifier, a microphone, and an earphone. The person who needs a higher sound intensity can clip the microphone to the television set (or radio) and adjust the volume on the amplifier as desired. Similar hardwire amplification systems can be used in other settings. For example, health care workers, including physicians, nurses, and speech–language pathologists, may use them to communicate with patients in hospitals and clinics. Such devices make it possible to carry on a conversation with relatively low vocal loudness, thus assuring some degree of confidentiality while talking with a person who is hearing impaired. In a restaurant, a hardwire device may be placed on the table, which will then make it possible for the person with hearing impairment to listen to all of his or her companions.

Summary

- The audiologist's work, which includes hearing aid evaluation, selection and fitting of hearing aids, and counseling of the person who is hearing impaired and his or her family, is known as aural rehabilitation.

- Among the many models of hearing aids, the behind-the-ear and in-the-ear aids are popular. Recently developed hearing aids use the digital technology.

- Some individuals who are profoundly deaf may not benefit from hearing aids, but may be candidates for cochlear implants, which stimulate the hair cells in the cochlea, or the central auditory prosthesis, which stimulates the auditory nerve fibers at the brain stem level.

- People with hearing impairment need a program of further training and treatment for their communicative disorders after the fitting of a hearing aid or insertion of an implant. This program includes

  —auditory training to help the person get used to amplification and to make best use of it;
  —speech-reading to understand speech by watching the face of a speaker;
  —cued speech, which is speech accompanied by manual cues that suggest speech sounds;
  —training in the use of tactile aids, which help people understand speech by the sense of touch; and
  —the Tadoma method for those who are deaf and blind to help them understand speech by placing their hand on the face of the speaker.

- In verbal communication training, the disorders of speech, language, voice, resonance, and rhythm are treated with the help of amplification.

- The nonverbal means of communication for people who are deaf include the American Sign Language and finger spelling.

- The Rochester method combines oral speech with finger spelling.

- The total communication approach combines oral speech, signs, and finger spelling.

- Adults with hearing impairment may benefit from a variety of assistive listening devices, which include FM systems, infrared systems, signaling or alerting devices, text telephones (TTs), telecommunication devices for the deaf (TDDs), and hardwire devices.

Dialogue

Soon after learning about aphasia, Ms. Noledge-Hungry had decided to major in speech–language pathology. However, when Professor Speech-Wisely started his exciting and illuminating lectures on hearing and its disorders, audiology began to sound good.

N-H: Dr. Speech-Wisely, I found hearing very interesting because of its connection to speech and language. But it is exciting in its own right and quite a complex subject matter, too!

S-W: Certainly. Historically, in the study of hearing and its disorders, medicine, physics, physiology, and psychology have come together. In recent years, speech–language pathology, linguistics, electronics, education of the deaf, and other disciplines have joined the ranks.

N-H: But we began our discussion with physics of sound, called acoustics. Could you please summarize acoustics for me?

S-W: **Acoustics,** a branch of physics, is the study of sound. The basic facts you must remember are these. **Sound** is a physical event, the objective cause of hearing. The source of sound is a vibrating body; the vibrations are waves of disturbances in the molecules of air, gas, liquid, or a solid object. Do you remember what is a pure tone?

N-H: Yes. A **pure tone** is a tone of a single frequency. **Frequency** is the number of times a cycle of vibration repeats itself in 1 second. It also is called **hertz.**

S-W: Very good. Now, what is the relation between frequency and pitch? Also, what is the relation between intensity and loudness?

N-H: I think I remember. **Frequency** is physical, but **pitch** is perceptual. Similarly, **intensity** is physical, related to the amplitude of the signal, but **loudness** is perceptual. The term perceptual refers to sensations.

S-W: Right. The intensity is measured in **decibels.** The hearing loss also is measured in decibels. How much louder a sound needs to be made before a person can detect the sound is what you measure in testing hearing. Can you summarize the **anatomy** of the hearing mechanism?

N-H: I will try. The ear, the auditory nerve, and certain portions of the brain are the structures of importance. The **ear** is divided into the outer, the middle, and the inner sections. We can see the outer ear and most of the **external auditory canal;** it is separated from the middle ear by the **tympanic membrane.** The **middle ear** contains the ossicular chain of three tiny bones. The first one is the **malleus,** attached to the eardrum. The second bone is the **incus.** The third bone, the **stapes,** has its foot in the oval window that leads to the inner ear. The inner ear is filled with fluid and has the **cochlea,** which contains the hair cells that are connected to the acoustic or the eighth nerve endings. The **acoustic nerve** exits out of the inner ear through the **internal auditory meatus** and terminates in the brain stem. From there, auditory fibers go to various auditory centers of the brain, mostly in the temporal lobe.

S-W: Excellent, you deserve an A for that! You should remember the details of cochlea presented in the text: the basilar membrane, the frequency response, and so on. Hearing is possible because of **air conduction,** which is due to movement of sound through the medium of air that strikes the eardrum, and **bone**

conduction of sound, which is due to vibrations of the bones of the skull that directly stimulate the fluids in the cochlea. Now, tell me what it means to be hearing impaired.

N-H: Persons who are **hearing impaired** may be hard of hearing or deaf. The people who are **hard of hearing** have a hearing impairment, but they still can hear; they can speak and understand language with some difficulty. People who are **deaf** are not able to hear the normal conversational speech, and they have tremendous difficulty in acquiring oral language.

S-W: What about the types of hearing loss?

N-H: We have conductive, sensorineural, and mixed types of hearing losses. Then there also is the special type called the central auditory disorders.

S-W: Good. In **conductive loss,** the sound is not efficiently conducted to the middle or the inner ear. The inner ear is normal. In **sensorineural loss,** the sound is conducted as usual, but because of damaged hair cells, acoustic nerve, or both, most of the sound is not received by the brain. The **mixed loss** has both the conductive and sensorineural components. In **central auditory disorders,** the auditory nerve at the brain stem or the cortical auditory centers are not working properly because of lesions. Common causes of conductive loss include otitis media and otosclerosis. You must be able to describe these diseases and the many causes of sensorineural loss. Now, what do you know about audiology and audiologists?

N-H: **Audiology** is the study of hearing and its disorders. An **audiologist** is a hearing specialist who is trained to measure hearing loss, identify the type and the degree of loss, and select and recommend hearing aids. An audiologist also develops and implements aural rehabilitation programs.

S-W: Yes. But audiologists also are scientists who research hearing and its disorders. Some research audiologists work in laboratories and may not see clients; other research audiologists are clinicians who investigate problems of hearing, their measurement and diagnosis, and techniques of rehabilitation.

N-H: Isn't **audiometry** the actual measurement of hearing and its disorders?

S-W: True. It is done with an **audiometer,** which is an electronic instrument that generates pure tones, noise, and speech materials. The audiologist can increase or decrease the intensity of the stimulus. The tones can be presented at various frequencies. Both air conduction and bone conduction can be tested. **Speech audiometry** is used to test the level at which a person can detect speech and the level at which speech is understood. Discrimination between words also is tested.

N-H: I was fascinated by the automatic methods of testing hearing. **Immittance** and **electrophysiological audiometry** do not require a voluntary response from the person tested.

S-W: Yes. They are helpful in testing infants and others who cannot actively participate in getting their hearing tested. Remember the operant audiometry?

N-H: Yes, in **operant audiometry,** you condition a response to sound stimuli. But there also is hearing screening, right?

S-W: Right. A brief test of selected frequencies presented at a fixed intensity is called the **hearing screening test.** It identifies those with a potential problem who are then tested in greater detail. How are the results of a hearing test recorded and interpreted?

N-H: The audiologist records the results on a graph called an **audiogram.** It shows the frequencies tested and the thresholds for air conduction and bone conduction for both the ears. In conductive loss, air conducted thresholds are worse than normal; the bone conducted thresholds are normal. The loss is roughly the same for all frequencies. In sensorineural loss, both kinds of thresholds are depressed, but the loss tends to be greater for the higher frequencies than for the lower frequencies. In mixed loss, both air conduction and bone conduction are affected.

S-W: Very good. The **central auditory disorders** create difficulty in speech discrimination and comprehension, especially when the speech stimuli are distorted.

N-H: I guess most people do not realize how closely hearing and speech are related. Congenital hearing loss is a major cause of speech and language problems. The language of people with hearing impairment may be limited in vocabulary and grammar. The high frequency sounds they do not hear too well are misarticulated the most. People with hearing impairment distort, substitute, and omit speech sounds; they confuse voiced sounds with unvoiced and nasal sounds with non-nasal sounds.

S-W: And also, their voice quality is not normal; it is monotonous. Speakers who are deaf are especially hypernasal. Their rhythm is choppy. Because of the many severe problems, the rehabilitation of people who are hearing impaired, especially those who are deaf, is complex.

N-H: Isn't amplification one of the most important aspects of aural rehabilitation?

S-W: Yes, actually, **amplification** and **communication training with amplification** are the two most important aspects of rehabilitation. Amplification is provided by desk-model auditory trainers or small, wearable hearing aids. Hearing aids are electronic instruments that amplify sound and deliver sound to the external ear canal. A **tactile aid** is a special type that provides vibrotactile feedback.

N-H: I read about cochlear implants in a newspaper. They were saying that implants can cure deafness.

S-W: Some early claims of success with the cochlear implants were exaggerated. However, continued research and development in the implant technology justify the hope that cochlear implants will be a significant option for certain children who are born deaf.

N-H: I understand that **auditory training** is training in discrimination between different kinds of sounds, including speech sounds. But don't you soon move on to speech training?

S-W: Yes, we do. Mere auditory training may not help speech production. Therefore, it is necessary to train productive speech. Children who are severely affected need both language and speech production training. People who are deaf also are taught speech-reading so they can understand other people.

N-H: It is hard to imagine the problems of a person who is deaf and blind. I liked reading about the **Tadoma** method.

S-W: Yes. You should be able to describe Tadoma and its limitations.

N-H: The speech and language training with individuals who are deaf must be a difficult and prolonged process.

S-W: Yes, it is. I worked with a mother of a child who was deaf who repeatedly told me that she couldn't believe the amount of patience I had. But communication training with people who are deaf also is very rewarding! When a child who previously has made only noises and grunts says "Mama!" the first time in a language therapy session, both the clinician and the parents are thrilled.

N-H: What about the nonverbal communication? Isn't it used frequently by people who are deaf?

S-W: Yes. People who are deaf almost naturally acquire some form of sign language. The **American Sign Language** is used most commonly in the United States and Canada. **Finger spelling** may be used along with sign language. **Total communication** includes signs, speech, finger spelling, and gestures. Educators of the deaf disagree on whether the deaf should be taught sign language from the beginning or whether a serious attempt must be made to teach speech and language to every deaf child.

N-H: I found the description of assistive listening devices fascinating. Technology seems to be providing a variety of means of communication for adults with hearing impairment.

S-W: Indeed. You should know about FM systems, infrared systems, various alerting and signaling devices, text telephones (TTs), telecommunication devices for the deaf (TDDs), and hardwire devices that are used in watching televisions.

Outlook

N-H: You know, Dr. Speech-Wisely, I had decided to major in speech–language pathology until you started talking about hearing disorders in the class. Now I am not sure again! I like working with children, but I know I enjoy older people, too. I might like to be an audiologist.

S-W: Well, congratulations! This is what I have been hoping to hear from you. But you do not have a dilemma now.

N-H: What do you mean? I do not have to choose between speech–language pathology and audiology?

S-W: No, not right now! The specialized courses you take and the training you receive in audiology are typically offered at the graduate level. As an undergraduate student, you major in communicative disorders or speech and hearing, depending on the university. You take basic courses that give you a foundation for more advanced study in either speech–language pathology or audiology. Therefore, you have plenty of time to decide whether you want to be a speech–language pathologist or audiologist.

N-H: What do I study as a graduate student in audiology?

S-W: You will study hearing disorders in greater detail. You will take graduate seminars on diagnostic audiology, pediatric audiology, hearing aids, aural rehabilitation. You will gain a better understanding of the anatomy and physiology of hearing, acoustics, and electronics, among other topics.

N-H: The courses sound interesting and different. Can I observe the work of an audiologist?

S-W: Sure. You can observe our audiology clinic. You can talk to our audiologists about what they do. You can watch hearing assessment, hearing aid evaluation and fitting, and everything else our audiologists do.

N-H: What are some of the work places for an audiologist?

S-W: Most audiologists work in hospital speech and hearing departments or in association with otologists. They may have their own private practice in which they assess hearing problems in all age groups; they also may dispense hearing aids. Educational audiologists work in public schools where they monitor the hearing of children and develop and implement aural rehabilitation programs.

N-H: What about teaching and research?

S-W: Some audiologists with doctoral degrees devote their time to research and to teaching at colleges and universities. They work in various public and private research institutions. Audiologists research new techniques of testing hearing, diagnosing hearing disorders, and improving their diagnostic tests. They also do research on psychoacoustic and other scientific matters.

N-H: I am glad I do not have to decide on speech–language pathology or audiology right now. It would be tough. To complicate the matter further, there also is the education of the deaf as a separate profession, right? That, too, sounds very interesting to me.

S-W: Yes, deaf education is a related discipline that is both interesting and challenging. As a deaf educator, you work mostly in public schools. You typically teach the hearing impaired in a special classroom. You teach them communication as well as various academic subjects such as math or history.

N-H: Where are the deaf educators trained?

S-W: In some universities, deaf education is a program within the department of communicative disorders. In other universities, the program may be a part of the department of education. In any case, the deaf educator studies speech, hearing, and various methods of communication.

N-H: I think I will just wait and see!

S-W: That's good. I will see you soon.

Study Questions

1. Define acoustics.

2. What are the sources of sound?

3. Define a pure tone.

4. Describe sound waves.

5. What is a more recent name for cycles per second?

6. Define pitch. Describe its relation to frequency of vibrations.

7. What is amplitude? How is it related to loudness?

8. What are decibels?

9. Define hearing level (HL).

10. Describe the ossicular chain.

11. What two structures are connected by the eustachian tube?

12. What are labyrinths?

13. What is the function of semicircular canals?

14. Where do you find the organ of Corti? What does it contain?

15. Describe the energy transformation that takes place in the organ of Corti.

16. Describe the two branches of the acoustic nerve.

17. Give a brief description of the auditory development in children.

18. Distinguish between air and bone conduction of sound.

19. Distinguish between the hard of hearing and the deaf.

20. What is conductive hearing loss? What are some of its causes?

21. What are myringotomy and stapedectomy?

22. What is sensorineural hearing loss? What are some of its causes?

23. What is presbycusis?

24. What are central auditory disorders? How are they different from peripheral hearing problems?

25. Define audiology. What do audiologists do?

26. Give a brief description of an audiometer.

27. What is a hearing threshold?

28. What is assessed by bone conduction testing?

29. Define speech reception threshold.

30. What is acoustic reflex?

31. What is electrophysiological audiometry?

32. How do audiologists test hearing in infants? Describe at least two procedures.

33. What is hearing screening?

34. What is an audiogram? What does it show?

35. Summarize the speech and language disorders of people with hearing impairment.

36. Give a brief description of the components of a hearing aid.

37. What are cochlear implants? Who are candidates for them?

38. Give a brief description of the purposes and the procedures of auditory training.

39. What is speech-reading? Who needs training in speech-reading?

40. What is Tadoma? Who benefits from it?

41. Give a brief description of the oral speech training with people who are deaf.

42. Distinguish between American Sign Language, cued speech, finger spelling, and the Rochester method.

43. What are assistive listening devices? Why are they needed?

44. What is an infrared system? What are its components?

45. Describe how a text telephone is used by a person who is deaf and his or her communication partner who is hearing.

References

Alpiner, J. G., & McCarthy, P. A. (Eds.). (1993). *Rehabilitative audiology: Children and adults* (2nd ed.). Baltimore: Williams & Wilkins.

Alcorn, S. (1932). The Tadoma method. *Volta Review, 34,* 195–198.

ASHA Committee on Infant Hearing. (1988). Guidelines for the identification of hearing impairment in at risk infants age birth to 6 months. *Asha, 30,* 61–64.

Bench, R. J. (1968). Sound transmission to the human fetus through the maternal abdominal wall. *Journal of Genetic Psychology, 113,* 85–87.

Borden, G. J., Harris, K. S., & Raphael, L. J. (1994). *Speech science primer: Physiology, acoustics, and perception of speech* (3rd ed.). Baltimore: Williams & Wilkins.

Coplan, J. (1987). Deafness: ever heard of it? Delayed recognition of permanent hearing loss. *Pediatrics, 79,* 206–213.

Cornett, R. O. (1967). Cued speech. *American Annals of the Deaf, 112,* 3–13.

Greenberg, H. (1964). *I never promised you a rose garden.* New York: Holt, Rinehart & Winston.

Greenberg, J. (1970). *In this sign.* New York: Holt, Rinehart, & Winston.

Friedlander, B. Z. (1970). Receptive language development in infancy. *Merril-Palmer Quarterly of Behavior and Development, 16,* 7–51.

Hall, J. W., III. (1992). *Handbook of auditory evoked responses.* Needham Heights, MA: Allyn & Bacon.

Hull, R. H. (1997). *Aural rehabilitation.* San Diego, CA: Singular.

Kelly, B. R., Davis, D., & Hegde, M. N. (1994). *Clinical methods and practicum in audiology.* San Diego, CA: Singular.

Mahoney, T., & Eichwald, J. (1987). The ups and "Downs" of high risk hearing screening: The Utah statewide program. In K. Gerkin & A. Amochaev (Eds.), *Seminars in Hearing, 8,* 155–163.

Martin, F. N., & Clark, J. G. (2000). *Introduction to audiology* (7th ed.). Needham Heights, MA: Allyn & Bacon.

Moores, D. F. (1978). *Educating the deaf.* Boston: Houghton Mifflin.

Musiek, F. E. (1985). Application of central auditory tests: An overview. In J. Katz (Ed.), *Handbook of clinical audiology* (pp. 321–336). Baltimore: Williams & Wilkins.

Nicholls, G. H., & Ling, D. (1982). Cued speech and the reception of spoken language. *Journal of Speech and Hearing Research, 25,* 262–269.

Norton, S. J., Martin, M. C., Reed, C. M., Braida, L. D., Durlach, N. I., Rabinowitz, W. M., & Chomsky, C. (1977). Analytic study of the Tadoma method: Background and preliminary results. *Journal of Speech and Hearing Research, 20,* 574–595.

Proctor, A., & Goldstein, M. H. (1983). Development of lexical comprehension in a profoundly deaf child using a wearable, vibrotactile, communication aid. *Language, Speech, and Hearing Services in Schools, 14,* 138–149.

Shaw, S. D. (1994). Language and hearing impaired children. In V. A. Reed (Ed.), *An introduction to children with language disorders* (2nd ed., pp. 258–289). New York: Macmillan.

Smithdas, R. J. (1958). *Life at my fingertips.* New York: Doubleday.

Speaks, C. (1999). *Introduction to sound* (3rd ed.). San Diego, CA: Singular.

Stach, B. A. (1998). *Clinical audiology: An introduction.* San Diego, CA: Singular.

Upton, H. W. (1968). Wearable eyeglass speech-reading aid. *American Annals of the Deaf, 113,* 222–229.

Yost, W. A. (1994). *Fundamentals of hearing* (3rd ed.). New York: Academic Press.

Culture and Communication: Diversity and Disorders

Sandra Davis, a speech–language pathologist in an elementary school in a central California town, once told the following story:

We have a large Asian population settled in and around the town. Most of the people are from Laos and Vietnam. We have many Asian children attending our public schools. A major problem we face is a language barrier. There are practically no teachers or speech–language clinicians who speak the languages of Laos or Vietnam. Many children and their parents do not speak English or speak only limited English. And yet, our teachers have the job of educating them. And we, the clinicians have the job of treating those children who may have speech and language disorders. What is a speech or a language disorder in a child who speaks only limited English?

Classroom teachers often refer children whom they think have a disorder of communication to us for assessment and treatment. One day, a teacher referred to me a 7-year-old Laotian boy, saying that he had a communicative disorder. I talked to the teacher and found out the teacher's reasons for referral:

1. The child knew some English but did not talk much.

2. The child did not look at the speakers when they talked to him.

3. He gave only "Yes" or "No" types of answers and avoided eye contact.

4. He made frequent mistakes in sentence structures when he did say something.

I made an assessment of the child's language performance with the help of an interpreter who spoke both Laotian and English. I found out that the

(continues)

child simply did not know much English. He still was learning it. Therefore, he was making many grammatical mistakes. To the extent I could determine, the boy spoke Laotian fluently and appropriately; there was no evidence of a deficiency in the use of his first language.

I had learned from published research and my previous work with the Asian families that young children do not say much when a teacher talks to them and that it is normal for them to look away from the teacher. While speaking to authority figures such as teachers and parents, children are expected to be brief and to the point.

I consulted with the teacher and explained my findings and discussed the cultural differences in communication. I recommended that the boy receive lessons in English language and not the services of a speech–language pathologist. I did not think that the boy had a disorder of communication. He was just different.

Unfortunately, to many people, a difference is the same as a disorder. This chapter is about this important distinction. That distinction stems from a vast cultural diversity of human societies. Therefore, this chapter also is about the relationship between culture and communication. The complex relationship between culture and communication and the enormous diversity of cultures that create linguistic diversity affect the work of specialists in communicative disorders.

Language and Culture

Language is an important aspect of the total cultural practices of a society. Language is a vehicle to transmit cultural practices from one generation to the next. By talking about their family, social, political, and other traditions—describing what are appropriate behaviors and what are not in their society—parents transmit cultural practices to their children.

Culture and language are related in different ways. People who share a broadly similar culture may speak different languages; a single country with a general cultural background may have many languages. People who speak the same language might differ in certain cultural practices. The same language might have its variations depending on such factors as social class, geographic location, and the ethnocultural background of speakers.

To understand a language, its use, its diversity, and its disorders, it is necessary to understand the broader cultural context of that language. Initially, children acquire their language within their family structure, which is the basic cultural unit. Later, children elaborate their acquired language in broader social and educational contexts. Such broader contexts help expand the cultural influence on communication. Differing family backgrounds influence the patterns of communication children acquire. For example, in most Asian families, children are expected to listen more and talk less when interacting with adults, especially parents and teachers. Also, in Asian families, children are not isolated from most adult conversations as they often are in European American families. In some families, especially in extended Asian families, the language development of the child might receive more assistance from siblings than from parents. The act of talking is not equally valued in all cultures. In some cultures, including the American Indian and Asian cultures, silence is valued. In European American cultures, silence often is interpreted as having nothing to say.

Variations and deviations of language are context specific; often, what is acceptable in one culture may not be acceptable in another culture. The story of the Laotian boy described at the beginning of this chapter illustrates this. Therefore, specialists in communicative disorders have begun to study communication and its disorders within the context of the culture to which speakers belong.

Multicultural United States

Some societies are more homogeneous in cultural practices than others. For example, Japan is more homogeneous than Great Britain, Canada, India, or the United States. Nonetheless, most of the countries of the world are multicultural. Most societies are a mixture of varied cultural practices. This diversity is the greatest in countries that are homes for people who originally came from different parts of the world. Different religions, races, and ethnicities contribute to this diversity. The United States is a prime example of such diversity.

Historically, it has been believed that different people who immigrate to the United States lose much of their cultural practices and evolve into a single cultural group in this "melting pot." It is true that people who immigrate to a different country change in many ways. They learn many of the social, economic, political, and other practices of their new homeland. But it is not true that a melting pot creates a people of a single culture, even when the circumstances force them to use a single dominant language outside the home. People of different linguistic and ethnic backgrounds retain some of their original cultural practices, some people more so than others. Therefore, despite the melting pot notion, the United States is a multicultural country.

During the last few decades, the diversity of the U.S. population has been increasing rapidly. These changes have been more prominent in certain states than in others. Largely due to changing patterns of immigration, the U.S. population of the 21st century will be very different from the population of the 20th century. For example, 70% of immigrants came from Europe in 1940. But in 1992, only 15% came from there. In 1992, 37% of immigrants came from Asian countries and 44% came from Latin American and Caribbean countries. Projected from current trends, the number of nonwhite people of the United States will continue to increase until the year 2050. In California, the nonwhite population will be in majority by that time. Obviously, such demographic changes have profound implications for a profession that deals with people and their patterns of communication.

California, New York, Texas, and Illinois have a high percentage of nonwhite populations.

Multilingual United States

Most countries are multilingual; in fact, multiculturalism and multilingualism go together. It is common knowledge that countries like Canada, Switzerland, and India have two or more languages. All languages of all countries have dialectal variations.

People tend to think that the United States is a **unilingual** country, a country of a single language, English. People may believe so partly because the country uses a single official language, and the majority of people speak only English. Most bilingual and multilingual countries have two or more official languages. In such countries, the government documents might be written in all official languages. All children might be required to learn a second language. In the United States, children learn a second language only as a matter of choice. Nonetheless, and regardless of the single official language, the United States is a multilingual society.

People who speak two languages are **bilingual.** Those who speak more than two languages are **multilingual** or **polyglot.** The U.S. Bureau of the Census (1996) projects that by 2020, the Hispanic population in the United States will increase by 26.4% and the Asian and Pacific Islander population by about the same percentage. Such increases will create even greater linguistic diversity as these populations tend to be bilingual or multilingual.

A country or society of differing cultural practices is **multicultural,** and practically all societies are multicultural. According to one estimate, nearly half the world population is bilingual, and many of them are multilingual (Reich, 1986). In the United States, it is estimated that 18% of the population speaks a language other than English at home, which means that more than 42 million Americans are bilingual, and some of them are multilingual. Nearly half of this population does not speak English well; many do not speak English at all. It is estimated that roughly 20 million people in the United States do not have English proficiency (U.S. Bureau of the Census, 1996).

When whites become a new minority in California, most of these characteristics will change.

A majority of children and adults whose English proficiency is limited speak Spanish, an Asian language, or a Native American language. Because the majority of the population speaks English, people who speak other languages are considered the **linguistic minority.** However, though the term *minority* means numerically smaller than a comparative group, it also has acquired negative connotations that should be avoided (Battle, 1998). Minority does not necessarily mean disadvantaged; also, people who are a numerical minority in one place may be a numerical majority in another place. Historically, the minority status also is partly determined by ethnic, political, economic, and social reasons. Although there are exceptions, lack of political and economic power and low social status have been aspects of this minority status.

There has been a steady increase in the number of public school children belonging to linguistic minority groups. It was estimated that more than 6.6 million children of minority linguistic backgrounds with limited English proficiency are enrolled in the U.S. public schools (Waggoner, 1984). This number is on a steady increase. A majority of children with limited English proficiency are in California, New York, and Texas. Neither classroom teachers nor speech–language pathologists across the country are well prepared to provide adequate services to these children. The teachers find themselves teaching in a language their pupils do not understand. Most speech–language pathologists in the country are English-speaking monolinguals who face the difficult task of sorting out children who simply do not speak English from those who have a disorder of communication in the native language, in English, or in both. In recent years, linguists, educators, special educators, speech–language pathologists, and various federal and state government agencies have been concerned with the issue of bilingual education and clinical services.

Another important issue is the variations in the way English is spoken by different ethnic groups and people in different geographic locations. No language is spoken the same way by all members of that language community. Language use varies across people and geographic locations. Variations of a specific language are called its **dialects**. Each dialect may have its unique phonological, semantic, morphological, syntactic, and pragmatic characteristics. Speech–language pathologists are concerned with dialects of a language because of a need to make a distinction between normal variations of a language and its disordered production.

We first discuss native dialects of English language, including its American and a few international variations, along with African American English. We next discuss dialects of English that are due to a different primary language, followed by a discussion of Native American languages. The chapter will conclude with a discussion of bilingualism and the issue of dialectal differences versus communicative disorders.

Primary English Dialects

That English is more international in its scope than other languages is well known. It is often used as a vehicle of scientific and commercial exchange around the world. It is spoken in many countries, both as a primary or native language and as a second language. Consequently, English has many dialects, some primary and some secondary or non-native. That speakers of English who speak it as their second language have a dialect is readily understood. However, that native speakers of English, too, have dialects may not be that readily understood. The varied dialects of native English speakers are called primary English dialects in this book.

> A **primary English dialect** is spoken by those who speak English as their first and often the only language.

Dialects of a language are a strong reminder that the general rules of a language do not produce a uniform method of speaking a language. Each language is spoken somewhat differently by different subgroups of a linguistic community. The differences are more dramatic when a single language is spoken in different countries. The English language is a good example. Everyone knows that English is not spoken the same way in Britain, the United States, Canada, Australia, New Zealand, and other countries. However, the speakers from these countries can understand each other, sometimes with a bit of linguistic patience and amusement. But more important, English varies within those countries. As defined earlier, such variations of a language are the dialects of that language. American English has several dialects. One of them, an idealized form, is often called the Standard American English (SAE), which is spoken by a certain number of people and used in printing, national network television newscasts, and government communications. Each dialect has characteristic sound patterns including accents and typical expressions.

> **Dialects of secondary English** are those spoken by people who have a different primary language.

Dialectal differences are due to several interrelated factors. These include the geographic region, socioeconomic level, speaking situations, subgroup membership, bilingualism, and race or ethnicity.

Influence of Geographic Regions on Dialects

A major factor responsible for different American dialects is **geographic region.** People living in different regions tend to develop variations in language use and production. Lack of mobility and social isolation of people are the major causes of these different speaking styles. Based on geographic regions, specialists have identified 10 major dialects of American English: Eastern New England, New York City, Western Pennsylvania, Middle Atlantic, Appalachian, Southern United States, Central Midland, North Central, Southwest, and Northwest (Nist, 1966). These regional dialects are illustrated in Figure 11.1.

The variations of American English become less pronounced as we move from east to west. The dialects spoken by people in most of the central and western states are more similar compared to the dialects of the east coast and deep south (Tiffany & Carrell, 1977). Therefore, the dialect spoken in the central and western states is often described as General American English. This is the dialect most frequently heard on the radio and national television networks.

Influence of Socioeconomic Levels on Dialects

Dialects based on socioeconomic levels are less pronounced in the United States than in Britain and other countries. Nonetheless, dialectal differences are found between the people of lower and higher socioeconomic levels. Though unjustified, an individual's dialect might be used to make (typically negative) judgments about his or her social and cultural background.

Socioeconomic factors include social class, education, occupation, and income level of families and groups of people. Different social classes also tend to be divided geographically; rich and poor people tend to live in different areas of cities and regions. These variables tend to be correlated with race and ethnicity as well. People of certain races have historically suffered lower socioeconomic status and have lived in certain undesirable areas of cities and regions.

Societies that have marked socioeconomic classes show significant dialectal variations across those classes. In Britain, the dialects of the working class and the upper class contrast more than they do in the United States. In certain societies, a person belonging to the lower socioeconomic level often does not

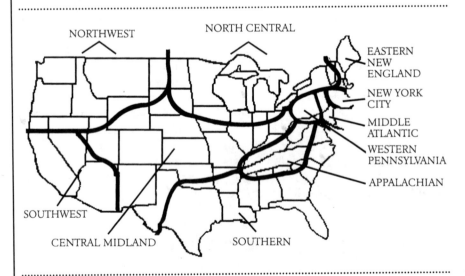

Figure 11.1. The major dialects of American English.

and even must not speak the dialect of those belonging to the upper socio-economic class. A servant may not speak the dialect of the master (Edwards, 1976).

A more liberal and yet degrading view of dialects based on socioeconomic classes is that an important part of the education of people in the lower socio-economic classes is the acquisition of the dialect of the upper class. In fact, George Bernard Shaw's play, *Pygmalion,* and the better known musical based on it, *My Fair Lady* (Lerner & Loewe, 1956), make it clear that the dialect of the educated and the affluent is the standard for the rest of the society. Upon meeting the poor and uneducated street flower girl Eliza Doolittle, Henry Higgins, the learned professor of phonetics, passes his judgment of her dialect (Lerner & Loewe, 1956, p. 109):

> Look at her—a pris'ner of the gutters;
> Condemned by ev'ry syllable she utters.
> By right she should be taken out and hung
> For the cold-blooded murder of the English tongue!

Influence of Speaking Situations on Dialects

Forms of language vary depending on the speaking situation. No speaker, regardless of the dialect used, speaks in the same manner in all speaking situations. Though not strictly a form of dialect, such variations contribute to the diversity of language use just as dialects do.

The speaking situation is a general term that includes the listener, the topic under discussion, the relation between the speaker and the listener, and other factors. Variations in language use that depend on speaking situations are called **registers.** A speaker of a language (and a particular dialect) typically masters several registers. One such register, mentioned in Chapter 5 on language acquisition and disorders, is **motherese,** or the speech directed to young children by mothers. Mothers simplify their speech to young children; use greater variability in pitch, with generally higher pitch; repeat often, and speak more fluently.

Other situation-bound language variations include formal and informal registers. Speakers use formal, more polite, and better structured language while talking in certain situations. Conversation between two individuals in church on a Sunday morning might be noticeably different from that between the same individuals in the afternoon when they drink beer and watch football. Speakers use less formal, more intimate, and less structured language in certain other situations. A lady's speech in a job interview is markedly different from her speech to her husband at home. Children's speech to teachers is different than their speech to friends.

Influence of Subgroup Membership on Dialects

Membership in a subgroup also is a basis of language variation. The age and the gender of the speaker are among the important subgroup membership variables that create language variation.

Although there is not much research information, language use is thought to vary across different age groups. The language of older people may be different than the language of younger adults, adolescents, and children. Listeners can distinguish a younger speaker from an older speaker by listening to samples of their audio-recorded speech. In many situations, a teenager does not speak like a 65-year-old person. The vocabulary, syntax, and vocal characteristics tend to differ across age groups.

Peer-group membership is another factor that affects the language variety of speakers, most noticeably that of the teenage speakers. This factor is closely related to age, but peer pressure seems to play a separate role in shaping the special kinds of teen dialects. Some closely knit adolescent groups have such characteristic dialects that we might describe them as **teenlects.** Parents may not understand them. Teens are especially active in inventing words or changing the standard meaning of words. As a result, the parents are constantly trying to figure out what the teen means. No matter how hard they try, the parents are usually behind the times and the teens. There are always teenlects, but particular forms do not last. They are more like trends in fashion. New varieties of teenlects keep replacing the old varieties.

> Gang languages are another example of dialects based on sub-group membership.

Much has been written about the influence of a speaker's gender on language variety. There is some evidence that men and women differ systematically in their use of language. Some authors have suggested the term **genderlect** to describe the characteristic patterns of speech thought to be influenced by the gender of the speaker (Kramer, 1974). As noted in Chapter 7, women's voices have a higher pitch than men's. This is mostly because men have larger laryngeal structures than women. However, some influence of the social gender role is not entirely ruled out. Women use a greater range of pitch variations in talking. Such variations often signal shades of emotional experiences that are not so characteristically expressed by men (Wardhaugh, 1976).

The gender differences are most prominent in the frequency with which women use certain words and phrases. Women are more likely than men to use (a) polite and euphemistic expressions (*Oh dear! My goodness!*); (b) words that are called intensifiers (*so, quite, vastly, such*); (c) certain kinds of adjectives (*adorable, lovely, cute*); (d) polite forms of speech in general; (e) greater and unusual variety of color terms (*magenta, chartreuse*); (f) devices that call attention to certain words in speech—the so called "italics" in speech; (g) hedging words (*kinda, sorta*); (h) tag-questions (*isn't it, don't you think?*); (i) the full forms of certain words (*fighting* instead of *fightin*); (j) fewer jokes; and (k) generally well-formed sentences (Lakoff, 1975). It is possible that some of these differences simply reflect stereotypic notions about gender differences. Nonetheless, some gender differences and stereotypes both seem to be real (Warren & McCloskey, 1993).

There is evidence that young boys and girls show differences in their use of language. In play situations, for example, a child playing the role of the mother uses more polite expressions (*Aren't you tired, honey?*), whereas the same child playing the role of the father uses more direct and authoritative expressions (*Go to bed now*). There is also evidence that parents and teachers speak differently to male and female children. Parents and teachers are more likely to use polite forms and requests while talking to girls (*Will you please . . .*) and more direct forms while talking to boys (*Pick it up*). It is possible that such differences and the traditional social perceptions of male and female roles in society are largely responsible for gender differences in language use. As the male and female roles in society change, it is possible that male and female speech differences will diminish.

African American English

A variation of the American English language that has received much scientific, political, and legal attention is **African American English (AAE)** (van Keulen, Weddington, & DeBose, 1998). Also known as **Black English (BE), Black English Vernacular, Black Dialect,** and **Ebonics,** it is often contrasted with the **Standard English (SE)** spoken by the majority of American English speakers. Currently, AAE is a native English dialect, because this dialect is not due to the influence of another language, such as Spanish or Chinese. Most individuals who use this dialect are monolingual English speakers. However, the dialect may have had its origin in a multilingual environment. That is, native African languages spoken by early Africans who were brought to the Americas may have influenced the evolution of a new English dialect. In any case, this dialect is now transmitted as a native dialect in the case of many African American children.

AAE is more prevalent among African Americans, but people of other races also use aspects of the dialect. Many rural white people, especially in the South, belonging to a lower socioeconomic status also use several expressions of AAE. Some educated people of higher socioeconomic status also use a few expressions of AAE. Reportedly, President Eisenhower used the typically black expression, "How long you been out?" (Williamson, 1972). It also should be noted that not all African Americans speak AAE. Many who do will have acquired the standard dialect as well. These speakers then code-switch depending on the speaking situation. They may use AAE in the company of those who speak that dialect and SE in the company of those who do not.

Popular and academic opinion in the past considered AAE a degenerate form of SE. However, scholarly study of AAE has shown that such an opinion is not valid. Rules of structure and usage can be extracted from AAE just as they are extracted from SE. For example, AAE uses such double negatives as "I have not seen no one." This is not a mistake but a predictable behavior in light of the AAE rule "that indefinites (e.g., *someone, something*) are negated with the verb. . . . This is a straightforward rule (so long as the listener also knows it), which is quite similar to one in Russian" (Warren & McCloskey, 1993, p. 222). Similarly, the AAE expressions "He be working" and "He working" have their rule-based justifications. The auxiliary *be* is used to express a more permanent and continuous state of affairs; it is omitted when the state of affairs is temporary. For example, when a man holds permanent employment and is currently working, the AAE expression is "He be working," but when a normally unemployed man is currently working on a temporary job, the expression is "He working." This is a logical and complex distinction that does not exist in SE (Warren & McCloskey, 1993).

In essence, AAE variations are not haphazard mistakes but are systematic and patterned behaviors. Just as we do not attribute Southern or Eastern or any other dialect to intellectual or biological reasons, we do not attribute AAE to such reasons. AAE is a product of historical, social, and cultural forces. Such is the case with every language and all of its dialects, including SE (Dillard, 1972; Taylor, 1983, 1986).

It must be remembered that AAE is not totally different from SE. A majority of the phonological, morphological, syntactic, and pragmatic rules are the same for AAE and SE. Naturally, how AAE varies from SE (or how the New York dialect differs from the Southern dialect) is of academic as well as

African American (AA) literature is an excellent source of AA culture and language; read works by Angelou, Hurston, and Morrison, among others.

practical interest. Though AAE variations can be found in all aspects of language, phonological and grammatical variations are prominent. A summary of some major characteristics follows.

Selected Phonological Characteristics of AAE

Omission of phonemes

- Omission of /d/ as in *don't:* "I 'on't know."
- Omission of /w/ as in *was:* "He 'as, too!"
- Omission of /l/ as in *always:* "a'ways"
- Omission of sounds in blends:

    omission of final /t/ as in *test:* "tes"

    omission of /k/ as in *desk:* "des"

Substitution of phonemes

- Substitution of /f/ for /θ/ as in *nothing:* "nofin"
- Substitution of /d/ for /ð/ as in *that:* "dat"
- Substitution of /n/ for /ng/ as in *walking:* "walkin"
- Substitution of /v/ for /θ/ as in *smooth:* "smoov"

Selected Grammatical Characteristics of AAE

- Plural /s/ omitted when a quantifier is used: "Give me ten dollar."
- Irregular past verbs not used: "He *come* yesterday."
- Regular past inflection *ed* omitted: "I pack up already!"
- Possessive /s/ inflection omitted when word order suggests possession: "Bring baby bottle."
- Use of a pronoun following a noun: "Uncle, *he* hungry."
- Use of *gonna* to indicate future tense: "He gonna go." (for *He is going to go.*)
- *Will* in the future tense (*will* + *be*) omitted: "She be home later." (for *She will be home later.*)
- Use of the singular present tense instead of the plural form: "You is a smart man!"
- Use of past tense *was* instead of its plural form: "You was helping me!"
- Omission of forms of *to be* (e.g., *is* or *are*): "She a nice lady!" or "They going to a movie."
- Use of double negation and use of *ain't* for *haven't, hasn't, am not, isn't, don't,* and *didn't:* "I ain't got none." (for *I don't have any*).
- Use of double modals: "I might could do it." (for *I might be able to do it.*)
- Substitution of *do* for *does:* "She do funny things."

Many sources offer excellent descriptions of AAE (Dillard, 1972; Kamhi, Pollack, & Harris, 1996; Roseberry-McKibbin, 1995; van Keulen, Weddington, & DeBose, 1998). A good understanding of the unique features of AAE is essential for a speech–language pathologist.

Primary English Dialects Around the World

To fully appreciate the varied primary or native dialects of English, one needs to take a linguistic around-the-world tour. Such a tour will quickly dispel the myth that English is spoken in one standard way, even by those who speak nothing but English. Historically, the oldest and the original native English dialect is that of Great Britain. As English settlers spread to other countries, including the United States, Canada, Australia, South Africa, and New Zealand, new native dialects of English emerged.

Read McCrum, Cran, and MacNeil (1992) for a fascinating story of the English language.

That any new dialect of English that is not the original British has been derided at one time or another is a historically telling fact. The American English in 1776 was very close to the British English. It was only as people from different parts of Europe arrived in the Americas and the settlers came in closer contacts with people of other races (e.g., American Indians and later African Americans) that a new dialect of English began to emerge in North America (McCrum, Cran, & MacNeil, 1992). In essence, American English had its roots in a multicultural–multiracial *immigrant* society. According to an authoritative source, the word *immigrant* used in the current sense is an American invention of 1789 (McCrum et al., 1992). In the latter part of the 20th century, the roots of American English acquired many new branches as immigration from varied parts of the world increased. But such sprouting of new branches is nothing new; it is only a continuation of the historical forces that helped establish the new Republic.

As American English evolved, the British, and even many Americans, thought that American English was inferior to British English. Similarly, the notion that British English is better than Canadian English, Australian English, New Zealand English, or South African English has been prevalent for many years (McCrum et al., 1992). But each of these native English dialects has its unique characteristics. The most obvious characteristic is phonological difference or accent. But equally important are words, phrases, slang, and other expressions that are unique to each variety of English.

Just like the **General American English,** there is a **General Canadian English** dialect. This dialect, prevalent west of Quebec, is based on urban middle-class speech. This dialect has its many rural variants, which may be sharply distinguished from the standard Canadian English. The urban middle-class Canadian English is said to be remarkably uniform from province to province (McCrum et al., 1992). Differences of dialects spoken in such geographically diverse provinces as Ontario, Manitoba, and Alberta are subtle.

The making of General Canadian English was largely influenced by the British loyalists (Americans called them "tories") who, after the American Revolution, fled the United States to the current region of Ontario in Canada (McCrum et al., 1992). However, Canadian English also is a product of the strong influence of Canadian French and to some extent the native Indian languages. Also, compared with American English, Canadian English retains many British English words (e.g., *tap* for *faucet, braces* for *suspenders,* and *porridge* for *oatmeal*). Some British, however, may think that Canadian English is distressingly Americanized (McCrum et al., 1992). An interesting fact is that Canadian English retains both American and British English features in word spelling and pronunciation. Their *colour* may be British, but their *center* (instead of the British *centre*) may be American (McCrum et al., 1992). Their articulation of such words as *progress* and *new* may be British, while that of *schedule* and *tomato* may be American. A distinctive feature of Canadian vowel production is the way the diphthong *ou* is changed to sound more like *oa* (e.g., the word *out* may sound more like *oat*).

From the late 1700s to mid-1800s, lands distant from Britain gave birth to new forms of English as the British empire expanded into such places as Australia, New Zealand, India, South Africa, Singapore, and Hong Kong. Several factors, including the specific linguistic background of people who immigrated to these countries and the influence of local languages, have shaped the variety of English that was eventually established in those countries. English spoken in India, Singapore, and Hong Kong were greatly influenced by varied local languages. On the other hand, English spoken in Australia, New Zealand, and South Africa bear certain similarities because the English, the Scots, and the Irish who immigrated there were roughly of the same background and generation (McCrum et al., 1992).

A main source of **Australian English** was the British English spoken in southern and eastern England. Early settlers of Australia were the British convicts who were deported from Britain. They hailed mostly from southern and eastern England, although some were from Scottish and Irish backgrounds. The language of the convicts came to be known as the "flash language," aspects of which may be preserved in the variety of English spoken by the aboriginal people of Australia. The initial European contact with the Australian aboriginal people resulted in a form of pidgin, a mixture of English and aboriginal languages. Even today, Australian English borrows many names of plants, birds, animals, and places from the aboriginal languages.

As the unique Australian English was being evolved, the American influence crept in. In the middle of the 19th century, the Australian gold rush attracted Californians who brought with them the linguistic Americanism to Australia. Thus the present-day Australian English, somewhat like Canadian English, contains an interesting mixture of British and American words and phrases. Thus, they may use both *elevators* and *lifts,* and turn a *tap* but not a *faucet;* they may fill their car with *petrol*—not *gas*—and drive it on a *freeway,* not a *motorway.*

Although there are shades of Australian English spoken in different parts of that immense and formidably varied country, it is more uniform than English spoken in Great Britain or the United States. Some linguists classify Australian English as *broad, general,* and *cultivated.* A third of the population speaks broad Australian, about half uses the general variety, and a small percentage uses the cultivated form, which is more like British English. Unlike the varieties of British English, Australian varieties are not based strictly on social class or occupation. And, unlike the varieties of American English, the Australian varieties are not based on regional differences (McCrum et al., 1992).

Ever since Australia opened its doors to emigrants from Asian countries, along with eastern and southern Europeans, Australian English has begun to be influenced by languages of the new immigrants. The so-called "new Australians" include Turks, Yugoslavs, Italians, Sri Lankans, and Asian Indians. Their native languages are likely to create new varieties of Australian English accents.

The origin of **New Zealand English** also is English of the urban working-class people from Britain. Therefore, New Zealand English and Australian

English share common elements, and many Americans may find it difficult to distinguish the New Zealand accents from those of Australia or Britain. The New Zealand English accent, though closer to the British, shares aspects of the three Australian dialects (general, broad, and cultivated). New Zealand English tends to emphasize the *wh* in such words as *when, why,* and *wheat.* Its /r/ is typically silent, although people with Scottish heritage living in the South Island of New Zealand tend to roll it (McCrum et al., 1992). Some New Zealanders tend to maintain an accent that is closer to their original British accent. New Zealand English is said to contain fewer slang expressions than Australian English.

New Zealand English borrowed words from the native languages of the islands, especially from the dominant Maori language. Native languages of New Zealand are different from those of the Australian aboriginal languages. For example, Maori language is related to Polynesian languages spoken in Tahiti, Samoa, and Hawaii. Just as they did in Australia, the British settlers borrowed words for plants, animals, flowers, and places from Maori language because they did not have English words for them. When faced with a choice, New Zealanders generally prefer the British to the Australian expressions, although many Australian words are a part of New Zealand English.

South African English is another native English dialect that varies from native English spoken elsewhere (e.g., Britain, Australia, New Zealand, or United States). South African English was shaped predominantly by the native British English of the settlers. However, it also was influenced by the native African languages and a language called Afrikaans, which is a variety of Dutch that was influenced greatly by the native African languages. The dominant African language that influenced both English and Dutch is Bantu, which is spoken by a majority of South Africans of African origin. Bantu is actually a group of languages that includes Swahili. Other African languages spoken in South Africa include Sotho, Nguni, Venda, and Tsonga.

In addition to native dialects, English has many non-native dialects that are due to bilingualism. When English is learned as a secondary language, new dialects emerge. In a multilingual and multicultural society, an understanding of these dialects is essential for a speech–language pathologist.

Secondary English Dialects

As noted so far, countries such as the United States, Canada, Great Britain, Australia, and New Zealand have primary (native) English dialects of speakers who do not speak any other language. In many other countries, English is spoken as a second language. In this text, dialects of English that are learned and used as second language are described as *secondary English.* A **secondary English dialect** is a variation of English largely due to the influence of a speaker's primary language, which is other than English.

Many ethnocultural groups in the United States speak English as a second language. The dialects of these groups are largely influenced by their primary language. Therefore, there are as many secondary English dialects as there are primary languages that create them.

People who speak secondary dialects of American English and whose primary language is a variety of **Spanish** constitute a large number. People with a Spanish background are often described as **Hispanic.** It is important to note that the term Hispanic does not refer to an ethnic or racial group; it refers to a *linguistic* background. Hispanics are a diverse group both racially and geographically. Hispanics are found in all shades of skin color and are distributed in North, Central, and South America and Europe. In the United States, Hispanics are a significant and growing minority. From 27 million in 1995, Hispanics have grown to 31 million in the year 2000 and are expected to increase to 63 million by the year 2030 (U.S. Bureau of the Census, 1996).

Spanish is now the second most common language spoken in the United States. Based on the geographic distribution of the speakers, linguists have described six major Spanish dialects spoken in the United States: Mexican and Southwestern United States; Central American; Caribbean; Highlandian; Chilean; and southern Paraguayan, Uruguayan, and Argentinean. There still are many more varieties, depending on the country of origin. In the United States, varieties of Spanish of the Mexican, Caribbean (especially Cuban), and Puerto Rican origin are spoken most commonly.

Read distinguished literary works by writers of Spanish background, including those by Marquez.

Secondary American English dialects of Hispanic origin are influenced by the characteristics of the particular variety of Spanish spoken by a specific Hispanic group. Speech–language pathologists in the United States who assess and treat people with communicative disorders need to know the particular variety of Spanish that influences their Hispanic clients. The clinicians also need to understand the general phonological, morphological, syntactic, and pragmatic characteristics of Spanish in general. Excellent sources are available to speech–language pathologists to understand the basic differences between English and Spanish language characteristics (Comrie, 1990; Kayser, 1995, 1998; Langdon & Cheng, 1992; Perez, 1994; Roseberry-McKibbin, 1995; Yavas & Goldstein, 1998; Zuniga, 1992).

Children who speak Spanish as their primary language at home and learn to speak English as a second language speak a dialect of English that might be described as Spanish-influenced English. This form of English dialect is most easily recognized by its phonological characteristics, although it has a few distinguishing grammatical characteristics as well. These characteristics are summarized in greater detail in Roseberry-McKibbin (1995).

Selected Phonological Characteristics of Spanish-Influenced English

- /t, d, n/ may be dentalized (i.e., these sounds may be produced by placing the tip of the tongue against the back of the upper central incisors).

- Final consonants may be devoiced (e.g., *doze* may sound more like *dose*).

- /b/ may be substituted for /v/ (e.g., *very* may sound more like *berry*).

- Stops may be deaspirated (i.e., release of little air in producing stop sounds).

- /ch/ may be substituted for /sh/ (e.g., *Shirley* may sound more like *Chirley*).

- /d/ may be substituted for /ð/ (voiced *th* sound) (e.g., *this* may sound more like *dis*).

- /t/ may be substituted for /θ/ (voiceless *th* sound) (e.g., *think* may sound more like *tink*).

- The schwa sound may be inserted before word-initial consonant clusters (e.g., *skate* and *spend* may sound more like *eskate* and *espend*, respectively).

- The word-initial /h/ may be silent (e.g., *hold* may sound like *old*).

- /j/ may be substituted for /ʤ/ (e.g., *Julie* and *joke* may sound more like *yuli* and *yoke*, respectively).

- /s/ may be produced more frontally (like the Spanish /s/).

- Several English consonants at the end of words may be omitted (this is because in Spanish only consonants /s/, /n/, /r/, /l/, and /d/ are used in the word-final position).

Selected Grammatical Characteristics of Spanish-Influenced English

- Adjectives may be inserted after the noun, with omitted auxiliary (e.g., *The house green*).

- The possessive *s* inflection may be omitted (e.g., *My mom hat is yellow*).

- The past tense /ed/ inflection may be omitted (e.g., *We walk yesterday*).

- Double negatives may be used (e.g., *I don't have no more*).

- The adverb may follow the verb (e.g., *He drives very fast his motorcycle*).

Asians are another linguistic minority group that is growing in the United States. The English dialect of the first-generation Asian emigrants varies tremendously because of the great variety of primary Asian languages. Emigrants from such Asian countries as India, Pakistan, Bangladesh, Sri Lanka, China, Thailand, Malaysia, Indonesia, Taiwan, Korea, and Japan constitute a diverse group with varied cultural and linguistic backgrounds. Because of the diversity of Asian languages, no single source is complete in its list of unique or contrasting features. Clinicians will have to consult several sources (Cheng, 1991, 1995; Roseberry-McKibbin, 1995; Shekar & Hegde, 1995, 1996).

Many Asian countries are multilingual. For example, India has 15 major languages, but almost 180 languages and 700 dialects are spoken in the country. English in India is a dominant second language and an auxiliary official language as well. Languages of the India subcontinent fall into two major linguistic families, Indo-European and Dravidian. Indo-European languages are spoken mostly in northern India and Dravidian languages are spoken mostly in southern India. Languages of the two families have freely borrowed from each other. Compared to English, Indian languages are phonetic in the sense that each alphabetic symbol stands for a specific sound. The words are pronounced precisely the way they are written. Therefore, the English sound system with fewer alphabetic symbols than sounds in the language and varied pronunciations of the same spelling creates difficulties for Asian Indian speakers.

Read some of the literary works by Asians writing in English, including Rushdie, Naipal, Tan, Masumoto, Roy, and Lahiri.

Chinese language has two main dialects, Cantonese and Mandarin. In their spoken form, the two dialects are mutually unintelligible, but they are intelligible when written because of a common graphic symbol system that substitutes for the alphabetic system of writing. The Chinese language does not contain consonantal blends, explaining the omission of sounds in blends when Chinese speakers speak English. Such speakers also may omit English final consonants in words (e.g., *offi* for *office*, *fi* for *fish*) because in the Chinese dialects very few consonants end words.

Native American Languages

In the United States and throughout the Americas, Native Americans are a significant group with a rich history of language variation. In the United States, Native Americans are an ethnocultural minority with about 2 million people, concentrated mostly in the western United States (U.S. Bureau of the Census, 1996). Native Americans belong to more than 500 tribal groups, each with a distinct cultural and linguistic heritage.

The languages of Native Americans vary greatly. These languages are spread from the northernmost part of Canada to the southernmost part of South America. Some 800 Native American languages have been identified. Experts believe that in North America alone, some 200 Native American languages may be spoken (Highwater, 1975). Because of their wide geographic distribution, many Native American languages are unrelated to each other. In addition, limited research on the Native American languages has made their linguistic classification controversial. These languages have been classified into a high of 60 families and a low of just 3 (Highwater, 1975; Peña-Brooks & Hegde, 2000). One American Indian Website lists 6 families of Native American languages: Eskimo-Aleut, Algonkian-Wakashan, Nadene, Penutian, Hokan-Siouan, and Aztec-Tanoan.

Unfortunately, the rate at which the Native American languages are transmitted to the younger generation is declining fast. Consequently, many Native American languages are now extinct, and many more are on the verge of extinction. Several Native American languages are spoken by less than 10 aged people. Younger Native Americans who do have a working knowledge of their language are English-speaking bilinguals.

Because of the variety of Native American languages, it is difficult to list their linguistic characteristics. Space will not permit a comparison of individual Native American languages with English. Also, Native American languages are undergoing significant changes. For example, there is the Old Blackfoot and a New Blackfoot, which is evolving. Some native languages have very few sounds. For example, the Arawakan language has only 17 phonemes (Peña-Brooks & Hegde, 2000). A few other features found in Native American languages contrast with those of English. For example, in American Indian languages vowels may be nasalized; some vowels may be voiceless (whispered); the same vowels may be lengthened or shortened to suggest different meanings; /k/ and /q/ may be contrastive (suggesting different meanings); and some consonants that are typically aspirated in English may be unaspirated (e.g., /p/, /t/, and /k/).

> Read a collection of stories written by Native American writers, such as the one edited by Witalec (1995) in the reference list.

Bilingualism

Bilingualism is an important source of language variation. Most bilingual speakers tend to speak their second language in a dialect popularly described as accent. This dialect is more likely to show when the second language acquisition is not simultaneous but sequential, although many children may be able to speak the second language with its native accent. The later the acquisition of the second language, the higher the chances of a dialect due to bilingualism.

The term *accent* is misleading because many native speakers of a language assume that they do not speak with an accent. All speakers speak with an accent; it just happens that a minority accent gets noticed among people who have a majority accent. *Dialect* is a more accurate term because it means language variation. It is believed that the first or the native language influences the acquisition and production of the second language. The second language speaker uses some of the sound and linguistic stress patterns of the native language while speaking the second language. Sounds that are absent in the first language may be omitted or mispronounced while speaking the second language. Peculiar grammatical features of the second language also might be omitted. The second language speaker may make syntactic errors as well.

Bilingual speakers, while in the company of similarly bilingual speakers, often switch back and forth from their first to second language. Such shifts in languages during the same conversational episode is called **code switching**. The term also applies to shifts in dialects within the same language. For example, an African American may switch from the Black English dialect to the Standard English dialect and back to the Black English dialect. A person from Texas may switch back and forth between the General American and Southern dialects.

Bilingual speakers tend to mix the two languages they speak, especially in informal conversations. Again, this is more likely to happen in the company of other similarly bilingual speakers. Such **language mixing** may involve words from the two languages used in a single sentence. Or, different sentences may be spoken in different languages. Certain topics may be more likely to be spoken in one language or the other. For example, bilingual children who receive instruction in the school in a second language may talk about personal or intimate topics in their first language but about academic subjects in their second language.

The Bilingual Child

There is a long-held belief that a bilingual child may not learn either language well. But this belief is not totally supported by research. During his or her second year, the bilingual child's rate of language acquisition may be somewhat slower than the normal, but eventually the bilingual child's dominant language proficiency matches that of monolingual children (Owens, 1996; Reich, 1986). The overall process of language acquisition in bilingual children is similar to that in monolingual children.

A child is bilingual because the mother and the father speak different languages. Often, one of the two parental languages is also the language of the surrounding community. For example, a child's mother may speak English and the father may speak German, but the family may live in an English-speaking community.

A child might be bilingual also because the parents speak one language but the surrounding community speaks another language. For example, the children of many recent immigrants from Laos and Vietnam to the United States find themselves in this situation. Whether or not the parents have proficiency in English, the children are likely to be exposed to both English and the family's native language.

Older children and adults may be bilingual because they have received formal instruction in high schools and colleges in a foreign language. Learning a foreign language later in life in an educational setting is different from young children's bilingual acquisition at home. Foreign language learners will have naturally acquired their first language. This chapter is not concerned with foreign language learning in educational settings.

Simultaneous and Sequential Bilingualism

A child can acquire two languages at the same time (**simultaneous bilingualism**) or one after the other (**sequential bilingualism**). At the beginning stage of simultaneous bilingualism, children do not seem to know that they are dealing with two languages, even when the two languages are different (Reich, 1986). When each of the parents talks exclusively in his or her language, the child seems to learn the two languages somewhat faster.

When the parents themselves switch languages and one of the languages is dominant in the environment, language mixing occurs (McLaughlin, 1998). The child's sentences contain words from both the languages. Words of the dominant language are more frequently used in sentences of the nondominant or weaker language. The child tends to avoid difficult words of the weaker language in favor of the comparable words in the stronger language. The rhythm and accent of one language might be used while speaking in the other language (Reich, 1986). Similar mixing can be evident in syntax as well. The child initially uses the word order and sentence structure of one language while speaking in both the languages. A mixture of the two can result in a syntax not found in either language.

Up to 2 years of age, bilingual children tend to have only one word for each object or event. The word may be from either language. Even when the children learn the two separate words for the same object, they soon drop one of the words. However, after the age of 2 years, when they presumably realize they are dealing with two languages, the children learn and retain both the words. The child who learns "Mommy's word" for an object asks for "Daddy's word" as well.

Eventually, the simultaneously bilingual child separates the two languages at all levels. Each is spoken with its own rhythm and accent. There is very little mixing of words and sentence structures. The child might be more proficient in one language than in the other, but both are functional and separate systems. The child can switch from one language to the other depending on the speaking situation.

The distinction between simultaneous and successive bilingualism is arbitrary. In successive bilingualism, the child has been monolingual for some time and begins to learn a second language after the 3rd birthday (McLaughlin, 1998; Owens, 1996; Reich, 1986).

Research shows that children are remarkably efficient at learning a second language in their new environment. A 3-year-old monolingual Malaysian child learned German so fast that by the age of 4, the child's new language was comparable to that of native German children of the same age. A 6-year-old Hungarian child learned French in 10 months and showed proficiency comparable to that of native 6-year-old French children. Several other examples of similar rapid learning of a second language have been documented (Reich, 1986). However, the possibility that such examples involve not the typical child but exceptionally talented children cannot be ignored. Nonetheless, many experts think that under age 7, most children can successfully acquire a second language in the natural environment of that language.

Does a child who sequentially learns a second language follow the same sequence as the monolingual child learning the same language? Experts disagree on the answer to this question, but there seems to be more evidence that sequential second language acquisition is similar to monolingual acquisition. The stages and sequence of learning a second language in early childhood are the same as those followed by a monolingual child (Hamers & Blanc, 1989; McLaughlin, 1998; Owens, 1996; Reich, 1986).

Summary

- Language use varies across individuals because of the influence of several factors including the geographic region, age, gender, race, and other personal characteristics of speakers.

- There are both native and non-native dialects of English as it is spoken around the world; cultural, geographic, ethnic, and other factors influence these dialects.

- African American English is a special variation of English with its own rules and some special vocabulary.

- Secondary dialects of English influenced by Spanish and other languages are becoming increasingly prevalent in the United States.

- No dialect is better than the other; dialects are just different forms of a language.

✐ Differences Versus Disorders

The traditional linguistic analysis, with its strict rules of sound combinations (phonology), word formations (morphology), word order and sentence structure (syntax), and word meanings (semantics) has often been misinterpreted to mean that there is but one standard set of rules for a given language formulation and production. The rules often are relative to a theoretical ideal or standard of the language. The particular variation considered the ideal may be spoken by people who live in prestigious geographic areas. In Britain, for example, the form of English spoken in London was considered *the* British English. The ideal may also be the form spoken by a majority of people, people in power, people of a particular race, people who are better educated, or people who are rich. The notion of an ideal may also evolve out of a combination of these and other factors. In the United States, such a combination seems to be responsible for the popularly held belief that there is a standard way of speaking American English.

The notion that each language has a standard form inevitably leads to a related but questionable notion that variations of a language are its degenerate, undesirable, or abnormal forms. Such a questionable notion is likely to be held by those who speak what is considered the standard form. Unfortunately, a few linguists, scholars of various disciplines, literary people, government officials, educators, and even speech–language pathologists have, at one time or another, perpetuated the notion that language variations are undesirable deviations from the correct, proper, and standard form.

People who speak a certain dialect may face many social, educational, and occupational barriers. Historically, the dialects of the middle-class white Americans have been the standard against which other dialects have been evaluated. The dialects of poor and less educated Americans regardless of race, and those of nonwhite races regardless of education and economic status, have historically been evaluated negatively. In schools and colleges, educators have shown biases in favor of what they think is the standard dialect. People who do not speak that dialect are thought to lack verbal skills, logical thinking abilities, and abilities to succeed in schools and colleges (Labov, 1970). Various employers are reluctant to hire people who speak nonstandard dialects. These people are more likely to be offered temporary and low-paying positions than those who speak the more generally accepted dialect (Terrell & Terrell, 1983).

Legal Challenges

In the 1970s, public, governmental, educational, and professional opinions about the dialects and bilingualism began to change. Two landmark court cases, one in California and the other in Michigan, were instrumental in forcing some of the changes (Taylor, 1986). In the first court case known as *Lau v. Nichols*, the residents of San Francisco's Chinatown argued that their children who did not speak English well were denied equal educational opportunity. The monolingual teachers who spoke only English were not helping children learn or understand the medium of instruction. The parents asked the court to order the school district to provide special assistance in English language by bilingual teachers. The parents' arguments were based on Title VI of the 1964 Civil Rights Act which stated,

> No person in the United States shall, on the ground of race, color, or national origin, be excluded from participation in, be denied benefits of, or be subjected to discrimination under any program or activity receiving federal financial assistance.

The school district argued that since it provided the same kinds of buildings, books, and curricula to all students within the district, it was in compliance with the provisions of the Civil Rights Act. On January 21, 1974, the U.S. Supreme Court ruled in favor of the Chinatown residents and stated that the schools that do not provide meaningful education for non-English speaking pupils are in violation of the Act.

In the second major case, African American parents who sent their children to Martin Luther King, Jr., School in Ann Arbor, Michigan, sued their school district and argued that the teachers did not appreciate African American English (AAE), and this created a barrier to academic success (Taylor, 1986). The parents did not ask for instruction in AAE; they wanted more sensitivity and understanding on the part of the teachers toward African American children's home language. The parents' argument in this case was based on Section 1703(f) of Title 20 of the U.S. Code which states,

> No state shall deny equal educational opportunity to an individual on account of his or her race, color, sex, or national origin by . . . (f) the failure of an educational agency to take appropriate action to overcome language barriers that impede equal participation by students in its instructional programs.

On July 12, 1979, the United States Eastern District Court of Michigan ruled that the Ann Arbor school district was in violation of Section 107(f) of Title 20 of the U.S. Code. The court required the school district to develop a plan for increasing the teacher understanding of AAE. Consequently, the school district developed a plan that included, among other things, in-service training to teachers on dialectal variations of languages and the history of AAE and its characteristics. Legal and professional experts consider this a landmark case that gave legal recognition to dialectal variations, especially AAE (Bountress, 1987).

The U.S. Congress has played a major role in passing several acts that promote equal educational opportunities to children of all linguistic and cultural backgrounds and children who have various handicaps, including those with disorders of communication. Significant among them is the Bilingual Education Act of 1968, the Education for All Handicapped Children Act of 1975 (P.L. 94-142) and its subsequent reauthorized version, including Individuals with Disabilities Education Act, and the Bilingual Education Act of 1976. Various codes, newer federal regulations, and various state regulations also have been instrumental in effecting positive changes in the country.

Dialects and the Speech–Language Pathologist

In the past, when scientific information about language variations was not available, speech–language pathologists might not have realized that a language difference is not the same as a language disorder. Therefore, many speech–language pathologists may have diagnosed a language disorder in a client who just happened to speak differently (Taylor, 1986). As the scientific information about language variation, the systematic and patterned nature of dialectal variations, and the relation between culture, communication, and ethnicity became well established, the profession of communicative disorders began to take a new look at the relation between language, culture, and ethnicity in the pluralistic American society. The profession began to address the issue of language differences versus disorders and to place clinical issues in the broader context of culture.

The American Speech-Language-Hearing Association (ASHA) has done a significant amount of work to promote better understanding among its members of language differences in culturally and linguistically diverse populations. ASHA now encourages course work on bilingualism, multiculturalism, and dialectal variations of the English language. It urges colleges and universities that train speech–language pathologists and audiologists to promote the idea that culture, communication, and its variations are interdependent and that no dialectal variation of a language is a deviation from some standard. Educational institutions also are urged to include adequate information on multiculturalism, bilingualism, and the educational and professional needs of the bilingual child. In fact, several universities and colleges now have special programs on bilingual–bicultural issues.

In recent years, ASHA has issued two position statements that are important in this context. The first statement concerns social dialects, and the second statement concerns the clinical management of communicative disorders in minority populations. In evaluating and treating language disorders in all populations, speech–language clinicians who are members of ASHA are expected to follow the guidelines established in these two position papers.

The position paper on social dialects makes it clear that "it is the position of the American Speech-Language-Hearing Association (ASHA) that no dialectal variety of English is a disorder or a pathological form of speech or language" (ASHA, 1987, p. 45). Speech–language pathologists must know the dialects of American English, including AAE, and English influenced by other languages (Spanish, Asian languages). A speaker of a particular dialect is not a candidate for clinical speech–language services unless there is a disorder within the dialectal system of the speaker. A child who speaks AAE, for example, is not a candidate for clinical services because of AAE; the child may be a candidate because within the AAE constraints, the child has a disorder of communication. In essence, failure to learn the verbal behaviors of the verbal community to which the child belongs, but not a failure to acquire the verbal behaviors of another verbal community, warrants clinical services.

Speakers of minority dialects may elect to learn the majority dialect but should not be forced to learn it.

The ASHA position paper recognizes that speakers of minority dialects may wish to acquire the dialect of the government, industry, mass media, sciences, and arts (ASHA, 1987). In such cases, a speaker of a particular dialect may choose to learn the dialect of the majority (or a dialect of any particular group, including a minority group). The speech–language pathologists can make themselves available to provide elective services to such a speaker. Speech–language pathologists can serve as consultants to teachers and other professionals on dialectal variations and modifications. Still, the priority is to treat people who exhibit disorders of communication.

ASHA also recognizes the clinical service needs of minority populations with disordered communication (American Speech-Language-Hearing Association, 1985). It is estimated that more than 3.5 million minority language speakers in the United States have a disorder of communication that is unrelated to their status as bilingual speakers. Unfortunately, not many speech–language pathologists have bilingual competencies. Most speech–language pathologists are monolingual English speakers. Therefore, the problem of assessing and treating communicative disorders of the minority language speakers is serious and currently without a totally satisfactory solution.

ASHA makes several recommendations. For bilingual speakers who have proficiency in English, the speech–language pathologists and audiologists can provide services in English. They can assess the use of English language and determine whether a disorder exists. If it does, the clinician may treat that disorder. However, to make a distinction between a disorder and a dialectal variation in English possibly due to the first language of the speaker, the clinician must know the basics of the minority language rules. The clinician must not make an assessment based on procedures that are unfavorable (discriminatory) to the client. For example, a language test that includes culturally unique items that the child is not familiar with because of his or her varied cultural background should not be used in assessing that child's language.

For individuals who have only a limited proficiency in English, but speak another language better, the clinical services must be provided in the primary (non-English) language. In other words, the client must receive services in the minority language. To do this, the clinician must be proficient in the minority language and should have knowledge about language acquisition and disorders in bilingual people. The clinician must be able to assess the minority language with nondiscriminatory procedures. Most speech–language pathologists who are monolingual are not able to fully serve these clients.

Finally, some clients are bilingual but limited in both the languages. They are communicatively disabled in every sense of the term. These individuals must be assessed in both the languages. Therefore, the clinician must know both the languages. In some cases, assessment might show that English is the dominant of the two languages. Treatment then can be given in English. Of course, some clients must be treated in their minority language because of its dominance.

In essence, if the disorder is in English, and the treatment must be offered in English, most clinicians are able to help the clients. A knowledge of cultural difference, dialectal variations, and nondiscriminatory procedures along with a general cultural sensitivity are still required. If the disorder is in the minority language, only a bilingual speech–language pathologist can provide the full range of services. To do the best under the circumstances, monolingual speech–language pathologists may use translators and interpreters. In all cases, the clinician can be a strong advocate of the minority language speaker. The clinician who cannot provide the needed services may seek services from other sources and agencies.

Currently, the culturally diverse populations are not receiving adequate services. The most adequate services are provided by bilingual clinicians who are proficient in both English and the client's primary language. ASHA hopes that more bilingual people and people of ethnic minority groups will enter the profession so that the bilingual and ethnic minority populations with communicative disorders will be served adequately.

> The need for bilingual speech–language pathologists is acute and is expected only to increase.

Myths and Stereotypes To Avoid

Professionals and otherwise educated citizens ought to avoid stereotypes about people and their cultures. Speech–language pathologists and audiologists, being human service professionals, have a special responsibility to understand the people they serve. This means that the professionals should learn authentic information about the people of different cultures they serve. An overzealous approach to cultures and cultural differences masks similarities between people. It is as important to know the similarities among people as it is to know the differences. Professionals should not presume that people have no common patterns of behavior just because they are of different ethnic, cultural, or geographic background. Currently, the emphasis is on understanding the diversity of cultures because it is the starting point. Eventually, a **science of multiculturalism** will identify cultural (and other) factors that make a difference in assessing and treating communication problems and factors that do not make a difference.

Until such a science of multiculturalism is developed, clinicians will have to work hard to avoid stereotypes about people, their cultures, and their patterns of communication. A lack of understanding of cultures, or a superficial understanding of differences among people, can promote stereotypic notions about people and their cultures. Some stereotypes to be avoided are summarized in Table 11.1.

Summary

- Language use varies across subgroups of a population that speaks the same language.

- Language variations are called dialects, which should not be confused with language disorders.

- All speakers speak with a dialect ("accent"), but the dialects of an ethnic or cultural minority may be evaluated negatively because of the false notion that there is only one correct way of speaking a language.

(continues)

Table 11.1

Stereotypes To Be Avoided About People of Different Cultural and Ethnic Backgrounds

Stereotypes	More Accurate Statements
People of different ethnic and cultural backgrounds are totally different.	People of different ethnic and cultural backgrounds are different in some respects and similar in other respects.
Individuals belonging to a particular cultural or ethnic group are totally similar.	There are great individual differences among members of particular cultural and ethnic groups; what holds good for the group as a whole may not hold good for individual members of that group. For example, not all African Americans are poor; not all African Americans speak AAE; some whites speak elements of AAE; not all Asian Americans are good in math; not all Asian Americans prefer to talk less; some whites talk less than some Asians.
The terms *multicultural* or *diversity* refer only to nonwhites.	The terms *multicultural* or *diversity* do not refer to any particular group; they refer to societies that contain multiple cultures, including European American cultures.
In all matters of scientific discussion and reporting, it is always necessary to identify the cultural or ethnic heritage of people involved.	Cultural or ethnic identity of people should be revealed only when necessary to understand the matter under discussion.
What holds good for members of a cultural group in their original country also holds good when the members migrate and live in a different country.	People who migrate to another country change to varying degrees, but they all change to some degree; they rarely are the same.
Members of each cultural or ethnic group need unique treatment techniques.	Maybe, maybe not; only controlled experimental research involving members of different cultural groups can tell.

- Those who speak a particular dialect may elect to learn another dialect; speech–language pathologists may help those individuals learn the chosen dialect.

- The primary professional concern of the speech–language pathologist is the remediation of disorders of communication.

- To adequately serve individuals of all ages in a multicultural, multiethnic, and multilingual society, clinicians should understand and appreciate the cultural, ethnic, and linguistic background and variation of their clients.

- Clinicians who diagnose and treat disorders of communication in bilingual people should be similarly bilingual.

- Clinicians who diagnose and treat disorders within a dialect should know the dialect; for example, to treat disorders within AAE, clinicians should know AAE.

Dialogue

By now, Ms. Noledge-Hungry is sure that she wants to major in speech–language pathology. As usual, she visits Professor Speech-Wisely in his office to talk about diversity and disorders of communication.

N-H: Dr. Speech-Wisely, I hadn't thought about language variation that much. During the first part of the course, we learned so much about the rules of language and its use that you almost begin to think that each language has but one form.

S-W: It is easy to get such an impression. The prevailing popular opinions may also foster such an impression. There are basic rules that apply across variations; there are some rules that are unique to particular variations. You must remember that the variations of a language, called **dialects**, are basically similar but different in certain specific respects.

N-H: Like the Southern English or the Eastern New England English or the African American English. All those varieties are essentially English.

S-W: Yes, African American English shares a majority of rules with Standard English, but it varies in some phonological, morphological, syntactic, and semantic respects. You should be able to give a few examples of African American English characteristics.

N-H: Although I hadn't realized it before, it makes sense to say that African American English is not a degenerate form of Standard English, and that it has its own rules and patterns. Some of its rules are more complex and signal differences in meaning that are not found in Standard English.

S-W: That's right. Also, it is good to have a general understanding of English as spoken in such diverse countries as Britain, South Africa, India, Hong Kong, New Zealand, Canada, and Australia. There are both **native dialects** and **secondary dialects** of English.

N-H: Spanish-influenced and Asian-language–influenced dialects of English are commonly heard in the United States. We hear the word *melting pot* a lot, but I found the viewpoint that the United States is not so much a melting pot as it is a country of people who have many cultural and linguistic backgrounds more appropriate.

S-W: As a future speech–language pathologist, it is an important point to be appreciated. Also, clinicians should have information on some of the common Native American languages.

N-H: Unfortunately, the Native American languages are dwindling. I was amazed that there are more than 800 Native American languages!

S-W: Yes. Now, define a bilingual and a polyglot.

N-H: People who speak two languages are **bilingual**. Those who speak more than two languages are **polyglot**.

S-W: Good. Most societies of the world are bilingual; many societies are polyglot. Technically, the U.S. population is polyglot; people speak English, several Native American Indian languages, Spanish, Asian, and many European languages. But those who have no proficiency or limited proficiency in English are considered a **linguistic minority**. Even those who have English proficiency but speak another language at home may be considered minority.

N-H: But the minority status is not due entirely to the smaller number of people. Lack of political and economic power, lower socioeconomic status, and ethnic background also may play a role in determining this status.

S-W: That is correct.

N-H: I found out that an amazing 18% of the population speaks a language other than English at home. While roughly 42 million Americans are bilingual, 20 million do not have adequate English proficiency.

S-W: More than 6.6 million children of minority background are enrolled in the U.S. public schools.

N-H: I thought that bilingualism was detrimental to a child's language ability. Research shows that it is not. Children can acquire two languages quite easily. When a child begins to learn two languages, it is called **simultaneous** bilingualism. It is **sequential** when the second language acquisition starts after age 3.

S-W: Also, the second language acquisition during early childhood is rapid. Most children studied have acquired a second language in less than a year. What are some of the factors that create different dialects of a language?

N-H: Geographic region, race, bilingualism, socioeconomic status, gender, age, and speaking situations all affect the use of language. There are at least 10 major American English dialects based on geographic region. I found both genderlect and teenlect interesting topics.

S-W: You should be able to describe the major dialectal variations of American English. You should also note that some variables are stronger than others. For example, geographic regions are a stronger variable than the gender of the speaker.

N-H: It is only in recent years that social scientists and professionals have concluded that language differences should not be confused with language disorders. All dialectal variations are natural variations of languages. There is no justification to make value judgments based on dialects.

S-W: That's correct. Nonetheless, people do make judgments about speakers based on their dialects. Employers and business establishments prefer people who speak the standard dialect. Educators may be prejudiced against pupils who speak a varied dialect. Both the scientific and the professional communities need to work more to educate people on this issue.

N-H: I appreciate the position taken by the American Speech-Language-Hearing Association. The Association says that dialectal differences are not disorders and should not be treated as such.

S-W: Yes. The Association also recognizes that some minority dialectal speakers may wish to learn the more commonly used dialect because it is to their advantage to do so. In such cases, the speech–language pathologists may be available to offer their services.

N-H: The clinicians should still consider treating the communicatively disabled their top priority.

S-W: Absolutely. And in the case of bilingual people who need clinical services in either their native language or English, speech–language pathologists must have proficiency in the native language. If the treatment can be provided in English, the need for the native language proficiency is minimal. If the treatment must be provided in the native language, the clinician must have complete proficiency in that language.

The Outlook

N-H: Dr. Speech-Wisely, I can speak Spanish fluently. I am fairly good at reading and writing in Spanish. I imagine it is an asset in the field of speech–language pathology.

S-W: Certainly! There is a great need for bilingual speech–language pathologists. The bilingual are among the least served segment of the population of communicatively disabled. Bilingual clinicians are in great demand and the demand can only be higher in the future.

N-H: Should I take some special courses to be a full-fledged bilingual clinician?

S-W: You might take additional courses on the structure of Spanish. You may want to keep your Spanish current all the time. You may also select a graduate program in speech–language pathology that offers a bilingual program.

N-H: So it is better to revive a second language if one was learned during the high school years and later forgotten.

S-W: Yes. Proficiency in one of the second languages more frequently spoken in the United States will be extremely useful to speech–language pathologists.

N-H: I might take some college courses in Spanish along with courses in speech–language pathology and audiology.

S-W: That is an excellent idea!

Study Questions

1. Distinguish between language difference and language disorder.

2. Distinguish between a bilingual and a polyglot.

3. Do social scientists believe that the United States is a unilingual country?

4. State three or more reasons why a group may have the status of a minority.

5. Distinguish between simultaneous and sequential bilingualism.

6. At what age does a bilingual child realize that he or she is dealing with two languages?

7. Define a dialect.

8. Describe at least three variables that contribute to the development of dialects of a given language.

9. Summarize the major characteristics of women's speech.

10. Give an overview of English as it is spoken around the world.

11. Distinguish between primary and secondary English dialects.

12. Describe at least four characteristics of African American English.

13. Describe the major phonological characteristics of Spanish-influenced English.

14. Summarize the two court cases that were described in the context of bilingual and African American English.

15. Summarize Section 1703(f) of Title 20 of the U.S. Code.

16. What is ASHA's position on social dialects?

17. What is ASHA's position on the communicative problems of the minority language speakers?

18. What is the meaning of elective treatment for dialectal differences? Does ASHA approve such services provided by its members?

References

American Speech-Language-Hearing Association. (1985, June). Clinical management of communicatively handicapped minority language population. *Asha,* pp. 29–32.

American Speech-Language-Hearing Association. (1987, January). Social dialect position paper. *Asha,* pp. 45–48.

Battle, D. E. (Ed.). (1998). *Communication disorders in multicultural populations* (2nd ed.). Boston: Butterworth-Heinemann.

Bountress, N. G. (1987). The Ann Arbor decision in retrospect. *Asha, 29,* 55–57.

Comrie, B. (Ed.). (1990). *The world's major languages.* New York: Oxford University Press.

Dillard, J. L. (1972). *Black English.* New York: Random House.

Edwards, A. D. (1976). *Language in culture and class.* London: Heinemann Educational Books.

Hamers, J. F., & Blanc, M. H. (1989). *Bilinguality and bilingualism.* Cambridge: Cambridge University Press.

Highwater, J. (1975). *Indian America.* New York: David McKay.

Kamhi, A. G., Pollock, K. E., & Harris, J. L. (1996). *Communication development and disorders in African American children.* Baltimore: Brookes.

Kayser, H. (1995). *Bilingual speech–language pathology: An Hispanic focus.* San Diego, CA: Singular.

Kayser, H. (1998). Hispanic cultures and language. In D. E. Battle (Ed.), *Communication disorders in multicultural populations* (pp. 157–195). Boston: Butterworth-Heinemann.

Kramer, C. (1974). Women's speech: Separate but unequal? *Quarterly Journal of Speech, 60,* 14–24.

Labov, W. (1970). Stages in the acquisition of standard English. In H. Hungerford, J. Robinson, & J. Sledd (Eds.), *English linguistics.* Atlanta, GA: Scott Foresman.

Lakoff, R. (1975). *Language and woman's place.* New York: Harper Colophon Books.

Langdon, H. W., & Cheng, L. L. (Eds.). (1992). *Hispanic children and adults with communication disorders.* Gaithersburg, MD: Aspen.

Lerner, A., & Loewe, F. (1956). *My fair lady.* New York: Chappell & Co.

McCrum, R., Cran, W., & MacNeil, R. (1992). *The story of English.* New York: Penguin.

McLaughlin, S. (1998). *Introduction to language development.* San Diego, CA: Singular.

Nist, J. (1966). *A structural history of English.* New York: St. Martin's Press.

Owens, R. W., Jr. (1996). *Language development: An introduction* (4th ed.). Needham Heights, MA: Allyn & Bacon.

Peña-Brooks, A., & Hegde, M. N. (2000). *Assessment and treatment of articulation and phonological disorders in children.* Austin, TX: PRO-ED.

Perez, E. (1994). Phonological differences among speakers of Spanish-influenced English. In J. E. Bernthal & N. W. Bankson (Eds.), *Child phonology: Characteristics, assessment, and intervention with special populations* (pp. 245–254). New York: Thieme.

Reich, P. A. (1986). *Language development.* Englewood Cliffs, NJ: Prentice Hall.

Roseberry-McKibbin, C. (1995). *Multicultural students with special needs.* Oceanside, CA: Academic Communication Associates.

Taylor, O. (1983). Black English: An agenda for the 1980s. In J. Chambers (Ed.), *Black English: Educational equality and the law.* Ann Arbor, MI: Karoma Press.

Taylor, O. (Ed.). (1986). *Nature of communication disorders in culturally and linguistically diverse populations.* Boston: Little, Brown.

Terrell, S., & Terrell, F. (1983). Effects of speaking Black English upon employment opportunities. *Asha, 25,* 27–29.

Tiffany, W. R., & Carrell, J. (1977). *Phonetics: Theory and application to speech improvement.* New York: McGraw-Hill.

U.S. Bureau of the Census. (1996). *Statistical abstracts of the United States: 1996* (116th ed.). Washington, DC: Author.

van Keulen, J. E., Weddington, G. T., & DeBose, C. E. (1998). *Speech, language learning and the African American child.* Needham Heights, MA: Allyn & Bacon.

Waggoner, D. (1984). The need for bilingual education—estimates for the 1980 census. *Journal of the Nation Association for Bilingual Education, 8,* 9.

Warren, A. R., & McCloskey, L. A. (1993). Pragmatics: Language in social contexts. In J. B. Gleason (Ed.), *The development of language* (pp. 195–237). New York: Macmillan.

Williamson, J. (1972). A look at Black English. *The Crisis, 78,* 169–185.

Witalec, J. (Ed.). *Native North American literary companion.* Detroit, MI: Visible Ink.

Yavas, M., & Goldstein, B. (1998). Phonological assessment and treatment of bilingual speakers. *American Journal of Speech-Language Pathology, 7,* 49–60.

Zuniga, M. E. (1992). Families with Latino roots. In E. W. Lynch & M. J. Hanson (Eds.), *Developing cross-cultural competence* (pp. 151–178). Baltimore: Brookes.

The Professions: Education and Organizations

- The American Speech-Language-Hearing Association
- State Regulation of the Profession
- The Road to Becoming a Professional
- Study Questions
- References

Whereas the study of human communication has a long history, the organized profession of communicative disorders is somewhat new. Human communication has been studied for centuries by philosophers who have speculated about the nature of language and thought; anthropologists and other scientists who have studied the origin of language; and psychologists and linguists who have studied the structure, function, and use of language. But the profession of communicative disorders is a creation of the 20th century.

At the beginning of the 20th century, there were no professionally trained speech–language pathologists or audiologists in the United States. There were no educational or professional training programs in the country. In Europe, the treatment of speech disorders was a domain of medicine. In the United States, it was the public schools that took a leading role in providing special teaching programs for children with communicative disorders. By 1910, Chicago public schools began to hire specialists who worked with children with disorders of speech. These specialists were called speech correction teachers (Paden, 1970) and worked mostly with children who stuttered or had disorders of articulation. Other disorders of communication began to be treated only much later.

In the early 1920s, the University of Wisconsin and the University of Iowa began to offer doctoral programs with an emphasis on speech disorders. Soon, other universities across the country instituted degree programs in speech disorders.

The professional education of specialists in communicative disorders has undergone many changes over the years. Most of these changes are due to phenomenal growth in the amount of research information concerning communication and its disorders. The organization to which the specialists belonged played a major role in shaping the education and the future of the profession.

The American Speech-Language-Hearing Association

Currently, the organization to which many of the specialists belong is known as the **American Speech-Language-Hearing Association.** But it was not always known by that name. When it was established in 1925 by a handful of people at the University of Iowa, it was called the **American Academy of Speech Correction** (Paden, 1970). It opened its membership to those individuals who were interested in the scientific study and treatment of speech disorders.

The professional organization has undergone several name changes. In 1927, the American Academy of Speech Correction was renamed the **American Society for the Study of Speech Disorders.** In 1934, it was changed to the **American Speech Correction Association.** In 1947, the organization was again renamed the **American Speech and Hearing Association (ASHA).** The addition of *Hearing* to the name of the association was a significant event. By this time, speech pathology's twin profession, audiology, was gaining much recognition. Because speech and hearing are so closely connected, the specialists in the two fields share a common base of knowledge and professional concerns. Therefore, they belong to the same organization.

The next name change came in 1978. The specialists treating communicative disorders were always involved in the study of language and treatment of language disorders in children and adults. However, their involvement became deeper and more focused in the 1960s and 1970s. To reflect the profession's involvement in language and its disorders more accurately, the Association was renamed the **American Speech-Language-Hearing Association.** However, the earlier acronym, ASHA, was retained.

The changing names of the professional organization parallels the changing names of the professionals themselves. Speech–language pathologists have been variously known as speech correction teachers, speech correctionists, speech therapists, speech teachers, speech pathologists, and speech clinicians. Currently, the term speech therapist is widely known. This term is not preferred by the specialists themselves or the national organization because therapists—physical therapists, for example—typically work under the supervision of a physician. Speech–language pathologists are not under medical supervision. The title currently preferred by the American Speech-Language-Hearing Association is **speech–language pathologist.** Although referring to practitioners of the profession, the title **speech–language clinician** is equally acceptable. Both the titles have been used throughout this book.

The specialists who are concerned with hearing, its disorders, and their assessment, and rehabilitation of people with hearing impairment have always been known as **audiologists.** However, audiologists who work in educational settings (e.g., public schools) may be known as **educational audiologists,** and those who work in the industrial sector are known as **industrial audiologists.**

ASHA has grown dramatically in recent decades. In 1935, the organization had less than 100 members. By the mid-1980s, the membership had increased to well over 40,000. At the time of this writing, the membership in ASHA is about 100,000 professionals, which includes speech–language pathologists, audiologists, speech and hearing scientists, and international affiliate members. Over 80% of ASHA members are speech–language pathologists. Less than 8% of the members are male, and only 7.5% of the members belong to ethnic minority groups. It is estimated that approximately 40,000 clinicians, the majority of whom work in public schools, are not members of ASHA.

Both the range of professional services and the professional organization are growing. Roughly 50% of clinicians who belong to ASHA work primarily in schools, mostly public schools. About 50% of ASHA members work in other professional settings including hospitals, outpatient clinics, rehabilitation institutes, institutes for people with mental retardation, nursing and extended care facilities, and private practice. A rapidly growing segment of the profession, however, is in private practice. About 45% of audiologists work in nonresidential health care facilities including offices of physicians and their own private clinics. Approximately 25% of audiologists are affiliated with hospitals. Both audiologists and speech–language pathologists work in universities and colleges, speech and hearing research laboratories, and government agencies. In addition, audiologists work in industries, prisons, and armed forces.

ASHA is a national scientific and professional organization located in the Washington, D.C. metropolitan area (Rockville, Maryland). ASHA's membership includes clinicians and scientists who study communicative behaviors and disorders. ASHA has several goals. The most important of them includes organized efforts to (a) ensure the quality of speech, language, and hearing services offered to the public; (b) stimulate the development of speech-language-hearing services to people who have communicative disorders; (c) encourage scientific study and research into the basic processes of communication, disorders of communication, and treatment of those disorders; (d) promote exchange of scientific and professional information through publications, conventions, and other continuing education activities; and (e) work with federal and state government agencies to protect the interests of both the consumers and professionals by advocating and supporting appropriate legislation and regulation.

One way of ensuring the quality of services rendered to the public is to make sure that speech–language pathologists and audiologists receive appropriate scientific and professional education. Another way is to periodically evaluate the clinical services offered by speech and hearing clinics. ASHA plays a major role in these two areas. ASHA is the recognized accrediting agent for college and university departments that offer master's degree programs in speech–language pathology and audiology.

ASHA has established standards of scientific and professional education in speech–language pathology and audiology. The standards include the kinds and variety of academic courses that must be offered and the amount and quality of clinical practice the student clinicians must have. Through its **Council on Academic Accreditation in Speech–Language Pathology and Audiology (CAA)**, ASHA accredits those master's degree programs in speech–language pathology and audiology that meet its minimum standards. The college or the university department that offers the master's degree program requests accreditation from ASHA. The CAA, which handles this request, sends a team of experts to the department. The team evaluates all aspects of the degree program including the quality and range of the academic course work, the qualifications of the teaching faculty, the certification status of the clinical supervisors, and the library and other support systems to see if the department meets ASHA's standards. The team makes an analysis of standards that are met and those that are not met by the university department and makes a report to the CAA. If the standards are met, the CAA, hence ASHA, formally accredits the department.

The **Professional Services Board (PSB)** of ASHA evaluates the clinical services a speech–language and hearing clinic offers. Upon receiving a request, a team of specialists chosen by PSB visits the clinic to evaluate its services. The team evaluates the basic physical facilities, the clinical equipment, the qualifications and the certification status of the clinicians, and the overall quality of the clinical services rendered to the clients. If minimal clinical standards are met, the PSB accredits the clinic. This accreditation of a speech and hearing clinic assures the public that the services they receive meet the clinical standards established by the national organization.

Find out from ASHA or from the department whether a degree program you are considering is accredited by ASHA.

When selecting a college or a university program in communicative disorders, students wish to make sure that the program is accredited by ASHA. To the student, ASHA accreditation means that the program meets the educational standards set by the national organization. It also means that the student, upon graduation with a master's degree in speech–language pathology or audiology, also will be able to receive the national clinical certificates from ASHA. A student who graduates from a university program that is not accredited by ASHA will not be certified. These clinical certificates are described in a later section.

ASHA plays a major role in promoting greater awareness in the public and government and legislative bodies about communicative disorders. As a professional and scientific organization, ASHA lobbies the U.S. Congress and many agencies of the federal government for better funding for research, recognition for speech–language and hearing services, and better protection for consumers of clinical services. ASHA seeks to give input to congressional committees that are considering various legislation that affects the profession of speech–language pathology and the clinical services the public receives.

ASHA publishes several journals that include scientific studies, clinical research, scholarly articles, and discussions of professional issues. Its main research journal is the *Journal of Speech, Language, and Hearing Research*. Its two journals, the *American Journal of Speech-Language Pathology* and the *American Journal of Audiology,* are devoted to clinical practice. *Language, Speech, and Hearing Services in Schools* is a journal concerned mainly with clinical services offered in public schools. ASHA's monthly publication, *Asha,* is devoted to the professional and administrative aspects of speech–language pathology and audiology. *Asha* also contains articles and news items related to professional issues, governmental and legislative matters that affect the profession, information on employment opportunities, and the governing activities of the organization. As you begin to take more advanced courses in speech–language pathology or audiology, you will start reading some of the articles in these journals. Among several other useful publications of ASHA, the *Guide to Graduate Education in Speech–Language Pathology and Audiology* is especially helpful to students who wish to select graduate programs in the country.

Membership in ASHA

Currently, the basic requirement for membership in ASHA is a **master's degree** with a major emphasis in speech–language pathology or audiology. However, a member who also provides clinical services or supervises clinical services must meet, or be in the process of meeting, requirements for the Association's clinical certification. Those who do not provide or supervise clinical services may retain membership in ASHA without holding its clinical certificate. For example, scientists who do research on speech, language, and hearing who meet the academic requirement may be members of ASHA without possessing one of the clinical certificates.

Students who have declared their major as speech–language pathology or audiology may become members of the **National Student Speech-Language-Hearing Association (NSSLHA)**, which is recognized by ASHA. NSSLHA maintains close ties with ASHA. NSSLHA membership is very valuable for students. The NSSLHA membership fees are roughly a quarter of the fees ASHA members pay. For this substantially reduced fee, the student members of NSSLHA receive all of ASHA's journals, which are important sources of scientific and professional information for both the graduate and undergraduate students. In addition, NSSLHA publishes its own journal, *Contemporary Issues in Communication Sciences and Disorders* (CICSD), which is distributed to the members.

Among its several other advantages, the student membership allows registration at the annual national conventions at reduced fees. Many college and university departments of communicative disorders have an active local chapter of NSSLHA. These local chapters sponsor guest lectures, raise funds for attending state and local conventions, and organize many professional events. The local chapters also organize social events, which give the students in the department opportunities to get better acquainted with other students and members of the faculty.

ASHA's Clinical Certificates

To ensure the quality of speech–language and hearing services offered to the public, ASHA developed two clinical certificates that are issued to its members who meet academic and clinical standards of the Association.

ASHA certifies speech–language pathologists and audiologists separately. The **Certificate of Clinical Competence in Speech–Language Pathology (CCC-SLP)** is issued to those who have the master's degree or its equivalent in speech–language pathology, have fulfilled clinical practicum and fellowship requirements, and have passed a national examination in speech–language pathology. The clinical practicum should include a minimum of 25 hours of supervised observation of services offered and a total of 350 hours of supervised clinical work with clients of all ages. The **Clinical Fellowship Year** (CFY) consists of additional, supervised clinical experience obtained after completing the graduate education. This may be 9 months of full-time (at least 30 hours a week), paid professional experience gained under the supervision of an ASHA certified speech–language pathologist. The clinical fellowship also may be completed in 36 months of part-time professional work (15 to 19 hours a week). The **Certificate of Clinical Competence in Audiology (CCC-A)** has similar requirements with the academic course work, clinical practicum, clinical fellowship, and a passing score on a national examination in audiology.

Graduate students can take the **National Examination in Speech–Language Pathology and Audiology (NESPA)** around the time they take a comprehensive examination for their master's degree. The NESPA can be taken any time thereafter as well. The Educational Testing Service (ETS) administers this test nationally. The ETS reports the scores of those who take the examination to ASHA and any other agency the student authorizes. For example, a state agency that licenses speech–language pathologists and audiologists also may receive the score.

ASHA's certificates are not legal documents comparable to a state license. However, they are recognized by most employers including hospitals, clinics, and universities throughout the country. Many state licensure laws were modeled after the ASHA requirements.

ASHA's Code of Ethics

Individuals who hold ASHA membership and clinical certification are committed to uphold the highest standards of clinical services. Treating individuals with communicative disorders is an ethical and socially responsible activity. Therefore, speech–language pathologists and audiologists who hold one of the certificates from ASHA are committed to its **code of ethics.**

The ASHA code of ethics (American Speech-Language-Hearing Association, 1994) contains the following four **ethical principles,** which direct and regulate the professional conduct of speech–language pathologists and audiologists:

1. Individuals (speech–language pathologists or audiologists) shall honor their responsibility to hold paramount the welfare of persons they serve professionally.

2. Individuals shall honor their responsibility to achieve and maintain the highest level of professional competence.

3. Individuals shall honor their responsibility to the public by promoting public understanding of the professions, by supporting the development of services designed to fulfill the unmet needs of the public, and by providing accurate information in all communications involving any aspect of the professions.

4. Individuals shall honor their responsibilities to the profession and their relationships with colleagues, students, and members of allied professions. Individuals shall uphold the dignity and autonomy of the professions, maintain harmonious interprofessional and intraprofessional relationships, and accept the profession's self-imposed standards. (pp. 1–2)

Every principle includes various rules of ethics that fully clarify its scope. Some of the rules under various principles include the following: Professionals must be well trained to provide services; must refer clients to other professionals when it is necessary; should not discriminate against clients on the basis of race, religion, gender, age, national origin, or sexual orientation; should not guarantee the results of treatment procedures; should not offer treatments of questionable validity; should protect the confidentiality of clients served; and should not misrepresent the profession to the public. These ethical principles make it clear that the professionals have an obligation to increase public knowledge about speech and hearing disorders and services. Also, through research and scholarly activities, professionals must strive to increase knowledge within the profession and share this knowledge with colleagues.

The code of ethics is an important document. The code regulates all aspects of a professional's conduct. Violation of the code has serious consequences, including the revocation of the clinical certificate and cancellation of membership in ASHA.

State Regulation of the Profession

State governments have laws and regulations that affect the work of speech–language pathologists and audiologists. Most states **credential** their speech–language pathologists and audiologists working in public schools. This credential is typically issued by the state department of education. Each state department of education has its own specifications that affect the educational training and professional practice of speech–language pathologists and audiologists who work in the public schools. However, most of the course work and clinical practicum experiences required by ASHA are also required to obtain a credential from a state department of education. Some state department regulations may require a few courses in education on the assumption that speech–language pathologists working in the schools must be familiar with certain educational methods and practices. A few states also combine a teaching credential with a credential in speech–language pathology. Such a credential requires more course work in regular and special education because the professional in this case is both a teacher and a speech–language pathologist.

Credentials issued by state departments of education are specific to that state's public school settings only. This certificate will not allow private practice, work in a hospital or clinic, or supervision of clinical practice in college speech and hearing centers. Professional settings other than public schools require either the ASHA certificate or the state licensure where one exists. An ASHA accredited university program in speech–language pathology and audiology requires both the ASHA certificate and the state license for its clinical faculty.

A majority of states have passed **licensure** laws to regulate the profession of speech–language pathology and audiology. There still are a few states that do not license speech–language pathologists and audiologists, although they may pass licensure laws in the future. A few states that do not have licensure laws regulate the work of speech–language pathologists and audiologists through registration or certification. Some states regulate audiologists in some way but not speech–language pathologists.

The state licensure is not the same as the state education department's credential, although both require similar course work and clinical practicum. Most state licensure laws are based on the requirements specified by ASHA. Therefore, by meeting the ASHA requirements, graduates in most states will also meet the requirements for the license to practice speech–language pathology or audiology. An important difference between the ASHA certificate and a state license is that the license carries the force of law within the state, but the certificate is issued by a professional organization and is nationally recognized (Lynch & Dublinske, 1986).

The state licensure is administered by a board (or a committee) created by the legislature. In different states, the boards are assigned to different state departments including departments of health, education, commerce, and consumer affairs (Lynch & Dublinske, 1986).

In the states that have licensure laws, speech–language pathologists and audiologists working in any setting other than public schools must have the appropriate license. These settings include hospitals, clinics and other health care facilities, private practices, rehabilitation institutes, and college and university clinics. Similarly, a license or ASHA's certificate is not enough to take a position in the public schools; the clinician must have the education department's credential. In fact, in a majority of states, a license or the ASHA certificate is not needed to work as a public school clinician; only the department of education's certificate is needed.

> Find out from your academic department whether your state has a licensure law.

The Road to Becoming a Professional

All this information about professional and governmental organizations and regulations can be overwhelming. As students move up the educational ladder, they learn about certain requirements at different times. Students select a particular state credential, license, and the ASHA certificate and find out what specific requirements must be fulfilled to obtain all three. The department of communicative disorders at the college or university will guide the student through the requirements and the paperwork.

All the certificates, credentials, licenses, other regulations, and code of ethics were no doubt developed to protect the public, who seek help for disorders of communication. Individuals who seek services know that a licensed, credentialed, or certified professional is qualified to provide the services. They also know that the professional is committed to ethical and responsible practice of his or her profession.

Equally important are the benefits of such regulations to the student and the eventual practitioner of the profession. By fulfilling the scientific and educational requirements, the student is assured of becoming a competent, confident, and independent professional who provides valuable service to members of the society. Prestige, professional status, and economic benefits also are associated with appropriate degrees, certificates, and licensure. Compared to a clinician who is not well prepared, a better educated and more competent clinician is able to meet greater challenges and to make more significant contributions to his or her chosen profession. Such a clinician also derives greater satisfaction from his or her work. Therefore, the regulations and requirements help professionals as much as they help consumers.

So far, three sets of requirements have been discussed: the requirements set forth by ASHA, those of state departments of education, and those from the state boards on licensure. To this is added what a university or college requires as a part of a program of study that must be completed before getting an undergraduate or a graduate degree in communicative disorders. Most colleges and universities require a broad general educational background before students begin their professional and scientific study in a given subject matter. During the first 2 years, most undergraduate students are busy taking courses on general education. They generally take an introductory course and perhaps a few basic courses in communication sciences and disorders during their freshman and sophomore years. In their junior and senior years, students concentrate on specialized courses in their field of study.

Most colleges and universities in the country design their graduate and undergraduate programs to meet the requirements of governmental and professional agencies. For example, an ASHA accredited university program in California certainly meets the requirements of ASHA, but it is very likely to meet the requirements of the California state licensure board as well. The university program is also likely to meet the requirements of the state department of education. Therefore, most students who graduate with a master's degree in communicative disorders from an accredited program in California might be simultaneously eligible for the state licensure, the ASHA certificate, and the educational credential. ASHA accredited programs in most other states follow a similar pattern.

Visit ASHA's Website (www.asha.org) for information on all aspects of professional education and practice.

It still is the responsibility of students to make sure that a university program they consider meets the requirements of a particular license or certificate that allows them to realize their professional goal. The previously mentioned ASHA's *Guide to Professional Education in Speech–Language Pathology and Audiology* lists all the accredited as well as nonaccredited programs throughout the country. This guide can be used in the initial selection of a graduate program in communicative disorders. After making an initial selection of one or more programs, the best course of action for the students is to discuss their educational and professional goals with a faculty advisor in the department. The students can then make sure that the university program they have selected meets their goals. With the help of their advisor, students plan their educational and clinical program. Throughout their educational career, students must keep in touch with the advisor to make necessary changes in the program. Such regular contacts with the faculty advisor will help students stay on the right track and complete the educational and professional requirements.

Typical Undergraduate Course Work

There are two types of undergraduate programs in the country. The first type is a **program in communicative disorders** (speech–language pathology and audiology). The second type is a **program in speech and hearing sciences.** Many courses are common to these two types of programs. The main difference between the two is that the program in communicative disorders tends to offer some clinical courses and may provide for limited clinical practicum experiences. In such a program, an undergraduate student might work with children and adults with communicative disabilities under the supervision of a certified and licensed speech–language pathologist or audiologist.

An undergraduate program in speech and hearing sciences focuses mostly on normal processes of speech, language, and hearing. In this type of program, very few, if any, clinical courses on disorders of communication are offered. Because such courses are prerequisites for clinical practicum, an undergraduate student enrolled in such a program cannot work with individuals with communicative disabilities.

At the undergraduate level, students typically do not major in audiology. Those who wish to be audiologists and speech–language pathologists take the same set of basic courses. Audiology and speech–language pathology tracks diverge at the graduate level. Even there, several courses are common to both the tracks.

All undergraduate programs offer certain basic courses. Even the undergraduate program in communicative disorders offers only a limited opportunity for clinical practice because there are several prerequisites that must be met before clinical courses and clinical practicum are taken. For example, the student must learn about the structure and function of the physical mechanism that makes speech and hearing possible. This involves taking a course on the anatomy and physiology of speech and hearing. The student then might take a course on phonetics, which is the science of production and perception of speech sounds. Most programs also offer a basic course on speech and hearing sciences, which includes acoustics (the study of sound), how the human vocal mechanism produces sound, how this sound is modified and articulated into speech sounds, and how listeners perceive speech sounds.

The next set of courses is likely to be concerned with articulation and language. A separate course serves as an introduction to articulation and its disorders. Another course focuses on what language is and how children acquire it. Beyond these courses, students might be offered a course each on language disorders, fluency disorders, and voice disorders. Many undergraduate programs in communicative disorders also offer a course on the assessment of speech–language disorders, in which such topics as case history, interview, standardized tests, language sampling, and other diagnostic procedures are discussed. Most undergraduate programs offer at least one course in audiology,

From your academic advisor, obtain a copy of required and elective courses in communicative disorders and compare them against ASHA's requirements.

which is concerned with hearing, its measurement, and its disorders. In addition, a separate course on hearing science, which explores the physics, physiology, and psychology of sound, might be offered.

Many courses in related disciplines are recommended for students in speech and hearing. Courses in psychology, including child psychology, learning theories, abnormal psychology, and the psychology of language offer useful information and broaden the perspective on communication, its development, and its disorders. Similarly, selected courses on genetics, neurophysiology, scientific methods, statistics, and linguistics might be recommended as optional courses. Because of the increasing use of computers in the clinical and research work in the sciences and professions of speech and hearing, it will be useful to take courses on electronics and computer science as well. If not formal courses on computer science, acquiring sophisticated skills in the use of computers will be helpful; some programs may require such skills.

Typical Graduate Course Work

A **master's degree** can be obtained in either speech–language pathology or audiology. Nonetheless, a few courses may be common to both degree programs. For example, in most programs, both involve a course on scientific methods and research. Courses on clinical and research instrumentation, statistics, administration of speech and hearing programs, and other specialized topics also might be common to both the specialties. Many speech–language pathology students take one or two courses in audiology. Similarly, audiology students take certain courses in speech–language pathology. Beyond that, the students in the two option areas specialize in their discipline.

Several courses at the graduate level parallel the courses taken at the undergraduate level. However, the graduate courses are more advanced, and the students learn more about the diagnostic, treatment, and research information regarding the various disorders of communication. It is typical for a graduate student to take an advanced course each on articulation, language, fluency, and voice, and study both the normal and disordered processes relative to these four basic dimensions of communication. In addition, several other specific disorders also might be the subject of separate graduate seminars. For example, separate seminars on cleft palate and associated disorders, aphasia, and speech disorders that have neurological bases are offered in many graduate programs. Finally, advanced courses on diagnostics or treatment methods also might be offered.

Audiology students take a seminar each on various aspects of hearing, its disorders, assessment, and rehabilitation. In a typical seminar in advanced audiology, sophisticated techniques of testing hearing and speech perception are taught. In a seminar in pediatric audiology, special problems of hearing and hearing assessment in children are discussed. In other seminars, hearing problems and their assessment in industrial workers (industrial audiology), electronics and instrumentation used in audiology, aural rehabilitation, hearing aids, and other topics might be discussed.

Students who wish to specialize in a given disorder or a certain aspect of the science or profession of communication can take additional and more advanced courses. Directed readings and independent studies give the student an opportunity to explore a given area or topic in greater detail. Both are done under the supervision of a faculty member and are tailored to meet the needs of individual students. Many graduate programs, especially those that have doctoral programs, offer more than one seminar on many topics or disorders of speech, language, and hearing. For example, a department may offer two or three seminars each on stuttering, cleft palate, voice, or advanced techniques of assessing hearing disorders. The student who wishes to specialize in one of the disorders might take advantage of such optional courses.

Finally, some graduate programs require a **thesis** of all graduate students, while other programs offer it as an option. A faculty member helps the student design and conduct a piece of research and supervises the thesis work. Typically, a committee of no less than three faculty members evaluates the thesis and conducts an oral examination in which the student presents the thesis and defends it. The committee then recommends its acceptance for the partial fulfillment of the requirements for the master's degree. The students who write a thesis find it extremely valuable because of the special knowledge they gain by their own research on a particular aspect of their discipline.

Those who do not write a thesis are required to take a **comprehensive examination.** Graduate students who have taken most of the required and optional courses take this examination. The examination covers the entire range of speech–language pathology. The students also often take an oral examination following the written comprehensive examination. Several sources as well as the NESPA are available to graduate students to prepare for this comprehensive examination (Payne & Anderson, 1991; Roseberry-McKibbin & Hegde, 2000).

Clinical Practicum

Some students cannot wait to start working with children and adults with communicative disorders. Others are a bit apprehensive about it. Some do not think much about it until they plunge into it; others think about it all the time. But most students find the clinical practicum exciting. It is through clinical practicum that students learn the techniques of their chosen profession (Hegde & Davis, 1999; Kelly, Davis, & Hegde, 1994).

Many programs do not offer clinical practicum to undergraduate students. In a program that does, undergraduate students who have had such courses as phonetics, speech and language development, articulation disorders, language disorders, and diagnostic methods are qualified to begin their clinical practicum. Graduate students, who will have taken most of the required courses necessary for clinical practicum, usually can begin their clinical practicum in their first semester.

Most college and university programs in communicative disorders maintain their own speech and hearing clinic on the campus. The primary purpose of such a clinic is to provide opportunities for the student clinical practicum. Of course, in this process, the clinic also provides valuable speech and hearing services to the community. The college and the university department might also have off-campus sites approved for clinical practicum. These include various speech and hearing clinics in the area.

The student clinician works under the direct supervision of a clinical supervisor who holds at least a master's degree in either speech–language pathology or audiology. In addition, the supervisor also holds the ASHA certificate in speech–language pathology or audiology and, where applicable, holds the state license as well.

The supervisor normally makes sure that the student clinician who treats a client has had an academic course on the disorder being treated. For example, a student who has had a course on articulation disorders, but no course on stuttering, may be assigned a client with articulation disorder but not one with stuttering. Most student clinicians work with two to three clients; each client is typically seen two times a week. The treatment sessions last 50 to 60 minutes. The clinical supervisor observes the treatment sessions through a one-way mirror and listens to the clinician–client conversations through an audio system installed for this purpose.

The supervisor makes sure that the student has an approved treatment plan for each client. The student clinician writes an entire treatment program or specific portions of a treatment program beforehand and gets it approved by the supervisor. The two discuss the details of the program and make necessary modifications. Throughout the semester, the student clinician and the supervisor hold meetings in which the client progress is reviewed and the clinician's performance is discussed and evaluated. The supervisor offers suggestions for improvement in the student clinician's performance.

To a limited extent, the supervisor may also participate in the treatment sessions to demonstrate certain treatment procedures, to explain the rationale of procedures being used to the client, and to generally counsel the client. The supervisor has the ethical responsibility to intervene whenever the student clinician is found to use inappropriate procedures or found to be ineffective.

The clinical practicum is an indispensable learning experience for the student. No doubt the student will make mistakes, but he or she will learn from them. By using effective treatment procedures, the student clinician sees systematic changes in the client's behaviors. A man who stuttered and has not been able to say much without embarrassing struggles and blocks begins to speak with relative fluency. The client now begins to face situations he had avoided all his life. He comes back and reports that for the first time in his life, he was able to talk fluently to his boss and that he was proud of himself. A child who has had no language begins to speak, and says "mommy" for the first time. No mother will fail to let you know what a moment of joy and satisfaction it was when she first heard that word from her child. A patient with aphasia who could not say his wife's name suddenly begins to call her by her name. The tears of joy are evident on both their faces. These are the moments when the clinician suddenly sees what a valuable and satisfying service he or she provided. These also are the moments of professional gratification.

Treatment changes the life of a client for the better. In turn, such changes have significant positive effects on the lives of people with whom they live and work. The clinician is the instrument of all such positive changes. This ability to touch the lives of many people is the heart of the profession of communicative disorders.

Finishing Up and Getting Started

After a certain amount of clinical experience at the college or the university speech and hearing center, the student clinician typically spends a semester working full time under supervision in a different clinical setting. This is the **clinical internship** (also called **externship**) required to complete the practicum requirements. The setting may be a public school, a hospital, a medical clinic, a private speech and hearing center, or a rehabilitation facility. This requirement is to give the student an opportunity to gain clinical experience in a variety of settings. Being a full-time involvement, internship also helps prepare the student for a professional position. The internship is usually done during the second and the final year of graduate study. Some students may opt to do two clinical externships, one in public schools and one in a medical setting, because the types of clinical experience gained in these settings are distinctly different. Public school externship is good to gain experience in assessing and treating communication disorders in children with little or no medical complications. Externship in medical settings, especially in adult rehabilitation facilities, is good to gain experience in assessing and treating communication disorders in adults and in the aging population that often are complicated by other medical problems (e.g., stroke, cancer of the larynx).

It is during the second year that the previously mentioned thesis is typically completed. Those who do not opt to do a thesis take their comprehensive examination. Upon completing all of the requirements of both the department and the university, the student is granted the master's degree in speech–language pathology or audiology.

Most state licensure and the ASHA national certificate require not only a master's degree along with required clinical practicum hours but also a passing score on the previously described national examination (NESPA) in speech–language pathology or audiology.

Before the new graduate who holds the master's degree is issued the license or the ASHA certificate, 9 months of paid, full-time professional experience are also required. ASHA calls this the **Clinical Fellowship Year,** during which the new graduate works under the supervision of a clinician who holds the certificate. The same experience also might fulfill the state licensure requirement when the supervisor also is licensed.

Upon completion of the clinical fellowship year, the master's degree holder is qualified to apply for the ASHA certificate and the state license. Those who wish to work in the public schools will get their school credential as soon as they graduate from the university. The graduate is now able to independently practice the profession of speech–language pathology or audiology.

What has been described is a basic and general outline of education and clinical training in communicative disorders. Regulations in each college or university and each state vary to a certain extent. In addition, the ASHA guidelines and state laws that affect the profession are frequently changed. Universities and colleges often revise their procedures and academic and clinical requirements. Therefore, as pointed out before, the student must be in constant touch with his or her faculty advisor, who will provide current and accurate information and guide the student in achieving his or her educational and professional goals.

The science and the profession of communicative disorders is a growing and vibrant discipline with a bright future. The discipline, partly because it is relatively new and partly because its identity is still evolving, offers many challenges and promises. Both the research scientists and professional clinicians find stimulating challenges in the discipline. The research information in the discipline has been exploding in recent years. Continued basic and clinical research is likely to produce more systematic knowledge and more effective clinical procedures to treat people with communicative disorders. Current students can be the future leaders who shape such exciting developments. More than anything, the science and the profession give a rare, challenging, and eventually gratifying opportunity to make a difference in the lives of people.

In many ways, successful treatment of communicative disorders restores the very essence of existence: social contact, the ability to touch and be touched, communication.

Study Questions

1. What does the acronym ASHA stand for?

2. When was the professional organization currently known as ASHA established?

3. What is the preferred title of people who provide speech and language services to individuals with communicative disabilities?

4. What is the title of people who specialize in hearing and its disorders?

5. Specify two goals of ASHA.

6. What does ASHA do to make sure that students enrolled in speech, language, and hearing programs are trained properly?

7. What does ASHA do to make sure that speech and hearing clinics in the country offer quality services to the public?

8. Why should a student prefer an ASHA-accredited college or university program in communicative disorders?

9. Who can become a member of ASHA?

10. What is NSSLHA?

11. What is CCC-SLP?

12. What is CCC-A?

13. How do state governments regulate the practice of speech–language pathology and audiology?

14. Typically, from whom should you obtain a certificate or a credential to work as a speech–language pathologist in a public school setting?

15. Typically, who or what agency issues a license to practice speech–language pathology or audiology?

▰▰▰▰▰ **References** ▰▰▰

American Speech-Language-Hearing Association. (1994). Code of ethics. *Asha, 36*(3) (March Suppl.), 1–2.

Hegde, M. N., & Davis, D. (1999). *Clinical methods and practicum in speech–language pathology* (3rd ed.). San Diego, CA: Singular.

Kelly, B. R., Davis, D., & Hegde, M. N. (1994). *Clinical methods and practicum in audiology.* San Diego, CA: Singular.

Lynch, C., & Dublinske, S. (1986). Licensure: The questions/The answers. *Asha, 28,* 33–36.

Paden, E. P. (1970). *A history of the American Speech and Hearing Association, 1925–1958.* Rockville, MD: American Speech-Language-Hearing Association.

Payne, K. T., & Anderson, N. (1991). *How to prepare for the N.E.S.P.A.: National examination in speech–language pathology and audiology.* San Diego, CA: Singular.

Roseberry-McKibbin, C., & Hegde, M. N. (2000). *An advanced review of speech–language pathology: Preparation of NESPA and comprehensive examination.* Austin, TX: PRO-ED.

Information About Communicative Disorders, Audiologists, and Speech–Language Pathologists

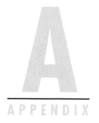

Information on disorders of communication, the professions of speech–language pathology and audiology, and the clinical and educational programs in the profession may be obtained by writing to the American Speech-Language-Hearing Association (ASHA), 10801 Rockville Pike, Rockville, Maryland 20852.

Many universities and colleges have degree programs in communicative disorders. These academic programs may be housed in a department of speech–language pathology and audiology, department of communicative disorders, or department of speech and hearing sciences. A majority of these departments administer a speech and hearing clinic where clients with communicative disorders are treated. Therefore, information on academic programs and clinical services also may be obtained by writing to these university or college departments.

In addition, information about available clinical services may be obtained from many hospitals and medical clinics that have a department of speech and hearing. Also, most larger cities have private speech and hearing centers that provide clinical services to people with communicative disorders. Such centers also will provide information on communicative disorders.

Audiologists and speech–language pathologists who maintain a business or professional address are listed under these titles in most telephone books.

Students and professionals can visit ASHA's Web site at www.asha.org. This Web site offers a variety of educational and professional information.

Glossary

A

Abducted. Open, drawn apart; as in *abducted vocal folds. See also* Adducted.

Acceleration/deceleration injuries. Brain injuries that result when the brain inside the skull moves back and forth because of a rapidly moving head that receives external force.

Accessory nerve XI. Classified as a cranial nerve, it is both a cranial and a spinal nerve that supplies the muscles of pharynx, soft palate, head, and shoulders.

Acoustic. Pertaining to sound.

Acoustic immittance. Transfer of acoustic energy; immittance may be measured as impedance (opposition to the flow of sound energy offered by the eardrum) or admittance (the ease with which the sound flows through the eardrum).

Acoustic nerve. Also known as the Cranial Nerve VIII, it conducts sound from the cochlea to the auditory centers in the brain.

Acoustic neuroma. A tumor that develops on the acoustic nerve, causing sensorineural hearing loss.

Acoustic reflex. A reflexive contraction of the tensor tympani and the stapedius muscles triggered by loud sounds and noises.

Acoustics. The study of sound; a branch of physics.

Acquired communicative disorders. Not inherited or congenital; a period of normal communication precedes the onset of an acquired disorder.

Acquired deafness. Deafness caused by various factors in a person who was born with normal hearing.

Action potentials. Electrical discharges of activated nerve cells.

Acute. A short and severe condition.

Addition. A form of articulation error; a sound that does not belong to a word is added ("cupa" for cup).

Adducted. Closed or nearly closed. As in *adducted vocal folds. See also* Abducted.

Afferent. Flow of information toward the cell body.

Affricates. A group of consonants with the characteristics of stops and fricatives.

African American English. A variety of English with its own phonologic, syntactic, semantic, and pragmatic rules; a part of the African American cultural heritage.

Agnosia. Difficulties some patients with aphasia have in recognizing common objects through sensory information (sight, sound, touch, feel). *See also* Auditory verbal agnosia; Visual agnosia.

Agrammatism. A major characteristic of patients with aphasia; omission of many grammatical elements, resulting in telegraphic speech.

AIDS dementia complex. A form of dementia with progressive intellectual and behavioral deterioration associated with acquired immonodeficiency syndrome (AIDS).

Air conduction. Sound traveling through the medium of air; air-conducted sound reaches the cochlea through the outer and middle ear.

Alexia. Reading problems due to brain damage.

Allophones. Variations of a phoneme.

Alveolar arch. A part of the mandible that houses the lower set of teeth.

Alveolar process. The outer edges of the maxillary bone (upper jaw) that house the molar, bicuspid, and cuspid teeth.

American Sign Language. A system of nonverbal communication that uses a set of hand and finger movements to express ideas and concepts.

Amplitude. Magnitude or range of movement of sound waves; the greater the amplitude, the louder the perceived sound.

Aneurysm. A sacklike bulging on the wall of a weakened artery; the bulge may rupture, causing cerebral hemorrhage.

Ankyloglossia. Limited movement of the tongue tip due to abnormally short lingual frenum; also known as tongue-tie.

Ankylosis. Restricted movement of a bone-joint due to disease.

Anomia. Difficulty in naming things, objects, and people; found in many patients with aphasia.

Anoxia. Lack or deficiency of oxygen; potential cause of brain damage.

Antecedent event. A stimulus presented *before* a target response is produced or attempted.

Anticipatory struggle theory. A theory that states that stuttering is a reaction of tension and speech fragmentation.

Aperiodic. Sound vibrations (or other events) that do not repeat themselves at regular intervals; aperiodic sound is perceived as noise.

Apert syndrome. A craniofacial abnormality due to premature fusing of different bones of the skull in the embryonic stage.

Aphasia. A language disorder due to brain damage or disease; a variety of difficulties in formulating, expressing, and understanding language.

Aphonia. Loss of voice.

Apraxia. A disorder of sequenced movement of body parts in the absence of muscle weakness or paralysis. *See also* Oral apraxia; Limb apraxia; Verbal apraxia.

Articulation. Movement; in speech, movement of the speech mechanism to produce the sounds of speech.

Articulation disorders. Problems in producing speech sounds.

Artificial larynx. A mechanical device that generates sound, which is articulated into speech by people whose larynx has been surgically removed.

Arytenoid cartilages. Two small, pyramid-shaped cartilages capable of various kinds of movements; the vocal folds move accordingly because of their attachment to the arytenoids.

Aspiration. A problem associated with swallowing disorders; entry of food into the airway.

Assessment. The process of identifying and describing a clinical problem.

Assistive listening devices. Instruments that help people with hearing impairment in various communicative situations.

Associated motor behaviors. Excessive tension, facial grimaces, and movements of hand, feet, and other body parts that are associated with stuttering.

Association fibers. Neural fibers that connect different parts of the brain in the two hemispheres.

Ataxia. Disturbed balance and abnormal gait caused by damage to the cerebellum.

Ataxic dysarthria. A speech disorder associated with ataxia. *See also* Dysarthria.

Athetosis. A neurological disorder characterized by slow, involuntary, writhing and wormlike movements.

Audible nasal emission. Noise of the gushing air as it escapes through the nose.

Audiogram. A graph that shows the results of various hearing tests.

Audiologist. A specialist in the study of hearing and in the assessment and rehabilitation of hearing impairment.

Audiology. The study and understanding of normal and disordered hearing and the rehabilitation of individuals with hearing impairment.

Auditory brain stem response audiometry. The technique of recording the electrical activity of the auditory nerve and the brain stem in response to various sound stimuli.

Auditory evoked potentials. The electrical impulses generated by the cochlea, the acoustic nerve, and the auditory centers of the brain in response to sound.

Auditory training. A rehabilitative process of training a person with hearing impairment to listen to amplified sounds, recognize their meanings, and distinguish one sound from the other.

Auditory verbal agnosia. Difficulty in recognizing the meaning of spoken words unless the objects the words name are shown.

Aural atresia. A completely closed external ear canal.

Aural rehabilitation. An educational process designed to improve the communicative abilities of people with hearing impairment; it includes auditory training, counseling, and speech–language therapy.

Auricle. The most visible part of the outer ear; also known as the pinna.

Auropalpebral reflex. A reflex response demonstrated by infants, who upon hearing a loud sound, quickly close their eyes; if the eyes are already closed, the infants tighten the eyelids.

Autism. A profound emotional and behavioral disorder characterized by lack of response to people and communicative disorders.

Autoclitics. Secondary verbal responses that help point out the causes of primary verbal responses.

Autonomic nervous system. A system of nerves divided into a sympathetic and a parasympathetic branch that control many involuntary functions of the body.

B

Babbling. The playful vocal sounds babies of 5 to 7 months produce when they are well fed, dry, and cheerful.

Basal ganglia. A structure deep within the brain which helps integrate motor impulses.

Baselines. Measures of a client's target behaviors before those behaviors are taught.

Basilar membrane. The floor of the cochlea, containing the organ of Corti and its several thousand hair cells that respond to sound.

Behavioral principles. Concepts and procedures of operant conditioning and learning.

Bernoulli effect. Increased velocity and decreased pressure when gasses or liquids move through a constricted passage.

Bifid uvula. A split uvula suggesting that there may be a cleft underneath the tissue covering the palate.

Bilabial. Involving both the lips; bilabial sounds are produced primarily by the two lips.

Bilateral. On both the sides; as in *bilateral cleft lip*, which means that there is an opening in the lip on both sides of the nose.

Bilingual. Of two languages; often refers to a person who can speak two languages.

Blissymbolics. A set of symbols developed by Charles Bliss; used in nonverbal communication.

Bone conduction. A process of conducting sound through bone vibrations.

Bound morpheme. A morpheme that cannot convey meaning by itself; for example, the regular plural *s* in the word *books*.

Brain stem. The medulla, pons, midbrain, diencephalon, and reticular formation.

Breathiness. The voice quality that results when the air escapes through partially open folds.

Broca's area. A center for motor speech control within the frontal lobe of the brain.

Broken word. A type of dysfluency; a silent pause within a word.

Buccinator. A large, flat muscle that makes up most of the cheeks.

C

Carrier symbols. A nonverbal means of communication in which geometric, abstract, and noniconic plastic symbols (chips) are used to communicate different words and to arrange sentences.

Cartilage. Tough connective tissue.

Cavity. A hollow space within the body; a structure within the body containing other structures.

Central auditory disorders. Complex language processing problems that are caused by a lesion or lesions in the central auditory system.

Central nervous system. The brain and the spinal cord.

Cerebellum. A structure below the brain and behind the brain stem that regulates equilibrium, body posture, and coordinated fine motor movements.

Cerebral arteriosclerosis. Hardening of the cerebral arteries, which become thickened.

Cerebral hemispheres. The two halves of the brain.

Cerebral palsy. Brain damage suffered during infancy or the prenatal period and the resulting paralysis and problems of physical growth, locomotion, communication, and sensory deficits.

Cerebrospinal fluid. A fluid that surrounds and cushions the cerebrum.

Cerebrum. The biggest of the central nervous system structures and the most important for speech, language, and hearing.

Chronic otitis media. The permanent rupture of the tympanic membrane with or without middle ear diseases.

Cineradiography. A method of taking motion pictures filmed through X ray of such internal organs as the velopharyngeal mechanism or vocal folds.

Circumlocution. Talking in an indirect and unnecessarily lengthy manner; a strategy some stutterers use to beat their stuttering on certain words by beating around the bush (avoid saying the feared word).

Class I malocclusion. Misalignment of some individual teeth while the two arches are normally aligned.

Class II malocclusion. The upper jaw is protruded and the lower jaw is retracted or receded.

Class III malocclusion. The upper jaw is receded and the lower jaw is protruded.

Clefts of the palate. Failure of the premaxilla to fuse with the maxillary bone and/or the failure of the palatine processes to fuse at the midline.

Cluster reduction. Omission of one or more consonants of a cluster ("tong" for "strong," for example).

Cluttering. A disorder of fluency characterized by rapid but disordered articulation, possibly combined with disorganized thought.

Cochlea. The main inner ear structure of hearing; it appears like the shell of a snail and is filled with a fluid called endolymph.

Cochlear implant. An electronic device that is surgically placed in the cochlea and other parts of the ear of a deaf person. The device delivers the sound directly to the acoustic nerve endings in the cochlea.

Code switching. Changing from one language to another during a conversation.

Commissural fibers. The fibers that connect the two hemispheres of the brain.

Communication. A form of social behavior; exchange of information.

Compensatory articulation. Correct or markedly improved production of sounds through unusual methods of articulation by a child with defective speech structures.

Complete cleft of the palate. Total separation of the two palatal shelves of the hard palate.

Complex tone. Two or more sounds of *differing* frequencies.

Concordant. The presence of a disorder, disease, or a trait in both the members of a monozygotic (identical) twin pair.

Conductive hearing loss. Diminished conductance of sound to the middle or inner ear due to abnormalities of the external auditory canal, the eardrum, or the ossicular chain of the middle ear.

Congenital disorder. A disorder noticed at the time of birth or soon thereafter.

Congenitally deaf. A person who is born deaf.

Consonant deletion. A phonological process that describes the omission of initial or final consonants of words; a problem of articulation.

Contact ulcers. Sores that develop on one or both sides of the posterior (back) end of the vocal folds.

Contralateral. Refers to the opposite side. *See also* Ipsilateral.

Cranial nerves. Nerves that emerge out of holes (foramina) in the base of the skull; they play a major role in speech production.

Cranial nerve VIII. *See* Acoustic nerve.

Craniofacial anomalies. Birth defects of skull and face.

Cricoarytenoid joint. A joint that connects the arytenoids to the cricoid cartilage that permits circular and sliding movements.

Cricoid cartilage. A cartilage of the larynx and also the top ring of the trachea.

Cricothyroid joint. A joint that connects cricoid with the thyroid cartilage; permits back-and-forth movements.

Cricothyroid muscle. A muscle that lengthens and tenses the vocal folds.

Criterion of performance. The level of accuracy (such as 90% correct) in the production of a target behavior taught in treatment.

Cross-sectional method. A research method in which many subjects, selected from different age levels, are studied simultaneously for a relatively brief duration. *See also* Longitudinal method.

Cued speech. Speech produced with manual cues that represent the sounds of speech; it supplements and improves speech reading.

D

Deaf. A person whose hearing loss typically exceeds 70 dB and cannot hear or understand conversational speech under normal circumstances.

Decibel. A basic unit used to measure the intensity of sound; it is one tenth of a Bell, the basic unit of measurement named after Alexander Graham Bell.

Decussate. To cross over; many auditory nerve fibers that come from one ear *decussate* to the opposite side of the brain.

Deep structure. In linguistic theory, the deep or the D-Structure primarily holds the rules of sentence formation.

Dementia. A general term used to describe progressive intellectual and behavioral deterioration associated with diseases of the nervous system in the aged; sometimes described as senile dementia.

Dementia of the Alzheimer's Type. Intellectual and behavioral deterioration associated with Alzheimer's disease; caused by such neuropathologies as neurofibrillary tangles, neuritic plaques, and granulovacuolar degeneration.

Denasalization. Substitution of an oral sound for nasal sounds ("mad" for *man,* for example); a problem of articulation.

Developmental aphasia. Also known as childhood aphasia, it is a failure to acquire language; the presumed cause is brain damage.

Developmental apraxia of speech (DAS). Disorders of articulation supposedly due to brain damage.

Diadochokinetic rate. The speed at which a speaker can repeat selected syllables (pa-ta-ka, for example).

Diagnosogenic theory. Wendell Johnson's theory, which says that stuttering begins only after parents mistakenly diagnose it in their child because of normal nonfluencies.

Dialect. Variations of speech within a specific language. Each dialect may have its own unique phonological, semantic, morphological, syntactic, and pragmatic characteristics.

Diaphragm. A thick muscle, shaped like a dome, separating the stomach from the thorax.

Diencephalon. A structure of the brain stem; it includes the thalamus and the hypothalamus.

Diphthong. A combination of two vowels.

Diplegia. Paralysis of either the legs or the arms.

Discordant. The presence of a disorder, disease, or trait in only one member of a pair of monozygotic (identical) twins.

Discriminative stimuli. People, objects, and physical settings that are associated with a reinforced response. Therefore, the response is more likely in the presence of its discriminative stimuli.

Distinctive features. Unique characteristics of a phoneme that distinguish one phoneme from the other.

Distortions. Imprecise productions of speech sounds.

Dizygotic twins. Fraternal twins formed out of two separate fertilized ova; genetically, they are no more similar than ordinary siblings.

Down syndrome. A genetically inherited condition of mental retardation.

Dysarthria. A group of speech disorders due to paralysis, weakness, or incoordination of speech muscles caused by central or peripheral nerve damage.

Dysfluencies. The many forms of interruptions that prevent the easy, effortless, and smooth flow of speech.

Dysphagia. Disorders of swallowing food or liquid, due to neurological problems (e.g., stroke, head injury).

Dysphonia. A general term that means a disordered voice.

E

Echoic. An imitative verbal response; the stimulus and the response sound the same.

Echolalia. Parrotlike repetition of what is heard; it is an early sign of autism.

Efferent nerves. Nerves that conduct impulses from the central nervous system to the peripheral organs.

Electrocochleography. A technique of measuring the electrical activity of the cochlea in response to sound.

Electromyography. A technique of sensing, amplifying, and recording the electrical activity of muscles.

Elicited responses. Reflexive responses triggered by stimuli; for example, the dilation of the pupil in response to light. *See also* Evoked responses.

Embolus. A blood clot, fatty materials, or an air bubble that forms a wedge-shaped obstruction of the blood flow (embolism); an embolus can cause a stroke.

Endolymph. A kind of fluid that fills the cochlea.

Endoscopes. Mechanical devices used to illuminate and examine internal organs by conducting light to and from an organ via thin fiberoptic tubes that are inserted either through the mouth (oral endoscopy) or through the nose (nasal endoscopy).

Epilepsy. A seizure disorder caused by an excessive electrical discharge of damaged or abnormal brain cells, resulting in convulsions in the body.

Esophagus. The flexible tube through which food reaches the stomach.

Etiology. The study of causes of diseases and disorders.

Eustachian tube. Also known as the auditory tube, it connects the middle ear with the nasopharynx and helps maintain a balanced air pressure within and outside the middle ear.

Evoked responses. Responses that are not imitated, not reflexive, but learned; they are produced in relation to various discriminative stimuli. *See also* Discriminative stimuli; Elicited responses.

Expansions. Elaborations of a child's utterance to make it longer and grammatically more correct.

Expressive oral language. Talking; language produced by speakers. *See also* Receptive language.

External auditory meatus. Also known as the ear canal, it is a muscular tube that resonates the sound that enters it.

External otitis. An infection of the skin of the external auditory canal.

Extrapyramidal system. A neural pathway that carries motor impulses from the brain to various muscles via several relay stations (hence also known as the indirect system). *See also* Pyramidal system.

Extrinsic muscles of larynx. Laryngeal muscles with at least one attachment to structures other than the larynx. *See also* Intrinsic laryngeal muscles.

F

Facial nerve VII. A cranial nerve that controls a variety of facial expressions and movements.

Fetal alcohol syndrome. A group of symptoms seen in children of chronically alcoholic mothers. The symptoms include brain damage, sensory disabilities, mental retardation, and often speech–language delay.

Fiberoptic endoscopy. *See* Endoscopes.

Finger spelling. A form of sign language in which the words are spelled in the air with fingers.

Fissures. Relatively deep valleys of the brain that form boundaries of broad divisions of the cerebrum. *See also* Gyrus.

Flaccid paralysis. Muscles that are too soft and flabby; it is caused by a lesion in the lower motoneuron.

Fluency. A characteristic of speech; fluent speech is easy, smooth, flowing, effortless, and devoid of excessive amounts of dysfluencies.

Foramina. An opening or hole.

Free morphemes. Those morphemes that can stand alone and mean something. *See also* Bound morpheme.

Frequency. In reference to sound, the number of times a cycle of vibration repeats itself within a second.

Fricatives. A category of speech sounds that are produced by severely constricting the oral cavity and then forcing the air through it.

Frontal lobe. The largest of the four lobes of the cerebrum containing the primary motor cortex and Broca's area that are especially important for speech production.

Fronting. A form of disordered articulation; sounds produced in the front of the mouth are substituted for those produced in the back of the mouth; a problem of articulation ("tome" for *come,* for example).

Frontonasal process. One of various bulges that develop during the 3rd week of embryonic growth; it develops into the nose, the central part of the upper lip, and the primary palate.

Functional disorders of communication. Disorders that do not have a demonstrable organic or neurologic cause.

Functional unit. A class or a group of verbal responses all of which share similar stimulus conditions and consequences.

Fundamental frequency. The average rate at which given vocal folds vibrate, or the lowest frequency component of a complex tone.

G

Genderlect. The characteristic patterns of speech thought to be influenced by the sex of the speaker.

Generalization. The production of untrained (new) behaviors following training of similar behaviors or the production of trained behaviors when shown new stimuli not used in training.

Gentle initiation of sound. A target behavior taught to stutterers to promote stutter-free speech; the speech sounds are started in a soft, easy manner.

Glides. A category of speech sounds that are produced by gradually changing the shape of the articulators.

Glossectomy. The surgical removal of the tongue and floor of the mouth.

Glossopharyngeal nerve IX. A cranial nerve that supplies the tongue and the pharynx.

Glottals. Sounds that are produced by keeping the vocal folds open and letting the air pass through it; because this results in friction noise, glottals are also fricatives.

Glottis. An opening that results when the vocal folds are abducted.

Grammatic morphemes. Small elements of grammar such as the plural *s* and the present progressive *ing;* they are also bound morphemes.

Granulovacuolar degeneration. Nerve cell degeneration due to small fluid-filled cavities containing granular debri.

Gyrus. A ridge on the cortex; the cortex has many gyri (plural).

H

Habitual pitch. Each person's typical vocal pitch; it varies within a range that contains the lowest and the highest note.

Hair cells. Hairlike structures (cilia) found on the Organ of Corti; they respond to sound vibrations.

Hard of hearing. Hearing impairment within the range of 25 dB and 75 dB; a person who is hard of hearing has some useful hearing.

Hard palate. The roof of the mouth and the floor of the nose.

Hardwire devices. Devices that include an amplifier, a microphone, and an earphone that physically connect a listener and a person with hearing impairment through wires; a variety of assistive listening devices.

Harshness. Roughness of voice; undesirable vocal quality due mainly to irregular vibrations of vocal folds.

Hearing level. The lowest intensity of a sound necessary to stimulate the auditory system.

Hearing science. The study of hearing, its anatomy and physiology, its perception and understanding, and its relation to communication.

Hearing screening. A brief testing procedure that separates people who have normal hearing from those who must be tested in detail (suspected to be hearing impaired).

Hemianopsia. Loss of vision in one half of the visual field in one or both eyes.

Hemiplegia. Paralysis of either the left or the right half of the body.

Hertz (Hz). The more recent name for *cycles per second.*

Hoarse. A voice quality that includes both breathiness and harshness.

Huntington's disease. A progressive neurological disease with neuronal loss in the frontal and parietal regions of the brain with such symptoms as involuntary, irregular, spasmodic movements of the limbs, neck, head, and facial muscles.

Hyoid bone. A U-shaped bone that floats under the jaw; the muscles of the tongue and various muscles of the skull, larynx, and jaw are attached to this bone.

Hyperkinesia. Increased (exaggerated) body movement.

Hypernasality. Excessive nasal resonance on non-nasal speech sounds.

Hypertelorism. Eyes that are too far apart in relation to the rest of the facial features.

Hypoglossal nerve XII. A cranial nerve that supplies the tongue.

Hypokinesia. Reduced range and force of muscle movements.

Hyponasality. Too little nasal resonance on the nasal sounds of a language.

Hypothalamus. A structure within the brain stem; it helps integrate the actions of the autonomic nervous system and controls emotional experiences.

I

Iconic symbol. A picture or a symbol that looks like the object it represents.

Idiopathic. Of unknown origin.

Incidental teaching. A procedure in which the naturally occurring opportunities for communication are used to teach language.

Incisors. The four upper front teeth housed in the premaxilla portion of the maxillary bone.

Incomplete palatal cleft. The partial fusing of the two palatal shelves of the hard palate.

Incus. The second and the middle bone of the ossicular chain in the middle ear. *See also* Malleus; Stapes.

Indirect laryngoscopy. The use of a small mirror placed in the throat by a laryngologist to view the laryngeal structures.

Infrared listening systems. An instrument that includes a transmitter that transmits messages on pulses of light and a receiver that receives those messages and delivers to the ears of people with hearing impairment; useful in large listening situations (e.g., concert halls).

Intensity. Magnitude of sound; the sounds that are perceived as louder are greater in intensity.

Interarytenoid muscles. Muscles between the arytenoid cartilages; they bring the vocal folds together (adduct).

Intercostal muscles. Muscles between the ribs.

Internal auditory meatus. The opening through which the auditory nerve exits the inner ear.

International Phonetic Alphabet. A set of phonetic symbols each of which stands for only one speech sound.

Intraverbals. A group of verbal responses that are stimulated by the speaker's own prior verbal responses.

Intrinsic muscles of the larynx. Muscles that begin and end within the larynx and include the thyroarytenoid, the cricothyroid, the posterior cricoarytenoid, the lateral cricoarytenoid, and the interarytenoid muscles. *See also* Extrinsic muscles of larynx.

Ipsilateral. On the same side of the body. *See also* Contralateral.

J

Jargon. Fluent but meaningless speech; seen in some aphasic patients.

L

Labiodental sounds. Sounds that are produced by the lips and teeth.

Labyrinth (of the temporal bone). A fluid-filled system of interconnecting canals and passages that houses structures of the inner ear.

Language. A system of symbols and codes used in communication; a form of social behavior shaped and maintained by a verbal community.

Language acquisition device (LAD). A presumed, innate mechanism thought to facilitate language acquisition in children.

Language assessment. A process of observation and measurement of a client's language behaviors; typically, it precedes the development of a language treatment program.

Language sampling. A procedure of recording a person's language behaviors under relatively normal conditions and, whenever possible, with the help of conversational speech; part of language assessment.

Language science. The study of the organized system of verbal and nonverbal means of communication.

Laryngeal trauma. Any type of injury to the larynx including those caused by automobile, snowmobile, and motorcycle accidents.

Laryngeal web. A thin membrane that grows across and closes some or most of the opening between the vocal folds.

Laryngectomee. A person who has undergone the surgical procedure called laryngectomy.

Laryngectomy. Partial or total removal of a diseased larynx.

Laryngitis. The inflammation of the membranes of the larynx.

Laryngologist. Medical specialist who treats throat problems.

Laryngopharynx. The structure above the larynx and below the oropharynx.

Larynx. A tubelike structure in the neck that includes various muscles along with the vocal folds, cartilages, and membranes.

Lateral cricoarytenoid. A muscle which brings the vocal folds together (an adductor).

Laterals. Sounds that are produced by letting the air escape through the sides of the tongue; English /l/ is a lateral.

Left neglect. Patients' tendency to ignore or forget the left side of the body; a symptom of right hemisphere syndrome.

Levator palatini. A pair of muscles that elevate the soft palate.

Limb apraxia. The inability of some patients to move one of their limbs when requested to do so.

Lingua-alveolar sounds. Sounds that are produced by raising the tip of the tongue to make a contact with the alveolar ridge, which is the place immediately behind the front teeth.

Linguadental sounds. Sounds that are produced by the tongue as it makes contact with the upper teeth.

Linguapalatal sounds. Sounds that are produced by the tongue as it comes in contact with the hard palate at the back of the alveolar ridge.

Linguavelar sounds. Sounds that are produced by the back of the tongue, which raises to make a contact with the velum (soft palate).

Linguistic (language) competence. A concept of Chomsky's theory; it is the innate and perfect knowledge of the rules of the universal grammar.

Linguistic (language) performance. A concept of Chomsky's theory; it is the actual production of language.

Linguistics. The study of language, its structure, and the rules that govern that structure.

Linguists. People who specialize in linguistics.

Liquids. Speech sounds that are produced with the least restriction of the oral cavity; also called semivowels; English /r/ and /l/ are liquids.

Loci. Locations; loci of stuttering are the particular locations within an utterance where dysfluencies and related behaviors occur.

Longitudinal fissure. A fissure that divides the cerebrum into a left and a right hemisphere.

Longitudinal method. A procedure of studying one or a few subjects for an extended period of time to document changes in selected aspects; children's acquisition of language may be studied longitudinally. *See also* Cross-sectional method.

Loudness. A perceived characteristic of sound; loudness is determined by the intensity of the sound signal; loudness of phonation or speech is determined by the degree of subglottal air pressure.

M

Malleus. The first bone of the ossicular chain located in the middle ear and attached to the tympanic membrane. *See also* Incus; Stapes.

Malocclusions. Deviations in the shape and the dimensions of the upper and lower jaw bones, positioning of individual teeth, and the relation between the two jaws.

Mandible. The lower jaw, which forms the floor of the mouth and houses the lower set of teeth.

Mandibular processes. Two of a number of bulges that develop during the 3rd week of embryonic growth; these processes result in the mandible, lower lip, and the chin.

Mandibulectomy. The surgical procedure of removing a diseased jaw.

Manner of articulation. The degree or type of constriction of the vocal tract while producing certain speech sounds.

Manual guidance. Any procedure in which the clinician uses his or her hands and fingers to guide and shape a correct response from a client.

Mastication. The act of chewing.

Maxillae. A pair of large facial bones that form a major portion of the hard palate and the upper jaw.

Maxillary processes. Two of a number of bulges that develop during the 3rd week of embryonic growth; they give rise to the face, mouth, cheeks, and sides of the upper lip.

Maxillectomy. The surgical removal of the upper jaw.

Mean length of utterance (MLU). The average length of a speaker's multiple utterances as measured in terms of morphemes.

Meatus. An opening or channel within the body.

Medulla. The uppermost portion of the spinal cord that enters the cranial cavity; it controls breathing and other vital functions of the body.

Melodic intonation therapy. A method of verbal rehabilitation of patients with aphasia who are taught to speak with a lyrical intonation.

Meniere's disease. A disease of the inner ear whose symptoms include spells of dizziness or vertigo, unilateral hearing loss, and tinnitus (various kinds of noise in the ear).

Meningitis. An infectious disease that destroys the layers of membrane (meninges) that cover the brain.

Microcephaly. A skull that is too small; a birth defect associated with mental retardation.

Micrognathia. An abnormally small jaw.

Midbrain. Also known as the mesencephalon, it is a narrow structure that lies above the pons and links the higher centers of the brain with the lower centers.

Mixed nerves. Fibers that carry sensory as well as motor impulses.

Modified airflow. A target behavior taught to stutterers to induce stutter-free speech; it includes inhalation of sufficient air and a slight exhalation before saying something and having enough air that is exhaled in a controlled manner throughout the utterance.

Monoplegia. Paralysis of only one limb.

Monozygotic (identical) twins. Two individuals formed out of a single fertilized egg, which splits into two; they are identical in genetic makeup.

Morpheme. The smallest meaningful unit of a language.

Morphology. The study of word structures.

Motherese. Speech directed to young children by mothers; motherese is simpler, more variable in pitch, repetitive, and more fluent than the speech directed to adults.

Moto-kinesthetic method. A procedure of teaching correct production of speech sounds; the clinician manually moves the articulators to provide motor and kinesthetic feedback to the client.

Motor nerves. Fibers that carry impulses for movement from the brain to the muscles.

Motor speech disorders. Also known as neurogenic speech disorders, they are caused by central or peripheral nervous system damage.

Mucoperiosteum. The thick layer of tissue that covers the hard palate.

Multilingual. Refers to "more than two languages," as in a *multilingual person* who speaks three or more languages.

Myoelastic–aerodynamic theory of phonation. Theory stating that vocal fold vibrations are due to air pressure, the difference between positive and negative pressure, and the elasticity of the muscles.

Myofunctional therapy. Treatment aimed at correcting tongue thrust.

Myringoplasty. Surgical repair of a perforated eardrum.

Myringotomy. A surgical procedure used to relieve pressure created by acute otitis media by making a small incision in the tympanic membrane.

N

Nasals. Speech sounds with nasal resonance added to them; they are produced while keeping the velopharyngeal port open.

Nasopharynx. The section of the pharynx that lies just behind the nasal cavities.

Nativism. An ancient philosophy asserting that much of human knowledge is innate.

Neologism. Creation of words that are meaningless to the listener; a frequent creation of some patients with aphasia.

Nervous system. An organization of nerves according to some structural, spatial, and functional principles.

Neuritic plaques. Degenerated minute areas of cortical or subcortical tissue associated with Alzheimer's disease.

Neurofibrillary tangles. Thickened, twisted, and looped neurofibrils of the brain that are associated with Alzheimer's disease.

Neurofibrils. Filament-like structures of nerve cell body, axons, and dendrites.

Neurologist. A medical specialist who diagnoses and treats disorders of the nervous system.

Neurons. Nerve cells that consist of three parts: a cell body, dendrites, and an axon.

Neurosis. A milder form of mental or psychological disorder; examples include phobia and anxiety.

Nonacceleration brain injuries. Brain injuries sustained by a stationary head when it is hit by an object.

Nonpenetrating brain injuries. Closed-head brain injuries in which the skull may or may not be damaged and there is no penetration of foreign objects into the brain.

Norms. The typical performance of a representative group of children on some test or measure.

O

Obturator. A prosthetic device used to cover the cleft of the hard palate and help achieve better velopharyngeal closure.

Occipital lobe. One of the four lobes of the cerebral cortex; it is located at the lower back portion of the head, just above the cerebellum. It is primarily concerned with vision.

Occlusion. The manner in which the upper and the lower dental arches meet each other.

Omission. An absence of a required sound in a word position.

Operant. A class of behaviors that can be increased or decreased by arranging certain consequences for them.

Operant audiometry. A method to establish hearing thresholds by conditioning voluntary responses to sound stimuli.

Operant conditioning. A procedure of creating, increasing, or decreasing behaviors by arranging certain stimulus conditions and immediate consequences.

Optimal pitch. The pitch judged to be the most comfortable, appropriate, and compatible for a particular person.

Oral apraxia. An inability to move the muscles of oral structures for nonspeech purposes.

Oral language. The production of speech sounds organized into a higher level of words and sentences that generate meaning.

Orbicularis oris. The muscle that makes up the lips.

Organ of Corti. The inner ear's structure of hearing; it contains the hair cells that respond to sound.

Organic disorders of communication. Disorders that are caused by some defect in the neurophysiological mechanism of speech.

Organic voice disorders. Deviations in voice due to structural problems in the phonatory mechanism.

Orofacial examination. A procedure to rule out gross organic problems of face and mouth that may be associated with disorders of communication.

Orthodontics. The study and treatment of deviations of dental structures.

Orthodontist. A dental specialist who moves the oral structures with the help of specially constructed devices.

Oscilloscope. An electronic device that converts electrical signals (such as those generated by speech) into visible patterns that are displayed on a monitor.

Ossicular chain. A set of three tiny bones (the malleus, incus, and stapes) found in the middle ear; the chain conducts sound to the inner ear.

Otitis media. An infection of the middle ear; it is a frequent cause of conductive hearing loss in children.

Otologist. A medical specialist who treats the diseases of the ear.

Otosclerosis. A disease in which spongy growth on the stapes of the middle ear reduces its mobility and causes conductive hearing loss.

Otospongiosis. The same as otosclerosis.

Oval window. An opening to, and a part of, the inner ear.

P

Palatine bone. A part of the hard palate.

Palatine process. The central, platelike portions of the maxillary bones; embryonically identified as the secondary palate, it forms the major portion of the roof of the mouth and the hard palate.

Palatoglossus. A muscle that lowers the soft palate.

Palatopharyngeus. A muscle that lowers the soft palate.

Palsy. Paralysis.

Papillomas. Tumors that grow on the airway and laryngeal structures including the vocal folds.

Paraphasia. Word substitution problem found frequently in people with aphasia who can talk fluently and grammatically.

Paraplegia. Paralysis of only the legs.

Parasympathetic. Refers to a branch of the autonomic nervous system that relaxes the body. *See also* Sympathetic.

Parietal lobe. One of the four lobes of the cerebral cortex; it lies behind the frontal lobe and integrates such body sensations as pain, touch, and temperature.

Parkinsonism. A degenerative disease of the nervous system whose symptoms include rigidity of posture, hand tremors, and speech disorders (hypokinetic dysarthria).

Parkinson's disease. A slowly progressing neurological disease in which the nuclei in the brain stem are degenerated, the sulci in the frontal brain region are widened, and dopamine production in the brain is reduced.

Part-word repetitions. A type of dysfluency; repeated productions of mostly the first sound or syllable of a word.

Pascal (Pa). A unit of sound pressure.

Penetrating brain injuries. Brain injury in which the skull is fractured and the meninges are torn.

Perilymph. The fluid that fills the canals that lie within the inner ear.

Periodic vibrations. A pattern of vibrations that repeats itself at regular intervals.

Peripheral hearing problems. Reduced hearing ability due to pathologies in the outer, middle, or inner ear (excluding the auditory nerve).

Peripheral nervous system. A collection of nerves that are outside the skull and the spinal column; it includes the cranial nerves, the spinal nerves, and portions of the autonomic nerves.

Pitch. Perceived differences in the fundamental frequency of vocal fold vibrations.

Pharyngeal flap operation. A surgical procedure to reduce hypernasality due to short velum; a muscular flap is raised from the back wall of the throat and attached to the soft palate.

Pharyngoplasty. A set of surgical procedures used to improve the functioning of the velopharyngeal mechanism by implanting various substances (including Teflon) into the pharyngeal wall to make it bulge.

Pharynx. The throat.

Phonate. To produce sound.

Phoneme. A group of speech sounds that are perceived as the same and that do not make a difference in meaning.

Phonemic paraphasia. A word substitution problem found in patients with aphasia; the substituted words sound like the correct words.

Phonetic placement method. A procedure of teaching a target sound by describing and demonstrating in front of a mirror how that sound is produced correctly.

Phonological disorders. Errors of many phonemes that form patterns or clusters.

Phonological processes. Many ways or patterns of simplifying difficult sound productions by omissions or substitutions.

Phonology. The study of speech sounds, sound patterns, and rules used to create words with those sounds.

Phrase. An utterance that is grammatically incomplete.

Phrase interjection. Inclusion of a phrase that does not add meaning or is not an integral part of an utterance.

Phrase repetition. A type of dysfluency; repetition of an utterance that is not a grammatically complete sentence.

Pinna. *See* Auricle.

Pitch. A sensation determined by the frequency of sound vibration; the greater the frequency, the higher the perceived pitch.

Place of articulation. One of three factors used to classify consonants; it refers to the place of articulatory contact or constriction.

Polyglot. People who speak more than two languages.

Pons. A structure that bridges the two halves of the cerebellum.

Positive reinforcement. A procedure of increasing a response by presenting something soon after that response is made; a frequently used positive reinforcer is verbal praise.

Posterior cricoarytenoid muscle. A muscle that pulls the vocal folds apart (an abductor).

Pragmatics. The study of the rules that govern the use of language in social situations.

Prefix. A morpheme added at the beginning of a base morpheme.

Prelingual. Refers to a period before the acquisition of language; as in *prelingually deaf.*

Premaxilla. The front portion of the maxillary bone.

Presbycusis. A common type of sensorineural hearing loss among the elderly.

Pressure. Force, distributed over a certain area.

Preverbal behaviors. Communicative behaviors that precede the production of words and phrases; babbling is the most significant of them.

Primary auditory cortex. An area within the temporal lobe concerned with hearing.

Primary English dialect. Dialects of unilingual English speakers.

Primary motor cortex. An area within the frontal lobe; it controls voluntary movement.

Primary palate. An embryonic structure from which the upper lip and the alveolar process evolve.

Probes. Procedures to determine if a target behavior taught by the clinician is produced without the clinician's feedback (reinforcement) in clinical and extra-clinical situations.

Prognosis. A statement about the future course of the disorder when certain steps are taken or when nothing is done.

Programmed learning. A method of mastering various skills by the systematic use of operant conditioning principles.

Projection fibers. Neural pathways to and from the brain stem and spinal cord on the one hand and the sensory and motor areas of the cortex on the other.

Pronoun reversal. A characteristic of children with autism who refer to themselves as "you," "he," or "she" and to other people as "I."

Prosody. Variations in rate, pitch, loudness, stress, intonation, and rhythm of continuous speech.

Prosopagnosia. Inability to recognize a familiar face; a symptom of right hemisphere syndrome.

Prosthesis. A device developed and fitted to compensate for missing or deformed structures.

Prosthodontist. A dental specialist who designs and fits devices that help improve the function of the oral structures.

Psychiatrist. A medical specialist who treats mental and behavioral disorders.

Psychoacoustics. The study of sound as a psychological experience of hearing.

Psychoanalysis. The study of mind and behavior as developed by Freud and his followers; it is also a method of treating neurosis by analyzing unconscious and repressed sexual urges that are transformed into psychological symptoms.

Psychogenic aphonia. The sudden loss of voice with no physiological or neurological cause.

Psychologist (clinical). A specialist who treats behavior disorders through psychological or behavioral (nonmedical) methods.

Psychosis. A severe form of mental or behavioral disorder, characterized by disorientation to time, place, and person; may also include hallucinations and delusions.

Psychotherapy. Treatment of psychological problems without the use of medication; the patient typically talks about his or her personal, emotional, and interpersonal problems during treatment sessions.

Punishment. A procedure designed to decrease the frequency of selected behaviors by arranging an immediate consequence for those behaviors.

Pure tone. A tone of single frequency.

Pyramidal system. A bundle of nerve fibers that originate in the motor cortex and travel to the brain stem; it is the primary pathway to carry impulses for voluntary movement. (Also called the direct system). *See also* Extrapyramidal system.

Q

Quadriplegia. Paralysis of all four limbs.

R

Rebus. A picture of an object or a person; a system of hand-drawn pictures used in nonverbal communication.

Receptive language. Understanding of what is said (spoken language).

Recurrent laryngeal nerve. A branch of the cranial nerve X (vagus); it moves down the chest cavity and then reverses its course back to the laryngeal area; innervates many intrinsic laryngeal muscles.

Referent theory of meaning. The view that the meaning of a word is the object, person, or the event the word refers to.

Register. A variation of language use depending on a particular speaking situation.

Reinforcer. An event that follows a response and thereby makes that response more likely in the future.

Resonance. Forced vibration of a structure that is related to the source of sound; vibration of cavities below and above the larynx (source of sound).

Response cost. A procedure of decreasing a wrong response by taking a reinforcer away from the child every time such a response is made.

Reticular activating system. A structure within the midbrain, brain stem, and upper portion of the spinal cord; the primary mechanism of attention and consciousness.

Rib cage. Also known as the thoracic cage, it is a cylinder-like structure of 12 ribs that houses vital organs including the heart and the lungs.

Right hemisphere syndrome. A symptom complex that results from damage to the right hemisphere and includes such symptoms as left-neglect, facial recognition problems, attentional deficits, disorientation, and certain communication deficits.

Rochester method. A means of communication that combines finger spelling and oral speech.

Root morphemes. Words that cannot be broken down into smaller units without destroying their meaning but to which other morphemes can be added.

S

Schweckendiek procedure. A surgical method of closing the cleft of the soft palate before closing the cleft of the hard palate.

Screening. A brief procedure that helps determine whether a person should be assessed at length.

Secondary English dialect. Dialects of bilingual or multilingual English speakers whose primary language is other than English.

Secondary palate. The same as the hard palate.

Semantic component. Refers to the meaning conveyed by words, phrases, and sentences.

Semantics. The study of meaning in language.

Semicircular canals. Structures of the inner ear responsible for maintaining balance (equilibrium).

Senile dementia. *See* Dementia.

Sensorineural hearing loss. Diminished hearing due to damaged hair cells of the cochlea or the auditory portion of the cranial nerve VIII. *See also* Conductive hearing loss.

Sensory nerves. Those cranial nerves that carry sensory information from a sense organ to the brain.

Septum. The structure that divides the nasal cavities.

Sequential bilingualism. Learning a second language after the first language has been mastered.

Serous otitis media. A disease of the middle ear, which is inflamed and filled with thick or watery fluid.

Signaling devices. Various instruments that alert people with hearing impairment to various signals (e.g., amplified telephone ringers or smoke alarms that flash light).

Silent nasal emission. Inaudible leakage of air through the nose during the production of non-nasal speech sounds.

Silent pause. A type of dysfluency; abnormally long silent durations within speech.

Silent prolongations. A type of dysfluency; tensed prolongation of an articulatory posture in the absence of voicing.

Simultaneous bilingualism. Learning two languages at the same time.

Soft palate. A flexible muscular structure at the juncture of the oropharynx and the nasopharynx; also known as the velum, it may be lowered to open the velopharyngeal port or raised to close it.

Sound. Waves of disturbance in the molecules of a gas, a liquid, or a solid created by the vibrations of an object; the sensation felt by the hearing mechanism due to those vibrations.

Sound prolongation. A type of dysfluency; unusually long durations of mostly the initial sounds of words.

Sound pressure level (SPL). A measure of the pressure of a sound; the intensity of a sound as expressed in terms of decibels at a certain sound pressure level.

Sound/syllable interjections. A type of dysfluency; addition of sounds or syllables that are not an integral part of an utterance.

Spastic dysphonia. A voice disorder caused by very tight closure (adduction) of the vocal folds and characterized by strangled, squeezed, choppy, harsh, and breathy voice.

Spastic paralysis. A form of paralysis due to lesions in the upper motoneurons characterized by too rigid muscles.

Spasticity. Increased tone or rigidity of muscles.

Speech. Production of phonemes; articulated sounds and syllables. *See also* Language.

Speech–language pathologist. A specialist in the study, assessment, and treatment of speech–language (communication) disorders.

Speech–language pathology. The study of human communication and its disorders, and assessment and treatment of those disorders.

Speech-reading. A method of understanding speech by looking at the face of the speaker; a skill used by people with hearing impairment to understand speech.

Speech reception threshold (SRT). The lowest level of hearing at which a person can understand 50% of the words presented.

Speech science. Study of speech, its anatomical and physiological bases, the formation and production of speech sounds, and perception and understanding of speech.

Spondee threshold. The lowest hearing level at which a person correctly identifies 50% of the spondee words.

Spondees. Standardized words of two syllables, both pronounced with equal stress and used to determine the speech reception threshold (SRT).

Spoonerism. The unintentional interchange of sounds in a sentence.

Stapedectomy. The surgical removal of a diseased or fixated stapes; a prosthetic device replaces the bone.

Stapedius muscle. A small muscle attached to the stapes in the middle ear; in response to loud sounds, the muscle normally contracts to stiffen the ossicular chain.

Stapes. One of the three bones of the ossicular chain in the middle ear. *See also* Incus; Malleus.

Startle reflex. An infant's automatic response to loud sound involving sudden movement that suggests a jumping response.

Stenosis. Narrowing of a body canal.

Stomodeum. The primitive mouth and nose created during the 3rd week of embryonic development.

Stops. Speech sounds that are produced by completely stopping the airflow; also known as stop-plosives.

Strabismus. A lack of coordinated movement of the two eyes because one of the eyes either deviates toward the nose (convergent) or away from it (divergent).

Stuttering. A disorder of fluency characterized by excessive amounts of dysfluency, tension, struggle, and related behaviors.

Subglottal air pressure. Air pressure below the vocal cords.

Submucous cleft. An opening in the palate covered by the mucous membrane.

Substitution. The production of a wrong sound in place of a right one.

Suffix. A morpheme added at the end of a word.

Sulcus. A shallow valley on the surface of the brain; the brain has many sulci (plural). *See also* Fissures.

Supplementary motor cortex. An area of the frontal lobe thought to be involved in the motor planning of meaningful speech.

Surface structure (the S-Structure). The actual arrangement of words in a syntactic order; the printed or spoken phrase or sentence.

Syllable. The combination of a consonant and a vowel.

Sympathetic. Refers to a branch of the autonomic nervous system that mobilizes the body for "flight or fight." *See also* Parasympathetic.

Synapse. The juncture at which neurons communicate with each other.

Synaptic cleft. The tiny gap between two neurons.

Syntactic problems. Difficulties in sentence construction.

Syntax. The arrangement of words to form meaningful sentences; a part of grammar.

T

Tactile speech-communication aids. Devices or methods that promote the comprehension of speech by means of touch.

Tacts. Verbal responses that describe and comment on things and events around the speaker.

Tadoma. A method by which a person who is deaf and blind places his or her hand on a speaker's face to feel the vibrations and thereby understand speech.

Telegraphic speech. Telegram-like speech that lacks such grammatical elements as the articles, prepositions, and conjunctions.

Temporal bone. That part of the skull that houses the middle ear structures.

Temporal lobe. One of the four lobes of the cerebral cortex; it contains the primary auditory cortex and Wernicke's area.

Temporomandibular joint. The joint between the mandible and the temporal bone.

Tensor palatini. A pair of muscles that stretch the soft palate.

Tensor tympani. A muscle in the middle ear that tenses the eardrum.

Text telephones. A telephone that allows the two communication partners to type in their messages, which are then displayed on a small screen so the person who is deaf can read them.

Thalamus. A part of the diencephalon, which lies in the brain stem; the thalamus integrates sensory information and relays it to various parts of the cerebral cortex.

Threshold of hearing. An intensity level at which a tone is faintly heard at least 50% of the time it is presented.

Thrombosis. The formation of a nontraveling blood clot that obstructs the flow of blood; a cause of stroke.

Thyroarytenoid muscle. An intrinsic laryngeal muscle that forms part of the vocal folds; it can shorten and tense the folds.

Thyroid cartilage. A large, butterfly-shaped cartilage that forms the frontal and side walls of the larynx.

Time-out. A procedure to decrease the frequency of an error response; every time an error response is made, a brief period of no reinforcement or silence is imposed.

Tomography. A computerized procedure of taking three-dimensional X-ray pictures of the body.

Tongue thrust. A pattern of deviant or reverse swallow in which the tongue pushes against the teeth.

Topic maintenance. A continued conversation on the same topic for an appropriate duration.

Total communication. A method of communication that simultaneously uses speech, manual signs, and finger spelling.

Trachea. A tube formed by a ring of cartilages leading to the lungs.

Transformation. In linguistics, a transformation is an operation that relates the deep and the surface structures and yields different forms of sentences; it is the arrangement and rearrangement of words to change sentence forms.

Traumatic brain injury. Injury to the brain sustained by physical trauma or external force applied to the head.

Traumatic laryngitis. Irritated and swollen laryngeal structures due to vocally abusive behaviors; associated with voice disorders.

Trigeminal nerve V. A cranial nerve that supplies many structures of the face; controls jaw and tongue movements.

Tympanic membrane. The thin, semi-transparent, cone-shaped eardrum, which is highly sensitive to sound.

U

Unilateral. One-sided.

Unilateral cleft. A cleft on one side of the alveolar ridge and the lip.

Unilingual. A person who speaks only one language.

Uvula. The small, cone-shaped tip of the velum.

V

Vagus nerve X. A cranial nerve the supplies many organs including the larynx, pharynx, base of the tongue, and external ear.

Veau–Wardill–Kilner procedure. A surgical method of lengthening the palate while closing a cleft.

Velocity. Quickness or speed of motion.

Velopharyngeal port. The structure that connects the oral and nasal passages; it may be closed or opened by various muscle actions.

Velum. The soft palate; formed by muscles that help raise or lower it.

Ventricles. The small spaces in the skull that are filled with cerebrospinal fluid.

Verbal apraxia. Difficulty in initiating and executing the movement patterns necessary to produce speech when there is no paralysis, weakness, or discoordination of speech muscles; thought to be due to the brain's disturbed motor planning.

Verbal paraphasia. A word substitution problem found frequently in patients with aphasia; the substituted words have meanings *similar* to the correct words.

Vestibular acoustic nerve VIII. A cranial nerve with two branches: the vestibular branch is concerned with the sense of balance and the acoustic branch with sound transmission.

Vestibular system. An inner ear structure containing three semicircular canals; the system is concerned with balance, body position, and movement.

Videofluoroscopy. A method of videotaping the functioning of an internal organ or system through X ray.

Visual agnosia. Difficulty in recognizing objects by looking at them; a patient with aphasia who has this difficulty must touch an object or hear the sound it makes to recognize it.

Visually reinforced head turn paradigm. A method to study speech perception in infants and young babies.

Vocal cords. A pair of thin muscles in the larynx whose vibrations are the source of voice.

Vocal fry. A quality of voice produced in slow, discrete bursts at an extremely low pitch.

Vocal nodules. Small, typically bilateral, nodes that develop on vocal folds and protrude from the surrounding cells; due to vocal abuse or misuse.

Vocalis muscles. The vibrating parts of vocal folds; also known as the thyroary-tenoid muscles.

Voicing. The presence of vocal fold vibrations in the production of speech sounds.

von Langenbeck operation. A surgical procedure of closing a cleft of the palate in which flaps of mucoperiosteum are raised, pushed toward the midline to close the cleft, and sutured.

W

Wernicke's area. A center in the temporal lobe thought to be responsible for both understanding and formulating speech.

Whole-word interjection. A type of dysfluency; adding words that are not an integral part of an utterance.

Whole-word repetitions. A type of dysfluency; repeated production of single words.

Index

About the Author

M. N. (Giri) Hegde is a professor of communicative sciences and disorders at California State University, Fresno. He holds a master's degree in experimental psychology from the University of Mysore, India, and a post-master's diploma in medical psychology from Bangalore University, India. His doctoral degree in speech–language pathology is from Southern Illinois University in Carbondale.

Dr. Hegde is a specialist in research methods, fluency disorders, language, and treatment procedures in communicative disorders. He has made many professional and scientific presentations to national and international audiences on a wide variety of topics in communicative disorders. He has published many research articles and over 18 books on a wide range of subjects in speech–language pathology. He has received numerous state and national professional accolades and honors, including the ASHA Fellow Award and the Outstanding Professor Award from California State University, Fresno.